BSAVA Manual of Canine and Feline Dermatology
fourth edition

Editors:

Hilary A. Jackson
ARPS BVM&S DVD DipACVD DipECVD MRCVS
RCVS Recognized Specialist in Veterinary Dermatology
The Dermatology Referral Service,
528 Paisley Road West, Glasgow G51 1RN, UK

Rosanna Marsella
DVM DVD DipACVD
Department of Small Animal Clinical Sciences, University of Florida,
Gainesville, FL 32610, USA

Published by:

British Small Animal Veterinary Association
Woodrow House, 1 Telford Way,
Waterwells Business Park, Quedgeley,
Gloucester GL2 2AB

A Company Limited by Guarantee in England
Registered Company No. 2837793
Registered as a Charity

ISBN 978-1-910443-80-4

The publishers, editors and contributors cannot take responsibility for information provided on dosages and methods of application of drugs mentioned or referred to in this publication. Details of this kind must be verified in each case by individual users from up to date literature published by the manufacturers or suppliers of those drugs. Veterinary surgeons are reminded that in each case they must follow all appropriate national legislation and regulations (for example, in the United Kingdom, the prescribing cascade) from time to time in force.

Printed in the UK by Cambrian Printers Ltd., Pontllanfraith NP12 2YA
Printed on ECF paper made from sustainable forests

**Save 15% off the digital version of this manual. By purchasing this print edition we are pleased to offer you a reduced price on online access at www.bsavalibrary.com
Enter offer code 21DERM15 on checkout**

Please note the discount only applies to a purchase of the full online version of the *BSAVA Manual of Canine and Feline Dermatology, 4th edition* via **www.bsavalibrary.com**. The discount will be taken off the BSAVA member price or full price, depending on your member status. The discount code is for a single purchase of the online version and is for your personal use only. If you do not already have a login for the BSAVA website, you will need to register in order to make a purchase.

Titles in the BSAVA Manuals series

Manual of Avian Practice: A Foundation Manual
Manual of Backyard Poultry Medicine and Surgery
Manual of Canine & Feline Abdominal Imaging
Manual of Canine & Feline Abdominal Surgery
Manual of Canine & Feline Advanced Veterinary Nursing
Manual of Canine & Feline Anaesthesia and Analgesia
Manual of Canine & Feline Behavioural Medicine
Manual of Canine & Feline Cardiorespiratory Medicine
Manual of Canine & Feline Clinical Pathology
Manual of Canine & Feline Dentistry and Oral Surgery
Manual of Canine & Feline Dermatology
Manual of Canine & Feline Emergency and Critical Care
Manual of Canine & Feline Endocrinology
Manual of Canine & Feline Endoscopy and Endosurgery
Manual of Canine & Feline Fracture Repair and Management
Manual of Canine & Feline Gastroenterology
Manual of Canine & Feline Haematology and Transfusion Medicine
Manual of Canine & Feline Head, Neck and Thoracic Surgery
Manual of Canine & Feline Musculoskeletal Disorders
Manual of Canine & Feline Musculoskeletal Imaging
Manual of Canine & Feline Nephrology and Urology
Manual of Canine & Feline Neurology
Manual of Canine & Feline Oncology
Manual of Canine & Feline Ophthalmology
Manual of Canine & Feline Radiography and Radiology: A Foundation Manual
Manual of Canine & Feline Rehabilitation, Supportive and Palliative Care: Case Studies in Patient Management
Manual of Canine & Feline Reproduction and Neonatology
Manual of Canine & Feline Shelter Medicine: Principles of Health and Welfare in a Multi-animal Environment
Manual of Canine & Feline Surgical Principles: A Foundation Manual
Manual of Canine & Feline Thoracic Imaging
Manual of Canine & Feline Ultrasonography
Manual of Canine & Feline Wound Management and Reconstruction
Manual of Canine Practice: A Foundation Manual
Manual of Exotic Pet and Wildlife Nursing
Manual of Exotic Pets: A Foundation Manual
Manual of Feline Practice: A Foundation Manual
Manual of Ornamental Fish
Manual of Practical Animal Care
Manual of Practical Veterinary Nursing
Manual of Practical Veterinary Welfare
Manual of Psittacine Birds
Manual of Rabbit Medicine
Manual of Rabbit Surgery, Dentistry and Imaging
Manual of Raptors, Pigeons and Passerine Birds
Manual of Reptiles
Manual of Rodents and Ferrets
Manual of Small Animal Practice Management and Development
Manual of Wildlife Casualties

For further information on these and all BSAVA publications, please visit our website: **www.bsava.com**

Contents

Contributors

Francesco Albanese
DVM
Private Veterinary Analysis Laboratory Mylav,
Milan, Italy

Zeineb Alhaidari
DVM DipECVD
Clinique Vétérinaire,
Cidex 248, RN 85, F-06330,
Roquefort-les-Pins, France

Natalie Barnard
BVetMed CertVD DipECVD MRCVS
EBVS® Specialist in Veterinary Dermatology, RCVS
Recognized Specialist in Veterinary Dermatology
Highcroft Veterinary Referrals,
615 Wells Road, Whitchurch,
Bristol BS14 9BE, UK

Emmanuel Bensignor
DrVet DipECVD DESV(Dermatology)
Registered Specialist in Veterinary Dermatology
Oniris Nantes Veterinary School and Veterinary
Dermatology Referral Service,
75003 Paris, 35510 Rennes-Cesson and
44000 Nantes, France

Darren Berger
DVM DipACVD
Iowa State University,
College of Veterinary Medicine,
1809 S Riverside Drive, Ames IA 50011, USA

Kerstin Bergvall
DVM DipECVD
Department of Clinical Sciences,
University of Agriculture, Uppsala, Sweden

Megan Boyd
DVM DipACVD
Animal Dermatology Center,
Studio City, CA 91361, USA

Mandy Burrows
BSc BVMS MANZCVS FANZCVS
Registered Specialist in Veterinary Dermatology
Animal Dermatology Clinic Perth, School of Veterinary
Medicine, Murdoch University, 6150 Western Australia

Karen L. Campbell
DVM MS DipACVIM DipACVD
MU Veterinary Health Center at Wentzville,
College of Veterinary Medicine, University of Missouri,
1092 Wentzville Parkway, MO 63385, USA

Cathy F. Curtis
BVetMed DVD MRCVS
RCVS Recognized Specialist in Veterinary Dermatology
Skin Specialist Vet Service,
Rooftops, Spring View Road, Ware,
Hertfordshire SG12 9LB, UK

Carla Dedola
DVM DipECVD
Clinica Città di Sassari,
Via Alghero 43, 07100 Sassari, Italy

Alison Diesel
DVM DipACVD
Texas A&M University College of Veterinary Medicine
and Biomedical Sciences,
College Station, TX 77843, USA

Jane M. Dobson
MA BVetMed DVetMed DipECVIM-CA(Oncology) FRCVS
European and RCVS Recognized Specialist in
Veterinary Oncology
Department of Veterinary Medicine,
University of Cambridge, Madingley Road,
Cambridge CB3 0ES, UK

Eva Espadale Reballi
DVM DipECVD MRCVS
EBVS® Specialist in Veterinary Dermatology, RCVS
Recognized Specialist in Veterinary Dermatology
Rutland House Referrals,
Abbotsfield House, 4 Abbotsfield Road,
Saint Helens WA9 4HU, UK

Lluís Ferrer
DVM PhD DipECVD
Veterinary School,
Universitat Autonoma de Barcelona,
Barcelona, Spain

Peter J. Forsythe
BVM&S DVD MRCVS
The Dermatology Referral Service,
528 Paisley Road West,
Glasgow G51 1RN, UK

Cecilia Friberg
DVM DipACVD DipECVD
Evidensia Södra Djursjukhuset Kungens Kurva,
Månskärsvägen 13, 14175 Kungens Kurva,
Stockholm, Sweden

Dunbar Gram
DVM DipACVD MRCVS
Department of Small Animal Clinical Sciences,
University of Florida,
Gainesville, FL 32610, USA

Patrick Hensel
Dr.med.vet DipACVD DipECVD(Dermatologie)
EBVS® Specialist in Veterinary Dermatology
Fachtierarzt für Allergien, Haut- und Ohrenerkrankungen
Tierdermatologie Basel, Emil Frey-Strasse 127,
CH-4142 Münchenstein, Switzerland

Hilary A. Jackson
ARPS BVM&S DVD DipACVD DipECVD MRCVS
RCVS Recognized Specialist in Veterinary Dermatology
The Dermatology Referral Service,
528 Paisley Road West,
Glasgow G51 1RN, UK

Anette Loeffler
PhD DVD DipECVD FHEA MRCVS
Royal Veterinary College,
Hawkshead Lane, Hatfield,
North Mymms, Hertfordshire AL9 7TA, UK

Dawn Logas
DVM DipACVD
Veterinary Dermatology Center
Maitland, FL 32751, USA

Katharine F. Lunn
BVMS MS PhD DipACVIM MRCVS
Department of Clinical Sciences,
NC State University College of Veterinary Medicine,
1052 William Moore Drive, Raleigh, NC 27607, USA

Rosanna Marsella
DVM DVD DipACVD
Department of Small Animal Clinical Sciences
University of Florida,
Gainesville, FL 32610, USA

Carly Mason
BVSc CertVD DipECVD MRCVS
Guide Dogs UK,
Southeast Region, UK

Karen A. Moriello
DVM DipACVD
School of Veterinary Medicine,
University of Wisconsin-Madison,
WI 53706, USA

Daniel O. Morris
DVM MPH DipACVD
School of Veterinary Medicine,
University of Pennsylvania, 3900 Delancey Street,
Philadelphia, PA 19104, USA

Ralf S. Mueller
Dr.med.vet DipECVD DipACVD FANZCVS(Dermatology)
Faculty of Veterinary Medicine,
Ludwig-Maximilians University Munich,
Veterinarstrasse 13, 80539 Munich, Germany

Tim Nuttall
BSc BVSc CertVD PhD CBiol MRSB MRCVS
RCVS Recognized Specialist in Veterinary Dermatology
Royal (Dick) School of Veterinary Studies,
University of Edinburgh, Easter Bush Campus,
Roslin EH25 9RG, UK

Manon Paradis
DVM MVSc DipACVD
Professor Emeritus
Department of Clinical Sciences,
Faculty of Veterinary Medicine, University of Montreal,
CP 5000, St-Hyacinthe,
Québec J2S 7C6, Canada

Sue Paterson
MA VetMB DVD DipECVD FRCVS
RCVS and European Specialist in Veterinary Dermatology
Virtual Vet Derms Telemedicine Service,
Kendal, UK

Rebecca Ricci
DVM PhD
*European Specialist in Veterinary and
Comparative Nutrition*
Department of Animal Medicine, Production and Health,
University of Padua, Agripolis, viale dell'Università 16,
35020 Legnaro (PD), Italy

Domenico Santoro
DVM MS DrSc PhD DipACVD DipECVD DipACVM(Bacteriology/
Mycology & Immunology)
Department of Small Animal Clinical Sciences,
University of Florida, Gainesville, FL 32610, USA

Manolis N. Saridomichelakis
DVM PhD DipECVD
Clinic of Medicine, Faculty of Veterinary Science,
University of Thessaly, Trikalon Str 224, GR-43132,
Karditsa, Greece

David H. Shearer
BVetMed PhD CertSAD PGCertVetEd FHEA CBiol FRSB DipRCPath
MRCVS
Vetcutis Ltd,
Holly House, Station Road,
Pulham St Mary, Norfolk IP21 4QQ, UK

Kathy C. Tater
DVM MPH DipACVD
Veterinary Information Network,
Davis, CA 95616, USA

Foreword

I was delighted and honoured both as a Past President of the BSAVA and as a Board Certified Veterinary Dermatologist to be asked to write the Foreword and contribute to the fourth edition of the *BSAVA Manual of Canine and Feline Dermatology*.

The last edition of the *BSAVA Manual of Canine and Feline Dermatology* was published in 2012 and, whilst at the time it provided an excellent reference source for a wide range of small animal dermatological conditions, the rapid advances in both the diagnosis and therapy of dermatological diseases have meant that this new edition has been completely updated to provide a go-to resource for busy primary care veterinary surgeons, nurses and veterinary students.

The editors, Hilary Jackson and Rosanna Marsella, must be congratulated for harnessing the combined expertise of a wide range of key opinion leaders within the global veterinary dermatology community, as well as contributing their own not inconsiderable wealth of knowledge to this new edition.

The initial chapters on the structure and function of the skin, together with a systematic approach to the investigation of skin disease, provide a firm initial grounding in dermatology. Subsequent chapters on clinical presentations, such as pruritus, scaling, papules and pustules, pigmentation and alopecia, form the main body of the text, which allows the time-pressed clinician to quickly access the appropriate information to help them identify and manage problems. Additional chapters focus on specific conditions such as otitis externa and media, and new to this edition are several excellent chapters dedicated to feline skin disease. The abundance of high-quality photographs of clinical signs, parasites and cytology are welcome, and the use of tables detailing differential diagnoses, together with clinical decision-making flow charts all enhance the usefulness of this text.

There is no doubt that this Manual should be on the bookshelf of every small animal clinic and veterinary hospital as an invaluable resource for veterinary professionals.

Sue Paterson
MA VetMB DVD DipECVD FRCVS
Director Virtual Vet Derms
BSAVA President 2019–20

Preface

Skin and ear diseases represent common problems in general practice. With many diseases, the cutaneous lesions have a similar appearance and thus it is important to embrace a logical approach when investigating a dermatological case, recognizing the importance of history and becoming familiar with the various point-of-care tests that can be used to inform therapeutic decisions. As the response to treatment largely depends on the correct identification of the primary disease, a systematic step-by-step approach is critical. The purpose of the *BSAVA Manual of Canine and Feline Dermatology* is to be an easy-to-read resource focused on the clinically relevant aspects of dermatological diseases.

This new edition retains the popular format from the third edition. The initial chapters review the basic structure and function of the skin and discuss a logical approach to history taking and the core investigative tests that can be performed. New to this edition is a separate chapter on skin cytology, which features many excellent images illustrating the cytology of common skin conditions that we hope will be useful to practitioners.

The introductory section is followed by chapters focused on a problem-oriented approach to common dermatological conditions. Here we have expanded the information on the approach and management of certain commonly seen conditions such as pyoderma, ear disease and atopic dermatitis. New to this edition is a chapter dedicated to the indications for allergy testing and the use of allergen-specific immunotherapy. There are also two separate chapters addressing feline dermatological conditions because, as we all know, cats are not small dogs.

The development and availability of new therapeutic options for pruritus warrants a standalone chapter in this new edition, alongside a separate chapter discussing the advantages and disadvantages of immunosuppressive therapy for autoimmune and immune-mediated diseases.

We are immensely grateful to all our authors for taking the time to share their expertise and knowledge in this new edition of the *BSAVA Manual of Canine and Feline Dermatology*. It is truly an international effort.

We would also like to thank the BSAVA Publications Team for all their patience and hard work pulling together this Manual during the COVID-19 pandemic.

We hope that you find this a useful edition to your practice library and that it proves a practical companion in your day-to-day practice.

Hilary Jackson
Rosanna Marsella
July 2021

Chapter 1

Structure and function of the skin

Eva Espadale and Domenico Santoro

The skin is the largest organ of the body and it is involved in a wide array of functions fundamental for homeostasis (Figure 1.1). Beyond acting as a physical barrier against external insults, the skin is also important as a thermoregulatory, sensory and immunological organ. Furthermore, because of the different regional requirements of this organ (e.g. ears, eyelids, lips, prepuce, nasal planum, footpads and claws), the skin has acquired specialized structures and functions. A consideration of these topics is beyond the scope of this chapter and the reader is referred to the relevant chapters later in the Manual. This chapter is mainly focused on providing a basic understanding of the structure and function of the skin and its role in the body's immune defence.

Mammalian skin is mainly composed of three layers – the epidermis, dermis and subcutis. These layers have different functions and will be treated separately in this chapter.

Function	Activities
Barrier	Controls loss of water, electrolytes and other molecules Excludes chemical, physical and microbiological agents
Sensation	Heat, cold, pain, itch, pressure
Thermoregulation	Insulation (hair coat), regulation of cutaneous blood supply, sweat gland function
Secretion	Epitrichial (apocrine), atrichial (eccrine) and sebaceous glands
Synthesis	Vitamin D
Motion/shape	Flexibility, elasticity and toughness
Storage	Electrolytes, water, vitamins, fat, carbohydrates, proteins, etc.
Indicator	General health, internal disease, physical and sexual identity
Immune regulation	Keratinocytes, Langerhans's cells, lymphocytes
Antimicrobial action	Lipids, organic acids, lysozymes, host defence peptides
Pigmentation	Prevents damage from solar radiation, and oxidation

1.1 Skin activities associated with homeostasis.

The epidermis

The outermost layer of the skin, or epidermis, is a stratified squamous epithelium overlying the basement membrane. The latter provides firm attachment of the epidermis to the dermis and allows the selective passage of molecules and cells between the two structures (see 'Basement membrane zone' below). The epidermis typically comprises four layers (Figure 1.2) that, from inner to outer, are:

- Basal layer (stratum basale, SB)
- Spinous layer (stratum spinosum, SS)
- Granular layer (stratum granulosum, SG)
- Horny layer (stratum corneum, SC).

In some body regions (such as the nasal planum and footpads), a fifth layer may be present. This is known as the clear layer or stratum lucidum or stratum conjunctum.

Each layer is composed of a single or few rows of cells, depending on the anatomical site. In general, the epidermis of cats and dogs is thin (two to three nucleated cell layers, not counting the horny layer) in areas of haired skin, ranging from 0.1 to 0.5 mm in thickness. The epidermis is thinnest on the abdomen, while the thickest epidermis is found on the footpads and nasal planum, where it may measure 1.5 mm.

The keratinocyte is the principal cell of the epidermis (approximately 85% of epidermal cell populations). The cytoskeleton of the keratinocyte is composed of actin filaments, keratin intermediate filaments and microtubules, which provide its structural strength. Keratin intermediate filaments are formed by bundles of keratin monomers typical of keratinized epithelia and highly abundant in the epidermis. In mammalian epidermis, type I (acidic) keratins and type II (neutral–basic) keratins form heterodimers via disulphide bonds. Specific keratins are found more prominently in various layers of the epidermis or in specific anatomical sites. For example, keratin 5 (K5) and K14 are mainly expressed in proliferating (basal) keratinocytes, whereas K1 and K10 are mainly expressed in differentiated keratinocytes, and K16 in highly proliferative epithelia such as palmoplantar epidermis or injured or stressed epithelia.

In the epidermis, the keratinocytes are joined together by several structures: desmosomes, tight junctions, Adherens junctions and gap junctions. In addition, modified desmosomes including hemidesmosomes and corneodesmosomes may be present. Desmosomes are composed of transmembrane proteins (desmogleins and desmocollins)

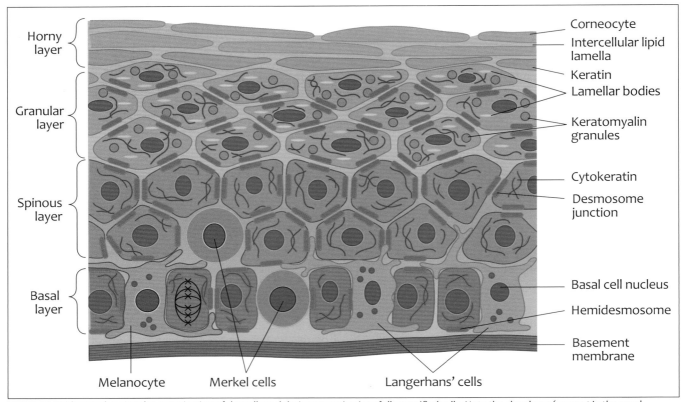

1.2 Epidermis showing the organization of the cells and their maturation into fully cornified cells. Note the clear layer (present in the nasal planum/footpads) would be interposed between the granular and horny layer.
(Redrawn after Patel, 2012)

and plaque proteins (desmoplakin, plakoglobin and plako-phillins), interconnected with intracellular keratin inter-mediate filaments that provide stability and strength. Defects in the structure of desmosomes result in various cutaneous pathologies (Figure 1.3). Tight junctions form continuous, zipper-like strings of cell junctions that seal the periphery of keratinocytes in the SG closely together and create a selective permeability barrier in the upper epidermis. Tight junctions are composed of transmembrane proteins (claudins and occludins) joined to the actin cyto-skeleton filaments by several plaque proteins (e.g. zonula occludens-1, -2, and -3). Tight junctions play an important role in regulating permeability of all epithelia, not just that of the skin. Any alteration in these structures can lead to a 'leaky' epithelium and increased movement of molecules. Corneodesmosomes are the main structural cell adhesion

Skin structure	Layer	Structure(s) affected	Structural defect	Disease	Species/breeds	Diagnostic considerations
Epidermis	Stratum corneum	Corneocyte formation	Filaggrin 1 and 2	Atopic dermatitis	Dogs (Labrador Retriever in the UK)	Clinical
			TGM1 mutation	Lamellar ichthyosis	Jack Russell Terrier	Clinical Histopathology
			K10 mutation	Epidermolytic ichthyosis	Norfolk Terrier	Clinical Histopathology Genetic test
			K16 mutation	Paw pad hyperkeratosis	Dogue de Bordeaux	Clinical Histopathology Genetic test
			SUV39H2 mutation	Nasal parakeratosis	Labrador Retriever	Clinical Histopathology Genetic test
		Intercellular lipids	Altered ceramide profile	Atopic dermatitis		Clinical
			PNPLA-1 mutation	Lamellar ichthyosis	Golden Retriever	Clinical Histopathology Genetic test

1.3 Diseases associated with known structural defects (genetic and acquired) in dogs and cats. The acquired defects are shown in **bold.** [a] Major autoantigen = antigen recognized by more than 50% of affected animals; [b] PAS stains perlecan present in the lamina densa; [c] Other minor autoantigens in canine MMP are BPAG1e and laminin 332 (previously laminin 5). BP = bullous pemphigoid; Dsc-1 = desmocollin-1; Dsg-1 = desmoglein-1; Dsg-3 = desmoglein-3; EB = epidermolysis bullosa; EBA = epidermolysis bullosa acquisita; EBS = epidermolysis bullosa simplex; HA = hyaluronic acid; H&E = haematoxylin and eosin; MMP = mucous membrane pemphigoid; MT = Masson's trichrome; PAS = periodic acid-Schiff; PKP1 = plakophillin-1; TEM = transmission electron microscopy; TGM1 = transglutaminase-1; VVG = Verhoeff van Gieson. (continues) ▶

Skin structure	Layer	Structure(s) affected	Structural defect	Disease	Species/breeds	Diagnostic considerations
Epidermis *continued*	Stratum corneum *continued*	Intercellular lipids *continued*	*NIPAL-4* mutation	Lamellar ichthyosis	American Bulldog	Clinical Histopathology Genetic test
			SLC27A4 mutation, gene encoding *FATP4*	Lamellar ichthyosis	Great Dane	Clinical Histopathology Genetic test
	Stratum granulosum and spinosum	Desmosomes	Defective calcium pump (mutation not identified)	Canine Darier disease	English Setter and crosses	Histopathology
			PKP1 mutation (plakophillin – 1 deficiency)	Ectodermal dysplasia and skin fragility (EBS, suprabasal)	Chesapeake Bay Retriever	Histopathology Immunohistopathology
			Autoantibodies against Dsc-1 (major canine autoantigen[a]) and Dsg-1 (minor)	Pemphigus foliaceus		Clinical Cytology Histopathology Immunohistopathology
	Basal/ supra-basal layer	Desmosomes/ hemi-desmosomes	**Autoantibodies against Dsg-3 and Dsg-1**	Pemphigus vulgaris		Clinical Histopathology Immunohistopathology
Basement membrane zone		Hemi-desmosomes	*PLEC* mutation, gene encoding for plectin	EBS basal	Eurasier Dog	Histopathology[b] Immunohistopathology TEM
			Autoantibodies against collagen XVII[c]	MMP	German Shepherd Dog (mainly), Poodle, cats	Clinical Histopathology Immunohistopathology
			Autoantibodies against collagen XVII	BP	Dogs (many breeds), cats	Clinical Histopathology Immunopathology
		Lamina densa	*LAMA3* mutation, encoding for the alpha-3 chain of laminin 332	Junctional EB	German Shorthaired Pointer	Histopathology[b] Immunohistopathology TEM Genetic test
		Anchoring fibrils in sublamina densa	*COL7A1* mutation, gene encoding for collagen VII	Dystrophic EB	Golden Retriever and Central Asian Shepherd Dog (mainly), cats (no confirmed mutation)	Histopathology[b] Immunohistopathology TEM
			Autoantibodies against collagen VII	EBA	Great Dane and German Shorthaired Pointer (mainly)	Histopathology Immunohistopathology
Dermis	Collagen fibres	Defects in collagen synthesis and bundle formation	Mutation in *COL5A1*	Ehlers-Danlos syndrome	Dogs, cats	Clinical (skin extensibility index) Histopathology (H&E, MT, VVG) TEM
		Increased collagen secretion	*ADAMTSL2* mutation	Musladin-Leuke Syndrome ('Chinese Beagle Syndrome')	Beagle	Clinical Genetic test
			FLCN mutation, gene encoding for folliculin	Renal cystadeno-carcinoma and nodular dermatofibrosis	German Shepherd Dog (mainly)	Histopathology Imaging Genetic test
	Matrix	Increased amounts of HA	*HAS 2* mutation, gene encoding hyaluronan synthase 2	Hereditary cutaneous hyaluronanosis (mucinosis)	Shar Pei	Clinical Histopathology (H&E, Alcian blue)
		Increased amount of amyloid	*MTBP* mutation	Shar Pei affected with autoinflammatory disease (SPAID)	Shar Pei	Clinical Histopathology (H&E, Alcian blue, Congo red)

1.3 (continued) Diseases associated with known structural defects (genetic and acquired) in dogs and cats. The acquired defects are shown in **bold.** [a] Major autoantigen = antigen recognized by more than 50% of affected animals; [b] PAS stains perlecan present in the lamina densa; [c] Other minor autoantigens in canine MMP are BPAG1e and laminin 332 (previously laminin 5). BP = bullous pemphigoid; Dsc-1 = desmocollin-1; Dsg-1 = desmoglein-1; Dsg-3 = desmoglein-3; EB = epidermolysis bullosa; EBA = epidermolysis bullosa acquisita; EBS = epidermolysis bullosa simplex; HA = hyaluronic acid; H&E = haematoxylin and eosin; MMP = mucous membrane pemphigoid; MT = Masson's trichrome; PAS = periodic acid-Schiff; PKP1 = plakophillin-1; TEM = transmission electron microscopy; TGM1 = transglutaminase-1; VVG = Verhoeff van Gieson.

junctions between corneocytes. They are mainly composed of the transmembrane protein corneodesmosin. Alterations in the expression and distribution of corneodesmosomes and tight junction proteins may play a role in the development and progression of human and canine atopic dermatitis.

In addition to their ability to function as a barrier, keratinocytes have significant immunological activity. Indeed, this cell type is responsible for the secretion of a variety of pro- and anti-inflammatory cytokines, interferons and host defence peptides (also known as antimicrobial peptides). Keratinocytes can also phagocytose bacteria and act as antigen-presenting cells, thus providing an important bridge between the innate and adaptive immunity of the skin.

Other cells present in the epidermis include:

- Melanocytes (approximately 5%)
- Langerhans' cells (3% to 8%)
- Merkel cells (approximately 2%), which are associated with tylotrich pads (see 'Cutaneous sensation and pruritus' below).

The origins and functions of cells in the skin are summarized in Figure 1.4.

Basal layer

The basal layer is a single row of columnar to cuboidal keratinocytes. These keratinocytes are produced by mitosis of a small number of stem cells in a process known as epidermal proliferation. Keratinocytes gradually migrate upwards into the outer layers of the epidermis and are ultimately shed as dead horny cells. During this process, the keratinocyte undergoes a complex series of metabolic events and morphological changes known as differentiation, to eventually form the SC (see 'Process of cornification' below).

Spinous layer

The spinous layer is composed of polyhedral to flattened cuboidal keratinocytes. In areas of haired skin, the spinous layer is one or two cells thick, but it becomes much thicker (up to 20 layers) at the footpads, nasal planum and mucocutaneous junctions.

The cells in this layer are called spinous cells because in conventional histological sections they appear to have spines. The spines are in fact desmosomes and other cell-to-cell adhesions crucial for providing mechanical stability and facilitating signal transduction within and between adjacent cells.

Granular layer

The cells of the granular layer are fusiform to flat in shape and are characterized by the presence of keratohyalin granules. Among others, these granules contain a precursor protein, profilaggrin, which, when dephosphorylated to filaggrin, is involved in the aggregation of the keratin bundles (see 'Process of cornification' below). The thickness of the SG is variable: it is one to two cells thick in areas of haired skin, and four to eight cells thick in non-haired skin.

Clear layer

Keratinocytes in the clear layer are fully differentiated and flattened, forming a compact, thin layer of dead cells. This layer is homogeneous, contains refractile droplets and is hyaline-like. Due to its high lipid content, the clear layer can be histochemically differentiated from the horny layer. This layer is mainly present in the footpads and, less developed, in the nasal planum.

Horny layer

The horny layer is the outer layer of terminally differentiated keratinocytes (corneocytes) that is constantly being shed, in a process known as desquamation. This layer is composed of thin, tightly packed corneocytes that are interconnected by corneodesmosomes and sealed together by an intercellular lipid matrix. The corneocytes have undergone structural and biochemical changes and are composed mainly of aggregated keratin bundles and filaggrin, within a cornified envelope that replaces the plasma membrane (see 'Process of cornification' below). The structure of the SC is often likened to a series of bricks (corneocytes) bonded by mortar (lipids) that holds the corneocytes together and provides a hydrophobic barrier.

Skin structure	Cell type	Origin	Function
Epidermis	Keratinocyte	Ectoderm	Barrier due to structure Immune response via production of cytokines and phagocytosis
	Langerhans' cell	Haemopoietic progenitor cells	Immune surveillance
	Melanocyte	Neural crest	Production of pigment, which protects from UV light, provides camouflage and allows sexual display in some species
	Merkel cell	Primitive epidermal cells	Slow adapting mechanoreceptors
Dermis	Fibroblast	Mesenchyme	Synthesis of extracellular matrix components Wound healing Production of degrading enzymes
	Dermal dendrocyte	Bone marrow	Antigen presentation Haemostasis Wound healing
	T lymphocyte	Bone marrow	Promotes cell-mediated and humoral immune response Generally CD3, alpha-beta positive
	Mast cell	Bone marrow	Involved in early immune response by releasing preformed granules and initiation of the process of inflammation
	Microvascular epithelial cell	Haemopoietic progenitor cells	Involved in immune response via the adhesion of effector cells, such as neutrophils, eosinophils, basophils and monocytes

1.4 Origin and functions of cells found in the epidermis and the dermis.

In canine skin, the SC is 12–15 μm in thickness and is composed of 45–52 layers; it is thicker in sparsely-haired areas. Its gradual desquamation is normally balanced by proliferation of the basal cells, which maintains a constant epidermal thickness. The SC content is generally 70% protein, 15% lipids and 15% water by weight, but these values vary by species, body location and other factors.

Process of cornification

Cornification is the process by which terminal differentiation of the epidermis occurs. This process results in formation of the SC. A basic understanding of this process is necessary, as genetic alterations that affect some of the specific steps described below are involved in the development of cutaneous diseases, such as ichthyosis and atopic dermatitis (see Figure 1.3). Cornification comprises four cellular events, the first of which is keratinization, followed by the synthesis of keratohyalin, formation of the cornified cell envelope, and ending in the generation of the lipid envelope.

Non-living corneocytes form through programmed cell death of viable keratinocytes of the SG. In the lower SG, the formation of keratohyalin granules occurs. Keratohyalin granules store several proteins needed for the structural changes that occur during the cornification process, including caspase-14, profilaggrin/filaggrin and loricrin. Particular attention should be given to filaggrin, a filament aggregating protein released from its precursor profilaggrin by caspase-14 and other enzymes. In the upper SG, keratinocytes start changing shape and collapse due to the compaction of the keratin intermediate filaments mediated by filaggrin. Filaggrin will eventually be further metabolized into natural moisturizing factors (urocanic acid and pyrrolidone carboxylic acid) and amino acids, which contribute to the hydration and acidic pH of the SC. Proper processing of filaggrin is essential for the dissolution of the nucleus and for effective skin barrier function. A deficiency of filaggrin or abnormal metabolism leads to decreased moisturizing factors and dry skin with defective skin barrier properties.

During this process, the flattening cells lose most organelles, including the nucleus, by autophagy. A cornified envelope forms on the inner surface of the corneocyte plasma membrane by deposition of a dense layer of proteins (loricrin, envoplakin, periplakin, involucrin, small proline rich proteins). To strengthen the corneocyte, transglutaminases (TGMs 1, 3 and 5) covalently cross-link keratin intermediate filaments, cornified envelope proteins and corneodesmosomes. Once the cornified envelope has formed, intercellular, non-polar lipids seal layers of corneocytes in the SC and form the major permeability barrier of the skin to water and environmental molecules. In addition to the barrier function, lipids play other important roles, such as temperature control regulating transepidermal water loss, regulation of cell cohesion, desquamation and epidermal proliferation/differentiation, and antimicrobial action.

The intercellular lipids are formed, stored and secreted by specialized organelles, lamellar bodies, found in the SG. During cornification, lamellar bodies fuse with the plasma membrane at the interface of the SG and SC and extrude their contents into the intercellular spaces. Secreted lipids undergo hydrolysis and enzymatic conversion into non-polar lipids, ceramides, free fatty acids, and cholesterol, and are arranged to form the extracellular lipid lamellae. Long fatty acid chains of omega-(acylated)-OH-ceramides, derived predominantly from linoleic acid, are covalently bound to cornified cell envelope proteins and form a cornified lipid envelope, which replaces the corneocyte plasma membrane and acts as a scaffold for the extracellular lipid lamellae. Once secreted, the intercellular lipids composition, by weight, is approximately 50% ceramides, 25% cholesterols and 10 to 15% fatty acids. These ratios are important for barrier function. Proper release and composition of lamellar granules is fundamental for the formation of normal lipid lamellae and an effective skin barrier. Decreased extrusion or altered composition lead to an impaired skin barrier and increased permeability of the skin.

Hair and its associated structures

Hair is an appendix essential to and characteristic of mammalian skin. Hair has a variety of functions: it provides a physical, antimicrobial and chemical barrier; it aids in camouflage, visual communication between animals and sexual dimorphism; and it disperses sebum and pheromones throughout the skin surface. Hair is also photoprotective. Furthermore, the length and density of the hair coat provides thermal insulation, while colour and glossiness play thermoregulatory roles. Specialized tactile hairs (sinus and tylotrich hairs) have been modified structurally to be able to perceive sensory stimuli (see 'Cutaneous sensation and pruritus' below).

The hair follicle and hair cycle

Hairs originate from the hair follicles formed during embryonic development by complex interactions between the mesenchymal and ectodermal cells. In general, no new hair follicles are formed after birth. Anatomically, the hair follicle is divided into three segments: the infundibulum, the isthmus and the inferior segment (Figure 1.5). Figure 1.6 summarizes the structure, characteristics and functions of the different hair follicle components.

Dogs and cats have compound follicles consisting of a larger diameter primary hair associated with an arrector pili muscle, a pilosebaceous unit and an epitrichial (formerly apocrine) sweat gland, accompanied by several secondary hairs; all hairs in a compound follicle leave the epidermis through the same opening (Figure 1.7). The ratio of primary to secondary hairs determines the different types of hair coat seen in different species and breeds. Primary hairs are shed all year around; secondary hairs are shed seasonally.

After the initial embryogenic follicular morphogenesis, the hair follicle is maintained by cycling through periodic stages of growth (anagen), regression (catagen), rest (telogen) and shedding (Figure 1.8). Ketogen is a recently introduced term to describe the 'empty' telogen follicles (i.e. telogen follicles that no longer contain a hair shaft). Each of these hair cycle phases has several sub-phases, with characteristic morphological features.

The hair cycle and thus the hair coat are controlled by a complicated interaction of both intrinsic and extrinsic factors, which is poorly understood. Intrinsic factors include growth factors and cytokines produced by the follicle itself, the dermal papilla and other (non-epidermal) cells (such as lymphocytes, macrophages, fibroblasts

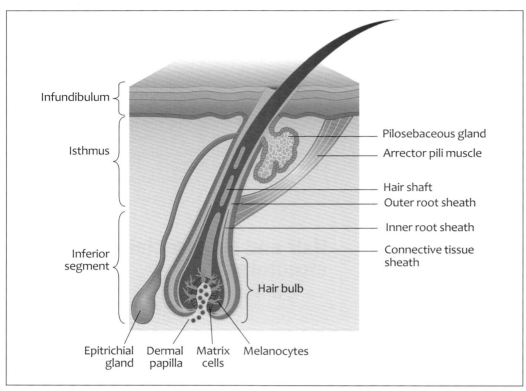

1.5 The hair follicle and its associated structures.
(Redrawn after Patel, 2012)

Infundibulum

Isthmus

Inferior segment

Pilosebaceous gland

Arrector pili muscle

Hair shaft

Outer root sheath

Inner root sheath

Connective tissue sheath

Hair bulb

Epitrichial gland   Dermal papilla   Matrix cells   Melanocytes

Structure	Characteristic	Function
Dermal papilla	Dermal fibrocytes embedded in extracellular matrix and containing nervous and vascular supplies	Induces follicular development Nourishes hair matrix
Hair matrix	Proliferative epithelial cells Melanocytes visible and active during anagen	Produce inner and outer root sheaths and hair shaft Produce and transfers pigment to hair shaft
Hair shaft: Medulla Cortex Cuticle	Consists of cuboidal cells absent in secondary hairs Pigment-containing cornified cells Outermost overlapping cornified cells	Insulation Bulk and strength of hair, hair colour Protects the cortex, provides glossiness or reflexivity
Inner root sheath (IRS): Cuticle Huxley's layer Henley's layer	Flat overlapping cells interlocking with hair cuticle 1–3 nucleated cells containing trichohyalin granules Single layer of non-nucleated cells also containing trichohyalin	Protects and supports the growing hair
Outer root sheath (ORS)	Covered by IRS below the isthmus; cells contain glycogen vacuoles; does not undergo keratinization In infundibulum undergoes normal keratinization; characterized by keratohyaline granules	
Basement membrane zone	Surrounds ORS, composed of fibrous tissue and glassy membrane	

1.6 Structure, characteristics and functions of hair follicle components.

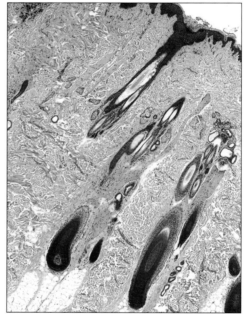

1.7 Microphotograph of a section of canine skin showing the compound follicular unit. (H&E stain; original magnification X40).
(Courtesy of Dr William Craft)

and mast cells) in the immediate environment. Major intrinsic factors regulating the hair cycle include:

- The wingless-related integration site (Wnt) signalling pathway that promotes stem cell activation and growth
- Notch signals important for stem cell differentiation into different cell lines
- Bone morphogenetic protein (BMP) and fibroblast growth factor 18 (FGF18), which regulate the repression of cycling.

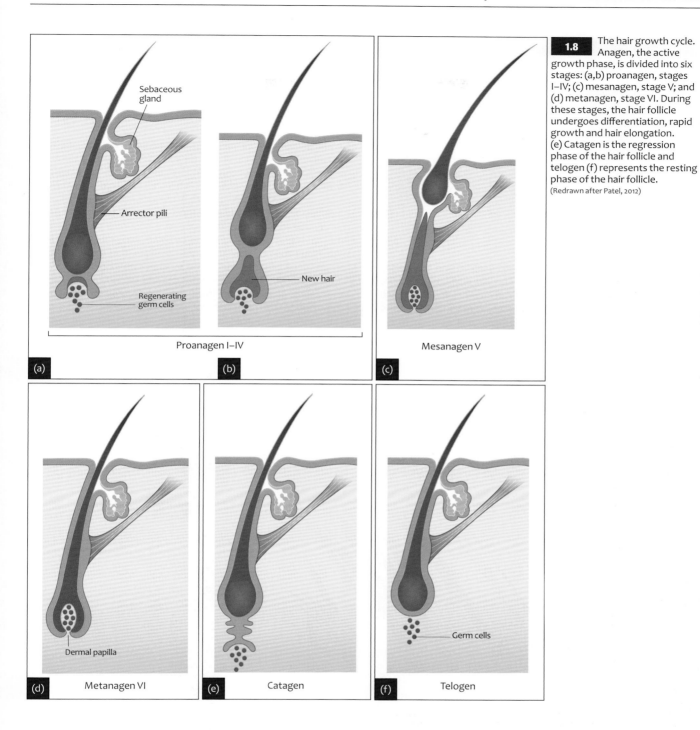

1.8 The hair growth cycle. Anagen, the active growth phase, is divided into six stages: (a,b) proanagen, stages I–IV; (c) mesanagen, stage V; and (d) metanagen, stage VI. During these stages, the hair follicle undergoes differentiation, rapid growth and hair elongation. (e) Catagen is the regression phase of the hair follicle and telogen (f) represents the resting phase of the hair follicle.
(Redrawn after Patel, 2012)

Extrinsic factors that influence the hair cycle include:

- Genetics
- General state of health
- Nutrition
- Hormones (thyroid hormones and growth hormone accelerate hair growth, whereas excessive amounts of glucocorticoids or oestrogens suppress it)
- Environmental factors.

Hair growth responds predominantly to photoperiod and, to a lesser extent, to ambient temperature. Hair replacement in dogs and cats is mosaic in pattern because neighbouring hair follicles are in different stages of the hair cycle at any one time.

Sebaceous glands

Sebaceous glands are simple alveolar glands that usually open through a duct into the infundibulum (pilosebaceous unit) located in the dermis. Their density and size depend upon anatomical site; they are most abundant around mucocutaneous junctions, in interdigital spaces, on the dorsal neck, rump and dorsal tail (tail gland, supracaudal organ, preen gland), and on the chin (submental organ). However, some sebaceous glands open directly on to the skin and are not associated with a pilosebaceous unit (free sebaceous glands). These are present in the eyelids (e.g. Meibomian glands). Sebaceous glands are absent from the nasal planum and footpads. Figure 1.9 lists the types and location of exocrine glands.

Location	Specialized gland	Type	Species
Skin	Atrichial/epitrichial Free and pilosebaceous	Sweat Sebaceous	Dog, cat Dog, cat
Eyelids	Moll's gland Meibomian (tarsal) Glands of Zeis (cilia)	Sweat Sebaceous Sebaceous	Dog, cat Dog, cat Dog, cat
Ears	Ceruminous	Sweat	Dog, cat
Perineum	Hepatoid (circumanal) Anal sac gland	Sebaceous Combined	Dog Dog, cat
Tail	Tail gland	Sebaceous	Dog, cat
Prepuce	Preputial glands	Sweat	Dog, cat
Footpads	Atrichial	Sweat	Dog, cat

1.9 Types and distribution of cutaneous exocrine glands in mammalian skin.

A single layer of basal cells (reserve cells) line the sebaceous lobules. These cells become progressively more lipidized and eventually disintegrate to form sebum toward the centre of the lobule (holocrine secretion). Sebaceous glands have an abundant blood supply and appear to be innervated. Secretion is thought to be controlled by both endocrine and non-endocrine factors; androgens cause hypertrophy and hyperplasia, while oestrogens and glucocorticoids have the opposite effect.

Sebum has both protective and behavioural roles. It keeps the skin soft and pliable, it provides the skin and hair with hydrophobic protection against overhydration, and it acts as a protective barrier against pathogens. Sebum also has an important antimicrobial action and ensures that the animal has a glossy coat; during periods of illness or poor nutrition, the hair coat may become dull due to inadequate sebaceous gland function. In addition, specialized sebaceous glands, such as the circumanal glands (perianal gland, also present in the skin of the prepuce and the dorsal and ventral aspects of the tail) and tail glands, are able to produce pheromones and thus play a role in behaviour.

Sweat glands

Sweat glands are simple or coiled tubular glands located in the superficial layers of the dermis. Those with a duct that opens into the infundibulum are referred to as epitrichial (formerly apocrine) glands, while those that have ducts opening directly on to the skin surface are known as atrichial (formerly eccrine) glands (Figure 1.10). Epitrichial glands are distributed throughout all haired skin, whereas atrichial glands are only found in the nasal planum and footpads. Specialized sweat glands are found in the ear canals (ceruminous glands) and in the eyelids (Moll's glands).

In general, epitrichial sweat glands do not appear to be innervated. It is thought that the production of adrenaline (epinephrine) and noradrenaline (norepinephrine) by adrenergic and cholinergic sympathetic nerve endings on the cutaneous blood vessels, or dopamine released by mast cells, transfers neurotransmitter substances such as adrenaline and noradrenaline to the gland. Atrichial sweat glands are richly supplied with cholinesterase-positive nerves.

Sweat protects the skin and its specialized structures, such as the eyelids and footpads, from frictional damage, maintains skin pliability and provides microbial defence through the presence of immunoglobulins, cytokines, transferrin and inorganic ions, such as sodium chloride. Contrary to humans and horses, sweat does not play a significant role in thermoregulation in cats and dogs.

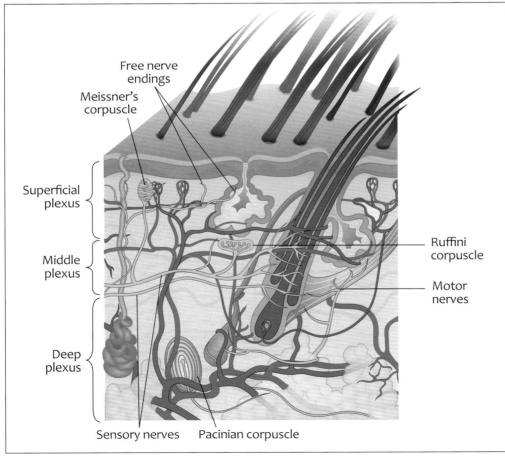

1.10 Components of mammalian skin, including epidermal structures (compound hair follicle and adnexal structures, free sebaceous gland, epitrichial sweat gland), blood supply, nerves and associated mechanoreceptors.
(Redrawn after Patel, 2012)

The basement membrane zone

The basement membrane zone (BMZ) is the interface between the epidermis and the dermis (Figure 1.11). This zone has many important functions, including:

- To ensure a firm attachment of the epidermis to the dermis
- To facilitate the transport of nutrients between the two structures
- To maintain epidermal proliferation and tissue architecture.

The components of the BMZ are the target of many genetic and immune-mediated diseases (see Figure 1.3). Thus, understanding the structure of the BMZ helps in understanding the clinical manifestations of many vesiculo-pustular diseases.

Ultrastructurally, the BMZ is composed of the following (Figure 1.12):

- The plasma membrane of basal cells
- The lamina lucida
- The lamina densa
- The sublamina densa.

Keratin intermediate filaments, formed by K5 and K14 heterodimers, connect the nuclear membrane of basal cells to hemidesmosomes. Hemidesmosomes are half-desmosomes and are located on the internal aspect of the basal side of SB keratinocytes; they are composed of inner plaque proteins (plectin and bullous pemphigoid antigen type 1 (BPAG1e, also called BP230)) and transmembrane proteins ($\alpha6\beta4$ integrin and bullous pemphigoid antigen

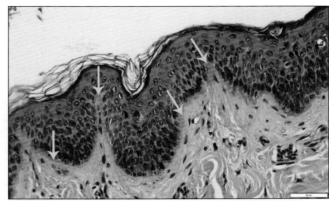

1.11 Microphotograph of a section of canine skin showing the basement membrane (arrowed). (Periodic acid-Schiff (PAS); original magnification X400)
(Courtesy of Dr William Craft)

type 2 (BPAG2, also called BP180) and collagen XVII). Anchoring filaments of the lamina lucida, composed of the extracellular domain of collagen XVII, connect the hemidesmosomes to anchoring fibrils. The lamina densa is composed of collagen IV, laminin (mainly laminin 5 (LAM332)), nidogen and perlecan, forming a tight network that acts as a filter to restrict the passage of molecules, but allows the movement of immune cells between the dermis and the epidermis. The sublamina densa is located below the lamina densa and is formed by anchoring fibrils, composed of collagen VII, which extend from the lamina densa to anchoring plaques in the superficial dermis. Focal adhesions (Figure 1.12) may also be seen, particularly during wound healing.

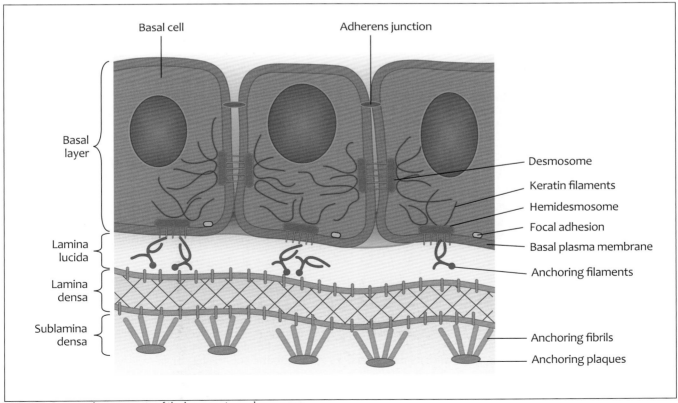

1.12 Structural components of the basement membrane zone.
(Redrawn after Patel, 2012)

The dermis

The dermis is the inner layer of skin. It has many functions, including maintaining body shape, absorbing the stresses associated with movement, modulating cell growth, wound healing, body temperature and body sensation, and contributing to body water storage. It is composed of insoluble fibres (collagen and elastic fibres) intermixed within a matrix of soluble polymers (glygosaminoglycans and proteoglycans), inflammatory mediators, cytokines and growth factors. The insoluble components of the dermis resist tensile forces, whereas the matrix resists and dissipates compressive forces. In addition, the dermis contains blood and lymphatic vessels, nerves and receptors, and cells (see Figure 1.4).

The superficial dermis is composed of fine, irregularly distributed, loose collagen fibres and a network of fine elastin fibres. Deeper in the dermis, the collagen is thicker and more dense and the fibres tend to run parallel to the skin surface; the elastin fibres are also thicker but less numerous.

Collagen

Collagen represents 90% of dermal fibres; it provides tensile strength and elasticity, but is also involved in cell migration, adhesion and chemotaxis. Collagen molecules have a triple helix structure comprising three polypeptide chains coiled around each other forming fibrils and are differentially stained by Masson trichrome staining. Glycine, proline and hydroxyproline are the amino acids most abundantly present in collagen molecules.

There are numerous (at least 28) genetically and structurally different types of collagen molecules in mammals. In mature individuals, the majority of dermal collagen is formed by types I (87%) and III (10%). Type V represents about the 3% of dermal collagen; it is found around blood vessels and helps determine the diameter of fully formed fibrils. Collagen XII and XIV are part of the recently discovered dermal FACITs (fibril-associated collagens with interrupted triple helices), which have also been found to influence the diameter of collagen fibrils.

Collagens are secreted by fibroblasts; the enzymes involved in their synthesis require iron, oxygen, copper and vitamin C. Collagen abnormalities mainly result from genetic defects and from deficiencies of vitamin C, iron and copper. Collagen synthesis is inhibited by glucocorticoids and retinoids, amongst others.

Collagenases, from the matrix metalloproteinase (MMP) family, are responsible for collagen degradation. Under normal conditions, fibroblasts are the main source of collagenases; however, inflammatory cells (neutrophils, eosinophils and macrophages) and keratinocytes can also produce collagenases under certain conditions, such as skin damage and wound healing.

Elastic fibres

Elastic fibres form a network throughout the dermis and are also present in the sheaths of hair follicles and in the walls of blood and lymphatic vessels. They are well visualized with Verhoeff van Gieson and Weigert elastin stains. Elastic fibres are composed of elastin and microfibrillar protein. Elastin is amorphous and in fully mature elastic fibres forms the core, surrounded by an envelope of microfibrils. The microfibrils are composed of type VI collagen and fibrillin. Microfibrillar material in the absence of elastin

is called oxytalan. When small amounts of elastin are present, it is called elaunin. In the superficial dermis, elaunin fibres are organized in an arcade-like arrangement. From these fibres, oxytalan fibres ascend almost vertically to terminate at the dermoepidermal junction and anchor to the basement membrane. Downwards, elaunin fibres join thick horizontal mature elastic fibres present in the deep dermis. Elastin is synthesized by fibroblasts and smooth muscle cells. Elastases are proteolytic enzymes capable of degrading elastic fibres.

Dermal matrix

The dermal matrix, previously termed dermal ground substance, is the gel found between the insoluble fibres (collagen and elastic fibres) and the dermal cells. It is composed primarily of water (plasma), glycosaminoglycans (GAGs) and proteoglycans along with other glycoproteins, mediators, cytokines and growth factors. GAGs and proteoglycans are best stained with Alcian blue, periodic acid-Schiff (PAS) and colloidal iron stains.

GAGs, also known as mucopolysaccharides, are long non-branched polysaccharides. Proteoglycans comprise a core protein covalently linked to GAG chains. In the skin, the main GAGs are hyaluronic acid (also known as hyaluronan), heparin sulphate, chondroitin sulphate A, dermatan sulphate and keratin sulphate. Although GAGs and proteoglycans account for only about 0.1% of the dry weight of skin, they can bind over 100 times their weight in water. Thus, they have an important water storage function, as well as a pivotal role in wound healing.

A critical (and the most abundant) cutaneous GAG is hyaluronic acid, which has multiple biological functions, including regulation of cell proliferation, activation of innate immunity and stimulation of sterile fever and inflammation. It is synthesized at the inner surface of the plasma membrane of fibroblasts by three glycosyltransferases (HAS 1–3); HAS 2 is usually the most active. A mutation located upstream from the *HAS 2* gene has been identified as the cause of hereditary cutaneous hyaluronanosis (mucinosis) and familial fever in Shar Peis (see Figure 1.3). Hyaluronic acid is degraded in lysosomes by hyaluronidases. Defects in some hyaluronidases result in the various animal mucopolysaccharidoses (it should be noted that only very rarely do patients present with cutaneous lesions).

Blood and lymphatic vessels
Blood supply

The skin has a well developed vascular supply. The cutaneous blood vessels (see Figure 1.10) are arranged in three intercommunicating plexuses of arteries and veins to form three networks:

- **Deep plexus:** at the base of the dermis, supplying the hair papillae and sweat glands
- **Middle plexus:** at the level of the follicular isthmus, supplying the sebaceous glands, arrector pili muscles and the mid-portion of the hair follicle
- **Superficial plexus:** just below the epidermis, giving rise to the superficial capillary network that supplies the epidermis, which is itself avascular.

The microcirculatory bed is composed of arterioles, arterial and venous capillaries, and venules. The majority of superficial dermal vessels are postcapillary venules. It is from here that inflammatory cells migrate across the vascular space into tissues during inflammation (endothelial cells develop gaps that result in increased vascular permeability). Arteriovenous anastomoses associated with thermoregulation are concentrated in the deeper parts of the dermis and are particularly common in the extremities. Control of blood flow in the capillaries is regulated by the contractile, fusiform pericytes that are aligned parallel to them.

Lymphatic drainage

The lymph vessels provide drainage for the interstitial tissue fluid from the dermis. They also drain microorganisms, topical products and drugs that have penetrated the epidermis and dermis, and channels them to the regional lymph nodes. Lymph vessels arise from capillary networks in the superficial dermis and around the hair follicles and drain into a subcutaneous lymphatic plexus. They differ from blood vessels being flatter and wider, with thinner and flatter endothelial cells and no contractile components.

Cutaneous sensation and pruritus

The skin is a major sensory organ; it has both somatic sensory and autonomic motor nerves (Figure 1.13). Somatic sensory nerves mediate sensations of touch, heat, cold, pressure, vibration, proprioception, pain and pruritus. Nerves of the autonomic motor system are associated with the hair follicle, cutaneous glands and arrector pili muscles.

Receptor	Sensory end organ	Function
Mechanoreceptors (corpuscular)	Pacinian corpuscle	Pressure and vibrations
	Merkel cells	Slow-adapting changes in pressure
	Meissner's corpuscle	Rapidly adapting pressure and velocity changes
	Ruffini's end bulb	Skin movement
Nociceptors	Free nerve endings	Itch and pain
Thermoreceptors	Free nerve endings	Warm and cold

1.13 Skin receptors and their functions.

Cutaneous nerves are located alongside dermal vessels; they are in close contact and interact with dermal cells, including mast cells, fibroblasts and keratinocytes. Neuropeptides released by cutaneous nerves (e.g. substance P, neurokinin A, vasoactive intestinal peptide) activate keratinocytes, mast cells and endothelial cells. In addition, keratinocytes and fibroblasts influence development of nerve fibres through the generation of neurotrophins (e.g. nerve growth factor). A plexus of nerves is present beneath the epidermis and free nerve endings can penetrate the epidermis itself (see Figure 1.10).

Pruritus

Pruritus is an unpleasant sensation that provokes the desire to scratch. In veterinary medicine, the definition should be extended to include the desire to chew, lick, bite and pull skin and/or fur. Pruritus is the most common clinical sign in dogs and cats with skin diseases and can have a dramatic impact on the quality of life of the patient, comparable with chronic pain. Although pruritus and pain are closely related, and there is an overlap of mediators and pathways between the two sensations, itch-specific nerve pathways have been demonstrated. Furthermore, the areas of the brain where pruritus and pain sensations are processed are different.

In the skin, pruritus begins with the release of mediators by keratinocytes, dermal leucocytes, mast cells and nerves. The mediators bind to receptors and stimulate free nerve endings located at the dermoepidermal junction and within the epidermis (intraepidermal nerve fibres, IENF). The IENF enter the dorsal root of the spinal cord and, after at least two neuronal synapses, transmit the signals to the brain via spinothalamic tract neurones. A significant pathogenic role of IENF in the pruritus associated with atopic dermatitis has been seen in human and animal models. In particular, the skin of atopic humans and dogs has an increased density of IENF compared with healthy skin, and for this reason, therapeutic approaches to reduce IENF are being evaluated.

Proteases, leucotrienes, prostaglandins, neurotropins, substance P, nerve growth factor, histamine and opioids are some of the itch mediators being targeted as potential therapeutic options. In addition, numerous cytokines are also known to exhibit pruritogenic effects. Of particular interest for their involvement in the pruritus pathway are interleukin (IL)-4, IL-31, IL-33 and thymic stromal lymphopoietin (TSLP). IL-31 is the target of the first therapeutic monoclonal antibody approved for use in dogs (lokivetmab), while anti-IL-4, -IL-13, -IL-33 and TSLP have been investigated in humans with atopic dermatitis and other pruritic skin diseases (for a more detailed explanation about the pathophysiology of pruritus, see Chapter 6).

Cutaneous immunology

The cutaneous immune system consists of resident and transient cells involved in both innate and adaptive immunity. The functions of the immune cells involved in cutaneous immunity are described in Figure 1.4.

The major immune cells involved in cutaneous immunity include keratinocytes, melanocytes, antigen-presenting cells (APCs, such as Langerhans' and dendritic cells), mast cells, lymphocytes and phagocytes (granulocytes and macrophages). As described above, keratinocytes are the main constituent of the epidermis; they not only function as a physical barrier, but also act as APCs and are a source of important inflammatory mediators. In fact, keratinocytes secrete many cytokines and chemokines that regulate the local immune response. In addition, keratinocytes are the major source of cutaneous host defence peptides, which are extremely important not only as first line of defence against microbes, but also as alarmins (danger signals) to activate an immune response in case of cellular damage.

Melanocytes are melanin-producing dendritic cells located in the basal layer of the epidermis. They produce two different types of melanin: eumelanin (black) and pheomelanin (yellow to red/brown). Melanin produced in the melanocytes is transferred to adjacent keratinocytes. Melanin has multiple functions in keratinocytes, including acting as free radical scavenger, absorbing ultraviolet light and binding to drugs. In addition, in mammals, it is also important in camouflage.

Langerhans' and dendritic cells are the most important APCs in the immune system. They are able to phagocytose, process and present antigens to naïve T lymphocytes, triggering a primary immune response. Although very similar morphologically, Langerhans' and dendritic cells differ in ontogenesis and location. The former are myeloid in origin and located in the epidermis, while the latter can be either myeloid or lymphoid in origin and are mainly located in the perivascular spaces of the superficial dermis. Immunophenotypically, Langerhans' cells express E-cadherin, but not CD4 and CD90, whereas dendritic cells are E-cadherin negative and positive for CD4 and CD90 antigens.

Mast cells are important immune cells involved in hypersensitivity reaction type I and allergies. Mast cells are mainly located in connective tissues (skin, gastrointestinal submucosa and the peritoneal cavity) and mucosae (alveoli and gastrointestinal mucosa). Connective tissue and mucosal mast cells differ in morphology, staining reaction, and T-cell-associated activation. Cutaneous mast cells are mainly associated with the superficial vascular plexus and adnexa. They contain darkly staining granules that, upon activation, secrete inflammatory mediators, including histamine, cathepsin G, proteases (tryptase and chymase), leucotrienes, prostaglandins and cytokines (e.g. IL-3, IL-4, IL-5, IL-13), into the surrounding tissues.

Key points

- In addition to being an effective physical barrier, the skin has an important immunological function
- Genetic and acquired structural defects of the skin can result in breakdown of the skin barrier, which predisposes secondary skin infections and, in the case of atopic dermatitis, allows for allergen penetration

---

References and further reading

Asahina R and Maeda S (2017) A review of the roles of keratinocyte-derived cytokines and chemokines in the pathogenesis of atopic dermatitis in humans and dogs. *Veterinary Dermatology* **28**, 16–e5

Bader HL, Ruhe AL, Wang LW et al. (2010) An ADAMTSL2 founder mutation causes musladin lueke syndrome, a heritable disorder of beagle dogs, featuring stiff skin and joint contractures. *PLoS One* **5**, e12817

Bauer A, Baterman JF, Lamande SR et al. (2019) Identification of two independent COL5A1 variants in dogs with Ehlers-Danlos Syndrome. *Genes* **10**, 731

Biggs LC and Mikkola ML (2014) Early inductive events in ectodermal appendage morphogenesis. *Seminars in Cell & Developmental Biology* **25–26**, 11–21

Bizikova P, Dean GA, Hashimoto T et al. (2012) Cloning and establishment of canine desmocollin-1 as a major autoantigen in canine pemphigus foliaceus. *Veterinary Immunology and Immunopathology* **149**, 197–207

Bønsdorff TB, Jansen JH and Lingaas F (2008) Second hits in the FLCN gene in a hereditary renal cancer syndrome in dogs. *Mammalian Genome* **19**, 121–126

Bønsdorff TB, Jansen JH, Thomassen RF et al. (2009) Loss of heterozygosity at the FLCN locus in early renal cystic lesions in dogs with renal cystadenocarcinoma and nodular dermatofibrosis. *Mammalian Genome* **20**, 315–320

Bowden PE, Henderson H and Reilly JD (2009) Defining the complex epithelia that comprise the canine claw with molecular markers of differentiation. *Veterinary Dermatology* **20**, 347–359

Cadieu E, Neff MW, Quignon P et al. (2009) Coat variation in the domestic dog is governed by variants in three genes. *Science* **326**, 150–153

Casal ML, Wang P, Mauldin EA et al. (2017) A defect in NIPAL4 is associated with autosomal recessive congenital ichthyosis in American Bulldogs. *PLoS One* **12**, e0170708

Credille KM, Barnhart KF, Minor JS et al. (2005) Mild recessive epidermolytic hyperkeratosis associated with a novel keratin 10 donor splice-site mutation in a family of Norfolk Terrier dogs. *British Journal of Dermatology* **153**, 51–58

Fletcher DA and Mullins RD (2010) Cell mechanics and the cytoskeleton. *Nature* **463**, 485–492

Gordon MK and Hahn RA (2010) Collagens. *Cell and Tissue Research* **339**, 247–257

Grall A, Guaguère E, Planchais S et al. (2012) PNPLA1 mutations cause autosomal recessive congenital ichthyosis in Golden Retriever dogs and humans. *Nature Genetics* **44**, 140–147

Holthofer B, Windoffer R and Troyanovsky S (2007) Structure and function of desmosomes. *International Review of Cytology* **264**, 65–163

Jagannathan V, Bannoehr J, Plattet P et al. (2013) A mutation in the SUV39H2 gene in Labrador Retrievers with hereditary nasal parakeratosis (HNPK) provides insights into the epigenetics of keratinocyte differentiation. *PLoS Genetics* **9**, e1003848

Kim HJ, Cronin M, Ahrens K et al. (2016) A comparative study of epidermal tight junction proteins in a dog model of atopic dermatitis. *Veterinary Dermatology* **27**, 40–e11

Leeb T, Eliane JM, Roosje P et al. (2017) Genetic testing in veterinary dermatology. *Veterinary Dermatology* **28**, 4–e1

Lloyd DH and Patel A (2012) Structure and function of the skin. *BSAVA Manual of Canine and Feline Dermatology*. BSAVA publications, Gloucester

Maja MS, Schulze K, Bergman W et al. (2009) The keratinocyte in epidermal renewal and defense. *Veterinary Dermatology* **20**, 515–532

Mauldin EA (2013) Canine ichthyosis and related disorders of cornification. *Veterinary Clinics of North America: Small Animal Practice* **43**, 89–97

Mauldin EA, Wang PP, Olivry T et al. (2017) Epidermolysis bullosa simplex in sibling Eurasier dogs is caused by a PLEC non-sense variant. *Veterinary Dermatology* **28**, 10–e3

Medeiros GX and Riet-Correa F (2015) *Epidermolysis bullosa in animals: a review*. *Veterinary Dermatology* **26**, 3–32

Metzger J, Nolte A, Uhde AK et al. (2017) Whole genome sequencing identifies missense mutation in MRBP in Shar-Pei affected with autoinflammatory disease (SPAID). *BMC Genomics* **18**, 348

Metzger J, Wöhlke A, Mischke R et al. (2015) A novel SLC27A4 splice acceptor site mutation in Great Danes with ichthyosis. *PLoS One* **10**, e0141514

Miller WH, Griffin CE and Campbell KL (2013) *Muller and Kirk's Small Animal Dermatology, 7th edn*. Elsevier Mosby, St. Louis, MO, USA

Moll R, Divo M and Langbein L (2008) The human keratins: biology and pathology. *Histochemistry and Cell Biology* **129**, 705–733

Muntener T, Doherr MG, Guscetti F et al. (2011) The canine hair cycle – a guide for the assessment of morphological and immunohistochemical criteria. *Veterinary Dermatology* **22**, 383–395

Nishifuji K and Yoon JS (2013) The stratum corneum: the rampart of the mammalian body. *Veterinary Dermatology* **24**, 60–e16

Olivry T and Chan LS (2001) Autoimmune blistering dermatoses in domestic animals. *Clinics in Dermatology* **19**, 750–760

Olivry T and Dunston SM (2015) Expression patterns of superficial epidermal adhesion molecules in an experimental dog model of acute atopic dermatitis skin lesions. *Veterinary Dermatology* **26**, 53–e18

Olivry T and Linder KE (2009) Dermatoses affecting desmosomes in animals: a mechanistic review of acantholytic blistering skin diseases. *Veterinary Dermatology* **20**, 313–326

Olivry T, Linder KE, Wang P et al. (2012) Deficient plakophilin-1 expression due to a mutation in PKP1 causes ectodermal dysplasia-skin fragility syndrome in Chesapeake Bay Retriever dogs. *PLoS One* **7**, e32072

Plassais J, Guaguère E, Lagoutte L et al. (2015) A spontaneous KRT16 mutation in a dog breed: a model for human focal non-epidermolytic palmoplantar keratoderma (FNEPPK). *Journal of Investigative Dermatology* **135**, 1187–1190

Ramírez GA, Rodríguez F, Herráez P et al. (2014) Morphologic and immunohistochemical features of Merkel cells in the dog. *Research Veterinary Science* **97**, 475–480

Santoro D, Marsella R, Pucheu-Haston CM et al. (2015) Review: pathogenesis of canine atopic dermatitis: skin barrier and host–micro-organism interaction. *Veterinary Dermatology* **26**, 84–e25

Spycher M, Bauer A, Jagannathan V et al. (2018) A frameshift variant in the COL5A1 gene in a cat with Ehlers-Danlos syndrome. *Animal Genetics* **49**, 641–644

Walko G, Castanon MJ and Wiche G (2015) Molecular architecture and function of the hemidesmosome. *Cell and Tissue Research* **360**, 529–544

Welle MM and Wiener DJ (2016) The hair follicle: a comparative review of canine hair follicle anatomy and physiology. *Toxicologic Pathology Journal* **44**, 564–574

Zanna G, Docampo MJ, Fondevila D et al. (2009) Hereditary cutaneous mucinosis in Shar Pei dogs is associated with increased hyaluronan synthase-2 mRNA transcription by cultured dermal fibroblasts. *Veterinary Dermatology* **20**, 377–382

Chapter 2

History, examination and initial evaluation

Kerstin Bergvall

Dermatology cases deserve proper attention and handling, as many skin diseases affect the quality of life of both the animal and the owner. In addition, many dermatological conditions require long-term management. A poorly managed patient might lead to owner frustration, high costs, severe complications and ultimately euthanasia of the animal, even though the disease in itself is not fatal.

Dermatology cases are often challenging. Many aetiologically different conditions can present similarly, thus a logical and thorough work-up is critical for successful management. Apart from this being time-consuming, the veterinary surgeon (veterinarian) needs to be skilled in client communication in order to obtain an accurate and relevant history, and to explain the diagnostic procedures needed to successfully handle the case. The owner might have seen a clinically similar case presentation online and may not be aware that many diseases can look very similar. It might, therefore, not be obvious to the owner that the diagnosis and treatment are not straightforward and that simplifying the procedure might lead to prolonged suffering and, ultimately, a more costly situation. If insufficient time is allocated, a structured and systematic work-up with the owner and the animal is not possible and the chances of making the correct diagnosis are decreased.

A list of possible differential diagnoses can be formulated based on the signalment, history and clinical findings on general and dermatological examination. Diagnostic tests are then chosen to verify or rule out these differential diagnoses. It is only when a definitive diagnosis is made that proper treatment protocols and a prognosis can be given.

Signalment

Signalment can help in formulating the list of differential diagnoses. There is a breed predisposition for many diseases that can aid in the diagnostic work-up. Breed predisposition can vary depending on geographical area and population. For example, Chow Chows, Akitas, Schipperkes, Newfoundlands, Border Collies, Dachshunds and German Shepherd Dogs are over-represented with the autoimmune, pustular to crusting disease pemphigus foliaceus. West Highland White Terriers, Boxers, Bull Terriers and Bulldogs are among breeds over-represented with atopic dermatitis. Nevertheless, such a list of breed predispositions has to be used with caution and it should be remembered that a given individual can have any disease (e.g. a pruritic West Highland White Terrier does not necessarily have to be atopic, but can be affected with sarcoptic mange and in a Chow Chow presenting with pustules and crusts, pyoderma still needs to be the top differential diagnosis). Breed predispositions for various dermatological conditions are not as distinct in cats as in dogs, but some diseases are more or less exclusively described in some breeds; for example, facial seborrhoea in Persian and Himalayan cats, ulceration of the nasal planum in Bengal cats and Malassezia dermatitis in the Sphynx and Devon Rex cats. There are also some genetically inherited skin diseases, such as hereditary nasal hyperkeratosis in Labrador Retrievers and Greyhounds, digital hyperkeratosis in Kromfohrländers, Dogue de Bordeaux and Irish Terriers, and hypotrichosis with short life expectancy in Birman cats. Genetic testing is available for a number of genetic diseases (Figure 2.1).

Breed of dog	Disease	Mode of inheritance	Mutation
American Bulldog	Ichthyosis	Autosomal recessive	NIPAL4
Bull Terrier, Miniature Bull Terrier	Lethal acrodermatitis	Autosomal recessive	MKLN1
Cavalier King Charles Spaniel	Keratitis sicca and ichthyosiform dermatitis	Autosomal recessive	FAM83H
Central Asian Shepherd Dog	Dystrophic epidermolysis bullosa	Autosomal recessive	COL7A1
Chesapeake Bay Retriever	Ectodermal dysplasia/skin fragilty syndrome	Autosomal recessive	PKP1
Chinese Crested	Ectodermal dysplasia	Autosomal dominant	FOXI3
Dachshund	Improper coat	Autosomal recessive	RSPO2
Dogue de Bordeaux	Digital hyperkeratosis	Autosomal recessive	FAM83G
English Springer Spaniel	Acral mutilation syndrome	Autosomal recessive	GDNF

2.1 Breeds for which genetic testing for inherited skin disease is available. (continues) ▶

Breed of dog	Disease	Mode of inheritance	Mutation
French Spaniel	Acral mutilation syndrome	Autosomal recessive	GDNF
Fox Terrier (Wire)	Improper coat	Autosomal recessive	RSPO2
German Shepherd Dog	Renal cystadenocarcinoma and nodular dermatofibrosis	Autosomal dominant	BHD
German Shorthaired Pointer	Junctional epidermolysis bullosa Acral mutilation syndrome	Autosomal recessive Autosomal recessive	LAMA3 GDNF
German Wirehaired Pointer	Improper coat	Autosomal recessive	RSPO2
Golden Retriever	Ichthyosis Dystrophic epidermolysis bullosa	Autosomal recessive Autosomal recessive	PNPLA1 COL7A1
Great Dane	Lamellar ichthyosis	Autosomal recessive	SLC27A4
Greyhound	Hereditary nasal parakeratosis	Autosomal recessive	SUV39H2
Griffon Bruxellois	Improper coat	Autosomal recessive	RSPO2
Havanese	Improper coat	Autosomal recessive	RSPO2
Irish Terrier	Digital hyperkeratosis	Autosomal recessive	FAM83G
Kromfohrländer	Digital hyperkeratosis	Autosomal recessive	FAM83G
Labrador Retriever	Hereditary nasal parakeratosis	Autosomal recessive	SUV39H2
Lagotto Romagnolo	Improper coat	Autosomal recessive	RSPO2
Lhasa Apso	Oculocutaneous albinism	Autosomal recessive	SLC45A2
Norfolk Terrier	Epidermolytic hyperkeratosis	Autosomal recessive	KRT10
Pekingese	Oculocutaneous albinism	Autosomal recessive	SLC45A2
Peruvian Hairless Dog	Ectodermal dysplasia	Autosomal dominant	FOXI3
Poodle	Improper coat	Autosomal recessive	RSPO2
Portuguese Water Dog	Improper coat	Autosomal recessive	RSPO2
Pyrenean Shepherd	Improper coat	Autosomal recessive	RSPO2
Shar Pei	Shar Pei auto-inflammatory disease (SPAID)	Autosomal dominant with incomplete penetrance	MTBP
Shih Tzu	Oculocutaneous albinism	Autosomal recessive	SLC45A2
Soft Coated Wheaten Terrier	Improper coat	Autosomal recessive	RSPO2
Viszla	Improper coat	Autosomal recessive	RSPO2
Xoloitzquintle (Mexican Hairless Dog)	Ectodermal dysplasia	Autosomal dominant	FOXI3
Breed of cat			
Birman	Hypotrichosis and short life expectancy	Autosomal recessive	FOXN-1

2.1 (continued) Breeds for which genetic testing for inherited skin disease is available.

Age can also make some diagnoses more or less likely (Figure 2.2). Diseases with clinical signs that present at birth include hereditary paw pad hyperkeratosis, ichthyosis and congenital forms of epidermolysis bullosa. Other conditions more likely to be seen in puppies compared with older dogs include juvenile cellulitis, cheyletiellosis and dermatomyositis. Demodicosis has to be considered in young dogs, especially those between 6 and 9 months of age, although it can be present in older dogs as well. Dogs with atopic dermatitis usually start to exhibit clinical signs between 6 months and 3 years of age. Food-responsive dermatosis (also known as food allergy or adverse food reaction) often starts before 1 year of age, but should not be excluded from the list of differential diagnoses in pruritic, older animals, as it can emerge at any age. A nodular, neoplastic disease that is not uncommon in young dogs is histiocytoma. This is in contrast to most other neoplastic diseases, which are more likely to occur in older animals. Hypothyroidism is a common condition in middle-aged and older dogs. Necrolytic migratory erythema and epitheliotrophic T-cell lymphoma are examples of diseases usually seen in elderly dogs. Young cats and kittens are susceptible to otoacariasis and dermatophytosis. Young cats are also over-represented with aural/pharyngeal polyps. On the other hand, paraneoplastic conditions such as thymoma-associated exfoliative dermatitis and alopecia in cats with pancreatic or bile duct carcinoma are seen almost exclusively in geriatric animals.

The colour of the dog can also be an important clue. Blue or fawn dogs can present with colour dilution alopecia, whereas black dogs can develop black hair follicle dystrophy. Cats with unpigmented ear pinnae carry the risk of developing squamous cell carcinoma (SCC) on the ear tips over time if they are exposed to the sun. Unpigmented skin is also a risk factor for actinic dermatosis and development of SCC in dogs after prolonged and repeated ultraviolet (UV) light exposure. Furthermore, the type of coat can be associated with certain conditions; for example, alopecia X and post-clipping alopecia occur in plush-coated dogs and abnormal cystic hair follicles arise in hairless breeds.

Age	Diseases
Birth to 4 months	Congenital hypotrichosis
	Cutaneous asthenia
	Dermatomyositis
	Dermoid cysts
	Digital hyperkeratosis (Irish Terrier, Dogue de Bordeaux, Kromfohrländer)
	Dystrophic epidermolysis bullosa
	Ectodermal dysplasia
	Food-responsive dermatosis
	Ichthyosis
	Impetigo
	Junctional epidermolysis bullosa
	Juvenile cellulitis
	Keratitis sicca and ichthyosiform dermatitis (Cavalier King Charles Spaniel)
	Lethal acrodermatitis
Before 1 year	Atopic dermatitis (between 6 months and 3 years)
	Colour dilution alopecia
	Demodicosis
	Facial dermatitis syndrome (Persian, Himalayan cats)
	Follicular dysplasia
	Food-responsive dermatosis
	Hereditary exfoliative lupus erythematosus (German Shorthaired Pointer)
	Hereditary nasal parakeratosis (Labrador Retriever, Greyhound)
	Histiocytoma
	Nasopharyngeal polyps (cats)
	Oral papilloma
	Otoacariasis (cats)
	Zinc-responsive dermatosis type 1 (Alaskan Malamute, Siberian Husky)
1 to 3 years	Alopecia X (hair cycle arrest: Pomeranian, Chow Chow, Keeshond)
	Atopic dermatitis (between 6 months and 3 years)
	Color dilution alopecia
	Food-responsive dermatosis (all ages)
	Histiocytoma
	Zinc responsive dermatosis (Alaskan Malamute, Siberian Husky)
Middle age to old	Cutaneous ulcerative lupus erythematosus (Collie and Shetland Sheepdog)
	Epidermal metabolic necrosis/hepatocutaneous syndrome
	Feline paraneoplastic alopecia
	Food-responsive dermatosis
	Hyperadrenocorticism
	Hypothyroidism
	Neoplastic diseases
	Nodular dermatofibrosis and renal cystadenocarcinomas

2.2 Examples of skin diseases with strong age predilection.

History

The history is an extremely valuable part of the work-up. The owner spends more time with the animal than the veterinary surgeon will ever do, and often has key information. The owner should be encouraged to be as precise as possible about the information they provide. Taking a good history requires time, and a skillful interview technique is needed to obtain the correct information from the owner. It is important to understand what the main complaint is and then acquire both a general and a dermatological history. The questions to be asked need to be adapted according to whether a dog or cat is being examined.

Information sheet

To avoid forgetting any important questions, it is useful to follow a history sheet (Figures 2.3 and 2.4). The owner can be asked the questions from the sheet, or the sheet can be given to the owner to complete in the waiting room. Sometimes it is better to send the sheet to the owner when the appointment is made and ask them to bring it along to the clinic. This allows owners to discuss the questions at home, without stress, which will likely result in a more complete and correct history. It is also possible to have the questionnaire on the clinic website and when booking the appointment, the owner can be advised to complete the form. In this case, the initial information will be available prior to starting the consultation and can be easily included in the patient's record.

Prior veterinary consultations

When the appointment is scheduled, it can be advisable to ask whether the animal has been seen by another veterinary surgeon and, if so, ask for a referral letter or request a copy of the records. This provides information regarding diagnostic tests that have already been performed, as well as treatments that have been previously administered; these are details that can be difficult for the owner to recall fully.

Duration of clinical signs

One very critical part of the dermatological history is the duration of the problem. A short history with a precise time of onset of pruritus is more likely in a dog with sarcoptic mange, whereas an allergic dog might have a longer history, progressively worsening signs and a less distinct time of onset. It is important to encourage the owner to be as precise as possible. A condition that has been going on for a long time may have lasted for 3 weeks, 6 months or 5 years. In addition, if the owner says 'It started when I got him', it should not be assumed that the condition began when the cat was a 12-week-old kitten; the owner may have adopted the cat when it was 2 years old. If the disease has been present for more than a year, it is important to know whether or not it is seasonal. Some diseases, such as atopic dermatitis, flea allergy and mosquito bite hypersensitivity, tend to be seasonal, whilst others occur all year round (e.g. food-responsive dermatosis). In climates where fleas or sand flies are endemic, it is important to know what form of flea control and sand fly protection has been used and the frequency of application of the products.

DERMATOLOGY CONSULTATION – DOG

Owner: .... Date: ....

Dog ID: .... Breed: ....

Age: .... Sex: ....

General information

How old was the dog when you got it? ....

Does your dog drink more than usual? ....

Does your dog urinate more than usual? ....

Does your dog eat with the same appetite as usual? ....

How many times per day does your dog need to go to the bathroom? ....

Does your dog have intestinal problems (vomiting, loose stool, gas)? ....

What does your dog eat, or put into the mouth?

    Food: ....

    Treats: .... Other: ....

What type of food and water bowl does your dog have? ....

Does your dog's relatives have any skin disorders? ....

Where does your dog sleep? ....

Are there any other animals in the household? ....

If so, how long have they been present? ....

Do any of them have skin disorders? ....

Does your dog spend time with dog walkers/at dog day care/kennel? ....

Does any person in contact with your dog have skin problems? ....

Does your dog have any other health problems, apart from skin related? ....

When was your dog last vaccinated? ....

When was your dog last dewormed? ....

Has your dog been abroad? (if so, where? when?) ....

HISTORY

Describe the problem: ....

At what age did your dog first show evidence of a skin problem? ....

Did it start suddenly or gradually? ....

Does your dog have   ☐ pruritus   ☐ skin lesions   ☐ coat changes: ....

                                  ☐ sneezing   ☐ running eyes? ....

If your dog is itchy (licks, chews, scratches), which came first, itching or skin lesions? ....

If your dog is itchy, how itchy on a scale 0–10? (0 = no itch; 10 = very severe itch) ....

Where are problems noticed?   ☐ Face   ☐ Paws   ☐ Ears   ☐ Neck   ☐ Back   ☐ Sides

                                  ☐ 'Arm pits'   ☐ Groin   ☐ Legs   ☐ Rear end   ☐ Tail

Is the problem constant or is it sometimes better (if so – when)? ....

Is there any seasonal difference? ....

Compared to when first noticed, is the problem?   ☐ worse   ☐ better   ☐ no difference?

How often do you bath your dog? ....

Which shampoo do you use if any? .... Moisturiser? ....

Is flea or tick prevention used? If so, what and how often? ....

Has any diagnostic test been done?   Test .... Result ....

                                       Test .... Result ....

                                       Test .... Result ....

Has any treatment been tried?

Medicine .... When? .... Dose? .... Effect? ....

Medicine .... When? .... Dose? .... Effect? ....

Medicine .... When? .... Dose? .... Effect? ....

2.3   Dermatological history form for a dog.

DERMATOLOGY CONSULTATION – CAT

Owner: .... Date: ....

Cat ID: .... Breed: ....

Age: .... Sex: ....

General information

Is your cat kept ☐ indoors ☐ outdoors ☐ both?

How old was the cat when you got it? ....

Does your cat drink more than usual? ....

Does your cat urinate more than usual? ....

Does your cat eat with the same appetite as usual? ....

How many times per day does your cat need to go to the bathroom? ....

What material is used in the litter box? ....

Does your cat have intestinal problems (vomiting, loose stool, defecating outside the litter tray)? ....

What does your cat eat?

    Food: ....

    Treats: .... Other: ....

What type of food and water bowl does your cat have? ....

Does your cat's relatives have any skin disorders? ....

Where does your cat sleep? ....

Are there any other animals in the household? ....

If so, how long have they been present? ....

Do they get along well? ....

Do any of them have skin disorders? ....

Does any person in contact with your cat have skin problems? ....

Any recent changes in the environment (new home, new family members)? ....

HISTORY

Describe the problem: ....

At what age did your cat first show evidence of a skin problem ? ....

Did it start suddenly or gradually? ....

Does your cat have ☐ pruritus ☐ skin lesions ☐ coat changes: ....

☐ asthma like symptons ☐ sneezing ☐ running eyes

    ....

If your cat is itchy (licks, chews, scratches), which came first, itching or skin lesions? ....

If your cat is itchy, how itchy on a scale 0–10? (0 = no itch; 10 = very severe itch) ....

Where are problems noticed? ☐ Face ☐ Paws ☐ Ears ☐ Neck ☐ Back ☐ Sides

                               ☐ 'Arm pits' ☐ Groin ☐ Legs ☐ Rear end ☐ Tail

Is the problem constant or is it sometimes better (if so – when)? ....

Is there any seasonal difference? ....

Compared to when first noticed, is the problem ☐ worse ☐ better ☐ no difference?

How often do you bath your cat? ....

Which shampoo do you use if any? .... Moisturiser? ....

Is flea or tick prevention used? If so, what and how often? ....

Has any diagnostic test been done? Test .... Result ....

                                  Test .... Result ....

                                  Test .... Result ....

Has any treatment been tried?

Medicine .... When? .... Dose? .... Effect? ....

Medicine .... When? .... Dose? .... Effect? ....

Medicine .... When? .... Dose? .... Effect? ....

2.4 Dermatological history form for a cat.

Pruritus

Pruritus can be caused by a variety of conditions and in many cases multiple factors are present concurrently that contribute to the pruritus. For the owner, pruritus is often considered to significantly affect both their own and their pet's quality of life. When investigating whether an animal is pruritic, it is important to ask explicitly whether it is scratching, rubbing, biting or licking, because some owners are not aware that biting or licking can be signs of pruritus. For cat owners, it is often not obvious that excessive grooming can reflect a pruritic behaviour, therefore this must be explained. If the animal is pruritic and has skin lesions, the owner should be asked whether the pruritus preceded the skin lesions or developed after the skin lesions became apparent. If the animal is pruritic everywhere, each body part should be asked about separately. To ascertain how severe the pruritus is, the owner can be asked to mark the level on a visual analogue scale (Figure 2.5). The pruritus scale can also be used later to aid in the evaluation of dietary trials and various treatment protocols. In such situations, asking the owner to keep a pruritus diary is often helpful.

10 ┐ Extremely severe/scratches constantly
Does not stop scratching whatever happens, not even in the consulting room (the animal needs to be held to stop scratching)

Severe pruritus for long periods
Scratches during night, while eating, playing, exercising or when being distracted

Moderate pruritus/scratches often
Can scratch during the night, but not while eating, playing, exercising or when being distracted

Mild pruritus/scratches rather often
Does not scratch while eating, playing, exercising or when being distracted

Mild pruritus/scratches only occasionally
Scratches slightly more than before the onset of the skin condition.

0 ┘ Normal – I do not think scratching is a problem to my animal

2.5 A visual analogue scale with descriptors for owner assessment of pruritus severity from 0–10 (Hill, 2002). Owners are asked to place a mark on the vertical line at the level representing the animal's degree of pruritus. This is then transformed by measurement into a score from 0–10. Owners should be reminded that rubbing, chewing or licking can be due to pruritus. For cat owners, it is important to include grooming behaviour as a sign of itching.

Gastrointestinal signs and dietary history

Gastrointestinal signs, including tenesmus, loose stool, mucoid faeces, haematochezia, vomiting, regurgitating and flatulence, can be associated with food-responsive dermatosis. Defecating three or more times per day has also been shown to be positively correlated with diet-associated disease. It is important to know what the dog or cat is being fed, as this information is crucial when evaluating metabolic problems and if a dietary trial is indicated. High intake of phytates or calcium can, for example, block the uptake of zinc and result in a zinc-responsive dermatosis. In cats, the high intake of unsaturated fatty acids found in certain types of food (oily fish) can lead to the development of pansteatitis. When asking about what the patient is eating, it is important to be very clear and ask about everything the animal is given. What treats are used? Does the animal receive any table scraps or supplements? Is the dog given rawhide chews? Does the dog have access to the cat's food bowl? Is any flavoured medication given to the animal? Is flavoured toothpaste being used?

Environment

Given that some diseases have a familial tendency (e.g. allergy, demodicosis, vasculitis, pattern alopecia, sebaceous adenitis, follicular dysplasia), it can be helpful to ascertain whether any of the relatives of the patient have skin disorders. In multi-pet households, if any other animals have clinical signs or lesions this should raise the suspicion for contagious conditions (e.g. ectoparasites or dermatophytosis). Other animals can also be important sources of re-infestation if they are not included in treatment protocols. Similarly, lesions on the owner can suggest zoonotic conditions, such as sarcoptic mange, flea infestation, cheyletiellosis or dermatophytosis.

For cats, it is important to know whether the animal is kept strictly indoors or has access to an outdoor area. Outdoor cats can come into contact with various animals, including rodents (reservoirs for cowpox) and other cats. They can also eat food not provided by the owner, which is important to remember if the cat has to be placed on a diet. Given that stress can induce excessive grooming behaviour and subsequent self-induced alopecia and skin lesions, questions regarding changes in the environment and how the presented cat and other animals in the household interact are important. For indoor cats, the risk of stress-induced stereotypical licking or scratching behaviour can be reduced by providing environmental enrichment (e.g. activity toys); providing a place to climb; considering where and how food is provided; and increasing number and cleanliness of litter trays. Urination or defecation outside the litter tray can also be an indication of stress and may help to define the cause of self-induced alopecia.

A travel history can also be a reason to include diseases that normally do not exist in the resident country; for example, leishmaniosis in a Scandinavian dog that has been to southern Europe.

Other clinical signs, diseases and medications

General information with respect to exercise intolerance, appetite, drinking habits, urinating and defecating is of relevance, especially in metabolic diseases. A loss of cycling in the bitch can also be associated with hormonal diseases such as hypothyroidism and hyperadrenocorticism. In addition, other systemic diseases, such as internal neoplasia, can manifest as cutaneous paraneoplastic syndromes. In cats, upper respiratory viral diseases can cause ulcerative facial dermatoses.

A complete drug history is essential. If the animal has received medical intervention to address the dermatological problem, information regarding the response to treatment is important; for example, some diseases tend to be more responsive than others to glucocorticoids. A lack of response to glucocorticoids may change the ranking of the differential diagnoses (e.g. the possibility of secondary pyoderma or *Malassezia* dermatitis should be considered). In addition, dogs with atopic dermatitis due to environmental allergens most commonly respond well to corticosteroids, whereas some animals with food-responsive dermatosis tend to be less well controlled. If the animal has received multiple (≥3) courses of antibiotics during the last year, the probability of the animal being a carrier of meticillin-resistant *Staphylococcus* should be considered and a bacterial culture and sensitivity test performed on the first visit. In addition, drug-induced or drug-triggered diseases exist. Vaccination and deworming can be associated with drug eruptions such as erythema multiforme and toxic epidermal necrolysis. Other examples include vasculitis (in the dog) and fibrosarcomas, which in cats can develop at the site of vaccination and are called post-vaccination sarcomas. Phenobarbital medication for epilepsy in the dog has been associated with liver damage and the subsequent development of necrolytic migratory erythema, and some antiparasitic topical spot-on formulations have been associated with drug-induced pemphigus foliaceus. Furthermore, before starting treatment, it is essential to know all the medication the animal is currently receiving to avoid combining drugs that might lead to side effects (for example, systemic non-steroidal anti-inflammatory drugs (NSAIDs) and corticosteroids) or where the combination needs dosage adjustment due to drug interactions (e.g. ciclosporin and antiepileptic medications).

General physical examination

Explaining to the owner what you are doing and why is essential to increase the chances of obtaining good compliance. A thorough general examination, including recording the rectal temperature, must be performed, as dermatological conditions can be associated with diseases in other organs. The general physical examination can, together with dermatological findings, point to certain diagnoses. Muscle atrophy, a distended abdomen and a palpably enlarged liver can be suggestive of hyperadrenocorticism. Muscle atrophy, lymphadenopathy, anaemia and lameness can indicate leishmaniosis. Bradycardia in an overweight patient with recurrent pyoderma is compatible with hypothyroidism. The general health of the animal can also be of critical importance when deciding upon or evaluating treatment protocols. For example, if a dog with uncontrolled allergic inflammation and pruritus at examination also has muscle atrophy of the hind limbs and the animal reacts with avoidance behaviour when manipulating the legs, orthopaedic problems can be present. Consideration should then be given to whether prescribing NSAIDs is indicated and, if so, it is preferable to avoid using corticosteroids. In cases of obesity and allergic dermatitis, the first choice for long-term control of allergic inflammation should not be oclacitinib or corticosteroids, as both carry the risk of further increasing the bodyweight.

Dermatological examination

The animal must be scrutinized systematically from nose to tail tip. The examination must be performed under good lighting and a veterinary nurse may be required to hold the animal. A muzzle or sedation may be needed if the animal is in pain. Furthermore, it is important to bear in mind that some skin infections can be zoonotic and gloves should be worn. Handling an infected animal can also carry a potential risk of a nosocomial infection; for example, by spreading meticillin-resistant staphylococci from one patient to another. Thus, hygiene routines need to be carefully monitored and this should include both hand hygiene and diagnostic instruments (Figure 2.6).

It is important to examine the ears (including otoscopy of both ear canals), the oral cavity, paws, ventral abdomen and hind limbs. Any deviations from normal skin, coat and mucosa should be carefully noted. A magnifying glass or dermatoscope (a pocket epiluminescence microscope that allows skin lesions to be viewed with high magnification and clarity; Figure 2.7) can be used to inspect lesions. A list of the type and location of lesions present, both primary and secondary, should be compiled. Figure 2.8 lists the nomenclature and definition of skin lesions and Figures 2.9–2.11 show examples of primary and secondary lesions. To be familiar with the correct terminology of

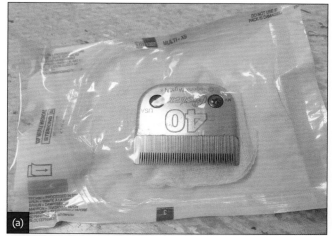

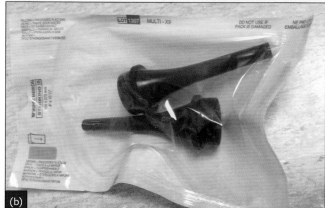

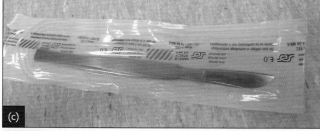

2.6 To avoid nosocomial infections far-reaching hygiene routines need to be utilized: autoclaved and sterile packed (a) clipper blades, (b) cones for the otoscope and (c) skin scraping blades.

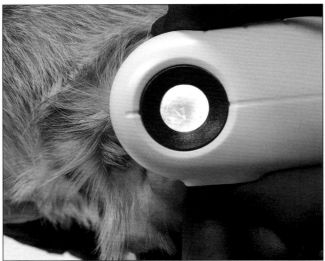

2.7 A dermatoscope is a practical hand-held tool that allows a close-up examination of skin lesions, with good light and 10X magnification.

Primary lesions	Definition
Macula	Non-palpable area of altered colour, <1 cm diameter
Patch	Macula ≥1 cm diameter
Papule	Solid elevation ≤1 cm
Nodule	Solid elevation ≥1 cm diameter
Plaque	Platform-like elevation
Vesicle	Blister ≤1 cm, filled with clear fluid
Bulla	Blister ≥1 cm
Pustule	Vesicle filled with pus
Tumour	Large mass
Wheal	Raised, oedematous area (pitting on pressure)
Can be primary or secondary	**Definition**
Alopecia	Loss of hair – spontaneous is primary, self-induced is secondary
Scale	Flakes of cornified cells
Crust	Dried exudate, containing blood/serum/scales/pus
Follicular casts	Accumulation of keratin and follicular material like a sock around the base of the hair shaft
Comedo	Hair follicle plugged with keratin and sebum
Hyperpigmentation	Increased pigmentation
Hypopigmentation	Decreased pigmentation
Secondary lesions	**Definition**
Collarette	Circular, peeling lesion (often remnant of pustule)
Scar	Fibrous tissue replacing damaged dermis/subcutis
Erosion	Epidermal defect, not beneath the basement membrane
Ulcer	Skin defect below level of the basement membrane
Fissure	Deep split
Lichenification	Thickening and hardening of the skin
Excoriation	Self-trauma

2.8 Nomenclature and definitions of skin lesions.

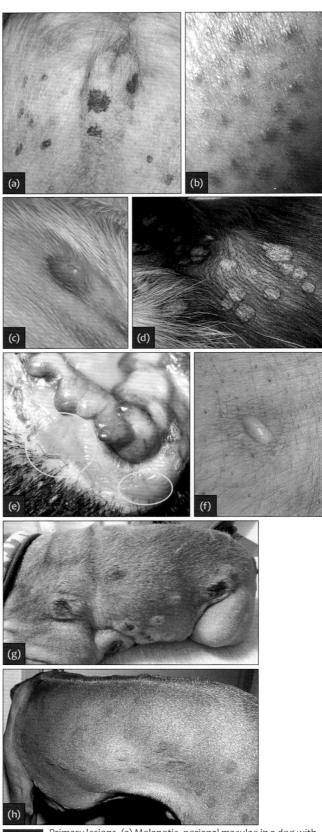

2.9 Primary lesions. (a) Melanotic, perianal maculae in a dog with a testicular tumour. (b) Papules. (c) Alopecic, erythematous nodule (mast cell tumour). (d) Plaque-formed lesions in a Border Collie with ciclosporin-induced lichenoid psoriasiform dermatitis. (e) Vesicle and bulla (circled) on the lip of a Great Dane with epidermolysis bullosa aquisita. (f) Large pustule in a dog with pyoderma and hyperadreno-corticism. (g) Nodules and tumours in an English Bulldog with non-epitheliotrophic lymphoma. (h) Wheal formation in a Rhodesian Ridgeback with urticaria.

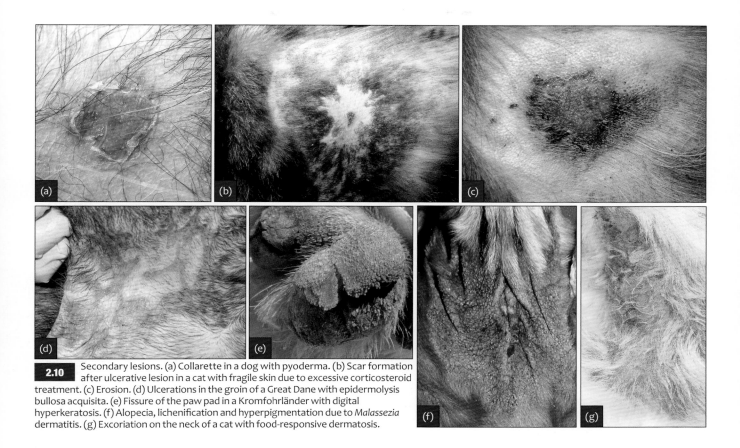

2.10 Secondary lesions. (a) Collarette in a dog with pyoderma. (b) Scar formation after ulcerative lesion in a cat with fragile skin due to excessive corticosteroid treatment. (c) Erosion. (d) Ulcerations in the groin of a Great Dane with epidermolysis bullosa acquisita. (e) Fissure of the paw pad in a Kromfohrländer with digital hyperkeratosis. (f) Alopecia, lichenification and hyperpigmentation due to *Malassezia* dermatitis. (g) Excoriation on the neck of a cat with food-responsive dermatosis.

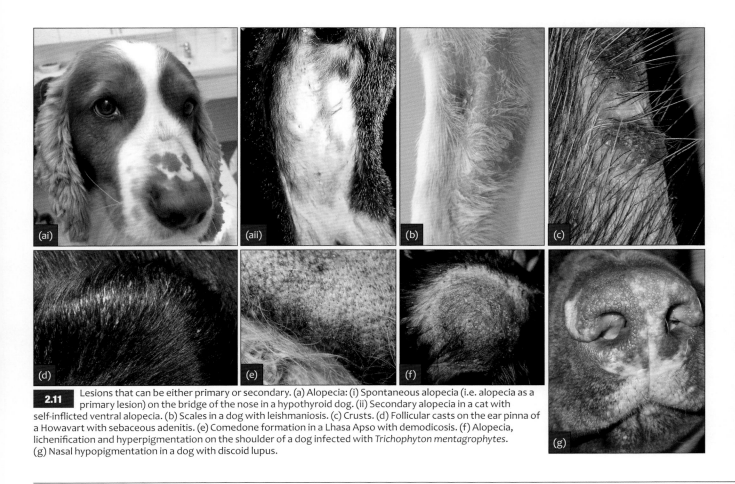

2.11 Lesions that can be either primary or secondary. (a) Alopecia: (i) Spontaneous alopecia (i.e. alopecia as a primary lesion) on the bridge of the nose in a hypothyroid dog. (ii) Secondary alopecia in a cat with self-inflicted ventral alopecia. (b) Scales in a dog with leishmaniosis. (c) Crusts. (d) Follicular casts on the ear pinna of a Howavart with sebaceous adenitis. (e) Comedone formation in a Lhasa Apso with demodicosis. (f) Alopecia, lichenification and hyperpigmentation on the shoulder of a dog infected with *Trichophyton mentagrophytes*. (g) Nasal hypopigmentation in a dog with discoid lupus.

lesions is important. Apart from understanding whether the patient's lesions are compatible with a certain condition, this is also fundamental when describing the animal to colleagues and pathologists if help is needed to proceed with the case. An inaccurate description might lead to an incorrect diagnosis with an inadequate response to therapy.

Primary lesions are more useful than secondary lesions for the formulation of differential diagnoses. Alopecia can be either primary (spontaneous) or secondary (self-induced due to scratching, rubbing, biting, licking or friction). One way to determine whether alopecia is primary or secondary is to pluck some hairs and place them under a microscope. If the tip of the hair is broken, it indicates that the alopecia or hypotrichosis was self-inflicted. If the tip is intact, the alopecia is primary (i.e. the hair is falling out spontaneously or not growing).

Diascopy can help determine whether bleeding (extravascular erythrocytes) or vasodilation is responsible for skin redness (Figure 2.12). There are also some inducible skin lesions that can develop in association with certain skin conditions or diseases (Figure 2.13).

A good tool to document the clinical findings is the digital camera. The pictures can be included in the patient's record and sent along with the referral letter to the pathologist if biopsy samples for histopathology are taken.

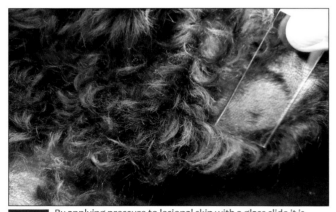

2.12 By applying pressure to lesional skin with a glass slide it is possible to discriminate between inflammatory, vascular and haemorrhagic or non-vascular (nevus) lesions. Haemorrhagic and non-vascular related lesions do not blanche on pressure.

Initial evaluation

Based on the owner's complaint, history and the clinical findings, a problem list should be generated. A list of the most likely differential diagnoses corresponding to each problem should then be made. The problem-based list of differential diagnoses should be discussed with the owner. Appropriate diagnostic tests should then be chosen to either verify or exclude those diagnoses and a diagnostic plan made together with the owner. Based on the results of the diagnostic tests, treatment options, costs and prognosis should be discussed.

It is important to ascertain the expectations of the owner. If the owner identifies any difficulties associated with carrying out the treatment plan, these should also be discussed. For example, if it is difficult to administer pills to a cat, can liquid medication be given instead? Is there any way to help with practical hints or tips on how to succeed with the treatment plan? Would a pill box be useful to remember to give medication on an every-other-day basis (azathioprine or corticosteroids)? A practical and informative demonstration of how topical treatments are carried out, as well as written information sheets, are valuable. If the animal has a treatable but not curable condition, the difference should be explained to the owner. Many dermatological conditions require a long term treatment protocol. The chance of success relies on the ability to build a treatment team together with the owner to care for the animal. The animal should be rechecked to evaluate the outcome of the treatment protocol and revisions made if necessary.

Key points
- Take a history of the evolution of the skin disease, as clinical features can change over time
- Consider the impact of the clinical signs on the animal's and owner's quality of life
- Take note of the animal's response to previous treatments, as this may be helpful in formulating a diagnostic work-up

Inducible phenomenon	Procedure	Skin condition association
Diascopy	Applying pressure with a glass slide to erythematous skin to determine if blanching occurs	Discriminating erythema due to blood vessel dilation (inflammation) from extravasated blood (bleeding, purpura)
Darier sign	Rubbing or stroking the skin induces wheal formation	Mastocytosis
Indirect Nikolsky sign or bulla spread sign (Asboe-Hansen or Lutz sign)	Applying pressure upon an intact bulla causes expansion into surrounding normal skin	Bullous pemphigoid, epidermolysis bullosa acquisita
Koebner (Köbner) phenomenon	Appearance of new skin lesions on areas of skin injury in otherwise healthy area	Perforating dermatitis
Nikolsky sign	Applying pressure with a finger on normal-looking skin causes epidermal separation producing an erosion	Pemphigus vulgaris
Pseudo-Nikolsky sign	Applying pressure with a finger cause epidermal separation but only in erythematous areas	Stevens-Johnson syndrome, toxic epidermal necrolysis

2.13 Inducible skin phenomena and their associations with various skin conditions.

Case example

An 8-year-old male, intact Tervueren (Belgian Shepherd Dog) with the complaint of pruritus was presented to the clinic. The owner estimated the pruritus score to be 5/10. Clinical examination revealed papules, crusts and collarettes on the lateral thorax, ventral chest and abdomen. The tail was sparsely haired and the dog had loss of primary hairs and spontaneous, symmetrical alopecia on the neck. A linear preputial erythema was noted. Heart rate, respiratory rate and rectal temperature were normal. Lymph nodes and testicles appeared normal upon palpation. A list of likely differential diagnoses, based on signalment, history and physical examination, and corresponding diagnostic tests was made (Figure 2.14).

Problem	Differential diagnoses	Probability	Diagnostic tests
Pruritus	Cutaneous infections (pyoderma, *Malassezia*)	Highly likely	Cytology, culture, response to treatment
	Ectoparasitosis	Likely	Flea combing, tape preparations and skin scrapings for direct microscopy, PCR test for scabies, anti-scabies IgG serology, response to treatment
	Allergy (food-responsive dermatosis/atopy/flea bite hypersensitivity)	Less likely (onset at an age too old for atopy, not living in flea endemic area, food-responsive dermatosis possible)	Food trial, exclusion of differential diagnoses, allergen specific IgE-testing (intradermal testing, serology), flea control
Papules/crusts/ collarettes	Cutaneous infections (pyoderma, dermatophytosis)	Highly likely	Cytology, culture, PCR test for dermatophytes, trichogram for direct microscopy
	Ectoparasitosis (scabies)	Likely (but no lesions on ear pinnae, elbows, hocks and no pinnal-pedal reflex)	Skin scrapings for direct microscopy, PCR test for scabies, anti-scabies IgG serology, response to treatment
Spontaneous, symmetrical alopecia on the neck/tail	Testicular tumour	Highly likely (linear preputial erythema)	Ultrasonography of testicles
	Hypothyroidism	Less likely (heart rate normal, rectal temperature normal, normal activity level, hairs were not easily epilated)	Routine bloodwork, evaluation of thyroid panel
	Hyperadrenocorticism	Less likely (no polyuria/polydipsia, no muscle atrophy, alopecia usually does not start at neck)	Urine cortisol:creatinine ratio, routine bloodwork, ACTH suppression test , LDD stimulation test, HDD suppression test, abdominal ultrasonography
	Alopecia X	Less likely (wrong breed)	Histopathology, rule out endocrine disease
	Telogen/anagen effluvium	Less likely (no history of severe disease/ cytotoxic therapy)	Trichogram, histopathology
	Cyclic flank alopecia	Less likely (wrong distribution, wrong breed)	Histopathology

2.14 Diagnostic plan for a pruritic Tervueren (Belgian Shepherd Dog) with symmetrical, spontaneous alopecia. ACTH = adrenocorticotropic hormone; HDD = high dose dexamethasone; IgE = immunoglobulin E; IgG = immunoglobulin G; LDD = low dose dexamethasone; PCR = polymerase chain reaction.

Superficial pyoderma and testicular neoplasia were considered highly likely. Bacterial pyoderma was diagnosed based on cytology findings. Ultrasonography of the testicles revealed a nodular lesion in the left testis. Abdominal ultrasonography did not detect any signs of metastasis. Haematology was within normal limits. After using an antibacterial shampoo every second day for 3 weeks, the pruritus score decreased to 2/10 and papules, collarettes and crusts were no longer detected. The dog was admitted for surgery and neutered. Histopathology revealed a Sertoli cell tumour in the left testis. Four months later the dog was normal and the hair had started to regrow.

In this case, the secondary pyoderma induced pruritus, which was the reason for bringing the dog to the clinic. A thorough clinical examination revealed indications of a testicular tumour, presumably the underlying cause of the pyoderma. The diagnosis and treatment interventions led to a complete remission for this patient.

References and further reading

Gross TL, Ihrke PJ, Walder EJ and Affolter VK (2008) *Skin Diseases of the Dog and Cat: Clinical and Histopathologic Diagnosis, 2nd edn.* Blackwell Science, Oxford

Hill PB (2002) *Small Animal Dermatology: A Practical Guide to Diagnosis.* Butterworth-Heinemann, Oxford

Hnilica KA and Patterson AP (2016) *Small Animal Dermatology: A Color Atlas and Therapeutic Guide, 4th edn.* WB Saunders, Philadelphia

Miller WH, Griffin CE and Campbell KL (2012) *Muller and Kirk's Small Animal Dermatology, 7th edn.* WB Saunders, Philadelphia

Noli C, Foster A and Rosenkrantz W (2014) *Veterinary Allergy.* Wiley-Blackwell, New Jersey

Patel A and Forsythe PJ (2008) *Saunders Solutions in Veterinary Practice: Small Animal Dermatology*, ed. F Nind. WB Saunders, Philadelphia

Rybnícek J, Lau-Gillard PJ, Harvey R and Hill PB (2009) Further validation of a pruritus severity scale for use in dogs. *Veterinary Dermatology* **20**, 115–122

Chapter 3

Core investigation and laboratory techniques

Sue Paterson

The initial investigation of any skin case should start with a thorough general and dermatological history and clinical examination, including an assessment of the skin. Once these have been performed, the attending clinician should be in a position to compile a list of differential diagnoses, after which the selection of core investigative techniques can be made. Whilst textbooks, including this Manual, will produce lists of the most appropriate techniques to be performed for different skin conditions, skin cases often present with combinations of different clinical lesions, so it is important to be flexible in the approach to problems and adapt the investigation to suit each individual case.

Equipment

Basic equipment

The author would recommend having all of the basic equipment needed to perform core investigations in one place in a veterinary dermatology 'toolbox' (Figure 3.1). This means that it can be easily located and taken to a consulting room or a minor procedures area by a veterinary surgeon (veterinarian) or a nurse to perform investigative tests. The contents of the box are low cost and easily obtainable and should be checked and topped up daily. In addition, a hand lens may be useful. This allows close examination of: primary skin lesions such as papules and pustules; some of the larger ectoparasites, such as fleas, lice and *Cheyletiella* mites; the parasitic larval stages of *Trombicula autumnalis*; and ectoparasite eggs from lice and *Cheyletiella* spp.

- Liquid paraffin
- Scalpel blades (No. 10)
- 4 m Scotch® tape
- Twin frosted microscope slides
- Cover slips
- Cotton wool swabs
- Bacteriology swabs
- Flea comb
- Sterile toothbrushes
- Fine pair of mosquito forceps
- 2 ml, 5 ml and 10 ml syringes
- Chinagraph pencil

3.1 Typical contents of a dermatology 'toolbox'.

Otoscope

An otoscope is an essential piece of diagnostic equipment and should be used to examine the ear of any animal showing signs of otitis or pruritus directed at the head or face, particularly where self-inflicted trauma leads to lesions such as 'hot spots' (areas of acute moist dermatitis) on the side of the face. It is important that the otoscope is maintained adequately with a well charged light source and used with either disposable otoscope cones or freshly sterilized cones between patients to prevent cross contamination. Otoscopic examination allows visualization of the ear canal and tympanic membrane, which is essential when selecting therapy. It also aids in the diagnosis of ear mite infestations and the presence of foreign bodies, such as grass awns, within the ear canal. Where the ear is painful, the animal should be sedated and given appropriate analgesia to allow a proper examination of the ear, or should be admitted for examination under general anaesthetic. Video-otoscopic examination of the ear offers significant advantages to hand-held otoscopy. Video-otoscopy provides superior illumination and allows the clinician to produce images for reference for patient records and to show the owners the condition of their pet's ear. Video-otoscopy allows the performance of diagnostic techniques, such as pinch biopsy and fine-needle aspiration, as well as the collection of cytology samples. Minor surgical procedures can also be performed via the working channel, such as flushing of the external ear canal and middle ear, and traction or laser removal of polyps. Deep ear flushes are crucial for cases of otitis media and should only be performed in patients that are intubated to prevent accidental aspiration pneumonia.

Wood's lamp

A Wood's lamp emits ultraviolet (UV) light at a wavelength of approximately 365 nanometers and can be used to detect the presence of dermatophyte species that fluoresce. Dermatophytes that are known to fluoresce include *Microsporum canis*, the most common dermatophyte identified in dogs and cats, together with *M. distortum*, *M. audouinii*, *M. equinum* and *Trichophyton schoenleinii*. A World Association of Veterinary Dermatology (WAVD) consensus paper revealed that the typical apple green fluorescence seen on hairs infected with *M. canis* is positive in 90–100% of cases (Moriello *et al.*, 2017); the paper also reported that a Wood's lamp has a positive predictive value of 90% and a negative predictive value of 94%. Reasons for failure to make an accurate diagnosis of *M. canis* infection with a Wood's lamp are listed in Figure 3.2.

False-negative diagnosis

- Inadequate or poorly maintained lamp
- Lack of magnification of the lesions
- Failure to allow the lamp to warm up before use (allow at least 5 minutes)
- Poor patient compliance
- Poor technique, including lack of appropriate training in its use
- Treatment of pet with systemic antifungal drugs. Topical drugs, such as enilconazole or lime sulphur, do not destroy fluorescence

False-positive diagnosis

- Fluorescence of the skin or scale rather than the hairs
- Fluorescence due to the presence of topical medication
- Fluorescence due to bacterial infection

3.2 Reasons for false-negative and false-positive diagnoses using a Wood's lamp to identify *Microsporum canis*.

Dermoscope

Dermoscopy has recently been described as a non-invasive technique to diagnose skin lesions in dogs and cats. A dermoscope allows illuminated magnification of the skin and has been used extensively in human dermatology over the last 20 years to investigate follicular diseases. Several papers have been published describing its use in the investigation of alopecic disease in the cat, including dermatophytosis (Scarampella *et al.*, 2015).

In-house diagnostic techniques

Coat brushing

Technique

Coat brushing can be performed using a toothbrush, fine-toothed comb or small plastic hair or scalp brushes (Denman). Collected material can be examined using a hand lens and/or transferred on to a slide for microscopy. If microscopy cannot be performed immediately, samples should be placed into a sterile pot to prevent ectoparasites escaping. A wet paper test is a modified form of coat brushing where the material from the animal's coat is brushed on to the wet paper. Live fleas can be easily visualized and flea faeces can be seen as streaks of blood.

Findings

Coat brushing samples may reveal superficial parasites such as adult lice, *Cheyletiella* spp. and their eggs, and fleas and flea faeces

Hair plucking (trichography)

Technique

Trichography is the microscopic examination of plucked hairs. Hair plucks are useful to assess the tips and shafts of the hairs and the hair bulbs. To perform a hair pluck, the hair should be grasped firmly between the finger and thumb and epilated in the direction of hair growth. A small pair of artery forceps may be used to grasp the hairs but can cause crush artefact on the hair shaft (Figure 3.3). To avoid this, drip tubing may be applied to the jaws of the forceps. Where hair plucks are used to identify dermatophytes, infected hairs (*M. canis* only) can be examined with a Wood's lamp, then plucked. Hairs can then be mounted in mineral oil, compounded chlorphenolac, blue-black ink or potassium hydroxide (KOH) 10–20% to help highlight fungal elements, before microscopic examination.

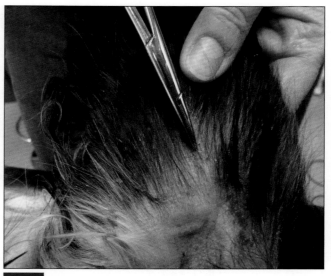

3.3 Artery forceps can be used to pluck hair.

Findings

Trichography may reveal anagen bulbs (round) or telogen bulbs (spear-shaped) (Figure 3.4). Common abnormalities include: frayed and fractured hair shafts (self-induced trauma; Figure 3.5) and parasites (*Cheyletiella* spp. eggs on hairs (Figure 3.6), follicular *Demodex* mites parallel to deep hair shafts (Figure 3.7)). Dermatophyte-infected hairs appear frayed and distorted (low power), fungal hyphae are seen within the hair shaft and arthroconidia (spores) are visible surrounding the hair shaft (high power).

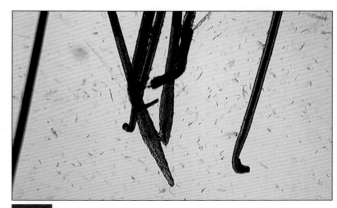

3.4 Anagen and telogen bulbs on a hair pluck.

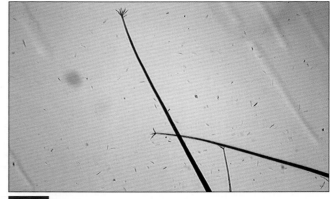

3.5 Frayed hair tips due to self-inflicted trauma.

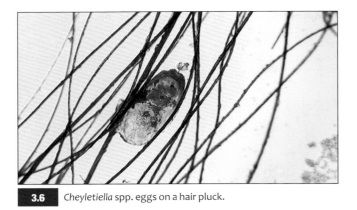

3.6 *Cheyletiella* spp. eggs on a hair pluck.

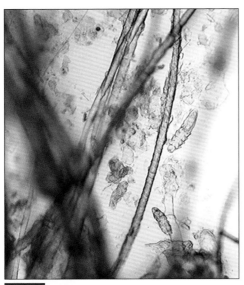

3.7 *Demodex* mites found parallel to the hair shaft on a hair pluck.

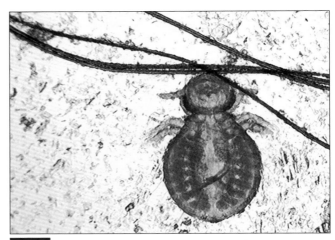

3.8 Adult *Trichodectes canis* (canine biting louse) on a tape strip.

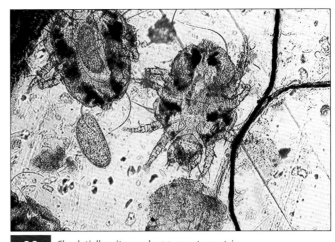

3.9 *Cheyletiella* mites and eggs on a tape strip.

Adhesive tape impression smears (acetate strips)

Acetate strips of coat

Technique: Samples may be taken using clear 4 m Scotch® tape. The sticky side of the tape is repeatedly pressed on to haired areas of the coat to collect material. Where animals are pruritic, this is best applied to inaccessible areas (e.g. the back of a cat's neck) to avoid loss of material due to grooming activity. The tape can be applied sticky side down directly on to the microscope slide for examination. As the tape acts as a cover slip, the sample can also be examined under high power (X100 in oil immersion).

Findings: Samples may reveal superficial living parasites such as adult lice (Figure 3.8) and their eggs, *Cheyletiella* spp. and their eggs (Figure 3.9), *Trombicula autumnalis*, *Otodectes cynotis*, and fleas and flea faeces.

Acetate strips of skin

Technique: Samples are taken with clear 4 m Scotch® tape as this holds its shape well when stained. The tape should be pressed firmly on to the area of skin to be examined (e.g. an area of erythema or superficial erosion) and gently rubbed with a thumb nail to ensure good contact of the tape with the skin. The tape should then be looped on to the microscope slide with the sticky side outermost (Figure 3.10) and immersed in stain. A modified Wright-Giemsa stain, such as Diff-Quik®, is suitable. Once stained, the tape can be carefully inverted with the adhesive slide downwards on to a microscope slide for examination. Note: it is important to ensure that stain bottles are checked, cleaned and replaced regularly (e.g. once weekly) to ensure the stain does not become contaminated with microorganisms, which may give false-positive results.

Findings: Samples may reveal bacteria and yeast (e.g. *Malassezia* spp.), as well as cellular infiltrates, which may be inflammatory or neoplastic. Occasionally, surface parasites such as *Demodex* spp. may be seen.

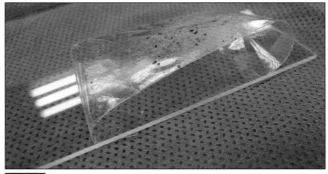

3.10 Tape strip from skin, looped on to slide ready for staining.

Acetate tape strips of squeezed skin

Technique: This technique is an effective way to identify *Demodex* spp. The sensitivity of this technique has been considered comparable to deep skin scrapings and it is less traumatic compared with traditional deep skin scrapings. For these reasons, it is used for sensitive areas. The skin is gently squeezed between the finger and thumb to extrude material, and the tape is pressed on to the area to collect a sample, which can then be examined microscopically.

Findings: Samples may reveal *Demodex* mites, larvae and eggs.

Direct and indirect impression smears
Direct impression smears

Technique: Direct impression smears are suitable for any exudative lesion (e.g. erosions, ulcers, furuncules, pustules or the underside of crusts). Samples from an intact pustule can be collected by gently rupturing the pustule using a sterile 25 G needle; the contents can then be pressed on to a microscope slide. For exudative lesions, the microscope slide can be pressed directly on to the lesion (Figure 3.11). A sterile 25 G needle can be used to express fluid from non-exudative lesions. The sample may be air dried or carefully warmed to fix it (e.g. using a hair dryer or hand drier). The slide is then stained using a modified Wright-Giemsa stain (Diff-Quik®) and gently rinsed across the reverse of the slide and dried again. The sample should be examined on low power (X10 objective) initially to select areas for close inspection subsequently on high power (X40) or under oil immersion (X100).

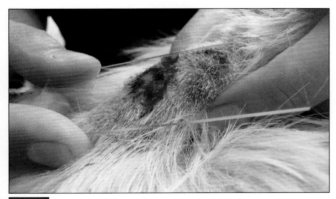

3.11 Direct impression smear from an exudative lesion.

Indirect impression smears

Technique: Indirect impression smears are best taken with a cotton swab from areas of ulceration and exudation, where a direct impression smear is difficult due to the location. Suitable areas include inaccessible ulcers (e.g. intertriginous lesions), a sinus or otic discharge. The swab should be gently rolled along the microscope slide, heat fixed and then stained as detailed above. Two samples should be taken from the ear canal. One sample can be prepared as other impression smears by heat fixing and staining. The second sample can be prepared and examined without heat fixing and staining to assess for ectoparasites. Examination of the sample should follow a logical progression from low to high power (see 'Direct impression smears' above).

Findings: Samples from the skin and ears may reveal bacteria and yeast (e.g. *Malassezia* spp.), as well as cellular infiltrates, which may be inflammatory or neoplastic. Parasites such as *Demodex* spp. and *Otodectes cynotis* may also be seen.

Superficial and deep skin scrapes
Superficial skin scrapes

Technique: Superficial skin scrapes remove the most superficial levels of the stratum corneum. If the hair coat is thick, then hair may be gently clipped to access the surface of the skin. Scrapes are taken using a No. 10 scalpel blade into either liquid paraffin or 10% potassium hydroxide. Site selection will generally depend on the case but the dorsum is the most common site to identify surface browsing parasites. The skin may be moistened either with liquid paraffin (if it is being used as the mounting material) or with water (if potassium hydroxide is being used) to ensure that the scraped material remains adherent to the scalpel blade. The scalpel should be held perpendicular to the skin and the scraping should be performed in the direction of the hair coat to collect material on to the blade. This can then be scraped into mounting material (liquid paraffin or 10% potassium hydroxide) on a microscope slide. Figure 3.12 details the advantages and disadvantages of each mounting material. A cover slip should then be applied to facilitate microscopic examination of the sample.

Deep skin scrapings

Technique: Deep skin scrapings remove the full thickness of the epidermis to create capillary ooze (Figure 3.13). The technique is identical to that used for a superficial skin scraping, only the depth of scrape differs. Site selection is important for a deep skin scraping. Multiple samples should be taken from non-excoriated predilection sites, such as the extensor aspect of the hock and elbow and the periphery of the ear pinnae, to identify *Sarcoptes scabiei*. Scrapes should be taken from non-excoriated areas of comedone formation to identify *Demodex* spp. The skin should be gently squeezed to express the mites from the follicles and scraped in the direction of the hair coat.

Findings: Figure 3.14 provides information on the best techniques to identify ectoparasites. Superficial skin scrapings may reveal parasites such as lice, *Cheyletiella* spp. and their eggs, *Trombicula autumnalis*, *Otodectes cynotis* and fleas. Deep skin scrapings may reveal *Notoedres*, *Sarcoptes* (Figure 3.15) and *Demodex* spp. (Figure 3.16).

Liquid paraffin	Potassium hydroxide (5–10%)
Mites are preserved and their motility can be used to identify them on a section	Mites are killed at high end of the concentration and are therefore immotile on sections
Where samples are not examined immediately, the mites may curl up making examination more difficult	Mites remain well preserved and samples can be examined some time after they have been taken
Not toxic to the skin of the patient and the investigator	Caustic to the skin of patient and the investigator
The sample is not cleared so skin debris can make identification of ectoparasites difficult	Potassium hydroxide will clear the sample within 30 minutes, making visualization of ectoparasites easier

3.12 Advantages and disadvantages of the different mounting materials.

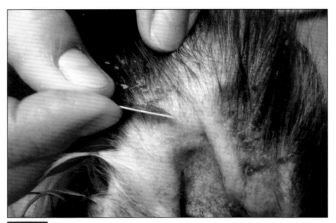

3.13 Deep skin scraping from an ear pinna showing capillary ooze.

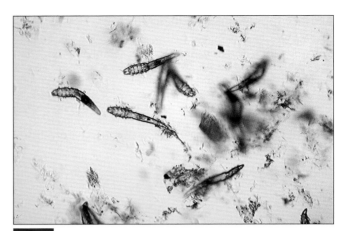

3.16 *Demodex canis* mites from a deep skin scraping.

Disease	Ectoparasite	Most important diagnostic tests
Sarcoptic mange (scabies)	*Sarcoptes scabiei*	Deep skin scrape
Notoedric mange	*Notoedres cati*	
Cheyletiellosis	*Cheyletiella blakei*	Coat brushing, acetate tape impressions and superficial skin scrapes. Eggs of *Cheyletiella* and lice can be identified on hair plucks
	Cheyletiella yagsuri	
	Cheyletiella parasitovorax	
Pediculosis (lice)	*Trichodectes canis*	
	Linognathus setosus	
	Felicola subrostratus	
Trombiculiasis (harvest mites)	*Trombicula autumnalis*	
Otoacariasis (ear mites)	*Otodectes cynotis*	Indirect impression smear of ceruminous discharge. Acetate tape impression smears or superficial skin scrapes of coat to pick up ectopic infestations
Demodicosis (demodectic mange)	*Demodex canis*	Deep skin scrapes, hair plucks, acetate tape impression smears of squeezed skin
	Demodex injai	
	Demodex cati	
	Demodex gatoi	

3.14 Best diagnostic techniques to identify each ectoparasite.

Fine-needle aspiration

Technique

Fine-needle aspiration is most suitable for nodular lesions, especially those associated with neoplastic and pyogranulomatous disease. Samples are collected using a 21–23 G needle attached to a 2 or 5 ml syringe. Most animals tolerate conscious sample collection, but samples can also easily be taken during other procedures. The lesion should be sterilized with spirit and immobilized between the finger and thumb. The needle can then be inserted into the lesion, whilst pressure is applied to the plunger to create negative pressure (Figure 3.17). The needle is gently repositioned within the lesion without removing it, to draw up as much material as possible. The pressure on the needle should be released before it is withdrawn. Sampling should be stopped if blood enters the hub of the needle. The needle should then be removed and the plunger withdrawn to fill the syringe with air. The needle is then replaced and the contents of the needle expressed on to a clean microscope slide. The material may be gently smeared, if necessary, and dried and stained as detailed for impression smears. The slide should be scanned initially on a low power (X4 or X10) to identify areas of interest before using high power (X40) or oil immersion (X100).

Findings

Fine-needle aspirates may reveal cellular infiltrates, which can be inflammatory or neoplastic. Where lesions are infected, bacteria and yeast may also be present in the samples.

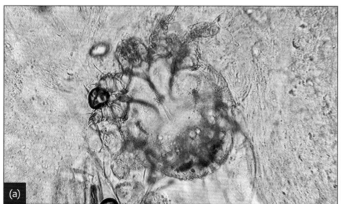

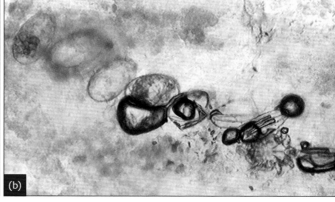

3.15 (a) *Sarcoptes scabiei* mite and (b) *Sarcoptes scabiei* mite eggs from a deep skin scraping.

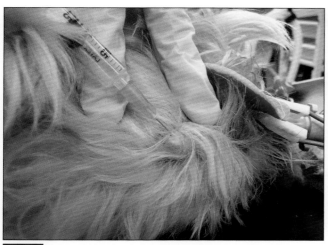

3.17   Fine-needle aspiration of a nodular lesion on a dog.

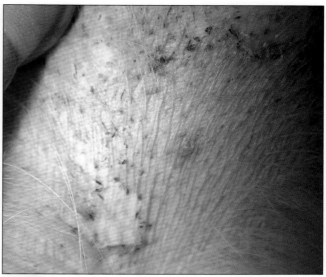

3.20   Superficial pyoderma lesions. Only the primary pustule is suitable to be sampled for culture.

Culture

Bacterial culture

Technique

Bacterial culture is not necessary in all cases of infection (Figures 3.18 and 3.19). Many cases can be identified on the basis of cytology and treated successfully with topical therapy (Beco *et al.*, 2013). Lesion selection is key in successfully culturing and identifying pathogenic bacteria. Where possible, samples for bacterial culture should be taken from a primary pustular lesion (Figure 3.20); more chronic secondary lesions, such as epidermal collarettes and areas of crusting, often reveal contaminants. A pustule should be ruptured using a sterile 25 G needle and the contents absorbed on to a sterile transport swab. Some authorities recommend the use of an alcohol wipe on the skin before sampling, but this can lead to false-negative results if the alcohol penetrates the pustule. Samples for culture should be submitted to a diagnostic laboratory. All submissions should include a complete clinical history, including the site of sample collection, so that an appropriate antibiotic susceptibility panel can be used. Where possible, the laboratory should undertake detailed identification of the bacteria isolated, especially if a multiple drug resistant isolate is suspected.

- Non life-threatening infection
- First episode of skin disease
- Clinical lesions are consistent with a surface or superficial pyoderma
- Cytology is consistent with staphylococcal infection
- There is no reason to suspect resistance

3.18   Situations where culture is not indicated and topical treatment may be adequate (Beco *et al.*, 2013).

- Life-threatening infection where the first antibiotic should be correct
- Clinical lesions of deep pyoderma
- Clinical signs and cytology are not consistent with each other
- Rod-shaped bacteria are found on cytology
- Infection has failed to respond to empirical therapy
- Antibiotic resistance is likely (several courses of antibiotics, non-healing wound, postoperative or nosocomial infection, owner or animal recent health care contacts)

3.19   Situations where culture is always necessary (Beco *et al.*, 2013).

Findings

Culture may identify the bacterial pathogen and its drug susceptibility. In most canine skin cases, coagulase-positive *Staphylococcus pseudintermedius* is the pathogen isolated.

Fungal culture

Technique

Three techniques can be used to obtain samples for dermatophyte culture: hair coat brushings, hair plucking and acetate strip sampling. Figure 3.21 describes other ways to diagnose dermatophytosis. Hair coat brushings and acetate strip sampling appear to be the most useful techniques. Coat brushing can be performed with sterile carpet squares or Denman brushes but, in practice, a new sterile toothbrush is the easiest way to take a hair coat brushing. Lesions should be brushed vigorously to collect material, which should be stored and when necessary posted in a paper bag rather than plastic to avoid overgrowth of commensal organisms. In the practice laboratory, the toothbrush can be inoculated directly into a fungal culture medium. Sabouraud's dextrose agar (SDA) and dermatophyte test medium (DTM) are suitable growth media. SDA encourages the development of typical fungal growth characteristics, e.g. reverse pigmentation and macroconidia, which are not usually seen on DTM. DTM incorporates a pH colour indicator that changes from yellow to red in the medium within 10 days, triggered by the production of alkaline metabolites, as early dermatophyte growth uses protein nutrients from the medium. Colour change after 10 days is usually caused by contaminants. DTM plates are often used in practice in-house laboratories as a quick method to identify dermatophytes; however, they are prone to both false-positive and false-negative results, so should be interpreted with care. External reference diagnostic laboratories often provide the most consistent results.

Findings

Typical reverse pigmentation and typical dermatophyte colony morphology on SDA; yellow to red colour change <10 days on DTM.

Technique	Comments
Wood's lamp examination	Identifies the typical apple green fluorescence of *Microsporum canis*-infected hair shafts. Other small animal dermatophytes (e.g. *Trichophytom mentagrophytes*) do not fluoresce
Dermoscopy	Dermatophyte-infected hairs in cats include opaque, slightly curved or broken hairs with a homogenous thickness ('comma hairs'), and hairs with a corkscrew or coiled appearance
Direct examination of hair and/or scale	Samples may be mounted in chlorphenolic, mineral oil or potassium hydroxide. Stains, such as lactophenol cotton blue and Indian ink, can be added to the mounting medium to improve visualization of fungal elements
Fungal culture	Samples for culture may be obtained by hair coat brushing (toothbrush), hair plucking or by acetate strip sampling. Sabouraud's dextrose agar (SDA) and dermatophyte test medium (DTM) are suitable growth media. SDA encourages the development of typical fungal growth characteristics, e.g. reverse pigmentation and macrocondia. DTM relies on a colour change from yellow to red in the medium, within 10 days, due to a pH change triggered by early dermatophyte growth
Polymerase chain reaction (PCR)	A positive PCR indicates the presence of dermatophytes but not that there is an active infection. It is probably best employed in combination with other tests
Biopsy	Not a useful diagnostic tool for dermatophytosis as very insensitive. False-negative results are very common. Histopathology with special stains may be useful for nodular lesions

3.21 Diagnostic techniques to identify dermatophytes (Moriello *et al.*, 2017).

Skin biopsy

Skin biopsy is useful for many different skin conditions. Samples should ideally be taken within 3 weeks for any dermatosis that is not responding to appropriate therapy. Biopsy is usually performed under light sedation and local analgesia. If a local anaesthetic is used it should not contain adrenaline (epinephrine), as this can distort vascular changes within the sample. Where footpads, periocular areas and the nasal planum are to be sampled, a general anaesthetic is preferable.

The indications for biopsy and use of each technique are detailed in Figures 3.22 and 3.23, respectively. Primary lesions, such as pustules, papules and vesicles, should be sampled wherever possible as they provide the most information about the underlying disease process. Chronic secondary lesions, such as lichenification, rarely provide diagnostic information. Punch, wedge and excisional biopsies can be performed. With the exception of excisional biopsies, multiple full thickness skin biopsy samples should be taken to provide the pathologist with a range of material; lesional and non-lesional skin should be included. Glucocorticoids should be withdrawn for 2–3 weeks before biopsy, and bacterial infection should be controlled to prevent distortion of the histopathological pattern. Where haired skin is to be sampled, hair should be gently clipped or cut with scissors. The skin should not be cleaned prior to sampling.

Samples for histopathology should be immersed in 10 times their own volume of 10% buffered neutral formalin; tissue samples for culture should be placed in sterile saline. Small and thin biopsy samples should be attached to cardboard or a tongue depressor for 20 to 30 seconds before immersing in formalin to ensure they do not warp.

- Neoplastic or suspected neoplastic lesions
- A nodule, ulcer or non-healing wound
- Vesicular and pustular lesions
- Skin lesions that develop suddenly, are severe or unusual
- Suspected conditions where therapy is expensive, hazardous or of an extended duration
- Skin lesions that develop during the course of therapy or lesions that are not responding to apparently rational therapy
- Any case where initial diagnostic tests suggest it is a dermatosis diagnosed by biopsy (e.g. sebaceous adenitis, immune-mediated disease)

3.22 Indications for taking a biopsy sample.

Biopsy type	Indications
Punch biopsy	• Primary lesions, where the whole lesion can be included • Alopecic areas, where a range of different sites, including an alopecic area and the junction of an alopecic area with unaffected skin, should be sampled
Wedge biopsy	• Deep lesions and ulcerated lesions (such as those seen with vasculitis), where the biopsy needs to extend down into the panniculus • Ulcers or depigmenting lesions, where the junction between normal and abnormal skin needs to be included • Areas such as the periocular skin, footpads and ear pinnae, where suturing and scarring may be more problematical and a linear wound will suture more easily
Excisional biopsy	• Larger samples than incisional or punch biopsies required • Small or deep lesions, tumours and nodules and where lesions are likely to be disturbed by punch biopsy (e.g. vesicle)

3.23 Indications for each biopsy technique.

The wound may be cleaned then sutured or stapled after biopsy collection. The sample should be submitted with a full signalment, complete history and a list of differential diagnoses to an experienced dermatopathologist.

Punch biopsy

Samples should be collected using a disposable 4, 6 or 8 mm sharp biopsy punch. In most cases, 6 or 8 mm punches should be used, but where sensitive or difficult to suture areas (e.g. footpad or nasal planum) are to be sampled, a small diameter punch (4 mm) may be better. The punch should be placed over the entire primary lesion and rotated in a single direction to cut through the tissue. Shearing damage to the sample (which can make interpretation more difficult) will occur if the punch is rotated backwards and forwards, or a blunt punch is used. Once the punch has been used, the core of tissue can be gently lifted from the skin using a fine needle. A scalpel blade can be used to cut the column of skin away from the underlying tissue. The hole can then be closed with a single stitch or staple. A line should be drawn on the sample in the direction of the hair coat in order to aid the pathologist.

Wedge or incisional biopsy

A scalpel blade is used to cut a wedge of skin, which is usually taken across a lesion edge to include both normal and abnormal skin. The direction of the ellipse should be with the long axis across the junction of normal and abnormal tissue. An indelible skin marker may also be used to ensure the pathologist is aware of the correct direction of cut when processing the samples. Once cut, the wedge may be removed in the same way as a punch biopsy and the wound sutured. Incisional biopsy wounds require several sutures.

Excisional biopsy

An ellipse of tissue is excised using a scalpel blade or fine tipped scissors (Figure 3.24) to remove a whole lesion. The sample should include the lesion with a section of normal skin so that the margins of the lesion can be assessed. It is useful to draw a line on the skin surface from the normal to the abnormal tissue, together with an explanatory note on the submission form, so that the laboratory technician can orientate the sample appropriately before it is cut for staining and examination.

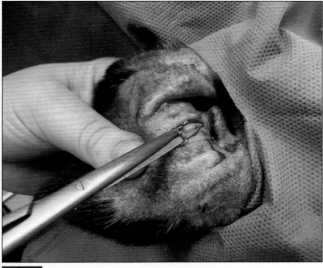

3.24 Excisional biopsy is preferable for larger lesions.

Faecal examination

Faecal examination can be useful in some situations. Faecal flotation can be useful to detect ectoparasites (including *Demodex* spp., *Sarcoptes scabiei*, *Cheyletiella* spp. and fleas) that have been ingested by the animal through licking or chewing. These parasites will often traverse the gastrointestinal tract and can be identified by standard faecal flotation techniques. Other indications for faecal examination are listed in Figure 3.25.

- Suspected allergy to endoparasites
- Cutaneous larva migrans in hookworm infestations
- When diarrhoea is a concurrent finding on examination
- To identify ectoparasites that have been ingested through grooming (e.g. *Sarcoptes scabiei*, *Cheyletiella* spp., fleas, lice, free living forage mites)
- As part of the investigation of a malabsorption syndrome

3.25 Indications for faecal examination in dermatology cases.

Key points

- Many core dermatological tests can be carried out in house and should be considered in all patients with skin disease
- Skin biopsy is most useful when lesions are unusual or not responding to routine treatment
- Primary lesions are the best areas to biopsy
- Bacterial culture and sensitivity is indicated when cytology supports a diagnosis of pyoderma but there is poor response to appropriate therapy

References and further reading

Barillas OF, Bajwa J, Guillot J and Arcique A (2019) Comparison of acetate tape impression, deep skin scraping, and microscopic examination of hair for therapeutic monitoring of dogs with juvenile generalized demodicosis: a pilot study. *Canadian Veterinary Journal* **60**, 596–600

Beco LE, Guaguere C, Lorente Mendez C *et al.* (2013) Suggested guidelines for using systemic antimicrobials in bacterial skin infections (1): diagnosis based on clinical presentation, cytology and culture. *Veterinary Record* **172**, 72–78

Moriello KA, Coyner K, Paterson S and Mignon B (2017) Diagnosis and treatment of dermatophytosis in dogs and cats: Clinical Consensus Guidelines of the World Association for Veterinary Dermatology. *Veterinary Dermatology* **28**, 266–e68

Scarampella F, Zanna G, Peano A *et al.* (2015) Dermoscopic features in 12 cats with dermatophytosis and in 12 cats with self-induced alopecia due to other causes: an observational descriptive study. *Veterinary Dermatology* **26**, 282–e63

Chapter 4

Cytology

Francesco Albanese

This chapter describes the cytological features of common non-neoplastic skin diseases and aims to correlate them with the clinical lesions in a problem-oriented approach centred on the primary skin lesions. Pustules, papules, plaques and nodular dermatitis, which may be associated with draining tracts, are common non-neoplastic lesions seen in dogs and cats. Cytology is a very important and commonly used diagnostic tool to determine the inflammatory cells present and, in many cases, infectious agents which are involved in their pathogenesis. In addition, cytology can be an invaluable tool in determining the contribution of *Malassezia* and/or bacteria to a disease process such as atopic dermatitis. A detailed description of sample collection is provided in Chapter 3. It should be noted that cytology can be diagnostic but that for some diseases a skin biopsy is needed to provide a definitive diagnosis.

Skin surface cytology

An increase in the number of bacteria and/or *Malassezia* on the skin is a common finding when the skin barrier is compromised by disordered cornification or inflammation. This is often termed bacterial or *Malassezia* overgrowth. Colonization often contributes significantly to the underlying disease process and may be associated with the development or exacerbation of pruritus. Samples from affected skin should be obtained using tape or a direct impression smear. A description of common findings can be found in Figure 4.1; examples of bacterial overgrowth and *Malassezia* dermatitis are given in Figures 4.2 and 4.3, respectively.

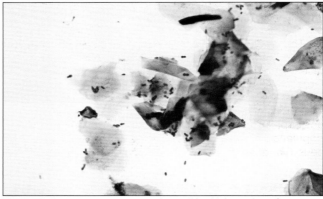

4.2 Cocci and rod-shaped bacteria, both free and on the surface of anucleate keratinocytes. (Diff-Quik® stain)

4.3 Numerous corneocytes along with a high number of peanut-shaped *Malassezia* spp. (Diff-Quik® stain)

Disease	Aetiology	Cytology findings
Bacterial overgrowth	An increase in bacteria on the skin in the absence of neutrophils often associated with atopic dermatitis	Numerous cocci (or rods) free or on the surface of corneocytes (Figure 4.2)
Malassezia dermatitis	Often associated with intertriginous areas, where an increase in humidity, lipid secretions or inflammation promote growth	Numerous bilobate budding yeasts (Figure 4.3)
Bacterial/*Malassezia* otitis	Primary ear disease results in predisposing/perpetuating factors, which favour microbial growth	Numerous bacteria (rods/cocci) and/or *Malassezia*. It may be associated with an inflammatory exudate (see Chapters 19 and 20)

4.1 Cytological findings associated with common secondary skin and ear infections in dogs and cats.

Papular diseases

Sample collection and interpretation

Papules can be inflammatory (infectious or sterile) or neoplastic. Cells from papules can only be collected using a slide imprint technique. It may be necessary to remove any surface crust. Since papules are very small, cytology specimens are often poorly cellular and haemorrhage is frequently present, thus some slides may not be diagnostic. In the case of papular leishmaniosis, lesions are larger than normal papules (papular-nodular lesions) and cytology allows to collect a large amount of inflammatory cells along with a variable number of amastigotes. It can be difficult to differentiate some sterile pyogranulomatous diseases, such as sterile pyogranuloma syndrome, from papular canine leishmaniosis on cytology, as often few amastigotes are present in the latter case. A higher number of plasma cells may support a diagnosis of protozoal disease. Figure 4.4 details the cytological findings associated with papular diseases; examples are given in Figures 4.5 and 4.6.

Pustular diseases

Pustules are very common lesions in dogs, but are rarely seen in cats. In both species they readily rupture due to the thinness of the epidermis. Cytology of an intact pustule can be important in determining the aetiology of the skin disease. By far the most common pustular skin disease in pets is bacterial pyoderma. Furthermore, a variable number of nucleated keratinocytes from intermediate epidermal layers (acantholytic cells or acantholytic keratinocytes) can be seen. In these cases, the acantholysis is secondary to the proteolytic enzymes released by the staphylococci (Nishifuji *et al.*, 2008). Cytology of samples collected from follicular and interfollicular pustules usually has similar diagnostic features. In addition to neutrophils and bacteria, occasional corneocytes derived from the roof of the pustule are found.

The most common sterile pustular disease in dogs and cats is pemphigus foliaceus. In this autoimmune skin disease, non-follicular pustules range from medium to large in size (Olivry and Linder, 2009). The disease process attacks the adhesion between keratinocytes, thus many acantholytic keratinocytes are seen. Pustules may contain eosinophils, in addition to neutrophils, in about half the population of dogs and cats affected by pemphigus foliaceus (Vaughan *et al.*, 2010). Rarely, a sterile non-follicular

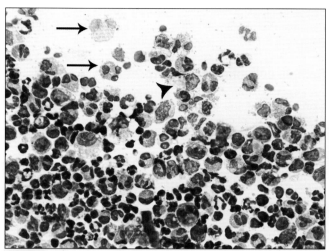

4.5 Miliary dermatitis. There are numerous eosinophils (arrowed) and some macrophages (arrowhead) in this sample obtained from a cat with feline eosinophilic dermatitis. (Diff-Quik® stain)

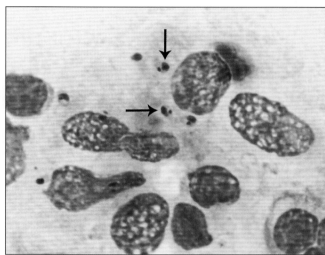

4.6 Canine leishmaniosis. The amastigotes can be recognized by the oval silhouette and the presence of an oval violet nucleus and a dark blue rod-shaped kinetoplast (arrowed). (Diff-Quik® stain)

pustulosis has been documented in dogs with leishmaniosis, in which an immune-mediated mechanism, probably triggered by protozoa antigens, has been speculated (Colombo *et al.*, 2016). Although the clinical presentation can mimic pemphigus foliaceus, the cytological and

Disease	Aetiology	Cytology findings
Superficial pyoderma	*Staphyloccus intermedius*, multifocal papules	Few degenerate neutrophils with intracelluar cocci
Miliary dermatitis	Ectoparasites, feline atopic skin syndrome, food-responsive dermatosis (also known as food allergy or adverse food reaction)	Eosinophils, variable numbers of macrophages and mast cells, rare basophils (Figure 4.5)
Mosquito bite hypersensitivity	Mosquito bites on the pinnae, bridge of the nose and muzzle (cats)	Eosinophils, occasional macrophages or basophils. Similar to miliary dermatitis
Benign papular mastocytic hyperplasia (urticaria pigmentosa-like)	Presumed mastocytosis, fine papules on trunk, often linear on abdominal skin. Rare in Sphynx and Devon Rex cats	Few well differentiated mast cells and eosinophils
Papular leishmaniosis	*Leishmania* protozoa. Puppies most often affected. Systemic signs absent and serology (antibodies/polymerase chain reaction) negative	Lympho-histo-plasmacytic inflammation. Amastigotes are recognizable by their oval shape (1–2 x 2–5 µm in size) and by the presence of a hyperchromatic rod-shaped structure, which represents the kinetoplast (Figure 4.6)

4.4 Cytological findings associated with various papular diseases.

histopathological findings are not compatible with this disease; the pustule is largely full of segmented neutrophils and there are very few or no acantholytic keratinocytes.

Sample collection and interpretation

An intact pustule should be ruptured and a direct impression smear of the contents made. Figure 4.7 details the cytological findings associated with pustular diseases; examples are given in Figures 4.8 to 4.10.

Disease	Aetiology	Cytology findings
Superficial pyoderma/ bacterial folliculitis	*Staphylococcus pseudintermedius* (dog)	Karyolysis (swollen and hypo-chromatic nuclei with loss of lobe segmentation), long streaks of nuclear material and intra-cytoplasmic cocci (Figure 4.8); few acantholytic keratinocytes
Pustular demodicosis	Staphyloccoci, *Demodex* mites	As above, with variable numbers of mites/eggs (Figure 4.9)
Pemphigus foliaceus	Autoimmune disease	Segmented neutrophils with well preserved nuclear lobes along with a variable number of round to polygonal keratinocytes, with central nucleus and deep blue cytoplasm (Figure 4.10)

4.7 Cytological findings associated with various pustular diseases.

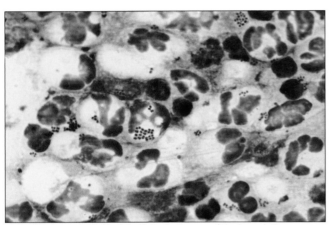

4.8 Bacterial folliculitis. Note that many of the karyolytic neutrophils are filled with staphylococci. (Diff-Quik® stain)

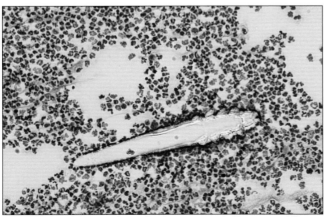

4.9 An adult *Demodex canis* mite accompanied by neutrophilic inflammation. (Diff-Quik® stain)

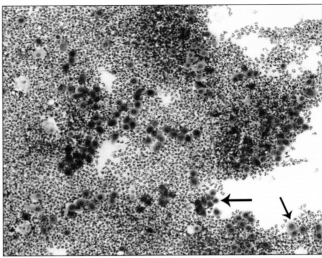

4.10 Pemphigus foliaceus. Note the numerous segmented neutrophils and rounded or polygonal acantholytic keratinocytes (arrowed). (Diff-Quik® stain)

Draining sinus tracts

Sinus tracts arise from a deep inflammatory process, which may affect the dermis, subcutis or both. Furunculosis is seen when the hair follicules rupture due to bacterial, fungal or parasitic (*Demodex*) infection. As a result, hair shaft fragments, sebum and infectious agents are released into the dermis. This may also occur with some less common sterile skin disorders. As keratin is a foreign body, a severe pyogranulomatous reaction is observed. Although present in cases of furunculosis, bacteria are not easily detected on cytology.

Sample collection and interpretation

A direct impression smear may be obtained, but in order to avoid being contaminated by surface bacteria, a fine-needle aspirate may be preferable. Figure 4.11 details the cytological findings associated with diseases that cause draining tracts and ulceration; examples are given in Figures 4.12 to 4.16.

Nodules and plaques

Skin nodules can arise from neoplastic or inflammatory processes. Inflammatory lesions can be infectious or sterile. It should be noted that in many of these conditions draining tracts may also be present.

Infectious lesions

Bacterial infections: The most common bacterial species involved in deep skin infections is *Staphylococcus* (see 'Draining sinus tracts' above). Less commonly, other bacteria such as *Nocardia*, *Actinomyces* or mycobacteria may be involved. These lesions can present with discrete nodules and are sometimes associated with draining tracts. The presence of filamentous bacteria on cytology warrants culture of the affected tissue and histopathology with specific stains. Since the cell wall of mycobacteria does not absorb standard dyes, achromatic linear rod-shaped areas (negative staining) are usually present (Figure 4.17). An acid-fast stain, such as Ziehl–Neelsen (ZN), colours the microorganisms bright red (Figure 4.18).

Disease	Aetiology	Cytology findings
Deep pyoderma	Often staphyloccoci. Other opportunistic bacteria may also be involved in chronic cases	Degenerate neutrophils, vacuolated and epithelioid macrophages, multinucleated giant cells, chronic lesions include lymphocytes and plasma cells (Figures 4.12 and 4.13)
Demodectic furunculosis	*Demodex* mites and usually bacteria as above	Similar cytology as above. *Demodex* mites may be seen
Eosinophilic furunculosis	Acute onset, aetiology unknown. Presents with papules/nodules, which progress to ulcerated plaques/nodules and draining tracts often around the face and ears	Variable number of macrophages, epithelioid macrophages and multinucleated giant cells, along with a high number of eosinophils and a variable amount of keratin (corneocytes and/or hair shafts) (Figure 4.14)
Juvenile cellulitis (Figure 4.15) and sterile granulomatous/ pyogranulomatous sydrome (SGPS) (Figure 4.16)	Juvenile cellulitis is an uncommon disease in puppies in which lesions are mainly localized on the face, eyelids, nose and pinnae Young dogs usually have significant lymphadenopathy, joint pain and fever. A similar syndrome is recognized in adult dogs SGPS is a rare immune-mediated disease characterized by multiple papular nodules or nodules, especially on the face and pinnae	Juvenile cellulitis: numerous histiocytes (macrophages and epithelioid macrophages) along with many segmented neutrophils SGPS: despite the name of the disease (sterile pyogranuloma), lesions are more commonly granulomatous; there are very few or, more often, no neutrophils present; lymphocytes are the cytological hallmark of this syndrome in most cases (lympho-histiocytic inflammation)

4.11 Cytological findings associated with diseases that cause draining tracts and ulceration.

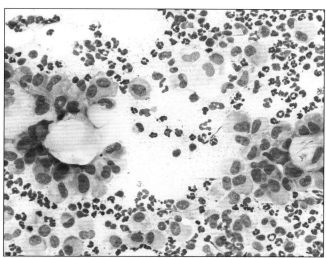

4.12 Pyogranulomatous inflammation. Note the epithelioid macrophages are surrounding large groups of corneocytes (endogenous foreign bodies).

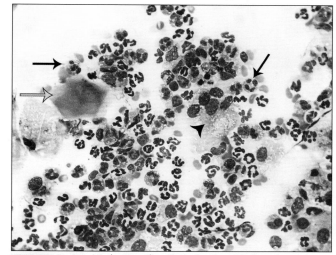

4.14 Eosinophils (arrowed), activated macrophages and multinucleate giant cells (arrowhead) in a dog with eosinophilic furunculosis. The involvement of the hair follicles is confirmed by the presence of corneocytes (yellow arrow). (Diff-Quik® stain)

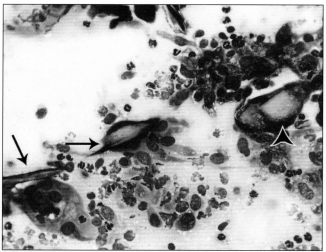

4.13 Pyogranulomatous inflammation in a dog with deep pyoderma. The free hair shaft fragments present following follicular rupture have been phagocytized by giant cells (arrowed) and intracytoplasmic corneocytes (arrowhead). (Diff-Quik® stain)

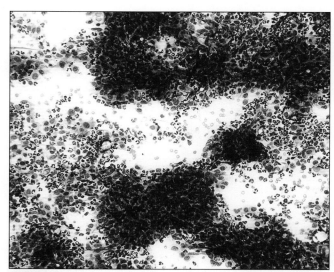

4.15 Pyogranulomatous inflammation in a case of juvenile cellulitis. Note the presence of large groups of epithelioid macrophages (granulomas) evident at low magnification. (Diff-Quik® stain)

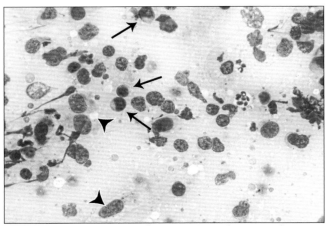

4.16 Lympho-histiocytic inflammation in sterile pyogranuloma syndrome. Note that the numerous lymphoid cells (arrowed) and macrophages (arrowheads) mainly have bare nuclei. (Diff-Quik® stain)

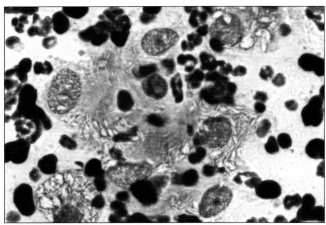

4.17 Macrophages with intracytoplasmic bacterial rods. As the cell walls of mycobacteria do not absorb routine stains, the bacteria appear clear (negative staining). (Diff-Quik® stain)

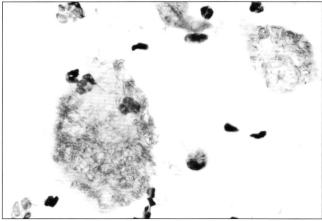

4.18 Feline leprosy. At high magnification the mycobacteria, which appear red due to Ziehl–Neelsen staining, are clearly visible. (Diff-Quik® stain)

Fungal infections: Although uncommon, dermatophyte infections may present as a kerion in dogs. Nodules are the consequence of a severe pyogranulomatous inflammation, resulting from infected hair shafts in the dermis due to folliculitis and furunculosis. In diagnostic samples, round to oval arthroconidia of 2–5 μm in size and surrounded by a thin clear halo are observed (Figure 4.19). Less frequently, segmented hyphae can also be present. In cases where the fungal infection is not detected with routine cytological stains, special stains such as periodic acid-Schiff (PAS) and Grocott's methenamine silver (GMS) can be used in order to stain the fungal bodies magenta and black, respectively.

Dermatophytic pseudomycetomas occur uncommonly in cats. It is an atypical granulomatous infection of *Microsporum canis* in the dermis and panniculcus. The formation of tissue grains seen with this infection is unusual for dermatophytosis.

Cryptococcus is a dimorphic fungus that has a characteristic yeast-like appearance once in the tissues (Figure 4.20). As with all fungi, special stains such as PAS and GMS are required to stain the cell wall. A few drops of India ink on wet squashed slides can greatly enhance the large unstained wall on a black background.

Phaeohyphomycosis is an infection caused by a group of dematiaceous (pigmented) fungi, which involves the skin and subcutaneous tissues of dogs and cats. *Alternaria alternata*, *Curvularia* spp., *Phialophora verrucosa* and *Fonsecaea* are the most commonly isolated fungi (Abramo *et al.*, 2002; Beccati *et al.*, 2005).

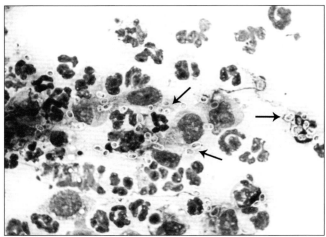

4.19 Dermatophytic kerion. The spores (arthroconidia) are easily recognizable as round to oval microorganisms with a thin clear halo (arrowed). (Diff-Quik® stain)

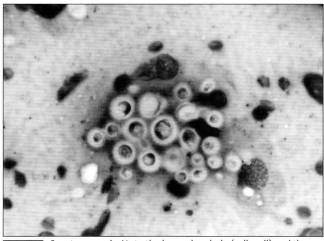

4.20 Cryptococcosis. Note the large clear halo (cell wall) and the typical narrow-based budding. (Diff-Quik® stain)

Protozoal infections: Single or multiple cutaneous/subcutaneous nodules are observed in dogs infected with *Leishmania infantum* and rarely in cats.

Parasitic infections: *Dirofilaria repens* is a filarial nematode found in certain parts of Europe. It is transmitted by mosquitoes and cycles through carnivores. The adults live in the subcutaneous tissues and can form nodules associated with a granulomatous inflammation. The presence of adults and microfilaria supports a patent infection (Albanese *et al.*, 2013).

Sample collection and interpretation: Samples should be collected from fresh exudates by direct impression smear or fine-needle aspiration. If tissue grains are present, these should be collected and a squash preparation on the slide prepared. Figure 4.21 details the cytological findings associated with infectious causes of diseases that result in nodules and plaques; examples are given in Figures 4.22 to 4.24.

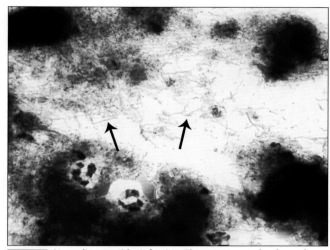

4.22 *Nocardia asteroides* infection. There are many slender and filamentous bacteria clearly evident at the periphery of the grains (arrowed). (Diff-Quik® stain)

Disease	Aetiology and clinical signs	Cytology findings
Bacterial nodule (*Nocardia*, *Actinomyces*)	Often arise as a result of animal bites or traumatic injury to the skin. Nodular swellings are often accompanied by multiple draining tracts	Filamentous, slender and often branched bacteria (Figure 4.22), which may be concentrated in grains that are cytologically recognizable as an amorphous basophilic material immersed in neutrophilic and macrophagic inflammation. Gram/acid-fast stains needed to further identify bacteria
Bacterial mycetoma (botriomycosis)	Nodules and draining tracts	Large clusters of non-filamentous bacteria (rods and cocci), both free and phagocytized by karyolytic neutrophils and macrophages. They may be recognizable on cytological specimens
Mycobacteria	Clinical lesions are characterized by single or multiple nodules, often ulcerated and with draining tracts. The clinical picture varies with the organism and species affected	Cytology also varies with the pathogen. In some cases, there is a paucity of organisms. A pyogranulomatous exudate is present. Bacteria are unstained and may be extracellular or contained within macrophages (see Figures 4.17 and 4.18)
Dermatophyte pseudomycetoma	Single or multiple nodules and plaques, often ulcerated and containing yellowish–white grains. Most commonly reported in Persian cats, occasionally other breeds and rarely dogs	Marked pyogranulomatous inflammation with numerous neutrophils, macrophages, epithelioid cells and giant cells arranged around grains formed by immune complexes deposited on fungal elements (Splendore–Hoeppli reaction); seen as an amorphous deep blue material
Kerion	Usually single nodules, often located on the nose or muzzle in dogs	Cell-rich exudate composed of segmented neutrophils, vacuolated macrophages, epithelioid macrophages and a variable number of eosinophils. Lamellar keratin and/or hair shafts fragments infected by fungi (see Figure 4.19)
Cryptococcus spp.	Usually present in cats; single or multiple nodules, sometimes ulcerated and mainly localized in the nostrils and on the skin of the nose, face, head and extremities	Fungal bodies are associated with numerous macrophages, epithelioid macrophages and giant cells; there are usually few neutrophils. Fungi are round or oval, 4–20 μm in size, with a round/oval nucleus and a characteristic clear achromatic mucopolysaccharide capsule that does not stain with the common rapid Romanowsky-type dyes. The large clear halo together with the typical narrow-based unipolar budding (teardrop appearance) are two cytological hallmarks of cryptococcosis (see Figure 4.20)
Leishmaniosis	*Leishmania* protozoa	With nodular leishmaniosis, samples are usually rich in amastigotes and inflammatory cells comprise macrophages and epithelioid macrophages, numerous plasma cells and a variable number of lymphocytes
Phaeohyphomycosis	Saprophytic free-living environmental fungi. Affects dogs and cats. Nodular lesions develop at the site of contaminated traumatic wounds often on the face or limbs	Granulomatous/pyogranulomatous inflammation with numerous neutrophils, macrophages, epithelioid macrophages and multinucleated giant cells; a few lymphocytes and plasma cells may also be present. Fungi vary in morphology from septate and branched hyphae of different lengths to yeast-like round/oval bodies, sometimes with a thick wall. In some cases, black pigmented fungi are easily recognizable on cytological examination (Figure 4.23)
Dirofilariasis	*Dirofilaria repens*; single or rarely multiple subcutaneous nodules of different sizes, sometimes associated with pruritus	Adult nematodes and microfilariae may be collected by fine-needle aspiration. Neutrophils, macrophages and a scarce number of eosinophils may be present (Figure 4.24)

4.21 Cytological findings associated with infectious causes of diseases that result in nodules and plaques.

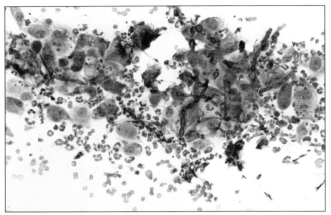

4.23 Phaeohyphomycosis characterized by pigmented septate and branched hyphae. Note the black fungal bodies phagocytized by epithelioid macrophages and giant cells. (Diff-Quik® stain)

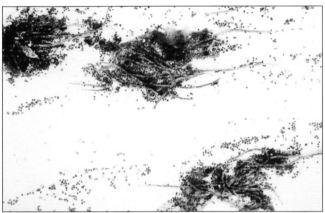

4.24 *Dirofilaria repens* larvae and the associated pyogranulomatous inflammation. (Diff-Quik® stain)

Sterile lesions

A number of uncommon sterile cutaneous disease processes may be seen. In many cases, it is important to rule out an infectious aetiology.

Sample collection and interpretation: Fine-needle aspiration is usually indicated to collect samples for diagnosis. Figure 4.25 details the cytological findings associated with sterile causes of diseases that result in nodules and plaques; examples are given in Figures 4.26 to 4.32.

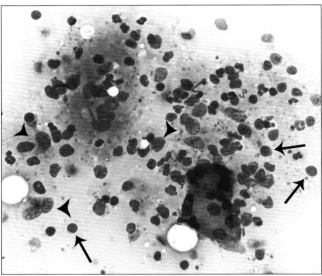

4.26 Histiocytosis. Note the large number of lymphocytes (arrowed) and histiocytes (arrowheads). (Diff-Quik® stain)

Disease	Aetiology and clinical signs	Cytology findings
Reactive histiocytosis	Affects middle-aged to older dogs. Nodules may be localized to the face and limbs or be more generalized. A systemic variant affects Bernese Mountain Dogs	Cytology may be unrewarding. Good quality specimens are characterized by histiocytes with oval, folded or kidney-shaped nuclei and large pale cytoplasm; the cytoplasm is often indistinct. A large number of lymphocytes is constantly present (Figure 4.26). Few plasma cells and neutrophils may also be detected
Calcinosis	Single to multiple firm papules or plaques often with an irregular shape	Calcium salts can vary from eosinophilic to basophilic coarse granules, or can be characterized by a large amount of achromatic irregular amorphous material surrounded by epithelioid macrophages, multinucleated giant cells and reactive fibroblasts (Figures 4.27 and 4.28). An inflammatory component characterized by neutrophils may be present
Eosinophilic granulomas/ plaques	Polymorphic nodules and plaques, often ulcerated. Common in cats and associated with pruritic skin disease. Less common in dogs, where they are usually found in the oral cavity	A large number of eosinophils and macrophages seen along with a variable amount of neutrophils and mast cells (Figure 4.29). In some cases, histiocytic giant cells arranged around amorphous, acellular and intensely basophilic material (degenerate esinophils) may be present (Figure 4.30)
Sterile panniculitis	More commonly seen in dogs. It may be associated with an injection reaction, pancreatitis/pancreatic neoplasia or infectious agents. A sterile immune-mediated multifocal panniculitis is reported in dogs	At low magnification, the cytological examination reveals a lipid background comprising many roundish or elongated oval droplets of fat of different sizes, with a variable amount of intermingled inflammatory cells (Figure 4.31). At high magnification, macrophages with cytoplasm filled with lipid microvacuoles, which gives the cells a typical foamy appearance, are visible
Xanthomatosis	Disorders of lipid metabolism. Multiple areas of alopecia and white–yellow papular nodules or small plaque/nodules	Large macrophages and multinucleated giants cells with a cytoplasm filled with small and overlapping lipid vacuoles that give the cells a typical foamy appearance are visible (Figure 4.32). There are few or no neutrophils present, and a variable amount of lymphocytes can be detected. To comfirm the lipid content of the vacuoles, an Oil Red O stain can be used; lipids stain bright red
Plasma cell pododermatitis	Swelling of one or multiple footpads in cats, may be ulcerated. Cause unknown	Poorly cellular; few plasma cells and lymphocytes are usually collected. In some cases, a variable number of Mott cells and active plasma cells filled with large and irregular vacuoles (Russell bodies) are visible. With ulcerated lesions, samples can be complicated by bacteria; in these cases, neutrophils and macrophages can dominate the cytological population

4.25 Cytological findings associated with sterile causes of diseases that result in nodules and plaques.

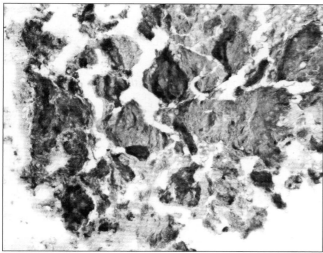

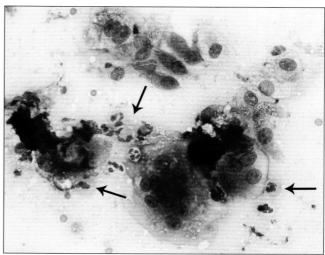

4.27 Acellular mineral salts collected by fine-needle aspiration from a mineralized nodular digital lesion in a German Shepherd Dog. Note the violet colour and amorphous nature of the material. (Diff-Quik® stain)

4.30 Eosinophilic plaque/granuloma. Giant cells are arranged around the amorphous basophilic material, which represents the 'eosinophilic mush' (necrotic eosinophilic foci). Numerous eosinophils are also visible (arrowed). (Diff-Quik® stain)

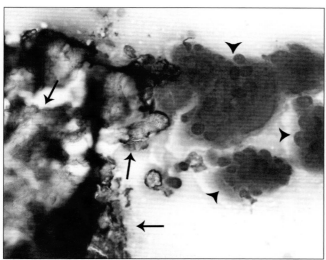

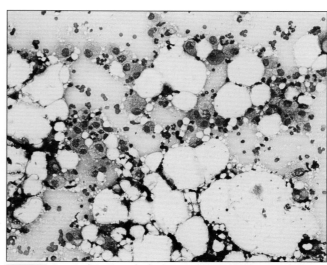

4.28 Calcinosis cutis. Note the numerous acellular, amorphous, achromatic and violet-stained mineral salts (arrowed) that have been attacked by multinucleated histiocytes (arrowheads). (Diff-Quik® stain)

4.31 Panniculitis. Note the large round to oval lipid accumulations surrounded by pyogranulomatous inflammation. (Diff-Quik® stain)

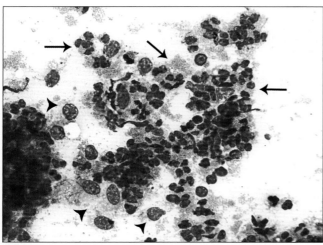

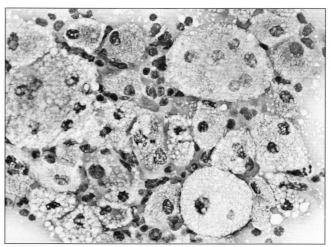

4.29 Eosinophilic plaque/granuloma. Note that numerous eosinophils (arrowed) and some macrophages (arrowheads) are visible. (Diff-Quik® stain)

4.32 Cutaneous xanthomatosis. Note the numerous large macrophages and giant cells with cytoplasm filled with lipid vacuoles, which gives the cells a 'foamy appearance'. (Diff-Quik® stain)

Key points

- Cytology requires practice but is indispensable to making an immediate therapeutic plan
- Cytology is invaluable in determining the role of secondary infections, such as bacteria and/or *Malassezia*, in a primary disease process
- For more complex diseases a skin biopsy may be indicated

Note on image magnification

Exact magnification of images in this chapter is not provided as it can vary with the combination of microscope and digital camera lenses used

References and further reading

Albanese F (2017) *Canine and Feline Skin Cytology: A Comprehensive and Illustrated Guide to the Interpretation of Skin Lesions via Cytological Examination*. Springer International Publishing, Switzerland

Albanese F, Abramo F, Braglia C *et al.* (2013) Nodular lesions due to infestation by *Dirofilaria repens* in dogs from Italy. Veterinary Dermatology **24**, 255–e56

Abramo F, Bastelli F, Nardoni S *et al.* (2002) Feline cutaneous Phaeohyphomycosis due to *Cladophyalophora bantiana*. *Journal of Feline Medicine and Surgery* **4**, 157–163

Banajee KH, Orandle MS, Ratterree W *et al.* (2011) Idiopathic solitary cutaneous xanthoma in a dog. *Veterinary Clinical Pathology* **40**, 95–98

Bardagi M, Fondati A, Fondevila D *et al.* (2003) Ultrastructural study of cutaneous lesions in feline eosinophilic granuloma complex. *Veterinary Dermatology* **14**, 297–303

Beccati M, Vercelli A, Peano A *et al.* (2005) *Phaeohyphomycosis* by *Phialophora verrucosa*: first European case in a cat. *Veterinary Record* **157**, 93–94

Colombo S, Abramo F, Borio S *et al.* (2016) Pustular dermatitis in dogs affected by leishmaniosis: 22 cases. *Veterinary Dermatology* **27**, 9–e4

Cornegliani L, Persico P and Colombo S (2009) Canine nodular dermatophytosis (kerion): 23 cases. *Veterinary Dermatology* **20**, 185–190

Doerr KA, Outerbridge CA, White DS *et al.* (2013) Calcinosis cutis in dogs: histopathological and clinical analysis of 46 cases. *Veterinary Dermatology* **24**, 355–e79

Gross TL, Ihrke PJ, Walder EJ *et al.* (2005) Eosinophilic furunculosis of the face. In: *Skin diseases of the dog and cat: clinical and histopathological diagnosis, 2nd edn.*, pp 450–453. Blackwell Science, Ames

Hobi S, Linek M and Marignac G (2011) Clinical characteristics and causes of pruritus in cats: a multicentre study on feline hypersensitivity-associated dermatoses. *Veterinary Dermatology* **22**, 406–413

Malik R, Smits B, Reppas G *et al.* (2013) Ulcerated and nonulcerated nontuberculous cutaneous mycobacterial granulomas in cats and dogs. *Veterinary Dermatology* **24**, 146–153, e32–e33

Malik R, Jacobs GJ and Love DN (2001) Cryptococcosis: new perspectives on etiology, pathogenesis, diagnosis, and clinical management. In: *Consultations in Feline Medicine*, ed. August JR, pp 39–50. WB Saunders, Philadelphia

Miller WH, Griffin CE and Campbell KL (2013) Sterile granuloma/pyogranuloma syndrome. In: *Muller & Kirk's Small Animal Dermatology, 7th edn.* pp 704–706. Elsevier, St. Louis

Moore PF (2014) A review of histiocytic diseases of dogs and cats. *Veterinary Pathology* **51**, 167–184

Nagata M and Ishida T (1997) Cutaneous reactivity to mosquito bites and its antigens in cats. *Veterinary Dermatology* **8**, 19–26

Nishifuji K, Sugai M and Amagai M (2008) Staphylococcal exfoliative toxins: 'molecular scissors' of bacteria that attack the cutaneous defense barrier in mammals. *Journal of Dermatological Science* **49**, 21–31

Noli C, Colombo S, Abramo F *et al.* (2004) Papular eosinophilic/mastocytic dermatitis (feline urticaria pigmentosa) in Devon Rex cats: a distinct disease entity or a histopathological reaction pattern? *Veterinary Dermatology* **15**, 253–259

Olivry T and Linder KE (2009) Dermatoses affecting desmosomes in animals: a mechanistic review of acantholytic blistering skin diseases. *Veterinary Dermatology* **20**, 313–326

Ordeix L, Solano-Gallego L, Fondevila D *et al.* (2005) Papular dermatitis due to *Leishmania* spp. infection in dogs with parasite-specific cellular immune responses. *Veterinary Dermatology* **16**, 187–191

Palmeiro BS, Morris DO, Goldschmidt MH *et al.* (2007) Cutaneous reactive histiocytosis in dogs: a retrospective evaluation of 32 cases. *Veterinary Dermatology* **18**, 332–340

Panich R, Scott DW and Miller WH (1991) Canine cutaneous sterile pyogranuloma/granuloma syndrome: a retrospective analysis of 29 cases (1976–1988). *Journal of the American Animal Hospital Association* **27**, 519–528

Ravens PA, Vogelnest LJ and Piripi SA (2013) Unique presentation of normolipaemic cutaneous xanthoma in a cat. *Australian Veterinary Journal* **91**, 460–463

Scott DW and Miller WH (2007) Juvenile cellulitis in dogs: a retrospective study of 18 cases (1976–2005). *The Japanese Journal of Veterinary Dermatology* **13**, 71–79

Vaughan DF, Hodgin EC, Hosgood GL *et al.* (2010) Clinical and histopathological features of pemphigus foliaceus with and without eosinophilic infiltrates: a retrospective evaluation of 40 dogs. *Veterinary Dermatology* **21**, 166–174

Vitale CB, Ihrke PJ, Olivry T *et al.* (1996) Feline urticaria pigmentosa in three related Sphinx cats. *Veterinary Dermatology* **7**, 227–233

Chapter 5

Dermatopathology

David H. Shearer

Dogs and cats presented for the investigation and treatment of skin disease can show a variety of clinical signs. The investigation into the cause of the dermatosis can be planned using a problem-solving approach based on the history and clinical signs present at examination (see Chapter 2). The cutaneous signs include pruritus, erythema, papules, pustules, alopecia, crusts, scales, erosions, ulcerations, nodules and pigment changes. One or more of these signs may be present and the balance of clinical features, along with the signalment and history, allows the dermatologist to create a list of differential diagnoses, plan diagnostic tests and/or prescribe treatment.

Gross lesions

Gross clinical lesions are divided into primary and secondary lesions, with some overlap between different types (Figure 5.1; see also Chapter 2). It is important to identify lesions accurately, to describe the lesions in the clinical notes, and to add the description to any pathology submission form(s). The interpretation of the histological features present in skin biopsy samples should be correlated with the presenting clinical signs, the exact body site from where the biopsy specimen was taken and the type of lesion present. A common assumption is that 'it looks bad, therefore it must be autoimmune'. Although some autoimmune dermatoses are severe, infectious agents are the most common cause of severe skin disease and biopsy may not always be rewarding in these cases. Furthermore, if there is an underlying disease compromising epidermal integrity, secondary infections are common and should be treated prior to taking samples for histopathology, as the inflammation associated with these infections can obscure more subtle histopathological findings. Occasionally, a benign presentation such as scaling

Primary	Primary or secondary	Secondary
• Macule/patch • Papule/plaque • Pustule • Vesicle/bulla • Wheal • Nodule • Tumour	• Alopecia • Scale • Crust • Follicular cast • Comedo • Pigment changes	• Epidermal collarette • Excoriation • Erosion/ulcer • Lichenification • Fissure • Callus • Scar

5.1 Gross skin lesions.

and alopecia in the older dog can be associated with neoplasia (i.e. epitheliotrophic lymphoma). In this case, the clinician often contacts the pathologist and asks, 'Are you sure that this is a neoplasm?'

Histological changes

If skin biopsy samples are indicated as part of the investigation of a skin disease, a few simple rules should be observed:

1. Remove hair; do not clean the biopsy site(s) or disturb surface crust. Any disturbed material should be included with the biopsy sample for examination.
2. In animals with generalized skin diseases, take multiple (ideally 6 mm) punch biopsy samples (between three and four is normal).
3. Biopsy primary lesions if possible, and, if lesion variation is present, submit representative samples and label accordingly (in different pots).
4. Try to get the opinion of a pathologist with specific expertise in skin pathology, e.g. a member of the International Society of Veterinary Dermatopathology (ISVD).

The gross appearance of the cutaneous lesions should correlate with the histological features and, in most cases, the microscopic features present should be predictable from the macroscopic lesions (Figure 5.2). If the histological features described by a dermatopathologist do not correlate with the gross appearance of the lesions, then it may be that of the multiple biopsy samples submitted only one of them contained the 'diagnostic' features required. Most lesions have a normal progression from formation to resolution or repair, and it is important to submit samples from various representative stages of the disease. Alternatively, the area containing the diagnostic features may have been lost during biopsy or processing; an example is the superficial crust or pustule in pemphigus foliaceus, which can be removed during preparation of the skin for biopsy or lost during histological processing (i.e. it separates from the skin). It is for this reason that the skin surface should never be cleaned before skin biopsy (see Chapter 3). In general, if the clinical features cannot be correlated with the dermatohistopathology report, then the pathologist should be contacted and the case discussed.

Clinical sign	Histological patterns
Pruritus	• Perivascular dermatitis • Nodular/diffuse dermatitis • Intraepidermal vesicular/pustular dermatitis • Folliculitis
Alopecia	• Atrophic dermatopathy • Perivascular dermatitis • Intraepidermal vesicular/pustular dermatitis • Folliculitis • Interface dermatitis
Scaling and crusting	• Atrophic dermatopathy • Folliculitis • Interface dermatitis • Nodular/diffuse dermatitis • Perivascular dermatitis • Intraepidermal vesicular/pustular dermatitis
Pustules	• Perivascular dermatitis • Intraepidermal vesicular/pustular dermatitis • Folliculitis
Ulcers	• Perivascular dermatitis • Interface dermatitis • Vasculitis • Intraepidermal vesicular/pustular dermatitis • Subepidermal vesicular/pustular dermatitis • Folliculitis/furunculosis • Panniculitis
Hyperpigmentation	• Perivascular dermatitis • Nodular/diffuse dermatitis • Folliculitis • Atrophic dermatopathy
Hypopigmentation	• Interface dermatitis • Nodular/diffuse dermatitis
Nodules	• Nodular/diffuse dermatitis • Folliculitis/furunculosis • Panniculitis • Vasculitis

5.2 Histological patterns associated with major clinical signs. Note that many of these patterns may be present concurrently.

When submitting samples, it is important to provide the signalment, give a brief history and describe the clinical features accurately on the submission form. The body sites from which the biopsy samples were taken should also be recorded. Microscopic anatomy of the skin varies between sites and the pathologist's interpretation of the histology may be affected by the exact sites of origin. Generally speaking, skin sections are examined by the pathologist initially under low power and before reading the clinician's notes on the submission form. This allows an unbiased assessment and interpretation of the histology. After examination under low power, the changes seen are categorized into a 'pattern' based on the analysis (Ackerman, 1978; Yager and Wilcock, 1994).

Examples of histological patterns include:

• Perivascular dermatitis (the 'dermatitis reaction')
• Interface dermatitis
• Vasculitis
• Nodular and/or diffuse dermatitis
• Intraepidermal vesicular/pustular dermatitis
• Subepidermal vesicular/pustular dermatitis
• Folliculitis/perifolliculitis/furunculosis
• Panniculitis
• Atrophic dermatopathy
• Metabolic dermatosis.

The biopsy sections are then examined in detail to identify specific dermatopathological changes, usually beginning with the epidermis, followed by the adnexae and dermis. The pathologist then makes an interpretation of the histological features in light of the clinical information provided. The pathologist's report usually includes a morphological diagnosis, aetiological diagnosis (if possible), description of the changes and a discussion of the findings (Figure 5.3). It should be emphasized that the histopathology may not provide a definitive diagnosis but should be interpreted in light of the signalment, history, clinical signs and any other clinicopathological information.

The pathology report should include a summary of the histological features present, a statement of the patterns seen, an aetiological diagnosis (if possible) and a commentary outlining the conclusions that can be made. A typical report might be set out as given below.

• **Morphological diagnosis:** This states the major and minor histological patterns present.
• **Aetiological diagnosis:** This is stated if a causative agent is seen in the sections examined.
• **Description:** This is a summary of the histological features seen and usually starts with the epidermis followed by the dermis and adnexae.

Comments: The pathologist states what can be concluded from the histological features and relates them to the clinical features. The pathologist should give a comment as to the clinicopathological correlation in this section and for this reason an accurate history and description of the gross changes is important

5.3 Dermatohistopathology report.

Common questions asked by clinicians

1. When should I perform a skin biopsy?
   • When routine diagnostic tests have been performed to rule out common diseases and the lesions have not resolved with rational therapy.
   • When the animal presents with unusual lesions.
2. Does current or recent therapy affect the histopathology?
   • Yes, we believe that some therapies do; in particular, glucocorticoids appear to affect the histological features even if the clinical signs are still present and the treatment has been recently withdrawn.
3. What are the effects of glucocorticoids?
   • They affect the hair follicle growth cycle, leading to telogenization of hair follicles.
   • They may affect the dermal collagen, leading to atrophy.
   • They may change the cell infiltrate within the skin. In particular, the number of eosinophils and even neutrophils may be reduced significantly.
   • The author suspects that glucocorticoids may remove or reduce the number of acantholytic keratinocytes present in cases of pemphigus foliaceus, even if crusts are still present clinically.
   • Both endogenous and exogenous glucocorticoids can have similar effects.
4. How long do I have to stop glucocorticoid therapy for?
   • We do not know because such studies have not been performed.
   • The longer the patient has received glucocorticoids, the longer their effect will persist following withdrawal (see Chapter 29).
   • In an ideal world, the skin should be biopsied before giving any (topical or systemic) glucocorticoid therapy.
   • If the animal has been on glucocorticoids, stop therapy for as long as possible before biopsy.

5. How do I choose which lesions to biopsy?
    *   Biopsy early, middle and late lesions in an attempt to provide information on the natural history of the disease. Early lesions are likely to be more diagnostic than late lesions.
    *   With ulcerative lesions, take samples at right angles to the edge of the ulcer in an attempt to reveal evidence of lesion pathogenesis.
    *   With tumours, the tumour edge and normal tissue should always be included because this allows assessment of the tumour's growth pattern and may impact on classification (benign versus malignant) and grading. It should be remembered that some benign tumours appear histologically anaplastic and malignant but are benign (e.g. canine plasmacytoma).

Basic dermatohistopathological changes

*   **Epidermal atrophy:** This is a reduction in the thickness of the epidermis. As a general rule, the thickness of the epidermis is inversely proportional to the hair density. This change is seen concurrently with alopecia and skin thinning.
*   **Acanthosis (epidermal hyperplasia):** This represents keratinocyte hyperplasia and various types are described. Acanthosis is seen in lesions with lichenification and inflammatory alopecia, typically in dogs with chronic dermatitis, pyoderma or *Malassezia* dermatitis.
    *   Regular acanthosis is a uniform increase in the stratum spinosum with no rete ridges.
    *   Irregular acanthosis has rete ridge formation and is the commonest form in the dog and cat.
    *   Psoriasiform acanthosis has regular rete ridge formation with or without club-shaped tips. This is rare in the cat and dog.
    *   Papillated acanthosis has folding and projection above the surface. This is acanthosis with upward proliferation of the dermis. It is a non-specific term.
    *   Pseudoepitheliomatous/carcinomatous acanthosis has an invasive appearance resembling squamous cell carcinoma. It occurs at the edge of ulcers.
*   **Crusts:** These are surface accumulations of squames, serum proteins, red blood cells and white blood cells. They are classified as serous, keratinous, cellular or haemorrhagic. Crusts often contain microorganisms such as bacteria, yeasts (*Malassezia*) and occasionally derma-tophytes. Crusts are most often seen in cases of pyo-derma, dermatophytosis and parasitic disease, but can be seen in the autoimmune disease pemphigus foliaceus.
*   **Hyperkeratosis:** This is an increase in the width of the stratum corneum. It can be orthokeratotic or parakeratotic, basket-weave or compact. Hyperkeratosis is seen grossly as scale or can form part of crusts.
    *   Compact hyperkeratosis is associated with chronic trauma.
    *   Orthokeratotic hyperkeratosis is an increase in the number of anucleate corneocytes.
    *   Parakeratosis is where there is retention of a pyknotic nucleus in the squames in the stratum corneum. It reflects increased cell turnover and a rapid response to injury. It occurs as a focal change either vertically (in episodic injury) or horizontally (in focal injury). Generalized parakeratosis is associated with zinc-responsive dermatosis and metabolic dermatoses.

*   **Hypergranulosis:** This is an increase in the thickness of the stratum granulosum, usually associated with compact hyperkeratosis due to chronic trauma. Areas of clinical lichenification can have hypergranulosis present on histology.
*   **Hypogranulosis:** This is a decrease in, or loss of, the stratum granulosum and is usually associated with parakeratosis.
*   **Papillomatosis:** Localized epidermal growth caused by papilloma virus infection. This is a specific term. These are usually exophytic lesions described as 'warts' but can be endophytic in verruca-like lesions.
*   **Dyskeratosis:** Premature, faulty keratinization, which can occur in the surface or adnexal epithelium. It can be a benign change seen in various dermatoses associated with abnormal keratinization or be associated with malignant lesions such as squamous cell carcinoma.
*   **Spongiosis:** Intercellular oedema in the epidermis, which gives the epidermis a spongy appearance. This change is usually associated with exocytosis of inflammatory cells and, if severe, it can lead to intraepidermal vesicle formation.
*   **Exocytosis:** The migration of inflammatory cells from the dermis into the epidermis and adnexae. It is usually associated with spongiosis.
*   **Intracellular oedema:** Intracytoplasmic vacuolation occuring in hydropic degeneration and ballooning degeneration of keratinocytes.
*   **Hydropic degeneration (vacuolar alteration/ liquefactive degeneration):** This refers to the presence of vacuoles within the stratum basale cells. This may lead to intrabasilar or subepidermal clefts. This change may be seen in diseases associated with ischaemic damage or an inflammatory attack directed at the basement membrane.
*   **Ballooning degeneration:** This type of degeneration is specifically seen in epidermal viral infections and is an extreme form of hydropic degeneration.
*   **Reticular degeneration:** Multilocular/intraepidermal vesicle formation associated with severe epidermal oedema. Severe keratinocyte swelling can also occur in metabolic dermatosis (superficial necrolytic dermatitis/ hepatocutaneous syndrome) or acute contact dermatitis.
*   **Acantholysis:** This describes the separation of keratinocytes. Primary acantholysis is separation of normal keratinocytes as seen in pemphigus foliaceus. Secondary acantholysis occurs as a result of damage to the keratinocytes and is seen in dyskeratosis, viral infections and in association with inflammatory cells in staphylococcal pyoderma.
*   **Pigment incontinence:** This refers to melanin that drops from the epidermis/adnexae into the dermis, where it is phagocytized by dermal monocytes/ macrophages. This is usually associated with stratum basale cell oedema. This is a feature of an interface dermatitis as seen in cutaneous lupus.
*   **Epidermal necrosis:** This can be caseous or coagulative. Caseous necrosis appears as an eosinophilic and basophilic mush. This is the most common and least specific form of necrosis and usually reflects trauma (especially scratching). Coagulation necrosis appears eosinophilic with pyknotic nuclei and the superficial dermis is often involved. Coagulative necrosis usually occurs as a result of physical damage (burning/freezing/chemical), ischaemia or immunological mechanisms. Lesions with epidermal necrosis present clinically with ulceration.

- **Necrolysis:** Describes epidermal coagulative necrosis with no dermal involvement and minimal inflammation (e.g. toxic epidermal necrolysis).
- **Apoptosis:** This is individual cell death and involves intracellular processes that require energy (compared with necrosis by oncosis, which is not energy dependent and occurs as a result of catastrophic cell damage). This can be a physiological or pathological process. These processes can be triggered in a variety of ways, one of which is cytotoxic attack by lymphocytes (satellitosis). Histologically, apoptosis appears as eosinophilic bodies that progress to be phagocytized by adjacent cells.
- **Satellitosis:** This refers to the appearance of cytotoxic lymphocytes surrounding an apoptotic cell; it indicates a cell-mediated immune response.
- **Civatte bodies:** These are apoptotic cells in the stratum basale of the epidermis.

Patterns used in dermatopathological interpretation

Perivascular dermatitis

In this pattern, there are prominent blood vessels (high endothelial venules), oedema of the dermis, and exocytosis of leucocytes into the dermis around the high endothelial venules (Figures 5.4 and 5.5). In addition to these dermal changes, there are epidermal changes that may reflect the aetiology or age of the lesions. The epidermal changes include acanthosis (hyperplasia), spongiosis, intracellular oedema (in the basal layer of an interface dermatitis), hyperkeratosis (basket-weave or compact), parakeratosis (focal or diffuse), epidermal necrosis (erosions/ulcerations) and crusts.

Perivascular dermatitis is further classified according to the vascular plexuses involved:

- Zone 1 (superficial dermal)
- Zone 2 (mid-dermal and perifollicular)
- Zone 3 (deep dermal).

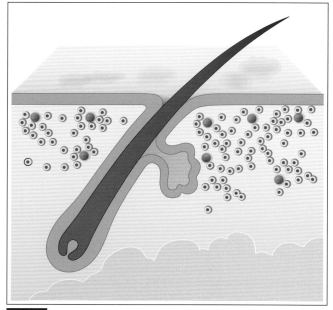

| 5.4 | Perivascular dermatitis (the 'dermatitis reaction'). |

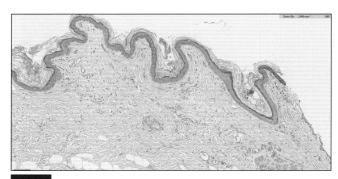

| 5.5 | Perivascular dermatitis in a canine skin sample. |

The type of cellular infiltrate (neutrophilic, lymphocytic or eosinophilic) may also reflect the aetiology or pathogenesis. An eosinophilic infiltrate tends to indicate type I hypersensitivity and a parasitic or allergic aetiology in the dog but may be less specific in the cat. This is a common reaction pattern, which is weak diagnostically.

Interface dermatitis

This reaction pattern describes a pathological process, which is focused on the dermal epidermal junction and the cells of the stratum basale. Degeneration of basal keratinocytes (Figure 5.6) with or without individual keratinocyte necrosis (apoptosis) occurs. Interface dermatitis is divided morphologically into cell-rich interface dermatitis (Figure 5.7) or cell-poor interface dermatitis (Figure 5.8). Pigment

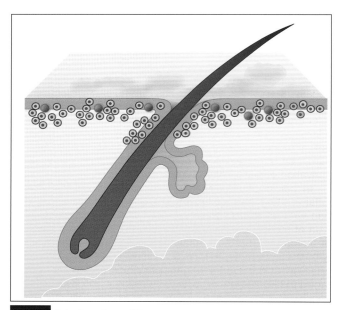

| 5.6 | Interface dermatitis. |

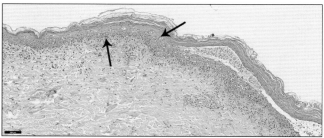

| 5.7 | Cell-rich interface dermatitis with single cell necrosis and satellitosis (arrowed) (cytotoxic dermatitis) in a canine skin sample. |

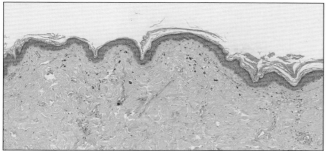

5.8 Cell-poor interface dermatitis (ischaemic dermatitis) in a canine skin sample.

incontinence, which represents pigment falling through the basement membrane of the epidermis and outer root sheaths, is a feature of interface dermatitis.

In cell-rich interface dermatitis, the cellular infiltrate is usually lymphocytic and spans the superficial dermis and epidermis or outer root sheaths of the hair follicles. Originally called a lichenoid reaction pattern (lichenoid dermatitis or lichenoid to interface dermatitis) after histological changes seen in the human skin disease lichen planus, dermatopathologists now call these changes a cell-rich interface dermatitis. If single cell necrosis and associated satellitosis by mononuclear cells is present in the sections, then the term cytotoxic dermatitis is used as a morphological diagnosis. The presence of single cell necrosis with satellitosis represents the binding of mononuclear cells to a keratinocyte and their induction of regulated cell death (apoptosis) through activation of death receptors and injection of granzymes. A cytotoxic dermatitis (cell-rich interface dermatitis with apoptosis and satellitosis) is seen in forms of cutaneous lupus, in which the apoptosis is mainly affecting the stratum basale cells and the toxic epidermal necrolysis – erythema multiforme (TEN-EM) spectrum. In cases which are on the TEN-EM spectrum, the apoptosis with satellitosis usually affects cells within the stratum basale and stratum spinosum. Hair follicles and surface epidermis can be affected by this process. In cases of toxic epidermal necrolysis, there are large areas of epidermal necrosis without a mononuclear infiltrate, which is thought to be the result of a cytotoxic process but mediated by cytokine activation of death receptors on the keratinocytes.

In cell-poor interface dermatitis there are few, if any, inflammatory cells present. There is vacuolar degeneration with or without necrosis, which is due to poor perfusion of the dermis epidermis. This pattern is seen in cases of ischaemic dermatopathy and most often is associated with the presence of vasculitis. The hair follicles are also affected and become degenerate, and are described as faded in histological reports.

Vasculitis

Vasculitis implies specific inflammation of the blood vessel walls. Histologically, there are tight perivascular cuffs of inflammatory cells (Figure 5.9), with evidence of degeneration of the vessel wall. In some circumstances there is necrosis of the inflammatory cells, represented by the presence of 'nuclear dust' (Figure 5.10). A variety of cell types can be seen in cutaneous vasculitis. This can be a difficult clinical and histopathological diagnosis, as not all blood vessels may be affected. Microhaemorrhages should alert the pathologist to the possible presence of vasculitis. Other changes that may be seen in vasculitis, include oedema, panniculitis, dermal necrosis and atrophy of the hair follicles.

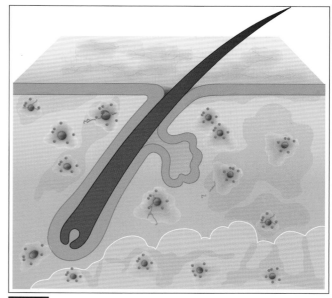

5.9 Vasculitis.

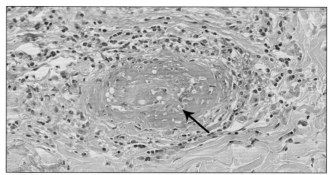

5.10 Cutaneous vasculitis in a canine skin sample. Note the degeneration of the blood vessel wall (arrowed) and nuclear debris with microhaemorrhage in the surrounding dermis.

Nodular/diffuse dermatitis

Nodular and diffuse dermatitis (Figure 5.11) are considered to be one pattern, but it is important to differentiate a disease centred on the hair follicles from non-follicular nodular dermatitis, as these patterns can vary in less common to rare diseases. The diffuse pattern reflects convergence of nodules (Figure 5.12). The cellular infiltrate gives some indication of the likely cause. A neutrophilic infiltrate occurs in response to pyogenic agents. Histiocytes/macrophages occur in response to foreign bodies and mycobacteria. The presence of both neutrophils and macrophages should alert the pathologist to the possibility of furunculosis. An eosinophilic nodular and diffuse dermatitis raises the possibility of a parasitic aetiology. A lymphocytic infiltrate can be seen with vaccine reactions and insect bites.

Intraepidermal vesicular/pustular dermatitis

Clefting that leads to vesicles or pustules within the epidermis (Figure 5.13) can occur as a result of spongiosis/epidermal inflammation (parasites or infection), acantholysis (due to infection or autoimmune disease), intracellular oedema and mechanical forces (friction). The clefts may be subcorneal (pemphigus foliaceus (Figure 5.14), pyoderma (Figure 5.15)), suprabasilar (pemphigus vulgaris) or

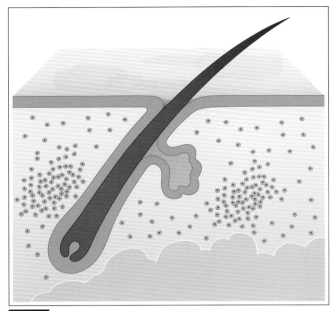

5.11 Nodular and/or diffuse dermatitis.

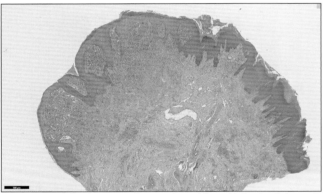

5.12 Nodular dermatitis due to a dermal fungal infection (*Alternaria* spp.) in a canine skin sample.

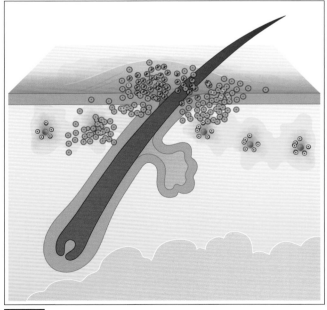

5.13 Intraepidermal vesicular/pustular dermatitis.

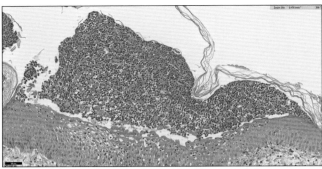

5.14 Subcorneal pustular dermatitis with acantholytic keratinocytes (pemphigus foliaceus) in a canine skin sample.

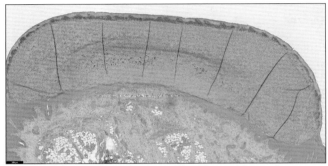

5.15 Subcorneal pustular dermatitis with no evidence of acantholytic keratinocytes, degenerate neutrophils and bacteria (bacterial pyoderma) in a feline pad skin sample.

may be with the follicular external root sheath (pemphigus foliaceus). A variety of cells can be present, including neutrophils (pemphigus foliaceus/pyoderma), eosinophils (pemphigus foliaceus/parasitic disease) and mononuclear cells (macrophages in bacterial pyoderma).

Subepidermal vesicular/pustular dermatitis

This is an uncommon pattern (Figure 5.16). It occurs with autoimmune diseases, such as bullous pemphigoid, thermal trauma (burns), severe dermal oedema, drug reactions (Figure 5.17) and severe interface dermatitis. It can also be a histological artefact.

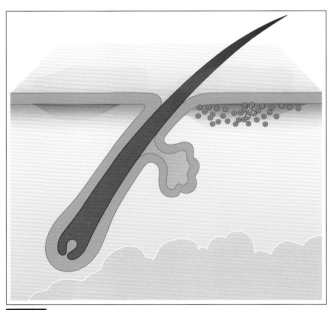

5.16 Subepidermal vesicular/pustular dermatitis.

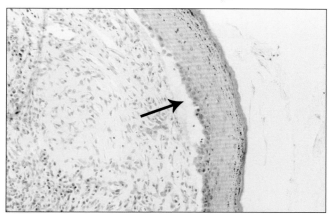

5.17 Subepidermal vesicular dermatosis (bullous drug reaction) (arrowed) in a canine pinna skin sample.

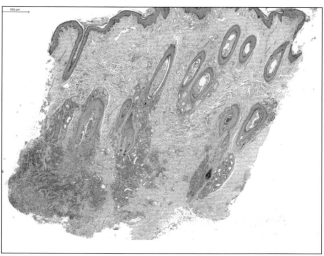

5.19 Folliculitis and furunculosis (deep bacterial pyoderma) in a canine skin sample.

Folliculitis/perifolliculitis/furunculosis

Inflammation associated with the hair follicles (Figure 5.18) can affect the perifollicular vascular plexus (perifolliculitis), the outer root sheath (mural folliculitis), the entire hair follicle (luminal folliculitis), the bulb (bulbitis), the sebaceous glands (sebaceous adenitis) or the epitrichial (apocrine) glands (hidradenitis). Furunculosis is identified by rupture of the hair follicle (Figure 5.19). The causes of follicular inflammatory disease include bacteria (polymorphonuclear neutrophils and plasma cells predominate), dermatophytes (lymphocytic folliculitis), demodicosis (typically a lymphoid mural folliculitis), parasites (mosquito/insect stings; eosinophilic folliculitis/furunculosis) and immune-mediated conditions (alopecia areata; lymphocytic bulbitis).

Panniculitis

Inflammation of the subcutaneous adipose tissue (Figure 5.20) can be septal or lobular. It can also be an extension of follicular disease. Histological examination may indicate the cause and pathogenesis (e.g. infectious agents, vasculitis or a foreign body may be apparent) (Figure 5.21).

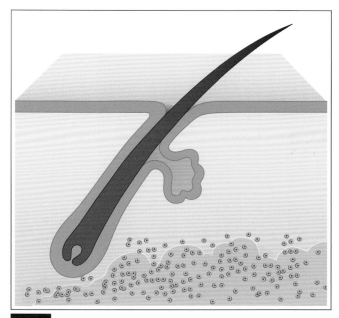

5.20 Panniculitis.

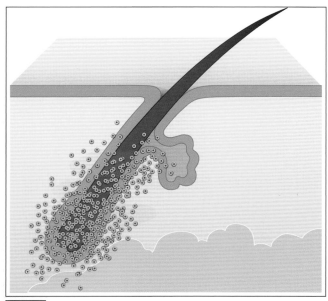

5.18 Folliculitis/perifolliculitis/furunculosis.

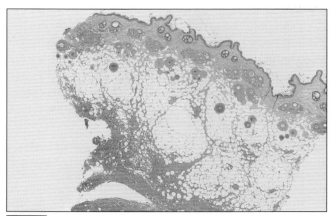

5.21 Panniculitis caused by vasculitis in a canine skin sample.

Atrophic dermatopathy

In this pattern there is atrophy of the epidermis, hair follicles and sebaceous glands (Figure 5.22). Orthokeratotic hyperkeratosis and follicular keratosis are usually present (Figure 5.23). Hairless telogen (kenogen) hair follicles are also a feature. In cases of hyperadrenocorticism, there may additionally be calcinosis cutis present. This pattern is seen with a number of endocrine dermatoses, which require a variety of hormonal assays to confirm their exact aetiology.

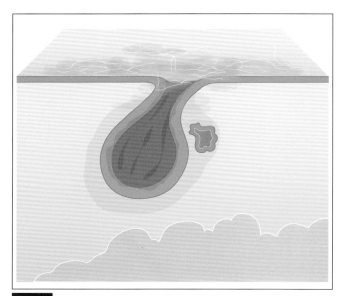

5.22   Atrophic dermatopathy (hair cycle slowing or arrest).

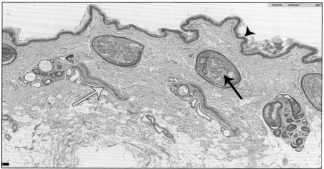

5.23   Atrophic dermatopathy in a canine skin sample. Follicular keratosis (black arrow); atrophied hair follicles (yellow arrow) and epidermal atrophy (arrowhead).

Metabolic dermatopathy

Metabolic dermatopaty (also known as superficial necrolytic dermatosis/hepatocutaneous syndrome) presents with a characteristic red (parakeratotic hyperkeratosis), white (epidermal pallor) and blue (acanthosis) colour in some areas of skin (Figure 5.24). It is important to note that this characteristic combination may be absent in some biopsy specimens, but is most often seen in samples from crusting pad lesions (Figure 5.25). Histopathology may be unrepresentative, especially in haired skin away from the pads. The pattern is rare and associated with end-stage hepatic disease or pancreatic neoplasia.

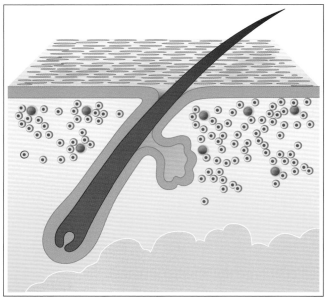

5.24   Metabolic dermatosis (parakeratotic hyperkeratosis, epidermal pallor and acanthosis; so-called red, white and blue).

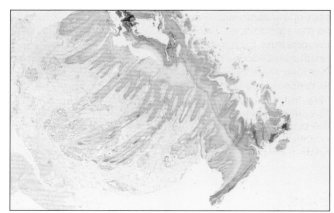

5.25   Metabolic dermatosis with characteristic red (parakeratotic hyperkeratosis), white (epidermal pallor) and blue (acanthosis) areas in a canine pad skin sample.

Key points

- Whenever possible, biopsy primary skin lesions and take multiple samples
- If bacterial infection is present treat this first
- Withdraw any anti-inflammatory treatment prior to taking skin biopsy samples

---

References and further reading

Ackerman AB (1978) *Histologic Diagnosis of Inflammatory Skin Disease. A Method by Pattern Analysis*. Lea & Febiger, Philadelphia

Goldschmidt MH and Shofer FS (1992) *Skin Tumours of the Dog and Cat*. Pergamon Press, Oxford

Gross TL, Ihrke PJ, Walder EJ and Affolter VK (2005) *Skin Diseases of the Dog and Cat. Clinical and Histopathological Diagnosis, 2nd edn*. Blackwell Science, Oxford

Scott DW, Miller WH and Griffin CE (2001) *Muller & Kirk's Small Animal Dermatology, 6th edn*. WB Saunders, Philadelphia

Yager JA and Wilcock BP (1994) *Colour Atlas and Text of Surgical Pathology of the Dog and Cat*. Mosby Year Book Europe, London

Chapter 6

An approach to pruritus

Kathy C. Tater

Pruritus is the sensation that leads to the desire to scratch. In veterinary medicine, patients typically use their paws and mouth to quell an itch. Thus, the veterinary medical definition of pruritus expands to include the desire to chew, lick, bite or rub at the skin. Pruritic skin diseases can be a diagnostic challenge to the clinician. Chronic pruritus typically results in the same set of secondary dermatological skin lesions in any patient, yet multiple conditions can act as the underlying trigger for the pruritus. Ignoring underlying causes of pruritus only results in a recurrence of the sensation when antipruritic medications are discontinued. The aim of this chapter is to present an approach to pruritus that helps the veterinary surgeon (veterinarian) investigate a pruritic patient. The emphasis is on diagnosing the underlying cause of the pruritus. Antipruritic therapies are reviewed briefly to enable the veterinary surgeon to select the most appropriate therapy for the management of pruritus.

Pathophysiology

An understanding of the pathophysiology of pruritus is at the core of the veterinary surgeon's ability to help the pruritic patient. For example, the knowledge that neurogenic pruritus can arise from nerve damage should lead the veterinary surgeon to conduct a thorough examination of the cervical region in a patient presenting with an acral lick granuloma on the forelimb. Likewise, the understanding that multiple pathways can be involved in the manifestation of pruritus should lead the veterinary surgeon to create a multimodal treatment plan to manage conditions such as atopic dermatitis.

The function of skin as both a sensory organ and an active immune organ (see Chapter 1) plays a key role in most pruritic patients. As a sensory organ, the skin has free nerve endings located at the dermoepidermal junction and within the epidermis (intraepidermal nerve fibres, IENF) that when stimulated lead to the perception of pruritus and other sensations. As an active arm of the immune system, the skin's various cells, including keratinocytes, leucocytes and mast cells, release pruritogenic chemical mediators (Figure 6.1). One pathway to pruritus is through direct stimulation of the IENF. Pruritus can also result from the activation of cellular receptors that stimulate transduction cascades, such as the Janus kinase–signal transducer and activator of transcription (JAK–STAT), mitogen-activated protein kinase (MAPK) and phosphatidylinositol 3-kinase (PI3K) signaling pathways.

Pruritogenic mediators
• Cytokines (interleukin (IL)-4, IL-13, IL-31)[a]
• Leucotrienes (LTB4)
• Peptides (endopeptidases, bradykinin, substance P, vasoactive intestinal polypeptides, neurotensin, secretin, encephalins, endorphins)
• Prostaglandins

6.1 Pruritogenic chemical mediators released by skin cells.
[a] This information comes from mice and people.

An understanding of these pruritic pathways and inciting stimuli underlies the veterinary surgeon's choice of medication for providing relief to the pruritic patient. For example, in atopic dermatitis, topical treatments containing ceramides may improve skin barrier function and thus decrease allergen penetration and subsequent allergen sensitization, leading to an inflammatory cascade and subsequent pruritus. The caninized monoclonal antibody, lokivetmab, targets the pruritogenic cytokine interleukin (IL)-31 and prevents it from binding to the cutaneous nerve receptors, thus preventing the sensation of pruritus. JAK inhibition is the mechanism of action for the antipruritic medication oclacitinib, and this leads to decreased activity of the pruritogenic cytokine IL-31 and the allergy and inflammation cytokines IL-2, IL-4, IL-6 and IL-13 (for more information on antipruritic medications, see Chapter 10).

Multiple factors influence the production and release of pruritogenic mediators, and more than one factor can contribute to a patient's pruritus. If the pruritic stimuli exceed a certain level, the dog or cat will show clinical signs. This concept is called the threshold phenomenon (Figure 6.2). Together, pruritic stimuli can have an additive effect in a patient. This concept is called summation of effect. Once the threshold is reached, clinical manifestation of pruritus ensues. The pruritic threshold varies from patient to patient and even within the same patient it can be modulated by additional factors such as stress, cold or heat. This is why a patient that was previously well controlled with one therapy may become symptomatic under stressful conditions.

Another important and common clinical scenario, which might push the previously well controlled patient to exhibit signs of pruritus, is the development of secondary cutaneous infections. It is worth noting that therapies, such as glucocorticoids and oclacitinib, are effective antipruritic agents, but through their anti-inflammtory action, they will predispose the patient to secondary infections.

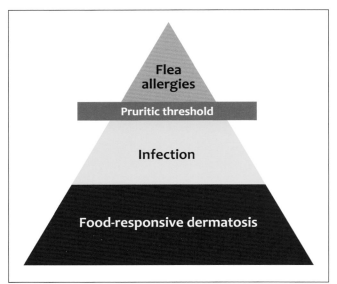

6.2 Pruritus is additive. When the threshold is exceeded, clinical manifestations of pruritus ensue. A practical example of these concepts can be seen in a dog or cat with both flea allergy and food-responsive dermatosis. The presence of both allergic stimuli results in a summation of the pruritic effect. Without the flea allergy, the dog or cat may be pruritic but comfortable overall with the food-responsive dermatosis, because the pruritic load is below the threshold of pruritus. When the client forgets to use a flea preventative, the additional pruritic stimulus from the fleas causes the pruritus to exceed the threshold, resulting in the dog or cat having a severe increase in itching.

Clinical approach

All aspects of the veterinary consultation (signalment and history, physical examination, diagnostic testing) yield clues to the underlying cause of pruritus. Given that many chronically pruritic patients develop the same set of secondary skin lesions no matter what the underlying cause, the signalment and history can be more important than the physical examination for making a diagnosis.

Signalment and history

Obtaining a thorough history (see Chapter 2) starts with a review of the patient's past medical record. This can usually be completed prior to the appointment if the animal is an existing patient of the practice. Most pruritic dogs and cats have been on multiple treatments for their pruritus. Knowledge of the patient's response or lack of response to these treatments can be important in achieving a diagnosis.

The patient's age when the pruritus began is important when prioritizing the differential diagnoses list. A common cause of pruritus is allergy, although it is very important not to assume that every itchy patient is allergic, as many other diseases can be responsible for pruritus. The typical age of onset for one form of allergy, atopic dermatitis, is 6 months to 3 years. In contrast, an allergy triggered by food may occur at any age. Certain dog breeds are more prone to pruritic conditions. Dogs with marked skin folds, such as Shar Peis and Bulldogs, can develop dermatitis within the skin folds (intertriginal dermatitis), which may be pruritic. However, it should be noted that in many brachycephalic dogs or obese animals, the manifestation of pruritus may be modified by conformation or the inability to reach affected sites.

Thus, a Bulldog with an intertriginous tail fold dermatitis may rub its dorsolumbar area or scoot along its perineum. Bassett Hounds have higher levels of *Malassezia* on the skin and this can manifest with variable pruritus.

It is important to allow sufficient time to obtain a thorough history (see Chapter 2). If the veterinary surgeon cannot devote the 15 minutes it usually takes to obtain a complete dermatological history, other veterinary team members should be empowered to take over this role. Any veterinary team member can be trained to ask a short list of key questions whenever a patient with pruritus is presented for an appointment (Figure 6.3). Alternatively, the client can fill out a written patient history form and the veterinary team member can review the responses with the client.

Client adherence is a core part of dermatology because various diagnostic tests (e.g. food trial for food-responsive dermatosis (also known as food allergy or adverse food reaction)) and nearly all treatments (e.g. topical therapy) take place at home. Whilst a large amount of information can be found in the patient's medical record, it is crucial to determine whether the recommended treatments were actually administered (i.e. was a food trial for food-responsive dermatosis actually performed or did the pet continue to receive treats during the food trial?). Ideally, the primary caretaker of the pet should accompany the animal to the appointment. If a client was not adherent with past veterinary recommendations, they should be asked why the recommendations were difficult to follow so that alternatives can be suggested.

Primary skin lesions (i.e. lesions that are the direct result of the underlying conditions causing pruritus) may not be present if some time has elapsed since the onset of pruritus. As the pruritic condition progresses, the distribution and type of lesions can change. The astute pet owner may be able to recall accurately how the pet looked at the onset of the pruritus. It can also be helpful to determine whether the pruritus was rapid or insidious in onset. For example, sarcoptic mange has a fairly acute onset, whilst pruritus associated with atopic dermatitis develops more slowly and can wax and wane.

Question	Information required
When did the signs (licking, chewing, scratching, head shaking) begin?	The client should be asked to state when the current episode pruritus began and also at what age the dog or cat first developed signs of pruritus
Any history of other skin or ear conditions?	Clients may not realize that signs of other skin or ear conditions (e.g. infection) can also be a sign of a pruritic condition
How severe is your pet's pruritus?	Clients can have varying opinions on what constitutes severe pruritus. It can be helpful to give examples of severe pruritus (e.g. patient is not able to sleep through the night due to pruritic behaviour) and to use a pruritus scoring system (asking clients to grade their pet's pruritus on a scale of 1–10, with 10 being severe)
What did the skin look like at the beginning?	If the client can remember what the pet looked like at the beginning, this may enable the veterinary surgeon to determine what primary skin lesions were initially present at the onset of pruritus
What have you used to treat the pruritus?	Clients may have tried a variety of products in an attempt to first manage the pruritus on their own

6.3 Key history questions for cases of pruritus.

Dermatological examination

Some causes of pruritus can be related to systemic disease. For example, *Malassezia* dermatitis or staphylococcal pyoderma can be secondary to systemic diseases such as endocrinopathies. Accordingly, a full evaluation of a pruritic patient involves both a comprehensive general physical examination and a dermatological examination. The patient should first be observed for its general attitude and for any signs of pruritus while taking a history. Pruritus may be suppressed during the visit to the veterinary practice if the patient is stressed or anxious.

A nose to tail dermatological examination should then be performed. Excellent lighting is mandatory because the dermatological examination is primarily visual. Magnifiers can be helpful for identifying small and subtle skin lesions. It is also strongly advised to have a veterinary assistant restrain the patient so that a thorough examination can be performed; the head should be kept still during the otoscopic examination and the patient should be lifted up or rolled on to its back or side to examine the ventrum. The ears, ear margins, mucocutaneous junctions, mucosae, interdigital region, claws, paw pads, axillae and inguinal area should all be examined. Areas of haired skin should have the hair parted so that the skin can be seen fully. The hair may need to be clipped in some long-haired patients to visualize the skin adequately.

Excoriations, salivary staining other than in the perioral area, and broken hairs are all consistent with pruritus. Dogs that chronically chew at themselves may also have worn incisors and canine teeth. Alopecia is a common dermatological lesion. Self-induced alopecia, or alopecia due to pruritic behaviour, needs to be differentiated from spontaneous alopecia. Spontaneous alopecia does not occur secondary to pruritus, but is caused by a primary follicular problem. Spontaneous alopecia often has a patchy, moth-eaten appearance or well demarcated lesions. Self-induced alopecia occurs in areas of skin where dogs and cats can easily lick, chew and scratch at their fur. In cats, this can be surprisingly symmetrical (as seen on the flanks) and have clearly defined borders. The skin may not look inflamed. It should not be assumed that a cat with symmetrical alopecia has an endocrine abnormality; this would be very rare.

Initial manifestations of pruritus may be erythema and excoriations but then alopecia and chronic lichenification and hyperpigmentation will develop. The presence of papules, pustules and epidermal collarettes are consistent with a superficial pyoderma. The presence of comedones with alopecia is consistent with demodicosis and should prompt the veterinary surgeon to obtain deep skin scrapes to evaluate this differential diagnosis.

The distribution of pruritus and of the skin lesions can be just as important as the type of skin lesions in obtaining a diagnosis. For example, in canine atopic dermatitis, the areas affected are typically the ears and the flexural surfaces of the skin and ventral abdomen, whilst canine flea allergy dermatitis typically affects the caudodorsal region. Figures 6.4 and 6.5 list the clinical signs and lesion distribution for some common pruritic dermatoses of the dog and cat.

Disease	Lesions	Distribution	Additional information
Flea allergy dermatitis	Papules, macules, alopecia, erythema, lichenification, hyperpigmentation, excoriations, fibropruritic nodules	Multiple sites but especially caudal dorsum	Can be present even without any visible fleas or flea dirt
Sarcoptic mange	Papules, macules, erythema, alopecia, crusts, excoriations	Pinnae, elbows, flanks	Severe and sudden pruritus
Demodicosis due to *Demodex canis*	Comedones, alopecia, hyperpigmentation, erythema, follicular casting	Any site with haired skin	Secondary pyoderma typically results in pruritus
Cheyletiellosis	Scaling, alopecia, erythema	Dorsum, generalized	
Superficial pyoderma	Papules, epidermal collarettes, alopecia	Any site with haired skin	Secondary to other conditions
Pediculosis	Alopecia, scales, crusts, debris on fur	Dorsum, generalized	
Atopic dermatitis	Papules, erythema, alopecia, excoriations, lichenification, hyperpigmentation, otitis externa	Flexural surfaces (e.g. caudal carpi and tarsi, axillae, inguinal region), periocular, perioral, ear canal, generalized	
Food-responsive dermatosis	Papules, erythema, alopecia, excoriations, lichenification, hyperpigmentation, otitis externa	Flexural surfaces (e.g. caudal carpi and tarsi, axillae, inguinal region), periocular, perioral, ear canal, generalized	Patients may have gastrointestinal signs, such as soft stool, frequent bowel movements
Malassezia dermatitis	Erythema, brown debris, lichenification, hyperpigmentation	Flexural surfaces (e.g. caudal carpi and tarsi, axillae, inguinal region), paws and nail folds, neck, perioral	Secondary to other conditions
Acral lick dermatitis	Firm alopecic plaque with central ulceration	Limbs, tail, hips	
Contact dermatitis	Erythema, papules, hyperpigmentation, lichenification, erosions	Hairless areas, paws, ventrum, muzzle	
Seborrhoea	Scaling, follicular casting, greasy hair coat	Pinnae, dorsum, flanks, paws	Secondary infection typically results in pruritus
Pemphigus foliaceus	Papules, pustules, crusts, alopecia, erythema, erosions	Head, pinnae, generalized, paw pads	Lesions develop before the onset of pruritus. Lesions on the head are usually bilaterally symmetrical

6.4 Clinical signs and lesion distribution for common pruritic dermatoses of the dog.

Disease	Lesions	Distribution	Additional information
Flea allergy dermatitis	Papules, macules, alopecia, erythema, lichenification, hyperpigmentation, excoriations, miliary dermatitis, eosinophilic granulomas	Multiple sites but especially caudal dorsum	Can be present even without any visible fleas or flea dirt
Otodectic acariasis	Otitis externa, excoriations, miliary dermatitis	Head and neck, ears, generalized	
Demodicosis due to *Demodex gatoi*	Alopecia, hyperpigmentation, erythema, mild scaling	Any site with haired skin but especially the forelimbs, flanks, caudal dorsum	
Notoedric acariasis	Papules, crusts, excoriations, alopecia, erythema	Head and neck, generalized	Severe pruritus and crusting
Cheyletiellosis	Scaling, alopecia, erythema	Dorsum, generalized	
Dermatophytosis	Alopecia, erythema, miliary dermatitis	Any site with haired skin	
Pediculosis	Alopecia, scales, crusts, debris on fur	Dorsum, generalized	
Mosquito bite hypersensitivity	Papules, erythema, crusts, excoriations, exudation	Head, muzzle, pinnae	Uncommon in indoor only cats
Atopic dermatitis	Papules, erythema, alopecia, excoriations, lichenification, hyperpigmentation, otitis externa, miliary dermatitis, eosinophilic granuloma	Flexural surfaces (e.g. caudal carpi and tarsi, axillae, inguinal region), periocular, perioral, ear canal, generalized	
Food-responsive dermatosis	Papules, erythema, alopecia, excoriations, lichenification, hyperpigmentation, otitis externa, miliary dermatitis, eosinophilic granuloma	Flexural surfaces (e.g. caudal carpi and tarsi, axillae, inguinal region), periocular, perioral, ear canal, generalized	Patients may have gastrointestinal signs, such as soft stool, frequent bowel movements
Malassezia dermatitis	Erythema, brown debris, lichenification, hyperpigmentation	Flexural surfaces (e.g. caudal carpi and tarsi, axillae, inguinal region), paws and nail folds, neck, perioral	Secondary to other conditions, may be more common in immunosuppressed cats
Eosinophilic granuloma	Firm alopecic plaque with erosion and/or ulceration	Oral mucosa, limbs, ventrum	Secondary to other conditions
Contact dermatitis	Erythema, papules, hyperpigmentation, lichenification, erosions	Hairless areas, paws, ventrum, muzzle	
Pemphigus foliaceus	Papules, pustules, crusts, alopecia, erythema, erosions	Head, pinnae, nail folds, generalized	Lesions develop before the onset of pruritus. Lesions on the head are usually bilaterally symmetrical

6.5 Clinical signs and lesion distribution for common pruritic dermatoses of the cat.

Diagnostic tests

To clients, tests may appear unnecessary for determining the cause of the pruritus. Clients can easily see the skin lesions themselves, and this can mislead them into thinking that the underlying cause of the pruritus should be obvious to the veterinary surgeon. The reality is that diagnostic tests are especially important when evaluating pruritus because most pruritic skin diseases result in similar skin lesions. Although allergies are a common cause of pruritus, they are not the only one. Likewise, although various effective anti-pruritic medications are available, skipping over cutaneous diagnostic tests in favour of only symptomatic therapy may lead to animal and client harm (e.g. failure to diagnose an antibiotic-resistant bacterial infection) or, ultimately, client frustration at the failure to diagnose an underlying problem.

Diagnostic tests should be selected after formulating a list of differential diagnoses: the most likely causes of pruritus should be investigated first. Differential diagnoses should be prioritized based upon the results of the rest of the consultation (i.e. the history taking and examination). Figures 6.6 and 6.7 present an overview of a diagnostic approach for the pruritic dog and cat.

Skin scrapings

It is never wrong to perform multiple skin scrapings on a pruritic dog or cat. Ectoparasites are a common cause of pruritus and many can be diagnosed with skin scrapings.

Establishing the presence of an ectoparasite enables the veterinary surgeon to prescribe an effective treatment for the pruritus. Missing such a diagnosis may result in many unnecessary diagnostic tests being carried out, additional cost to the client and the continuation of the pruritus.

Ectoparasite therapy trial

It is never wrong to consider a trial course of a parasiticide (see Chapter 8) in a pruritic dog or cat. Flea infestation is a common cause of pruritus, but fleas are often not found on the animal. A reduction in pruritus after treatment with an anti-flea medication would be consistent with this diagnosis. Scabies mites (*Sarcoptes scabei var. canis*) are found on skin scrapings in only a small percentage of dogs that have sarcoptic mange. Therefore, trial therapy with an anti-sarcoptic parasiticide is indicated in any dog suspected of having scabies, even if the skin scrapings are negative. *Demodex gatoi*, the short-bodied *Demodex* mite of cats, causes pruritus and may not always be present on skin scrapings. A decrease in pruritus after a trial course of weekly lime sulphur dips, which are effective against this mite, could be consistent with feline demodicosis.

Skin cytology

Skin cytology can be used to diagnose common causes of pruritus such as *Malassezia* or bacterial dermatitis. This technique should routinely be performed in pruritic animals.

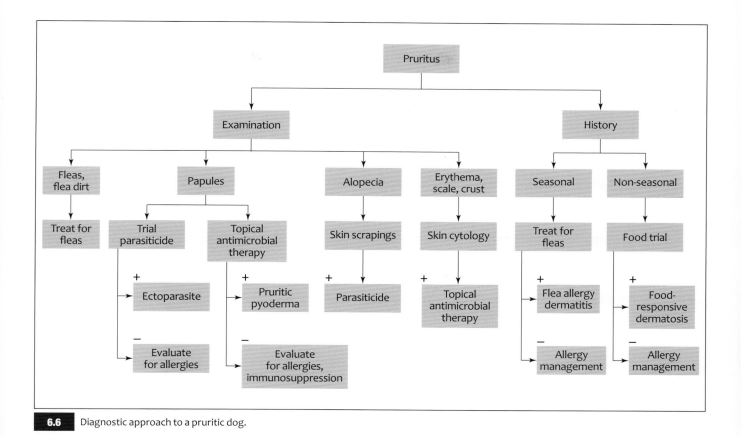

6.6 Diagnostic approach to a pruritic dog.

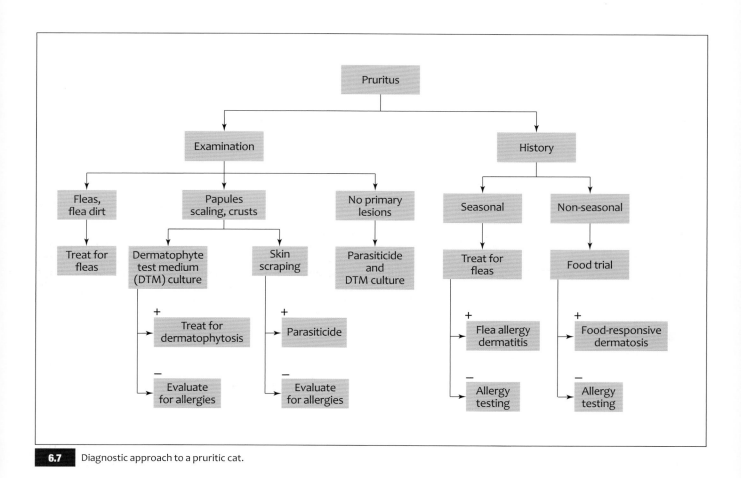

6.7 Diagnostic approach to a pruritic cat.

Intact pustules can be ruptured with a 25 G needle and the contents smeared on to a slide and examined to determine whether there are bacteria or inflammatory cells present. Tape strips of the skin surface should also be examined (see Chapters 3 and 4).

Dermatophyte evaluation

While most dogs and cats with dermatophytosis are not pruritic, a dermatophyte infection evaluation (see Chapter 12) may be indicated in some patients with pruritus. Clinical signs of dermatophytosis include alopecia and broken hairs. Since most pruritic cats have these signs, dermatophytosis is often a differential diagnosis. Dermatophytosis should also be considered for dog breeds that are prone to this infection, such as Yorkshire and Jack Russell Terriers.

Faecal examination

Faecal examination through a flotation test can diagnose some surface-dwelling ectoparasites such as *Demodex gatoi* or *Cheyletiella* if those parasites have been swallowed in the course of grooming. Faecal examination can also reveal endoparasites, such as hookworms, which can cause pruritic dermatitis.

Food trial

Dogs and cats with year-round pruritus should be evaluated for a food-responsive dermatosis. Food-responsive dermatoses cannot be diagnosed using an allergy test. Instead, they need to be investigated by implementing a food trial. A diet containing novel ingredients should be used for the food trial. Novel ingredients can be identified by obtaining a thorough diet history for the patient. Alternatively, a diet containing hydrolysed proteins can be used. It is important to realize that hydrolysed diets may not diagnose all cases of food-responsive dermatosis, as they are primarily developed to target type I hypersensitivity to food. The diet should be fed for several weeks with no other foods or flavoured medications. A decrease in pruritus whilst on the food trial followed by an increase in pruritus after reintroducing food items is diagnostic for a food-responsive dermatosis (see Chapter 9).

Intradermal or serological allergy testing

These tests should only be used in patients that have been clinically diagnosed with atopic dermatitis and where other causes of pruritus have been ruled out. This is discussed in detail in Chapter 11. Likewise, there is no clinical or diagnostic validity for so-called allergy tests that utilize other samples such as saliva or hair. Allergy tests are used to help the veterinary surgeon select allergens for the formulation of allergen-specific immunotherapy. The patient's environment and pattern of pruritus are also important factors in the selection of allergens for immunotherapy formulation.

Skin biopsy

Biopsy of chronically self-traumatized skin with secondary skin lesions usually will not identify the cause of pruritus and, in general, is not useful in the diagnostic work-up of a pruritic patient. Biopsy may be helpful if primary skin lesions are present, or in animals with uncommon pruritic dermatoses that are failing to respond to routine treatment, such as epitheliotrophic lymphoma in the older patient, or to diagnose a condition such as a primary seborrhoea. Skin biopsy is also sometimes necessary to diagnose demodicosis in some thick-skinned dogs such as Shar Peis. If a biopsy is performed, multiple sites containing the primary skin lesions should be sampled. These samples should then be submitted with a detailed dermatological history to a dermatopathologist.

Complete blood count and general chemistry profile

Blood tests should be performed as part of a comprehensive evaluation of the patient's general health if a systemic condition is suspected. Otherwise, blood tests are unlikely to identify the underlying cause of the pruritus and other diagnostic tests, such as skin scrapes, skin cytology and an ectoparasiticide trial may provide more information.

Treatment trial

Antipruritic medications (see Chapter 10) are sometimes used as part of the diagnostic work-up for a pruritic patient. In patients with multiple co-existing skin conditions, such as atopic dermatitis and a pyoderma, treatment of the pyoderma followed by re-examination may be needed initially to determine which condition is the key contributor to the patient's overall level of pruritus, and antipruritic medications are best avoided. However, if the pruritus is severe and must be controlled pending the response to other therapies, such as a food trial, then a short-term course may be prescribed. In addition, antipruritic therapy may be needed if the client will not allow diagnostic tests to be carried out and instead wants a treatment to manage the clinical signs. However, they should be reminded that the treatment is only managing the pruritus and not addressing the underlying condition. This will hopefully minimize the client's frustration if the pruritus recurs after discontinuation of the treatment.

Key points

- There are multiple mediators that can activate intraepidermal nerve fibres
- The threshold for pruritus can be reached by a summation of internal and external factors
- A logical approach, which involves initially evaluating for common diseases, such as parasites and secondary infections, is indicated for each patient

---

References and further reading

Metz M, Grundmann S and Ständer S (2011) Pruritus: an overview of current concepts. *Veterinary Dermatology* **22**, 121–131

Miller WH, Griffin CE and Campbell KL (2013) *Muller and Kirk's Small Animal Dermatology, 7th edn.* WB Saunders, Philadelphia

Steinhoff M, Bienenstock J, Schmelz M *et al.* (2006) Neurophysiological, neuroimmunological, and neuroendocrine basis of pruritus. *Journal of Investigative Dermatology* **126**, 1705–1718

Chapter 7

Ectoparasite infestation – clinical presentation

Cathy F. Curtis

Insecta

Fleas

Ectoparasite infestation is a relatively common cause of skin disease in domesticated animal species, and the most frequently observed offender in both dogs and cats in the UK is the cat flea (*Ctenocephalides felis felis*). In a survey of over 4000 animals carried out in the UK (Bond *et al.*, 2005), the cat flea represented 93.2% and 98.9% of the fleas found on dogs and cats respectively. This ancient parasite is probably one of the most ubiquitous worldwide, having been isolated from over 50 different host species. Conversely, individual host species, such as the domestic dog, can be infested by a variety of flea species (e.g. the dog, hedgehog, rabbit, poultry and even the human flea), demonstrating the truly polyxenous nature of this parasite, which undoubtedly contributes to its survival.

Biology

Ctenocephalides felis felis is a brown, wingless insect of approximately 3–4 mm in length (Figure 7.1), its life cycle being an example of complete metamorphosis comprising oval, larval, pupal and adult stages. Adult *C. felis felis* acquire a host and rapidly start feeding on blood taken directly from capillaries, with females commencing egg-laying within 24–36 hours of this first blood meal and following multiple matings. Once adult fleas have established themselves on a host, the movement rate to an

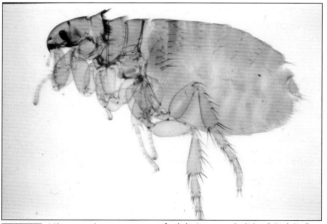

7.1 Microscopic appearance of adult *Ctenocephalides felis felis* flea from a Domestic Shorthaired cat. (Original magnification X100)

uninfested host is low (3.7%) (Franc *et al.*, 2013). Host grooming, particularly in cats, appears to be a significant mortality factor, and studies have shown that cats can remove up to 17.6% of their flea burden daily (Hinkle *et al.*, 1998). The mean longevity of fleas on the host is 7.8 days and an average of 38.4 eggs are laid per day. Most eggs fall from the host's coat within 8 hours and the developing first stage larvae emerge a few days later, depending on environmental temperature and relative humidity, with optimal conditions being approximately 27°C and >53% humidity, respectively (Thiemann *et al.*, 2003).

The first larval instar (L1) moults twice to L2 and L3. All three stages are negatively phototactic and positively geotactic; hence, they accumulate deep in the carpet pile or in cracks between floorboards, particularly in areas where animals rest, as they rely on faecal blood and flea eggs as a source of nutrition (Shryock and Housemann, 2006). The third larval instar spins a silk cocoon, pupates and becomes a pre-emerged adult. At 26.6°C, adult females and males emerge from the cocoon 5–8 days and 7–10 days after pupation respectively (Hudson and Prince, 1958), although it should be noted that emergence is delayed at lower temperatures. This temperature-dependent mechanism, coupled with a reduced metabolic rate and the protective effect of the cocoon, allow the pre-emerged adults to survive for several weeks to months within the cocoon until a time when environmental conditions are favourable and a suitable host is in the vicinity. The major triggers for emergence are carbon dioxide and mechanical pressure. The emerged adults locate their host using visual and thermal detection systems and experimentally have been shown to be attracted to light (particularly intermittent sources) and heat. Air currents and carbon dioxide generated by a passing host stimulate jumping behaviour and despite a preference for dogs and cats, adult *C. felis felis* will also feed on humans (Figure 7.2).

Pathogenesis

Although flea infestation is common, some dogs and cats will develop a flea bite allergy. In these animals, pruritus in response to flea bites can be intense. Type I (immediate and type IV (delayed) hypersensitivity reactions have been described in response to flea saliva, plus late phase immunoglobulin (Ig)E and cutaneous hypersensitivities in the dog (Miller *et al.*, 2013a). In one canine study, IgE was shown to bind to at least 15 different flea components in sera from allergic dogs and, more recently, the 18-kD protein Cte f1 was identified as a major allergen in flea

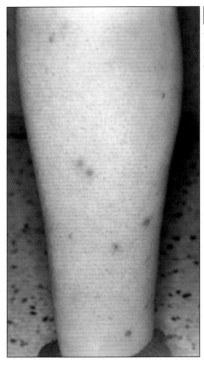

7.2 Lower leg of a person living in a cat flea-infested house; note the multiple papules developing as a result of the fleas' bites.

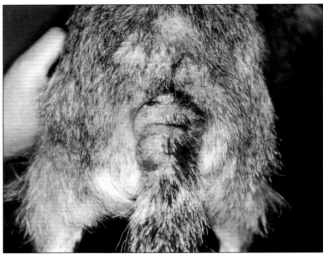

7.3 Caudodorsal rump of a Border Terrier with chronic flea bite hypersensitivity. Note the degree of alopecia, hyperpigmentation and lichenification.

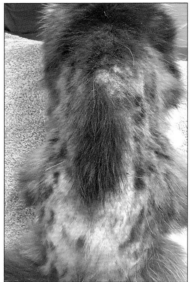

7.4 Symmetrical, self-induced alopecia of the dorsum and rump of an 8-year-old Domestic Longhaired cat with flea bite hypersensitivity.

saliva (McDermott *et al*., 2000). In one experimental model, dogs exposed continuously to fleas were found to have higher flea antigen-specific IgE values compared with those being intermittently exposed and they did not develop immunotolerance. All dogs in the study that were exposed to fleas developed clinical lesions, which differs to the findings of a similar study in cats, in which only the continually exposed subjects developed lesions. The agreement between serological IgE titres and intradermal test reactivity to crude flea antigen in both canine and feline studies was good. Furthermore, a number of studies have demonstrated that both methods of testing have a role to play in the diagnosis of flea bite hypersensitivity in dogs and cats, although it should be remembered that these tests should always be used as part of, and not the sole focus of, any allergy work-up (see 'Diagnosis' below)

Clinical approach

The feeding activity of fleas, during which protein fractions in their saliva are injected into the dermis, can result in moderate to marked pruritus characterized by papules, self-induced alopecia and erythema, typically affecting the dorsum, rump (Figures 7.3 and 7.4), caudal ventral abdomen and caudal thighs in hypersensitive canine and feline hosts. Allergic dogs and cats may develop focal, ulcerated or eroded lesions at the flea feeding sites (Figure 7.5), or more generalized, crusted papules. In dogs, these papules principally affect the dorsum and caudal thighs; whereas, in cats the distribution is along the dorsum and is often referred to as miliary dermatitis (Figure 7.6). Additionally, in cats other reaction patterns associated with pruritus such as diffuse, truncal or symmetrical alopecia, head and neck pruritus or lesions of the eosinophilic granuloma complex (EGC), namely eosinophilic plaques, linear granulomas and indolent/rodent ulcers, may also be observed. It should be noted that, although EGC lesions may be manifestations of flea allergy, they have also been linked to other immunological aberrations.

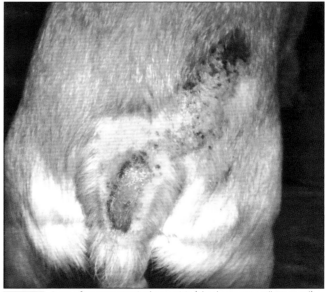

7.5 Area of pyotraumatic dermatitis (also known as a 'hot spot') on the right dorsal rump of a Labrador Retriever as a consequence of reactivity to a flea bite.

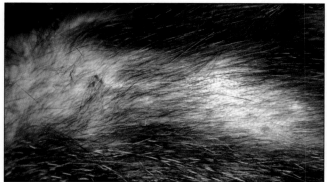

7.6 Close-up view of miliary dermatitis and alopecia on an adult Shorthaired cat, secondary to flea allergy dermatitis.

Clinical disease can be seasonal (i.e. typically Spring through to Autumn) or present all year round if climatic and environmental conditions are optimal. It should be noted that in northern countries, non-seasonal disease can result from fleas surviving in household environments. In addition to dermatological disease, fleas may transmit other pathogens, including the tapeworm *Dipylidium caninum* and, of greater concern, *Rickettsia felis*, *Bartonella* spp. and *Haemoplasma* spp., with 14% of 662 dogs and 812 cats in one UK study being shown to be polymerase chain reaction (PCR)-positive for at least one of the latter three pathogens (Abdullah *et al.*, 2019).

The implications of these findings are significant for both other pets and humans. *Ctenocephalides felis felis* has long been known to feed off humans (particularly in the absence of a feline or canine host) and the systemic diseases spread by fleas are significantly more serious than the more typical pruritic, erythematous wheals most commonly found on the feet, ankles and calves of people inhabiting an environment where a flea-infested pet lives/ has lived. Prophylactic measures to control fleas remain the best approach to prevent flea-related disease. There are many effective, long-lasting and safe insecticides commercially available (see Chapter 8 for further information).

Diagnosis

All six life cycle stages and the insect's faecal material are visible to the human eye; therefore, a detailed, direct examination of the hair coat via coat brushings (either on to white paper or a table top) or of the animal's bedding for adult, oval, larval or pupal forms should always be performed, as this is often rewarding. If fleas or flea faeces are not observed, but a flea bite allergy is suspected on the basis of the history and clinical signs, then a parasiticidal trial should be undertaken (see Chapter 8). This should include treatment of the primary pet, in-contact animals and the environment.

Where flea allergy dermatitis is suspected, serological testing may be considered. In recent years, a specific enzyme-linked immunosorbent assay (ELISA) has been developed, which detects circulating levels of anti-flea saliva IgE using the IgE receptor (FCεR1α) for primary capture of antibody (Stedman *et al.*, 2001). When compared with an intradermal test, the Heska Corporation claim sensitivity and specificity rates of 78% and 91% in dogs, and 87% and 71% in cats, respectively (McCall, 1997ab). It should be noted that most laboratories offering serum allergy testing will include flea allergen in their allergen panel, but methods of detection of IgE will vary between companies.

Another diagnostic option is the use of whole flea or purified flea saliva extracts in an intradermal test, which induces positive, immediate type I hypersensitivity reactions in both dogs and cats, and delayed reactions in approximately 30% of dogs (Figure 7.7). This is often quoted as the 'gold standard' test because at least 90% of dogs and cats with clinical and historical features of flea bite hypersensitivity will develop positive test results. However, positive reactions can be seen in 24% and 36% of clinically normal household dogs and cats, respectively (Moriello and McMurdy, 1989; Kunkle *et al.*, 2000), thus reducing the specificity of this test.

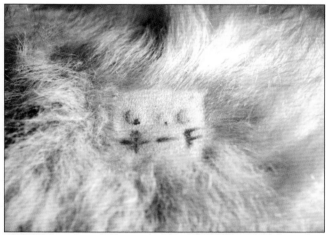

7.7 Intradermal skin test showing an immediate positive reaction to flea allergen (F) in a Golden Retriever with flea bite hypersensitivity. Controls are 1/10 histamine solution (+) and saline (–).

Lice

Lice are small, wingless, parasitic host-specific insects and infestation is known as pediculosis. There are two suborders:

- **Anoplura** (sucking lice) – mouthparts are adapted for sucking the blood of the host. Only one species of louse is commonly seen in domestic animals, *Linognathus setosus* (Figure 7.8), which affects dogs
- **Mallophaga** (biting lice) – generally feed on skin cells and hair. Biting lice affect both dogs (*Trichodectes canis*; Figure 7.9) and cats (*Felicola subrostrata*; Figure 7.10).

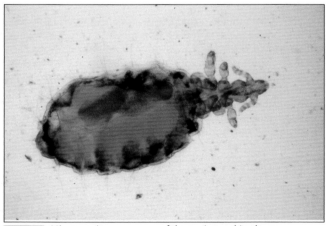

7.8 Microscopic appearance of the canine sucking louse, *Linognathus setosus*. (Original magnification X100)

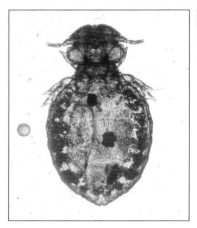

7.9 Microscopic appearance of the canine biting louse, *Trichodectes canis*. (Original magnification X100)

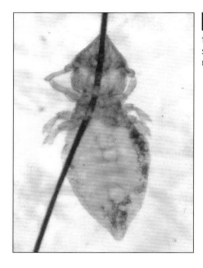

7.10 Microscopic appearance of the feline biting louse, *Felicola subrostrata*. (Original magnification X100)

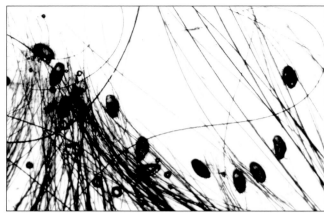

7.11 Microscopic appearance of a hair plucking suspended in liquid paraffin, showing multiple louse eggs cemented on to the hair shafts. (Original magnification X100)

Pathogenesis and clinical approach

Pediculosis can induce pruritus in the host and is most commonly seen in juvenile, elderly and debilitated animals. The movement and feeding action of both suborders of louse cause irritation, but in addition to this, heavy infestations of sucking lice can lead to anaemia, particularly in puppies and small dog breeds. *Trichodectes canis* can act as an intermediate host to the dog tapeworm *Dipylidium caninum*, and the reaction to bites from *Felicola subrostratus* can resemble miliary dermatitis in cats.

Diagnosis

Adult lice are usually a mid-brown colour and several millimetres long. These, and their empty white egg cases (nits), are visible to the naked eye, so a diagnosis can often be made by direct dermatological examination of the coat and skin, particularly in heavy infestations. If the species of louse needs to be identified, they can be captured with a scalpel blade coated in liquid paraffin, or caught on a piece of acetate tape, prior to microscopic examination. Alternatively, hair suspected of harbouring louse eggs can be plucked from the coat, suspended in liquid paraffin and examined microscopically under low power (Figure 7.11)

Biting insects

A small number of biting insect species (e.g. blackflies, horseflies, stable flies, mosquitoes and midges) can cause skin disease in small animals, but in the UK and northern Europe these insects are rarely responsible for the transmission of disease. However, climate change and the relaxation of intercontinental pet travel restrictions could result in the spread of more exotic insect vectors, such as Phlebotomine sandflies (see below), and clinicians need to be aware of these diseases and remain vigilant with respect to their detection.

Pathogenesis and clinical approach

The major differential diagnoses for fly bite dermatitis are:

- Flea bite hypersensitivity
- Sarcoptic mange
- Superficial pyoderma
- Pediculosis.

Fly bites are rarely witnessed by the owner, unless a swarm attacks their pet. Multiple blackfly bites have been known occasionally to kill animals (Miller *et al.*, 2013b), but individual fly bites typically cause only focal dermatitis, with a varying degree of pruritus, depending on the sensitivity of the animal. These are generally seen in regions where there is less protective hair, such as the pinnae and face. Mosquito bites usually result in pruritic papules, but a hypersensitivity to mosquito saliva has been described in cats, and affected animals develop papulocrustous lesions on the pinnae and crusting on the bridge of the nose (Nagata and Ishida, 1997). An uncommon, acute onset intensely pruritic facial dermatosis, known as eosinophilic folliculitis and furunculosis (EFF), has been described in dogs (Curtis *et al.*, 1995; Figure 7.12); it has been potentially attributed to fly bites, but this has never been proven.

Of greater concern is the protozoal disease leishmaniosis, caused mainly by *Leishmania infantum*, which is transmitted by sandflies belonging to the genus *Phlebotomus* (Old World) or *Lutzomyia* (New World). This serious, potentially fatal, zoonotic disease affects mainly dogs, but is occasionally seen in cats. The incubation period is months to years, hence asymptomatic 'carrier' animals may be an undetected reservoir of infection for protracted periods of time. It is most common in Mediterranean countries and Central and South America but, in recent years, reports from North America and northern Europe have increased and two separate incidences of leishmaniosis in UK dogs that have not travelled abroad have recently been reported (McKenna *et al.*, 2019; Wright and Baker, 2019). In a recent review, the true incidence of this disease in the UK was

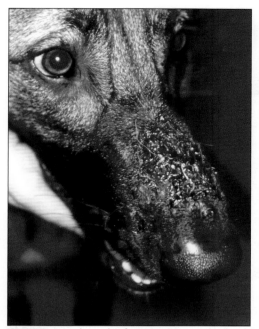

7.12 Dorsal muzzle of a young German Shepherd Dog with ulceration typical of eosinophilic folliculitis and furunculosis, presumed to be caused by a fly bite.

reported to be considerably higher than clinicians may realize, so it should be considered a significant differential diagnosis in dogs with appropriate systemic and/or dermatological signs, particularly if they originate from or have travelled abroad (Walker, 2019). The full range of clinical signs of leishmaniosis is variable and beyond the scope of this chapter, so readers are encouraged to consult appropriate texts on the subject (see also Chapter 30).

Diagnosis

Occasionally, owners may observe flies on their pets, but fly bite-induced dermatitis would generally be a tentative diagnosis based on the history and clinical suspicion. Skin biopsy specimens harvested from animals with suspected mosquito bite hypersensitivity or EFF may have histopathological features consistent with these dermatoses. Skin tests with mosquito extracts can be performed in cats with suspected mosquito bite hypersensitivity; immediate and delayed hypersensitivity reactions have been observed (Nagata and Ishida, 1997).

Acari

Sarcoptic mange

Biology

Sarcoptic mange (sarcoptic acariasis, scabies) is a non-seasonal pruritic skin condition caused by infestation with the mite *Sarcoptes scabiei*. *Sarcoptes scabiei* belongs to the family Sarcoptidae and is a globose mite with short legs, measuring 200–400 μm (Figure 7.13a). The mite has four stages to its life cycle: ovum, six-legged larva, eight-legged nymph and eight-legged adult. The duration of this life cycle, from ovum to ovum, is 14–21 days, depending on environmental conditions. Males and females mate on the surface of the skin, then the gravid females penetrate into the epidermis to form burrows, into which their eggs

are laid. Faecal pellets (scybala) may also be seen within the tunnels and, if identified, can be used to confirm a diagnosis (Figure 7.13b). Once hatched, the larvae and nymphs excavate their way back to the skin surface to mature and find mates. These mites are obligate parasites, but can survive for limited periods away from the host, hence environmental acaricidal control, in addition to on-animal treatment, is warranted in an outbreak of the disease (see Chapter 8).

Pathogenesis

Sarcoptic mange affects many mammalian species and the variant *S. scabiei* var. *canis* occurs commonly in canidae. In contrast, sarcoptic mange due to the canine mite is rare in the cat and relatively few reports of feline sarcoptic mange appear in the veterinary literature. These cases are often associated with concurrent systemic disease (e.g. feline immunodeficiency virus (FIV); Curtis *et al.*, 2019).

Human and canine studies have shown that mites can penetrate the skin within 30 minutes of exposure; feeding, oviposition and deposition of faeces within the skin exposes the host to mite allergens, which in the majority of infested dogs induces both humoral and cell-mediated immunological responses (Bornstein and Zakrisson, 1993; Arlian *et al.*, 1996). These defence mechanisms can lead to spontaneous resolution of the disease after a few months, but most dogs develop a moderate to intensely pruritic dermatosis, which initially affects the pinnal margins, elbows, hocks and ventrum and can eventually progress to

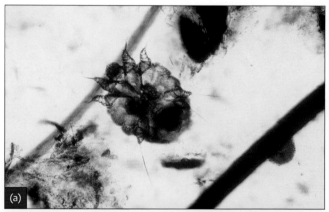

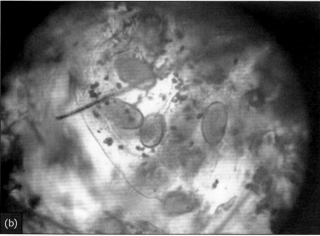

7.13 Microscopic appearance of *Sarcoptes scabiei*. (a) Adult mite in liquid paraffin. (Original magnification X100) (b) Ova and faeces (scybala) of *Sarcoptes scabiei* in liquid paraffin. (Original magnification X400)

BSAVA Manual of Canine and Feline Dermatology

involve the entire body surface (Figure 7.14). Similarly in cats, infestation can initially be localized to, for example, the head and pinnae (Figure 7.15), but in time, can generalize to affect the trunk and tail (Figure 7.16).

As a rule, sarcoptic mange is highly contagious. However, it is important to note that scabies cannot be ruled out if there is only one affected dog in a multiple-dog household. The development of clinical signs can be due to a variety of factors, including the parasitic load, the closeness of the contact and the development of a hypersensitivity reaction to the mites. Indirect infestation via fur or fomites has been reported, but the majority of mites are transmitted by direct contact with an infested dog or fox.

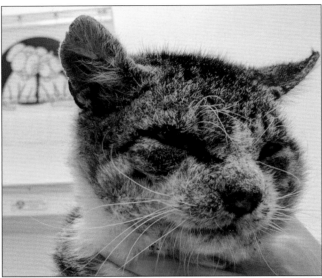

7.15 Feline sarcoptic mange in a mature Domestic Shorthaired cat. Note the crusting over the face and ears, similar to lesions that develop in dogs (see also 'Notoedric mange').

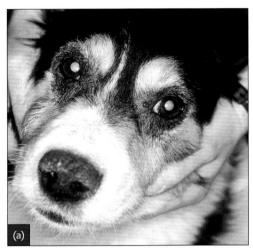

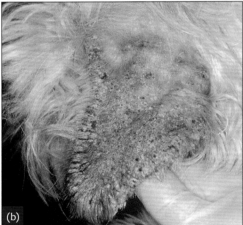

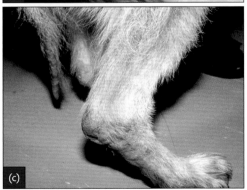

7.14 (a) Bilateral periocular alopecia, erythema and lichenification in an adult male crossbreed dog with sarcoptic mange. (b) Left pinna of a male Lhasa Apso with advanced sarcoptic mange. Note the marked degree of hyperkeratosis and scaling, particularly around the pinnal margin. (c) Hocks of an adult male German Shepherd Dog affected by sarcoptic mange.

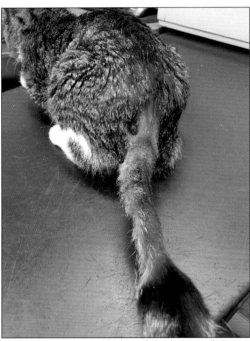

7.16 Crusting and scaling of the dorsum of a Domestic Shorthaired cat with feline sarcoptic mange. Note the hair loss from the tail due to self-trauma.

Clinical approach

The major differential diagnoses for sarcoptic mange are:

- Flea bite hypersensitivity
- Atopic dermatitis
- Food-responsive dermatosis (also known as food allergy or adverse food reaction)
- Superficial pyoderma
- *Malassezia* dermatitis
- Demodicosis
- Cheyletiellosis
- Pemphigus foliaceus
- Dermatophytosis.

One of the most useful facets of the diagnostic approach is the history provided by the owner. Sarcoptic mange can affect dogs of any age or breed and there is no known sex predilection. The classic historical feature of the disease is the sudden onset of intense pruritus in one or more localized areas, which enlarges with time. As mentioned above, typical sites affected initially in both dogs and cats are the periocular skin, pinnal margins, elbows and hocks, but over time, the lesions may become generalized. In common with other infectious and ectoparasitic skin diseases, the lesions are often asymmetrical, which differentiates them from allergic and immune-mediated dermatoses.

All dogs (and potentially also cats, if they are exhibiting clinical signs) in contact with an infested individual should be treated simultaneously to limit the opportunity for cross- and re-infestation, and an acaricide should also be applied to the environment. Furthermore, owners should be informed that they could contract sarcoptic mange from their dog, although provided the animal is treated appropriately, the infestation is usually self-limiting in humans.

Diagnosis

The definitive diagnosis of scabies relies on direct visualization of mature or immature mites and/or their eggs and faeces in either skin scrapings, skin biopsy specimens or faecal samples. Skin scraping is practised most frequently, using the following technique:

1. Place a few drops of liquid paraffin on the surface of a microscopy slide.
2. Dip the cutting edge of a No. 10 scalpel blade into the liquid paraffin, to aid the adherence of the dislodged skin and crust to be removed.
3. Gently scrape the area being tested repeatedly with the blade, in the direction of hair growth (to optimize sample collection), until the underlying skin develops capillary ooze (demonstrating that the superficial dermis has been reached).
4. Mix the dislodged skin/scale into the liquid paraffin on the microscope slide.
5. Cover with a coverslip (to prevent the mites from escaping, as they are still very motile and can 'swim' out of the paraffin if left uncovered).
6. Examine the slide at low power and any areas of interest at medium power.

It should be borne in mind that even with good technique and experienced lesion selection, Sarcoptid mite detection rates can be as low as 20%, so in situations where mites elude detection, serum samples from suspected cases can be submitted for detection of circulating anti-*Sarcoptes* IgG by ELISA. This test was initially developed in Sweden (Bornstein and Zakrisson, 1993) and independent testing has reported sensitivity and specificity rates of 83% and 92%, respectively (Curtis, 2001). False-negative results are therefore still possible, and false-positive results can be obtained in atopic dogs that are sensitive to house dust mites, as cross-reactivity between house dust, sarcoptic and storage mites has been demonstrated in dogs with atopic dermatitis (Virchow and Bigler, 2004). It should be noted that serum testing is only useful in dogs where the disease has been present for at least 3–4 weeks, allowing an antibody response to develop. If the clinician is still suspicious of sarcoptic mange, a scabicidal therapeutic trial should be performed.

Cheyletiellosis

Cheyletiellosis is typically a mild, albeit very contagious, dermatosis caused by *Cheyletiella* spp. mites living on the skin surface. Cheyletiellidae are relatively large (500 x 350 μm), white, 'fiddle-shaped' Acari with legs that protrude beyond their body margins and terminate in hair-like setae. The most distinctive feature is a pair of crescent-shaped hooks on the accessory mouthparts (Figure 7.17a).

Pathogenesis and clinical approach

Cheyletiellid mites feed on tissue fluid and lymph obtained by piercing the epidermis with a stylet-like chelicerae. Following mating, adult females lay eggs which they bind to the hairs of the host with a silken thread (Figure 7.17b). When shed, these eggs can act as an environmental reservoir of infestation. These mites are obligate parasites but are capable of surviving away from the host for at least 10 days in suitable environmental conditions. In addition to direct transmission, infestation may occur indirectly via fomites such as leads, grooming tools or even other, larger ectoparasites such as fleas, lice and flies.

Cheyletiella yasguri is the species isolated most frequently from dogs, but as a family Cheyletiellidae are not believed to be host-specific and may readily transfer between dogs, cats and rabbits. However, it should be noted that *C. blakei* is most frequently isolated from cats and *C. parasitovorax* is most commonly associated with rabbits.

Cheyletiellosis is primarily a dorsally distributed disease characterized by pruritus, mild erythema and excessive scaling (Figure 7.18). In cats, papulocrustous lesions may

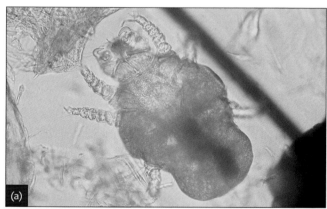

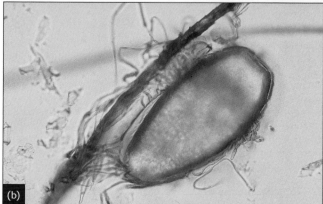

7.17 Microscopic appearance of *Cheyletiella* spp. (a) Mite harvested from a canine skin scraping, suspended in liquid paraffin. Note the distinctive crescent-shaped hooks on the accessory mouthparts. (Original magnification X100) (b) Ovum in liquid paraffin. Note the thread attaching the egg to the hair. (Original magnification X400)

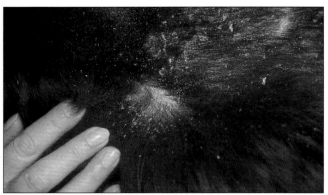

7.18 Severe scaling and erythema in an adult Newfoundland with cheyletiellosis.

also develop; thus, cheyletiellosis is a differential diagnosis for feline miliary dermatitis. Pruritus is variable, ranging from absent to moderately severe, and young animals usually exhibit more obvious clinical signs than adults. In dogs, infestation may lead to pyotraumatic dermatitis, so 'hot-spot' cases with concurrent dorsal or truncal scaling should be screened for the mite. An asymptomatic carrier status also exists, and this should be borne in mind when tackling problem cases in which repeated re-infestation and zoonotic transmission occurs (Figure 7.19).

The major differential diagnoses for cheyletiellosis are:

- Flea bite hypersensitivity
- Pediculosis
- Atopic dermatitis
- Food-responsive dermatosis
- Superficial pyoderma.

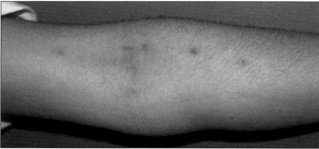

7.19 Papular lesions on the forearm of the owner of a dog infested with *Cheyletiella* mites.
(Courtesy of M Paradis)

Diagnosis

The simplest diagnostic test is to sit or stand the animal on a dark surface and, using the hand, a brush or a flea comb, dislodge some of the scale from the skin surface. On closer inspection, the scale may appear motile as a result of mite activity; this is the origin of the alternative name of the disease, 'walking dandruff'. More accurate methods of diagnosis involve harvesting mites and eggs using adhesive acetate tape preparations or skin scrapings. An adhesive acetate tape preparation can be made using the following technique:

1. Apply the sticky surface of a piece of acetate tape repeatedly along the dorsum of a scaly animal.
2. Apply the acetate tape, sticky side down, directly to the surface of a glass microscope slide.
3. Examine the slide (at X40 magnification) for evidence of mature/immature mites and eggs.

To improve detection rates, care must be taken to collect samples from the skin surface and not just the distal ends of the hairs. Despite being present in large numbers in the majority of cases, it should be remembered that *Cheyletiella* can sometimes be difficult to detect; in two separate studies, investigators failed to recover mites in 15% of infested dogs and 58% of infested cats (Paradis and Villeneuve, 1988; Paradis *et al.*, 1990). Therapeutic trials with reliable acaricides are therefore indicated in suspected cases. It is important to treat all in-contact animals (as some may act as asymptomatic carriers), to treat past the life cycle (by approximately 3 weeks) and to consider the persistence of the parasite in the environment.

Trombiculidiosis

Of the several hundred different species of Trombiculidae (chigger) mites that have been recognized, only a handful cause disease in humans and animals. *Neotrombicula autumnalis* (harvest mite, berry bug) and *Eutrombicula alfreddugesi* (North American chigger mite) are the most familiar pathogenic mites in Europe and North America, respectively.

Pathogenesis and clinical approach

Only the larval stages of Trombiculidae are parasitic to mammals (Figure 7.20); the remainder of the life cycle is completed in the environment, with the nymphal and adult stages feeding on vegetable matter. Canine and feline (and occasionally human) infestations are therefore seasonal, with the majority of cases occurring between June/July and November, although there has been one reported case of an atypical feline *Trombicula* larval infestation in January (White *et al.*, 2001). Other larval chigger mites reported to cause skin disease in small animals are: *Walchia americana*, which was isolated from a domestic cat in North America (Lowenstine *et al.*, 1979); *Leptotrombidium subquadratum*, which can cause canine and human pruritus in South Africa during the summer months (Heyne *et al.*, 2001); and *Helenicula miyagawai* in Japanese cats (Takahashi *et al.*, 2004). *Straelensia cynotis* is distinguished by its intrafollicular habitat and has been reported in rural and hunting dogs in southern France, northern Spain and Portugal (Ramirez *et al.*, 2009).

The major differential diagnoses for trombiculidiosis are:

- Atopic dermatitis
- Food-responsive dermatosis
- *Malassezia* dermatitis
- Pododemodicosis.

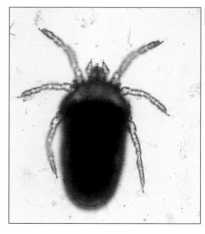

7.20 A six-legged *Neotrombicula autumnalis* larva harvested by skin scraping and suspended in liquid paraffin. (Original magnification X100)

All Trombiculidae cause papular to papulocrustous lesions at their feeding sites, which tend to be concentrated interdigitally or along the ventral abdomen. Eutrombiculid and Neotrombiculid larvae, which appear as red-orange 'specks', can also affect the ears and have a particular preference for the marginal pouch (also known as 'Henry's pocket') (Figure 7.21). Most infestations are asymptomatic, but some parasitized animals become extremely pruritic and, in extreme cases, wheals can develop at the site of mite attachment. *Straelensia cynotis* infestation has been reported to cause a pruritic, nodular dermatitis, particularly affecting the head and dorsum.

Diagnosis

Whenever trombiculidiosis is suspected, direct examination of the coat and particularly the predilection sites is warranted, as the mites are visible to the naked eye. If the mites remain undetected, suspicious lesions should be scraped or even biopsied because the immune reaction of the host may wall-off or 'encyst' the mite (Bourdeau *et al.*, 2000), making them detectable only by deep scrapings or histopathological examination. *Straelensia cynotis* mites are typically detected histopathologically.

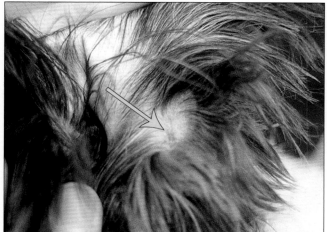

7.21 Left ear of a mature Shih Tzu bitch showing the presence of an accumulation of red-orange *Neotrombicula autumnalis* larvae (arrowed) in the cutaneous marginal pouch (also known as 'Henry's pocket').

Otoacariasis

Otoacariasis (otodectic mange) is caused by *Otodectes cynotis* (known colloquially as the ear mite), which belongs to the family Psoroptidae. The mite is white, with long legs that protrude beyond the body, and a terminal anus. *Otodectes* is an obligate parasite that inhabits the vertical and horizontal ear canals of dogs and cats and is capable of surviving for several weeks to months away from the host (Larkin and Gaillard, 1981).

Pathogenesis and clinical approach

O. cynotis is non-burrowing and lives on the surface of the ear canal lining. In cats, mite feeding has been shown to induce a reaginic hypersensitivity response in some individuals, which may subsequently develop tolerance to the mite's salivary proteins (Powell *et al.*, 1980). Infested cats may also demonstrate skin test reactivity to environmental mites such as *Dermatophagoides* spp. and *Acarus siro*,

although this cross-reactivity appears to abate once the ear mite infestation is cleared (Saridomichelakis *et al.*, 1999). This finding should be borne in mind when cats (and potentially dogs) present with ear/head pruritus as a predominant clinical sign, which could be mistakenly diagnosed as atopic disease.

The major differential diagnoses for otodectic mange are:

- Bacterial or *Malassezia* otitis
- Sarcoptic mange
- Atopic dermatitis
- Food-responsive dermatosis
- Foreign body reaction.

Animals infested with *Otodectes cynotis* most commonly develop otitis externa, characterized by vertical and horizontal canal erythema and a dark brown, ceruminous otic exudate (Figure 7.22). Secondary bacterial or fungal (i.e. *Malassezia*) otitis is reasonably common. In addition to otitis externa, 'ectopic' infestations of the head, neck, tail head and, rarely, the trunk can occur when mites escape the ear canals (Scott and Horn, 1997). Papulocrustous lesions (miliary dermatitis) may also be observed. Puppies and kittens appear to be most susceptible to otoacariasis as older animals may acquire immunity. Zoonotic infections have been reported (Herwick, 1978; Suetake *et al.*, 1991; Lopez, 1993), with mites typically producing pruritic papular lesions on areas of the body that have been in contact with the infested pet.

Diagnosis

Otodectes cynotis are motile, relatively large (400–500 μm), pearly white mites that are visible to the naked eye. An auroscopic examination may reveal gross evidence of otoacariasis. Alternatively, a sample of cerumen may be removed gently from the ear using a cotton swab and smeared on to a glass slide. The sample is then mixed with liquid paraffin and enclosed by a coverslip for microscopic examination at low power magnification (X40). The examination should reveal evidence of mature/immature mites and ova (Figure 7.23).

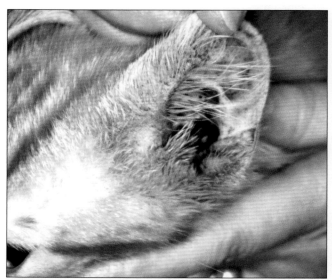

7.22 Kitten with ceruminous otitis caused by otodectic mange. Note the accumulation of dark cerumen in the vertical canal orifice.

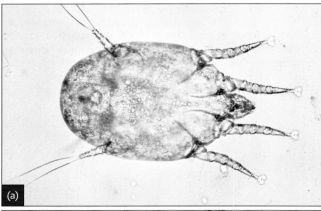

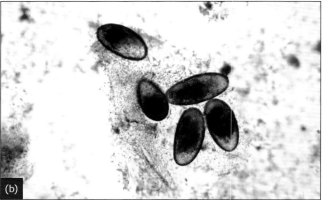

7.23 Microscopic appearance of *Otodectes cynotis*. (a) Larval mite suspended in liquid paraffin. (Original magnification X100) (b) Ova. (Original magnification X400)

Notoedric mange

Notoedres cati is a globose mite belonging to the family Sarcoptidae. It is primarily responsible for feline notoedric mange (feline 'scabies', although this term can also be applied to cats infested with *Sarcoptes scabiei* mites) but has also been isolated from foxes and rabbits and, more recently, a dog residing in Italy (Leone, 2007). Case reports are sporadic and outbreaks are reported most commonly in North America, central continental Europe and India.

Pathogenesis and clinical approach

The major differential diagnoses for notoedric mange are:

- Flea bite hypersensitivity
- Sarcoptic mange (rare in cats)
- Atopic dermatitis
- Food-responsive dermatosis
- Dermatophytosis
- Demodicosis
- Pemphigus foliaceus (rare).

The appearance and distribution of the lesions are very similar to those described for canine sarcoptic mange. Typically, papulocrustous lesions develop on the pinnae and then spread to the face and neck, with the feet and perineum being affected subsequently owing to the curled sleeping position adopted by cats. Left untreated, scale and crust develop at the affected sites and the lesions can become generalized. The associated pruritus is intense and affected areas rapidly become self-traumatized.

Diagnosis

Unlike *Sarcoptes* spp. mite infestations, *Notoedres* spp. mites are typically present in large numbers and are usually easy to find in skin scrapings suspended in liquid paraffin and examined under a microscope. It should be noted that in comparison with *Sarcoptes* spp., *Notoedres* spp. mites are smaller, have concentric striations over the body and a dorsal (rather than a terminal) anus.

Demodicosis
Canine

The majority of canine demodicosis cases are caused by the mite *Demodex canis* (Figure 7.24), which was first described in the mid-1800s (Leydig, 1859) and, in the case of the female mite, measures up to 300 μm in length. In the 1980s and 1990s, two additional species of demodectic mite were isolated from dogs: *Demodex cornei* (Scarff, 1988; Chesney, 1999), which has a short tail and overall length of up to 148 μm (Figure 7.25); and *Demodex injai* (Hillier and Desch, 1997; Desch and Hillier, 2003), which is the longest of the mites, at up to 368 μm (Figure 7.26). All three mite species inhabit the hair follicles and, occasionally, the sebaceous glands, although *Demodex cornei* is thought to occupy a more superficial position within the skin. Rarely, mites have been isolated from other sites within the body, for example, the urinary bladder, lungs, intestinal wall, lymph nodes and body fluids such as blood and urine, but this is believed to be a consequence of lymphatic drainage.

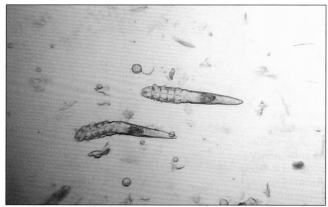

7.24 Adult *Demodex canis* mites suspended in liquid paraffin. (Original magnification X40)

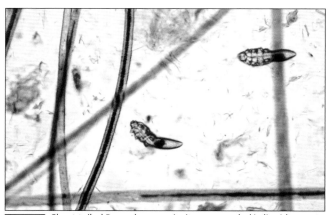

7.25 Short-tailed *Demodex cornei* mites suspended in liquid paraffin. (Original magnification X40)

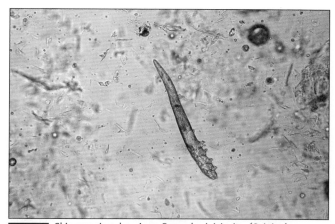

7.26 Skin scraping showing a *Demodex injai* mite. (Original magnification X100; oil immersion)

Feline

Three species of demodectid mites have also been isolated from cats: *Demodex cati* (up to 220 μm in length, similar in appearance to *D. canis*); *Demodex gatoi* (up to 115 μm) (Figure 7.27); and a third, as yet un-named species, which was originally reported in the 1980s, but which has only relatively recently been confirmed as a separate species (up to 174 μm) (Ferreira *et al.*, 2015). *D. cati* and the un-named mite reside in the hair follicles and have been reported to co-exist in the same host; *D. gatoi* is unique, in that it inhabits the superficial layers of the stratum corneum. In the UK, demodicosis would be classified as an uncommon condition in cats, compared with dogs.

Pathogenesis and clinical approach

Normal transmission of demodectid mites is believed to occur in the first few days of the nursing period. During early lactation, mites transfer from the bitch's or queen's skin to the facial and pedal skin of the puppies and kittens as they feed. The mite is host-specific and, with the exception of its spread from bitch-to-puppy, it is not generally considered to be contagious between dogs. However, *D. gatoi* infestations are considered contagious and can be intensely pruritic (Saari *et al.*, 2009); this observation, coupled with the fact that some cats are thought to carry the mite asymptomatically, suggests that some individuals may be hypersensitive to the mite (Miller *et al.*, 2013b).

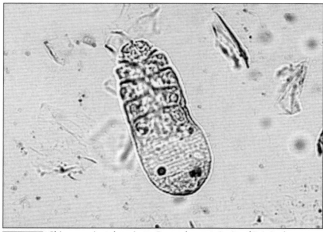

7.27 Skin scraping showing a *Demodex gatoi* mite. (Original magnification X100; oil immersion)
(Courtesy of K Tater)

In neonates, the complement of mites contracted from their mother is generally believed to be low and, in the majority of animals, mite populations remain low throughout life and clinical signs of infestation never develop. Individuals within the same litter can vary with respect to their tendency to develop signs of disease, however, and certain canine (e.g. West Highland White Terrier, various brachycephalic breeds) and feline (e.g. Siamese, Burmese and Cornish Rex) breeds are more susceptible to demodicosis than others. These observations have resulted in the hypothesis that affected individuals may have a *Demodex*-specific immune deficiency of differing severity, depending on whether they develop mild/localized disease (capable of spontaneous resolution) or chronic, generalized disease (see below).

Previous immunological studies in dogs suggested that this defect is most likely to be T-cell mediated, rather than a B-cell, innate or humoral immunity problem. More recent investigations have demonstrated that affected dogs have elevations in circulatory immunosuppressive cytokines (e.g. interleukin (IL)-10) and simultaneous reductions in pro-inflammatory cytokines (e.g. tumour necrosis factor-alpha (TNF-alpha)) compared with healthy controls, suggesting that the mites themselves can induce immunosuppression in their host, to facilitate their proliferation (Kumari *et al.*, 2017). To the author's knowledge, the immunological defects responsible for feline demodicosis are as yet unreported; however, it is interesting to note that *D. cati* infestations are commonly associated with a concurrent immunosuppressive disorder (e.g. FIV/feline leukaemia virus (FeLV) infection; diabetes mellitus; spontaneous or iatrogenic hyperglucocorticoidism, neoplasia), suggesting a relationship between the host's degree of immunocompetence and development of disease. With this in mind, detection of this mite species should alert the clinician to check the general health status of the patient.

Infestation with demodectic mites typically results in one of two major forms of disease: 'localized' or 'generalized'. Most cases of localized demodicosis occur in young animals, with a typical age of onset of 3–8 months in dogs. Mite overgrowth and the resultant follicular inflammation initially result in patchy hypotrichosis and alopecia, particularly of the face, forelimbs and feet (Figure 7.28).

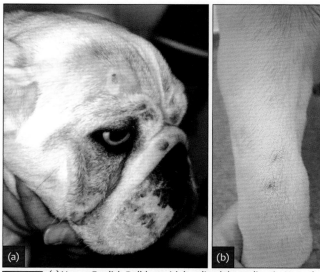

7.28 (a) Young English Bulldog with localized demodicosis. Note the alopecic, erythematous patches over the face. (b) The right forelimb of the same dog showing patches of hypotrichosis caused by demodicosis.

In cats, localized demodicosis is relatively rare and can also present as a ceruminous otitis externa (Figure 7.29). Pruritus is variable, but is generally absent to mild (with the exception of *D. gatoi* infestations in cats, which may be presented for generalized over-grooming or modest to severe self-trauma). The underlying skin may be erythematous ('red mange') and mildly scaly, and comedones may be observed. Truly localized demodicosis at a young age of onset will typically resolve spontaneously without treatment; however, it is recommended that these dogs are monitored for further generalization of the disease.

Generalized demodicosis also occurs in young animals but can develop at any age. As described above, certain breeds are predisposed, but any breed of dog or cat with a concurrent illness, or patients receiving immunomodulatory therapy (e.g. for allergic skin disease) or chemotherapy, could potentially develop demodicosis as a secondary phenomenon. Correction of the underlying disease or cessation of therapy may result in spontaneous resolution of the demodicosis.

Clinically, in generalized cases, the skin lesions are more widespread, severe and chronic and the alopecic patches described above can, with time, become mildly to moderately hyperpigmented, (with the exception of the feet, which in dogs may develop intense hyperpigmentation) (Figure 7.30). Some dogs with generalized demodicosis have pedal involvement, whereas in others the paws are affected, or may remain affected when other cutaneous lesions resolve. 'Pododemodicosis' can be very painful and affected dogs frequently lick at their feet and may exhibit a shifting lameness; the latter sign may help to distinguish between this disease and pododermatitis caused by a hypersensitivity disorder. It is worth noting that infestation with *Demodex injai* may result in a different clinical picture; affected dogs do not lose as much hair and the major clinical sign may be an often intense pruritus of the face or dorsum. The dorsal distribution may be accompanied by seborrhoea oleosa, particularly in terrier breeds, such as Border and Fox Terriers.

In canine patients, secondary pyoderma, which may be superficial and/or deep, is a common complication, particularly of generalized cases of demodicosis, hence epidermal collarettes, pustules and furunculotic lesions may be observed. In time, the disease can progress to affect large areas of the skin and the patient may become depressed and pyrexic, and may have regional lymphadenomegaly.

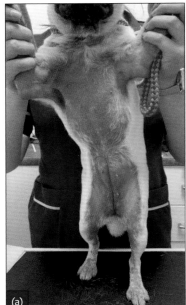

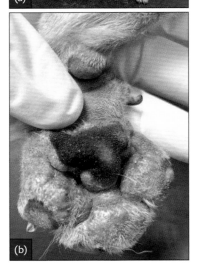

7.30 Generalized demodectic mange in a 7-month-old Pug. (a) Note the erythema, hyperpigmentation and alopecia over the ventrum and diffuse hypotrichosis of the distal hind limbs and feet. (b) Ventral aspect of the left forefoot of the same dog. Note that the digital and interdigital skin is swollen, erythematous and alopecic. Dogs with pododemodicosis are often lame (to distinguish them from dogs with pododermatitis caused by allergic skin disease, for example, which infrequently causes lameness).

Before the advent of modern, effective acaricides, some cases of generalized demodicosis were considered severe enough to warrant euthanasia.

Diagnosis

Skin scrapings are a reasonably reliable diagnostic technique for harvesting *Demodex* mites and their spindle-shaped ova (Figure 7.31), and can be performed in a similar way as described above for *Sarcoptes* mites. Given the follicularly-oriented habitat of most demodectid species, it may be useful to gently squeeze the skin prior to scraping, as this may help to 'express' mites from their follicles. Alopecic and comedone-rich areas may yield the most mites, as their activity is responsible for the folliculitis, hair loss and increased sebum production that causes these lesions. In the case of *D. gatoi*, a tape strip technique may be employed. The sticky side of a 5–7 cm piece of clear acetate tape can be pressed directly on to alopecic areas and then transferred to a microscope slide for examination. Diff-Quik® staining is employed by some clinicians, as this may highlight the mites, but they are visible microscopically at X40 magnification without stains. In difficult or aggressive patients, a trichogram (i.e. hair pluck) technique can be employed:

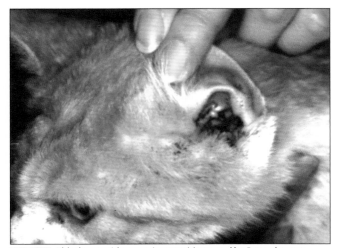

7.29 Elderly cat with ceruminous otitis caused by *Demodex* spp. mites; this cat had concurrent lymphoma and *D. cati* infestation, which, in the cat, is often associated with systemic disease.

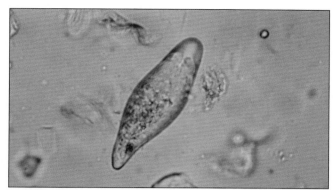

7.31 Microscopic appearance of a *Demodex canis* ovum; note its spindle-shaped form, which distinguishes it from many of the ovoid forms of other ectoparasite eggs. (Original magnification X400)

1. Grasp a few hairs with a small pair of forceps and epilate rapidly.
2. Suspend the hairs in a small amount of liquid paraffin on a microscope slide.
3. Cover with a coverslip.
4. Examine microscopically at X40 magnification.

This method is particularly useful for obtaining samples from dogs with painful pododemodicosis, as they often resent the restraint needed to take skin scrapings from these areas, and their resistance increases the risk of being cut with the scalpel blade. In some cases, sedation may be required to collect skin scrapes and trichograms. It is also possible to diagnose demodicosis histologically and, in most cases, the patient need only be sedated for the procedure, as opposed to anaesthetized. Local anaesthetic (0.5–1.0 ml aliquots) can be injected beneath the sites to be sampled and then, typically, a 6 mm biopsy punch is used to harvest plugs of skin suspected to be infested with mites. A competent pathologist should easily be able to spot mites within the hair follicles, sebaceous glands, or in surface keratin in the case of *D. gatoi*.

Ticks

There are approximately 800 species of tick recognized worldwide, the majority of which act as temporary ectoparasites. They are classified broadly into two categories:

- Argasid (soft) ticks
- Ixodid (hard) ticks.

Argasid ticks are generally found on wild animals, particularly birds, in warmer climates; whereas, ixodid ticks parasitize wild animals, livestock and domestic pets allowed access to the outdoors, and are endemic in the outside areas occupied by their hosts. Most tick species have a similar life cycle progressing through egg, larval, nymphal and adult stages, typically on three different hosts over a period of 1–3 years. Juvenile and adult ticks can survive for protracted periods of time in the environment whilst awaiting a host from which to suck blood, and in the winter can even hibernate (Miller *et al.*, 2013b).

Unfed ticks climb to the top of bushes in their 'quest' for a passing host, detecting them by means of the carbon dioxide they emit. They use hooks on their front legs to grab on to hair or clothing and after finding a place to settle, they use their outer mouthparts to pierce the skin, to allow penetration by the inner, barbed hypostome. A 'cement'–like substance, in addition to a mixture of anticoagulant, anti-inflammatory and anaesthetic compounds, all emanating from the salivary glands, are secreted into the attachment site via the hypostome. These help to optimize feeding by providing firm attachment, access to uncoagulated blood, manipulation of the host's immune defence mechanisms and detection avoidance by the host. Undisturbed, ticks typically feed for 3–7 days and once engorged, detach themselves to return to the environment to, in the case of larval and nymphal forms, progress to the next life cycle stage (Sonenshine and Anderson, 2014). Adults are thought to survive for 1–2 years. Typically, tick infestations peak in spring and autumn, but in years with favourable weather conditions, ticks may also be isolated from pets throughout the summer months (Bowman, 2009).

In Europe, species of the 'hard tick' genus *Ixodes* (e.g. *I. ricinus* (Figure 7.32), *I. canisuga*, *I. hexagonus*) are isolated most commonly from domestic pets, with occasional reports of *Haemophysalis punctata*, *Dermacentor reticulatus* and *Rhipicephalus sanguineus*. In a recent survey of ticks on UK dogs, the prevalence rates were:

- *I. ricinus* (sheep tick) = 89.2%
- *I. hexagonus* (hedgehog tick) = 9.8%
- *I. canisuga* (dog tick) = <1%
- *D. reticulatus* (marsh tick) = <1%
- *H. punctatea* (red sheep tick) = <1%.

However, when the ticks on 56 dogs that had travelled outside the UK within the previous 2 weeks were assessed, *I. ricinus* accounted for 67.4% (n=29), *R. sanguineus* (brown dog tick) for 30.2% (n=13) and *D. variabilis* (American dog tick) for 2.3% (n=1). The latter dog had been imported from the USA and the dogs infested by *R. sanguineus* had visited the Mediterranean, predominantly Cyprus and Spain (Abdullah *et al.*, 2016).

Whilst in the UK clinicians are familiar with the potential zoonotic risk of Lyme disease and anaplasmosis from *Ixodes* spp. ticks, increasing numbers of travelling pets, coupled with the relaxation of import requirements and quarantine regulations, mean that the threat of exotic diseases (such as babesiosis and ehrlichiosis) in UK pets and people has increased, as the organisms responsible can be transmitted by *Rhipicephalus* and *Dermacentor* ticks, and the survey demonstrates that these parasites are managing to make their way to the UK.

In the USA, *I. scapularis*, *I. pacificus*, *D. variabilis*, *D. andersoni*, *R. sanguineus* and *Amblyomma americanum* are amongst the most common species to be isolated from dogs and cats. In Australia, species belonging to the *Ixodes*, *Haemophysalis* and *Rhipicephalus* genera are found most frequently.

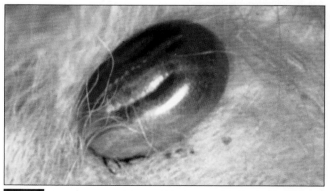

7.32 *Ixodes ricinus* tick attached to the skin of a dog.

Pathogenesis and clinical approach

Tick bites are irritating and can cause hypersensitivity reactions at the site of attachment (Figure 7.33). Inefficient attempts at their physical removal can inadvertently result in the mouthparts/head of the tick remaining embedded in the skin, leading to further irritation and potentially infection and abscess formation. Their major clinical significance, however, is the ability to transmit one of several debilitating and potentially fatal tick-borne diseases to wild and domestic animals and humans. Examples include Lyme disease (borreliosis), babesiosis, ehrlichiosis, bartonellosis, anaplasmosis and, in the USA, Rocky Mountain spotted fever (caused by *Rickettsia rickettsii*). In addition, some species of tick (e.g. *I. holocyclus* in Australia and *D. andersoni* and *D. variabilis* in North America) can cause paralysis and death of the host via the release of a neurotoxin from the tick's salivary gland during feeding.

In the UK, the most common tick-borne disease in humans and animals is Lyme disease, caused by the spirochaete *Borrelia burgdorferi* and transmitted by *Ixodes* species ticks. Clinical signs in dogs are typically acute arthritis and lameness in one or more joints, fever, lethargy and lympadenomegaly, which can wax and wane. Alarmingly, however, there have been recent reports of babesiosis (Holm *et al.*, 2006; Swainsbury *et al.*, 2016; Guthrie, 2017) and ehrlichiosis (Wilson *et al.*, 2013), with a few fatalities, in the south east of England, in dogs which had no travel history outside the UK. These diseases are usually carried by *Dermacentor* and *Rhipicephalus* tick species, respectively, which were not previously thought to be endemic in the UK.

Pockets of *D. reticulatus* infestation in outdoor spaces in Essex have been identified, with one survey revealing 14 of 17 ticks of this species were found to be positive for *Babesia canis* by PCR (Hansford *et al.*, 2016). Babesiosis is caused by the intraerythrocyte protozoa *Babesia canis* and typical signs include anorexia, haemoglobinuria, anaemia and thrombocytopenia; ehrlichiosis is caused by the rickettsia *Ehrlichia canis*, which results in lethargy, inappetence and pancytopenia. With these reports in mind, coupled with increased intercontinental pet movements and imports, it is crucial that veterinary surgeons (veterinarians) remain aware of the possibility of systemic tick-borne diseases, as these are unfortunately not as 'exotic' or rare as they once were.

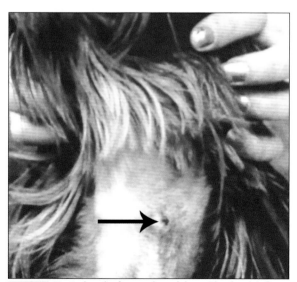

7.33 Ventral neck of a crossbreed dog with a focal, inflammatory reaction (arrowed) to a recently removed tick.

Diagnosis

Ticks are visible to the naked eye at all life cycle stages, so they can be found and identified by direct examination. Differences in the location of their anal and genial grooves and genital pores on their ventral surfaces can be used for species differentiation, in addition to the presence or absence of patterns on the dorsal scutum. Larval stages may be mistaken for lice, but microscopic examination (X40 magnification) can be used to differentiate between different ectoparasite species.

Key points

- When treating ectoparasitic infestations, it is crucial to be familiar with the life cycle of the parasite in question to ensure treatment protocols adequately cover all life cycle stages and, if appropriate, in-contact animals and the environment
- Fleas, and particularly ticks, can be reservoirs for organisms capable of causing serious animal and human diseases, and veterinary surgeons should familiarize themselves with their clinical signs
- Despite being considered part of the cutaneous flora, *Demodex* spp. mites can cause significant skin disease in some animals, and their presence may be associated with concurrent systemic disease

References and further reading

Abdullah S, Helps C, Tasker S *et al.* (2016). Ticks infesting domestic dogs in the UK; a large-scale surveillance programme. *Parasites and Vectors* **9**, 391–399

Abdullah S, Helps C, Tasker S *et al.* (2019) Pathogens in fleas collected from cats and dogs: distribution and prevalence in the UK. *Parasites & Vectors* **71**, 1–10

Arlian LG, Morgan MS, Rapp CM *et al.* (1996) The development of protective immunity in canine scabies. *Veterinary Parasitology* **62**, 133–142

Bond R, Mottram RL, Beugnet F *et al.* (2005) Survey of flea infestation in dogs and cats in the United Kingdom during 2005. *Veterinary Record* **160**, 503–506

Bornstein S and Zakrisson G (1993) Humoral antibody response to experimental *Sarcoptes scabiei* var. *vulpes* infection in the dog. *Veterinary Dermatology* **4**, 107–110

Bourdeau P, Degorce-Rubiales F, Breton C *et al.* (2000) Newly recognised manifestation of trombiculosis with epithelial encystment in 12 dogs. *Veterinary Dermatology* **11**, 26

Bowman D (2009) Arthropods. In: *Georgis' Parasitology for Veterinarians, 9th edn.*, pp. 5–83. Saunders Elsevier, St Louis

Chesney CJ (1999) Short form of *Demodex* species mite in the dog: occurrence and measurements. *Journal of Small Animal Practice* **40**, 58–61

Curtis CF (2001) Evaluation of a commercially available enzyme-linked immunosorbent assay for the diagnosis of canine sarcoptic mange. *Veterinary Record* **148**, 238–239

Curtis CF, Bond R, Blunden AS *et al.* (1995) Canine eosinophilic folliculitis and furunculosis in three cases. *Journal of Small Animal Practice* **36**, 119–123

Curtis CF, Bourdeau PJ, Barr PA *et al.* (2019) Use of the novel ectoparasiticide fluralaner in the treatment of feline sarcoptic mange. *Veterinary Record Case Reports* **7**, e000772. doi: 10.1136 /vetreccr-2018-000772

Desch CE and Hillier A (2003) *Demodex injai*: a new species of hair follicle mite (Acari: Demodecidae) from the domestic dog (Canidae). *Journal of Medical Entemology* **40**, 146–149

Ferreira D, Sastre N, Ravera I *et al.* (2015) Identification of a third feline *Demodex* species through partial sequencing of the 16S rDNA and frequency of *Demodex* species in 74 cats using a PCF assay. *Veterinary Dermatology* **26**, 239–245

Franc M, Bouhsira E and Beugnet F (2013) Direct transmission of the cat flea (*Ctenocephalides felis*) between cats exhibiting social behaviour. *Parasite* **20**, 49

Guthrie A (2017) Babesiosis confirmed in non-travelling dog by Herts vet. https://www.vetsurgeon.org/news/b/veterinary-news/archive/2017/10/09/babesiosis-confirmed-in-non-travelling-dog-by-herts-vet.aspx. Accessed 10 Nov 2017.

Hansford KM, Medlock JM, Swainsbury C *et al.* (2016) *Babesia canis* infection in questing ticks in Essex. *Veterinary Record* **178**, 323

Herwick RP (1978) Lesions caused by canine ear mites. *Archives of Dermatology* **114**, 130

Heyne H, Ueckermann EA and Coetzee L (2001) First report of a parasitic mite, *Leptotrombidium subquadratum* (Acari: Trombiculidae: Trombiculinae), from dogs and children in the Bloemfontein area, South Africa. *Journal of the South African Veterinary Association* **72**, 105–106

Hillier A and Desch CE (1997) A new species of *Demodex* mite in the dog. Case report. *Proceedings of the Annual Member Meeting of the American Academy of Veterinary Dermatology and the American College of Veterinary Dermatology* **13**, 118

Hinkle NC, Koehler PC and Patterson RS (1998) Host grooming efficiency for regulation of cat flea (Siphonaptera: Pulicidae) populations. *Journal of Medical Entomology* **35**, 266–269

Holm LP, Kerr MG, Trees AJ et al. (2006) Fatal babesiosis in an untraveled British dog. *Veterinary Record* **159**, 179–180

Hudson BW and Prince FM (1958) A method for large-scale rearing of the cat flea, *Ctenocephalides felis felis* (Bouché). *Bull World Health Organisation* **19**, 1126–1129

Kumari P, Nigam R, Singh A et al. (2017) *Demodex canis* regulates cholinergic system mediated immunosuppressive pathways in canine demodicosis. *Parasitology* **144**, 1412–1416

Kunkle G, Jones L and Petty P (2000) Immediate intradermal flea antigen reactivity in clinically normal adult dogs from South Florida, USA. *Veterinary Dermatology* **11**, 9–12

Larkin AD and Gaillard GE (1981) Mites in cats' ears, a source of cross antigenicity with house dust mites: preliminary report. *Annals of Allergy* **46**, 301–303

Leone F (2007) Canine notoedric mange: a case report. *Veterinary Dermatology* **18**, 127–129

Leydig F (1859) Haarsackmilbe des Hundes (*Demodex canis*) *Archiv für Naturgeschichte* **25**, 345

Lopez RA (1993) Of mites and man (letter to editor). *Journal of the American Veterinary Medical Association* **203**, 606–607

Lowenstine LJ, Carpenter JL and O'Connor BM (1979) Trombiculosis in a cat. *Journal of the American Medical Association* **175**, 289–292

McCall CA, Stedman K, Bevier DE et al. (1997b) Correlation of feline IgE, determined by Fcε RIα-based ELISA technology, and IDST to Ctenocephalides felis salivary antigens in a feline model of flea bite allergic dermatitis. *Compendium for the Continuing Education of the Practicing Veterinarian* **19**, 29–32

McCall CA, Stedman K, Penne SJ et al. (1997a) Fcε RIα-based measurement of anti-flea saliva IgE in dogs. *Compendium for the Continuing Education of the Practicing Veterinarian* **19**, 24–28

McCall CA (1997b) *Compendium for the Continuing Education of the Practicing Veterinarian* **19** (Suppl.), 29–32

McDermott MJ, Weber E, Hunter S et al. (2000) Identification, cloning, and characterization of a major cat flea salivary allergen (Cte f 1). *Molecular Immunology* **37**, 361–375

McKenna M, Attipa C, Tasker S and Augusto M (2019) Leishmaniosis in a dog with no travel history outside the UK. *Veterinary Record* **184**, 441

Miller WH, Griffin CE and Campbell KL (2013a) Hypersensitivity disorders. In: *Muller and Kirk's Small Animal Dermatology, 7th edn.*, pp. 363–431. Saunders Elsevier, Missouri

Miller WH, Griffin CE and Campbell KL (2013b) Parasitic skin disease. In: *Muller and Kirk's Small Animal Dermatology, 7th edn.*, pp. 284–342. Saunders Elsevier, Missouri

Moriello KA and McMurdy MA (1989) The prevalence of positive intradermal skin test reactions to flea extract in clinically normal cats. *Companion Animal Practice* **19**, 28–30

Nagata M and Ishida T (1997) Mosquito bite reactions in cats. *Veterinary Dermatology* **8**, 19–26

Paradis M, Scott DW and Villeneuve A (1990) Efficacy of ivermectin against *Cheyletiella blakei* infestation in cats. *Journal of the American Animal Hospital Association* **26**, 125–128

Paradis M and Villeneuve A (1988) Efficacy of ivermectin against *Cheyletiella yasguri* infestation in dogs. *Canadian Veterinary Journal* **29**, 633–635

Powell MB, Weisbroth SH, Roth L et al. (1980) Reaginic hypersensitivity in *Otodectes cynotis* infestation of cats and mode of mite feeding. *American Journal of Veterinary Research* **41**, 877–882

Ramirez GA, Altimira J, Garcia B et al. (2009) Clinical, histopathological and epidemiological study of canine straelensiosis in the Iberian Peninsula (2003–2007). *Veterinary Dermatology* **20**, 35–41

Saari SA, Juuti, KH, Joanna H et al. (2009) *Demodex gatoi*-associated contagious pruritic dermatosis in cats – a report from six households in Finland. *Acta Veterinaria Scandinavica* **51**, 40

Saridomichelakis MN, Koutinas AF, Gioulekas D et al., (1999) Sensitization to dust mites in cats with *Otodectes cynotis* infestation. *Veterinary Dermatology* **10**, 89–94

Scarff D (1988) Morphological differences in *Demodex* spp. *Proceedings of the Fifth Annual Congress of the European Society of Veterinary Dermatology*, p. 23

Scott DW and Horn RT (1997) Zoonotic dermatoses of dogs and cats. *Veterinary Clinics of North America* **17**, 117–144

Shaw SE, Kenny MJ, Tasker S et al. (2004) Pathogen carriage by the cat flea *Ctenocephalides felis* (Bouché) in the United Kingdom. *Veterinary Microbiology* **102**, 183–188

Shryock JA and Houseman RM (2006) Time spent by *Ctenocephalides felis* (Siphonatera: Pulicidae) larvae in food patches of varying quality. *Environmental Entomology* **35**, 401–404

Sonenshine DE and Anderson JM (2014) Mouthparts and digestive system: Anatomy and molecular biology of feeding and digestion. In: *Biology of ticks. Volume 1, 2nd edn*, eds DE Sonenshineand RM Roe. Oxford University Press, New York, pp. 122–162

Stedman K, Lee K, Hunter S et al. (2001) Measurement of canine IgE using the alpha chain of the human high affinity IgE receptor. *Veterinary Immunology and Immunopathology* **78**, 349–355

Suetake M, Yuasa R and Saijo S (1991) Canine ear mites *Otodectes cynotis* found on both tympanic membranes of an adult woman causing tinnitus. *Tohoku Rosat Hospital; Practicing Otology of Kyoto* **84**, 38–42

Swainsbury C, Bengston G and Hill P (2016) Babesiosis in dogs. *Veterinary Record* **178**, 172

Takahashi M, Misumi H, Urakami H et al. (2004) Trombuculidiosis in the cats caused by the bite of the larval trombiculid mite *Helenicula miyagawai* (Acari: Trombiculidae). *Veterinary Record* **154**, 471–472

Thiemann T, Fielden LJ and Kelrick MI (2003) Water uptake in the cat flea *Ctenocephalides felis* (Pulicidae: Siphonaptera). *Journal of Insect Physiology* **49**, 1085–1092

Virchow F and Bigler B (2004) Cross-reactivity between house dust, sarcoptic and storage mites in dogs with atopic dermatitis. *Veterinary Dermatology* **15**, 37

Walker C (2019) Letter to the Editor. *Journal of Small Animal Practice*; ID JSAP-2019–0402

White S, Rosychuck R and Fieseler K (2001) Clinicopathological findings, sensitivity to house dust mites and efficacy of milbemycin oxime treatment of dogs with *Cheyletiella* sp. infestation. *Veterinary Dermatology* **12**, 13–18

Wilson HE, Mugford AR, Humm KR et al. (2013) *Ehrlichia canis* infection in a dog with no history of travel outside the United Kingdom. *Journal of Small Animal Practice* **54**, 425–427

Wright I and Baker S (2019) Leishmaniosis in a dog with no history of travel outside the UK. *Veterinary Record* **184**, 387–388

Chapter 8

Ectoparasite infestation – treatment and prophylaxis

Lluís Ferrer

Ectoparasiticidal drugs

There are many drugs available for the treatment and prevention of ectoparasite infestations in dogs and cats. These are chemical compounds with different mechanisms of action and spectrum of efficacy and are administered either topically or systemically. Figure 8.1 shows the characteristics of the main ectoparasiticidal drugs.

Each pharmacological group and drug has a different activity profile. The action spectrum of the different products could be represented on an axis: at one end of the axis there are drugs with pure acaricidal activity (e.g. amitraz) and at the other end there are drugs with exclusively insecticidal activity (e.g. imidacloprid). Between these two extremes are the remaining ectoparasiticidal drugs, which combine acaricidal and insecticidal properties. Licensed and commercially available products often

contain a combination of two or more drugs with a complementary action spectrum, (for further information on individual drugs, the reader is referred to the *BSAVA Small Animal Formulary*).

The newest group of ectoparasiticide drugs added to the vademecum is the isoxazolines (fluralaner, afoxolaner, sarolaner, lotilaner). Isoxazolines have a broad insecticidal and acaricidal spectrum. They are non-competitive antagonists of gamma-aminobutyric acid (GABA) and L-glutamate receptors of the chloride channels of neurons and muscle cells. The binding of isoxazolines to the receptors blocks the transfer of chloride ions across the cell membrane, inhibiting the transmission of neuronal signals. Affected parasites are paralysed and die. Following oral administration, isoxazolines are rapidly absorbed into the blood and distributed throughout the whole body of the host, including the skin. Blood-sucking parasites (fleas and ticks) are

Pharmacological group	Drugs	Mechanism of action	Activity	Administration
Pyrethroids	Permethrin, deltamethrin, flumethrin	Opening of Na⁺ channels, inducing nerve cell membrane depolarization	Insecticide and acaricide	Topical: collar, spot-on solutions, aerosol sprays Environmental treatments
Phenylpyrazoles	Fipronil, pyriprole	Bind to GABA receptors leading to neuronal hyperactivity	Insecticide and acaricide	Topical: collar, spot-on solutions, aerosol sprays
Neonicotinoids	Imidacloprid, dinotefuran, nytenpyram	Agonists of nicotinic receptors of insects causing rapid spastic paralysis	Insecticide	Topical (imidacloprid, dinotefuran) Systemic (oral): nytenpyram
Macrocyclic lactones – avermectins	Moxidectin, selamectin eprinomectin	GABA-mimetic effect, binding to glutamate-gated chloride channels	Moxidectin is mostly acaricidal. Selamectin is insecticidal but also has acaricidal activity	Topical: (spot-on), but they are absorbed and act systemically
Macrocyclic lactones – milbemycins	Milbemycin	GABA-mimetic effect, binding to glutamate-gated chloride channels	Acaricide	Systemic (oral)
Macrocyclic lactones – spinosyns	Spinosad, spinetoram	Stimulation of nicotinic Ach receptors	Insecticide	Systemic (oral)
Isoxazolines	Afoxolaner, fluralaner, sarolaner, lotilaner	Selective inhibition of GABA and glutamate-gated chloride channels, leading to hyper-excitation and death	Insecticide and acaricide	Systemic (oral) Spot-on solutions (for cats and dogs)
Benzoylureas	Lufenuron	Inhibition of egg hatching and larval moulting	Insecticide (fleas)	Systemic (oral, injection)
Juvenile hormone analogues	S-methoprene, pyriproxyfen	Decrease prolificacy, egg hatching and last moult from larvae to pupae stage	Insecticide	Topical Environmental treatments (foggers, sprays)

8.1 Main ectoparasiticidal drugs. Ach = acetylcholine; GABA = gamma-aminobutyric acid.

killed during their blood meal. It is suggested that parasites living in the skin (*Cheyletiella*, *Sarcoptes*, *Demodex*) are also exposed to the drug and killed. Isoxazolines are selective for arthropod receptors (and not for the receptors of mammals) and therefore are very safe. In clinical trials, only mild and transient diarrhoea, vomiting, lack of appetite and drooling were recorded in <2% of dogs in the first days after treatment (Datz, 2018). However, adverse drug reactions involving neurological signs (tremor, ataxia, convulsions) have been reported sporadically in dogs treated with isoxazolines (Gaens *et al.*, 2019). The dog owner should be informed about possible adverse drug reactions after treatment with isoxazolines and an individual benefit-risk assessment must be performed. Particularly, isoxazolines should be used with caution in dogs with pre-existing epilepsy.

Ectoparasites affecting companion animals can be divided into two groups: ones that represent a continuous nuisance and a threat as vectors of pathogens; and ones that induce a disease and should be treated. Fleas, sandflies, mosquitoes and ticks belong to the first group. They may induce clinical signs, such as pruritus, hair loss or flea allergy dermatitis, but they represent a major threat as vectors of infectious agents (Figure 8.2). The control measures are based on both a curative effect (killing existing infestations) and a preventive effect (reducing risk of new infestations). For that purpose, long-acting formulations and continuous treatment are needed. In addition to the external antiparasitic action, it is important to note that regular protection will also indirectly reduce the risk of arthropod-borne diseases.

Mites such as *Sarcoptes*, *Notoedres*, *Cheyletiella*, *Otodectes* and *Demodex* are found in the second group. There are no prevention measures against these mites. Affected dogs and cats are treated following a veterinary diagnosis using formulations with an appropriate spectrum of activity. The current recommendations for the treatment and prevention of the main ectoparasites of the dog and cat follow in the sections below. It should be noted that licensing of these compounds for the treatment or prevention of ectoparasites on small animals will vary geographically and clinicians are urged to check the datasheets and use a locally licensed product where feasible.

Insecta

Fleas

Fleas are obligate ectoparasites that live and reproduce on the surface of the skin. Most eggs fall from the host's coat into the environment within 8 hours of being laid, where the immature larval and pupal forms develop. Most dogs and cats become infested by direct contact with another infested animal or when visiting an area with a high load of immature forms. Not all animals tolerate the presence of fleas in the same way: some may have only small lesions (papules or crusted papules) and minimal pruritus, whereas other animals develop an allergic reaction with intense pruritus and severe lesions, many of which are self-inflicted (see Chapter 7).

Ectoparasite	Pathogen	Disease	Vector	Prevention
Ticks	*Ehrlichia canis*	Canine monocytotropic ehrlichiosis	*Rhipicephalus sanguineus, Dermacentor variabilis*	Topical acaricides
	Anaplasma platys	Canine thrombocytotrophic ehrlichiosis	*R. sanguineus*(?)	Topical acaricides
	Anaplasma phagocytophilum[a]	Human and canine granulocytotropic ehrlichiosis	*Ixodes* spp.	Topical acaricides; systemic isoxazolines
	Borrelia burgdorferi[a]	Borreliosis (Lyme disease)	*Ixodes* spp.	Topical acaricides; systemic isoxazolines
	Babesia canis	Canine babesiosis	*Dermacentor reticulatus*	Topical acaricides; systemic isoxazolines
	Babesia vogeli	Canine babesiosis	*R. sanguineus*	Topical acaricides; systemic isoxazolines
	Babesia microti[a]	Human and canine babesiosis	*Ixodes* spp.	Topical acaricides; systemic isoxazolines
	Cytauxzoon felis	Feline cytauxzoonosis	*Amblyomma americanum*	Topical acaricides; systemic isoxazolines
	Hepatozoon canis	Hepatozoonosis	*R. sanguineus*	Topical acaricides
Sandflies	*Leishmania infantum*[a]	Canine and feline leishmaniosis	*Phlebotomus perniciosus* and other *Phlebotomus* spp.	Topical insecticides with repellent activity (deltamethrin, permethrin, flumethrin) in spot-on preparations or collars
Mosquitoes	*Dirofilaria immitis*	Heartworm disease	*Culex* spp., *Aedes* spp. (many species proven to be significant vectors)	Macrocyclic lactones (microfilaricides) to prevent disease. Topical insecticides with repellent activity to reduce mosquito bites
Fleas	*Bartonella henselae*[a] *Dipylidium caninum* *Rickettsia felis*[a] *Haemoplasma* spp.	Feline and canine bartonellosis Tapeworm infestation Flea-borne spotted fever Anaemia	*Ctenocephalides felis*	Topical insecticides Endoparasiticides

8.2 Main arthropod-transmitted pathogens to dogs and cats. [a] = Zoonotic disease.

A successful plan for the treatment of a flea infestation should include:

- Treatment of all affected and in-contact animals
- Prolonged treatment (i.e. a minimum of 6 months) to avoid re-infestation. Ideally, treatment should be maintained continuously
- Treatment of the environment in order to eliminate as many immature forms as possible.

Common dog and cat fleas are sensitive to most insecticides. Although resistance to some products has been demonstrated, most treatment failures are the result of non-compliance, short-term treatment or failure to treat all in-contact animals.

Treatment of the animal

Dogs and cats with evidence of flea parasitism should be treated immediately and continuously with an effective insecticide (adulticide).

There are numerous options with proven efficacy available commercially. Initially, the administration of a systemic insecticide with a rapid onset of action is advised.

- In the dog, nitenpyram, spinosad and the isoxazolines are excellent options. Nitenpyram has a very short duration of action and treatment should be either continued daily with this drug or a longer acting preparation administered. Spinosad and the isoxazolines should be administered every 4 weeks (with the exception of fluralaner, which should be administered every 12 weeks).
- In the cat, selamectin (either alone or in combination with sarolaner), fipronil combined with eprinomectin and fluralaner administered as a spot-on treatment are effective options.

There has been much discussion about whether systemic insecticides are appropriate for dogs and cats with flea bite hypersensitivity, as the effect of the drugs occurs after the animal has been bitten, potentially allowing an allergic reaction to flea saliva to occur. Whilst this is true, it is also the case that the severity of the disease depends on the patient's flea load and the number of bites. Furthermore, these highly effective insecticides reduce the number of fleas very quickly and clinical improvement is rapid.

An alternative to systemic insecticides are topical insecticides, such as spot-on preparations, sprays and slow-release collars:

- Pyrethroids (permethrin, deltamethrin, flumethrin), fipronil and imidacloprid are the most widely used and effective. However, it is important to note that most pyrethroids are toxic to cats and should never be used in this species
- Spot-on products usually last 4 weeks and it is very important not to reduce the frequency of application because the effectiveness and protection against infestation drop considerably. However, if the animal is being bathed regularly, then the frequency of application of spot-on products should be increased accordingly
- Spray and aerosol products have a shorter duration of action and are often used as a 'shock' treatment to eliminate fleas quickly after exposure; they should be combined with long-term treatment options to prevent new infestations.

Environmental treatment

In all cases, it is necessary to apply measures to reduce, or ideally eliminate, the immature forms (eggs, larvae, pupae) from the environment, as these stages comprise the bulk of the flea population. Routine cleaning can be very effective and it is recommended that vacuum cleaning of areas frequented by animals (especially armchairs, sofas, carpets and rugs), as well as washing or changing the animal's bedding, is carried out daily. However, in many cases, it is necessary to use an environmental insecticide (e.g. an aerosol spray containing an insect-growth regulator, such as S-methoprene or pyriproxygen, in combination with an adulticide, such as pyrethroid) to help eliminate the immature flea forms. The adulticide has a rapid onset of action against the larvae and adult fleas and can be effective for ≥2 months. Insect-growth regulators prevent normal development of the eggs, larvae and pupae and have residual activity for up to 12 months. Some spot-on products and collars contain insect-growth regulators; however, it should be noted that this is insufficient to treat a household infestation and environmental treatment is still required.

Sodium polyborate can be used to kill fleas by desiccation. The powder should be applied in the deepest part of the carpet in order to have a long-lasting effect despite vacuuming. This can be undertaken by professional pest control companies.

For outdoor environments, where the use of chemicals may not be ideal, it is possible to use biological treatments such as the application of 'beneficial nematodes' (Steinernema carpocapsae). These are non-pathogenic nematodes that feed off fleas and pose no harm to humans or pets. They are available commercially in the form of granules that can be sprayed around the outdoor area. These nematodes require moisture and protection from direct ultraviolet (UV) light.

An alternative approach is the use of diatomaceous earth, which physically disrupts the exoskeleton of fleas. Some environmental treatments can be toxic to domestic animals (e.g. small rodents, birds and fish), thus it is very important to strictly follow the instructions for use. In complicated cases (e.g. due to the size or characteristics of the house, or the severity of the flea infestation), employing a pest control company to design and implement an environmental treatment plan should be considered.

Lice

In most cases of pediculosis, treatment involves bathing the animal, thorough grooming (including removal of all thick hair mats and tags) and the application of an insecticide.

Both dog lice (Linognathus setosus, Trichodectes canis) and the common cat louse (Felicola subrostratus) are sensitive to most insecticides.

The best options for treatment are:

- Fipronil
- Imidacloprid
- Selamectin
- Isoxazolines (oral or topical application for dogs; topical application for cats).

All affected and in-contact animals should be treated. In addition, although lice do not survive for long in the environment, it is recommended that the home, bedding and grooming equipment are thoroughly cleaned.

Acari

Sarcoptic mange

Several ectoparasiticides are effective for the treatment of sarcoptic mange (sarcoptic acariasis, scabies) caused by *Sarcoptes scabiei* in the dog. These include pyrethroids, macrocyclic lactones (ivermectin, moxidectin, milbemycin, selamectin) and isoxazolines; amitraz has been used in the past, but is no longer available. Many dermatologists prescribe an oral isoxazoline together with selamectin or moxidectin as a spot-on application to achieve quick and effective results in the control of clinical signs. If the pruritus is very intense, an oral antipruritic therapy can be administered at an antipruritic dose (e.g. prednisolone at 1.0 mg/kg orally q24h or oclacitinib at 0.4–0.6 mg/kg orally q12h) for 7–10 days. Sarcoptic mange carries a good prognosis for a complete cure with effective treatment.

All in-contact animals should be treated, even if they do not present with clinical signs and the results of skin scrapings are negative, because some dogs have minimal clinical signs and a very low parasitic load. Although infestation occurs mainly by direct contact (from infested dogs or foxes), indirect transfer has also been reported. Mites have been shown to be capable of surviving away from the host for short periods of time (up to 3 weeks depending on environmental conditions). Consequently, the environment, including the animal's bedding and grooming equipment, should be thoroughly cleaned. Animals with sarcoptic mange should be prevented from coming into contact with other animals during the first two weeks of treatment, as the risk of contagion is high.

There is no preventive treatment for sarcoptic mange. Standard treatments for the prevention of flea and tick infestations do not prevent infestation with *Sarcoptes scabiei* and it is not uncommon to diagnose the disease in a dog that has been regularly treated with a spot-on ectoparasiticide or a pyrethroid impregnated collar.

Cheyletiellosis

Cheyletiella yasguri and *Cheyletiella blakei* can be treated with the same products reported effective against canine scabies (see above) and feline notoedric mange (see below), respectively. In the case of the dog, monthly application of a selamectin or moxidectin spot-on treatment or an oral isoxazoline are curative. In the case of feline cheyletiellosis, topical selamectin, a combination of selamectin with sarolaner or fluralaner are excellent options. All affected and in-contact animals, as well as the environment, should be treated.

Trombiculidiosis

Several spot-on ectoparasiticides (e.g. fipronil, milbemycin, moxidectin, eprinomectin, selamectin) are effective for the treatment of trombiculidiosis. If mites are found on an animal, they may also be removed with a topical ectoparasitic wash or dip. Following treatment, pruritus is usually controlled quickly, but in some cases a short course of prednisolone (1.0 mg/kg orally q24h) may be necessary. The parasitic larvae are a seasonal threat and are associated with rough vegetation, thus a logical approach would be to restrict access to the environment during periods of risk. Nevertheless, the application of an ectoparasiticide treatment every 14 days is usually effective in preventing new infestations.

Otoacariasis

Otodectes cynotis infestation is common in dogs and cats. The affected ears should be properly cleaned and treatment initiated for possible secondary infections (e.g. bacterial, *Malassezia*) that have been detected by cytology. There are various options available for the treatment of ear mites, including selamectin (alone or in combination with sarolaner for cats), moxidectin spot-on and any of the isoxazolines, which can be administered orally or topically for dogs or as a spot-on treatment for cats. All in-contact animals should be treated as asymptomatic carriers as they may be a source of re-infection.

Notoedric mange

The sensitivity of *Notoedres cati* is similar to that of *Sarcoptes scabiei* (see above) and thus similar drugs are effective for the treatment of feline notoedric mange and the rare cases of cats infested with *Sarcoptes scabiei*. In the past, topical products such as lime sulphur were used to treat notoedric mange; however, safer and more effective treatments such as macrocyclic lactones and isoxazolines are now available. Treatments with proven efficacy include selamectin (alone or in combination with sarolaner), the combination of eprinomectin with fipronil, the combination of moxidectin with imidacloprid and the isoxazolines (e.g. fluralaner, afoxolaner, lotilaner). These are all spot-on treatments that should be applied every 4 weeks (a minimum of three applications is recommended), with the exception of fluralaner, which should be administered every 12 weeks. In addition, it is important to note that most pyrethroids are toxic to cats and should never be used in this species. All in-contact animals should be treated and the environment, including bedding and grooming equipment, should be thoroughly cleaned. If treated properly, notoedric mange is a curable disease with a good prognosis.

Demodicosis

Dogs

The majority of cases of canine demodicosis are caused by *Demodex* canis, although infestations with *D. injai* and *D. cornei* may also be seen. The treatment is similar in all cases. Infestation with demodectic mites typically results in one of two major forms of disease: 'localized' or 'generalized'. There is consensus that no treatment is required for localized demodicosis, unless the lesions begin to progress towards generalized demodicosis.

Generalized demodicosis was considered an untreatable disease until the mid-1980s. However, since then several treatments have been shown to be effective, including oral ivermectin, subcutaneous doramectin, oral milbemycin, topical moxidectin and topical amitraz (no longer available). In recent years, isoxazolines have been demonstrated to be the best treatment option for canine demodicosis. Although large controlled randomized trials are lacking, several studies have demonstrated that fluralaner, sarolaner, afoxolaner and lotilaner, at doses recommended for the prevention of flea and tick infestations, are effective for the treatment of canine demodicosis (Mueller *et al.*, 2020). At the time of writing, there is no evidence indicating that any one of the four currently available isoxazolines has greater efficacy for the treatment of canine demodicosis.

Isoxazolines very rapidly control the mite overpopulation: after 1 month of treatment, there is a >95% reduction in mite population; and after 2 months of treatment, skin scrapings are usually negative. The lesions improve more slowly and a full clinical cure can take ≥3 months, especially in the case of adult-onset generalized demodicosis. Treatment should be maintained for at least 1 month following the resolution of lesions and until skin scraping samples are negative for *Demodex* (even mite fragments) 1 month apart. This is necessary because skin scrapings are sometimes not able to detect a low level of mites and the animal can look clinically normally before they have a negative sample. However, in the case of *D. injai* infestation, where mites are infrequently found, the use of skin scrapings to monitor the response to treatment may not be possible and the clinician should rely on the improvement of clinical signs.

It has been hypothesized that the rapid acaricide effect of isoxazolines allows the immune system of the dog to regain control of the *Demodex* population, reversing T-cell exhaustion. After treatment with isoxazolines, relapse is uncommon (probably <10%). However, to avoid any disease recurrence, it is advisable to maintain the treatment for at least a few months following parasitological and clinical cure.

In the case of adult-onset generalized demodicosis, the potential existence of an underlying systemic disease should be investigated and any treatment that may have predisposed the dog to demodicosis should be withdrawn. Other comorbidities, such as atopic dermatitis, may be present. A minimum database of a complete blood count, serum biochemistry (including hormone panels), urinalysis and thoracic and abdominal imaging should be performed. In some geographical areas it is also highly advisable to test for the presence of vector-borne diseases (e.g. leishmaniosis, ehrlichiosis).

Cats

Feline demodicosis can be caused by *D. cati*, *D. gatoi* or other *Demodex* species. The traditional treatment for feline demodicosis was the topical application of an acaricidal dip (e.g. 2% lime sulphur for weekly whole body dips for 6–8 weeks). More recently, macrocyclic lactones, especially ivermectin at a dose of 0.25 mg/kg orally q24–48h, have been shown to be effective for the treatment of feline demodicosis. Although these treatments are effective in the majority of cases, it should be remembered that they are unauthorized for this use and are therefore prescribed under the Cascade. Topical (spot-on) moxidectin/imidacloprid has anecdotally been reported to be effective in some cases of feline demodicosis, although treatment failures have also been noted.

Isoxazolines can also be used for the treatment of feline demodicosis. A few case reports have shown that fluralaner at the dose used to prevent fleas and ticks in dogs (25–35 mg/kg orally q90d) is effective in treating demodicosis caused by *D. cati* and *D. gatoi*. Considering the proven efficacy of the other isoxazolines (afoxolaner, sarolaner, lotilaner) against canine *Demodex* mites, it is very likely that they will also be effective in treating feline demodicosis. Some of the recent spot-on formulations developed for cats that contain fluralaner or sarolaner as active ingredients are probably the best options for the treatment of feline demodicosis. Nevertheless, it is important to note that these drugs are prescribed under the Cascade and that controlled studies are needed to demonstrate their efficacy.

In all cases of feline demodicosis, it is necessary to investigate the potential existence of an underlying disease that may explain the *Demodex* overgrowth and, where possible, treat it. In cases of demodicosis caused by *D. gatoi*, all in-contact animals should be treated due to the transmissible nature of the mite. Environmental treatment is not necessary.

Ticks

Ticks can be removed manually from dogs and cats by grasping them with tick removal devices, forceps or gloved fingers and applying slow traction until they are pulled free. Permethrin, deltamethrin and fipronil dips, sprays or concentrated drops may be applied to dogs if there is a heavy infestation and will provide short-term protection against re-infestation. However, it should be noted that most pyrethroids are toxic to cats and should never be used in this species.

There are also numerous products available to prevent tick infestation and, given their importance as vectors of infectious diseases, it is important that dogs and cats are protected throughout the year.

- Topical spot-on acaricides (e.g. pyrethroids, fipronil, moxidectin, eprinomectin, fluralaner) – these are very effective and those containing pyrethroids also have a repellent effect, reducing the number of ticks that manage to hook on to the skin. Those ticks that do manage to attach to the skin die and generally fall off within 24 hours. The problem with this form of topical application is that if animals have access to water or are bathed frequently, the concentration of the drug in the skin may be reduced and no longer protective.
- Collars with pyrethroids (deltamethrin, flumethrin) – these are also effective and continuously release the active ingredient. The collars are long-lasting (6–8 months) and are an easy option for pet owners. Collars containing flumethrin can be used with cats. The main disadvantage is the loss of the collars, which can be quite common.
- Oral isoxazolines – these have been proven to be very effective against most ticks, including *Rhipicephalus sanguineus*, *Dermacentor reticulatus*, *Ixodes ricinus*, *Ixodes hexagonus* and *Amblyomma americana*. They can be used alone or in combination with macrocyclic lactones in cats. Isoxazolines offer good protection even for animals with an active outdoor life or that are bathed frequently. As they are systemic products, oral isoxazolines only act after the tick has taken a blood meal and do not prevent attachment. However, they have a rapid onset of action, with tick death and detachment typically occurring within 12–24 hours. The transmission of infectious agents by ticks (e.g. *Borrelia burgdorferi*, *Anaplasma phagocytophilum*, *Babesia canis*, *Cytauxozoon felis*) requires attachment for at least 24–28 hours, in most cases, thus systemic isoxazolines are effective in preventing infection. Exceptions include *Ehrlichia canis* and *Rickettsia* spp. where transmission can occur after only a few hours of attachment; therefore, isoxazolines may have limited efficacy in preventing diseases caused by these agents.

However, it should be noted that due to the life cycle of the tick, the prevention of infestation is challenging. Most ticks have a three host life cycle, typically involving wild animals. New infestations remain possible, therefore, if the dog or cat continues to visit high risk outdoor areas. The exception is *Rhipicephalus sanguineus*, which can complete its entire life cycle on the dog. In cases of infestation with *R. sanguineus*, the environment should be treated with an effective acaricidal product as high numbers of the various life stages of the tick may be present in the animal's immediate surroundings. Thus, in practical terms, regular prophylactic treatment will minimize tick attachment, but 100% control is rarely achieved.

Key points

- Regular use of flea and tick prophylaxis is good practice. The practitioner should refine this treatment based on the geographical location and individual risks posed by the owner/pet lifestyle
- To maximize successful flea control, it is beneficial to alternate products with different mechanisms of action and to include products that contain insect-growth regulators to minimize the development of resistance and to disrupt the life cycle of the parasite at different stages
- Certain ectoparasites may be difficult to identify with routine diagnostic tests. If there is a high index of suspicion, then an appropriate parasiticidal trial should be undertaken

References and further reading

Allerton F (2020) *BSAVA Small Animal Formulary 10th edition, Part A: Canine and Feline*. BSAVA Publications, Gloucester

Beugnet F and Franc M (2012) Insecticide and acaricide molecules and/or combinations to prevent pet infestation by ectoparasites. *Trends in Parasitology* **28**, 267–279

Datz C (2018) Isoxazolines. *Plumb's Therapeutics Brief*, 65–67

Gaens D, Rummel C, Schmidt M *et al.* (2019) Suspected neurological toxicity after oral application of fluralaner (Bravecto) in a Kooikerhondje dog. *BMC Veterinary Research* **15**, 283

Long S (2019) Choosing treatment for dogs with generalized demodicosis – Isoxazolines or imidacloprid and moxidectin? *Veterinary Evidence* **4**, 1–17

Mueller RS, Rosenkrantz W, Bensignor E *et al.* (2020) Diagnosis and treatment of demodicosis in dogs and cats: clinical consensus guidelines of the World Association for Veterinary Dermatology. *Veterinary Dermatology* **31**, 5–27

Otranto D (2018) Arthropod-borne pathogens of dogs and cats: From pathways and times of transmission to disease control. *Veterinary Parasitology* **251**, 68–77

Chapter 9

Atopic dermatitis and food-responsive dermatosis

Ralf S. Mueller

- Allergen – an antigen that favours development of a hypersensitivity response.
- Allergy – a condition characterized by hypersensitivity responses to allergens.
- Atopic dermatitis – an allergic skin condition associated with a hypersensitivity response to allergens.
- Atopy – a genetic predisposition to develop a type I, immunoglobulin E (IgE)-mediated hypersensitivity to environmental allergens.
- Food intolerance – an abnormal physiological response to a food (pharmacological or metabolic reactions) or food poisoning.
- Food-responsive dermatosis (also known as food allergy or adverse food reaction) – a clinically abnormal response to a dietary constituent, which may involve an immune-mediated reaction to a specific dietary antigen.
- Hypersensitivity – an exaggerated response of the immune system to an antigen.

Canine atopic dermatitis is the most common manifestation of the atopic disease. Dogs may also develop atopic conjunctivitis and rhinitis, apparently triggered by environmental allergens. In most cases of canine atopic dermatitis, an allergen-specific IgE response is present; however, atopic dermatitis-like clinical signs may develop without detectable IgE. The reason for this is currently not understood. The term (atopic dermatitis-like) is used to refer to these cases. Furthermore, aberrations in the skin barrier and immune response can be demonstrated in some individuals. Thus, it is currently accepted that the term atopic dermatitis describes a clinical syndrome rather than one single disease, as the clinical signs of atopic dermatitis can be associated with multiple causes. This is a change from the originally accepted view of atopic dermatitis as being equated to an immediate hypersensitivity response to environmental allergens.

Food-responsive dermatosis encompasses both immunological and non-immunological reactions to elements in the diet, and may present as a clinically identical dermatitis. Owing to the similarity in clinical presentations, the International Committee on Atopic Disease in Animals has proposed that canine atopic dermatitis should be considered to be triggered by environmental or food allergens, or a combination of both. For practical purposes, it is useful to consider environmental atopic dermatitis, food-responsive dermatosis and flea allergic dermatitis as potentially co-existing problems. It is important to point out that food-induced dermatitis can also manifest in ways other than an atopic dermatitis-type presentation. It can manifest as hives, plaques and even as vasculitis. In many patients, the clinical presentation is indistinguishable from the classic atopic dermatitis triggered by pollen or dust mite allergens.

According to the allergic threshold principle, pruritus from several concurrent skin diseases may 'add up'. Factors that can exacerbate canine atopic dermatitis are often called 'flare factors'. For example, in a dog with bacterial pyoderma secondary to canine atopic dermatitis and flea allergic dermatitis, the resulting pruritus is from the combination of the dermatoses. Thus, it is extremely important for the successful management of atopic dermatitis to minimize the pruritus by addressing all the compounding concurrent triggers and secondary skin diseases.

Environmental atopic dermatitis

Pathogenesis

Historically, the route of allergen exposure in canine atopic dermatitis was presumed to be via the respiratory system, but there is now substantial evidence for both sensitization and elicitation via the epicutaneous route as well.

Presentation of the offending allergens to the T-cells by the Langerhans' cells leads to the preferential activation of T helper type 2 (Th2) cells, which secrete cytokines favouring the production of allergen-specific IgE antibodies. The IgE antibodies are bound to the surface of circulating basophils and tissue mast cells. When allergens cross-link the surface-bound allergen-specific IgE antibodies, degranulation of the cell occurs, with the subsequent release of inflammatory mediators. Preformed mediators stored within the granules include histamine, heparin and proteolytic enzymes. Other mediators, such as prostaglandins and leucotrienes, are synthesized and released subsequent to degranulation. In addition, the activation of Th2 cells leads to the release of interleukin (IL)-31, a pruritogenic cytokine. Pruritus then causes scratching, rubbing or licking and secondary traumatic lesions, such as excoriations, alopecia and lichenification. With chronic lesions, an exaggerated Th1 response and an increased release of interferon-gamma is seen.

Allergen-specific IgGd antibodies have been implicated in the pathogenesis of canine atopic dermatitis because they bind to the surface of mast cells, but their exact role in this condition is unclear. An impaired skin barrier is seen in dogs with atopic dermatitis. Whether this contributes to the cause or is a result of the disease possibly depends on the individual patient, similar to observations made in humans. An impaired skin barrier can result in increased absorption of allergens and further surface microbial colonization.

Strong breed predilections and limited breeding trials suggest that atopic dermatitis is a genetically inherited disease.

Differential diagnoses

The most common differential diagnoses for canine atopic dermatitis include:

- Superficial pyoderma (often concurrent with canine atopic dermatitis)
- *Malassezia* dermatitis (often concurrent with canine atopic dermatitis)
- Sarcoptic mange
- Contact irritant or allergic dermatitis
- Food-responsive dermatosis
- Trombiculosis
- Pododemodicosis.

Clinical approach

History

The presenting complaint in most dogs with atopic dermatitis is pruritus, although dogs occasionally present with a recurrent pyoderma that is completely responsive to antibiotics. Pruritus manifests as scratching, licking, rubbing and 'scooting'. Owners need to be questioned specifically about the behaviour of the dog to determine the extent of the disease.

- Clinical signs of atopic dermatitis are typically seen in dogs between 6 months and 4 years of age, although occasionally younger and older animals may be affected. This is very important to consider, particularly when the patient is moved to a warmer climate with more pollen exposure at a later time in their life.
- Seasonal pruritus is most commonly reported initially, but this may vary with the climate and environment in which the patient lives. Owners commonly report an increasingly longer period of pruritus every year, and after a few years many dogs are affected perennially.
- Most patients with atopic dermatitis without a secondary infection respond to glucocorticoids at anti-inflammatory doses (≤1 mg/kg of prednisolone).
- A breed predisposition to atopic dermatitis is recognized in the Boston Terrier, Boxer, Cairn Terrier, Chinese Shar Pei, Cocker Spaniel, Dalmatian, English Bulldog, English Setter, Fox Terrier, Golden Retriever, Irish Setter, Labrador Retriever, Lhasa Apso, Pug, West Highland White Terrier and Yorkshire Terrier. However, breed predispositions may vary with location.

Physical examination

Uncomplicated atopic dermatitis manifests as pruritus, which results in erythema, salivary staining, self-induced alopecia and excoriations at predilection sites (Figures 9.1 and 9.2). A primary papular eruption may also be seen. In chronic atopic dermatitis, lichenification and hyperpigmentation result (Figure 9.3). Bilateral otitis externa is common

- Axillae
- Carpal/tarsal regions
- Ears
- Face
- Inguinal area
- Interdigital areas
- Perianal area
- Ventral abdomen

9.1 Predilection sites for canine atopic dermatitis.

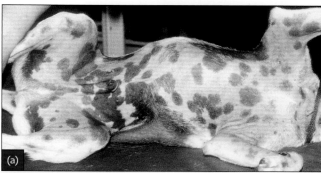
(a)

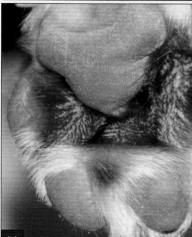
(b)

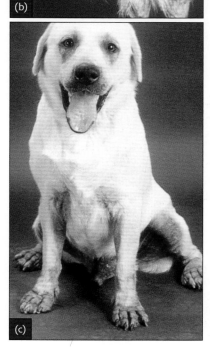
(c)

9.2 Canine atopic dermatitis. (a) Ventral erythema of the axillae, abdomen and groin in a crossbreed dog. (b) Interdigital erythema in a 3-year-old neutered Labrador Retriever bitch. (c) A 3-year-old male Labrador Retriever with typical clinical features of atopic dermatitis. Note the involvement of the paws, ventral abdomen and periorbital areas. Alopecia is secondary to self-trauma.

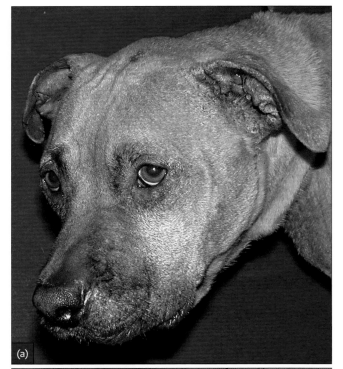

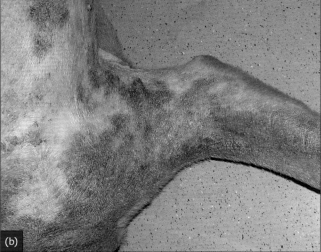

9.3 Lichenification and hyperpigmentation in a dog with chronic atopic dermatitis. Note the typical distribution of lesions. (a) Periocular region, muzzle and pinnae. (b) Axilla and inner forelimb.

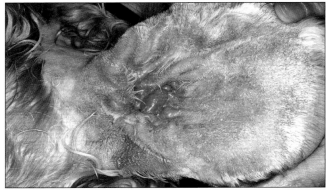

9.4 Chronic otitis externa in a 5-year-old Cocker Spaniel with atopic dermatitis.

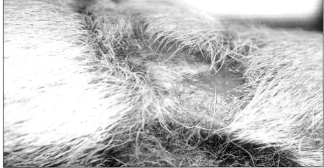

9.5 Focal acral lick dermatitis of the left foreleg of a 7-year-old German Shepherd Dog bitch with atopic dermatitis.

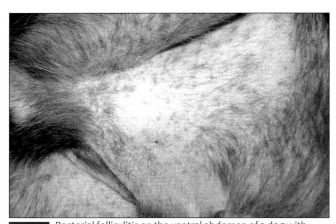

9.6 Bacterial folliculitis on the ventral abdomen of a dog with atopic dermatitis.

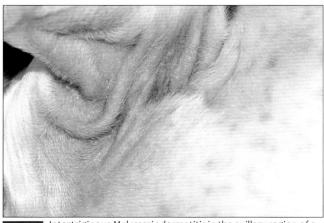

9.7 Intertriginous *Malassezia* dermatitis in the axillary region of a Beagle with canine atopic dermatitis.

and affects the concave pinna and vertical ear canal (Figure 9.4). In early stages, only pruritus and mild erythema of the ear canal may be noted. Occasionally, unilateral otitis externa can be seen. Atopic rhinitis and conjunctivitis may also occur concurrently with dermatological signs. Acral lick dermatitis (Figure 9.5) or pyotraumatic dermatitis ('hot spots') may also be a manifestation of atopic dermatitis.

Clinical signs of secondary bacterial infection may be present, such as papules, pustules, epidermal collarettes and crusts (Figure 9.6). *Malassezia*, another common secondary infection, tends to favour intertriginous regions such as the interdigital web (ventral and dorsal), axillae, facial folds, ventral neck and ear. This infection often manifests as erythema, greasy exudates and scaling (Figure 9.7). Malodour can be associated with both yeast and bacterial skin and ear infections.

Diagnostic tests

The diagnosis is usually based on the history, physical examination and exclusion of differential diagnoses. Various authors have generated criteria for the diagnosis of canine atopic dermatitis; the latest and most accurate is that published by Favrot *et al.* (2010) (Figure 9.8). Even if parasites are not found, trial therapy with parasiticides prior to a work-up for allergy is recommended. Secondary bacterial or yeast infections should be identified by cytology and treated. Typically, in canine atopic dermatitis, pruritus remains after these infections have resolved. A detailed approach to pruritus and to the presentation, diagnosis and management of ectoparasites and infections is covered elsewhere in the Manual.

- Onset of clinical signs in an animal <3 years of age
- Dog living mostly indoors
- Pruritus responds to glucocorticoids
- Pruritus *sine materia* at onset (i.e. no skin alterations)
- Affected front feet
- Affected ear pinnae
- Non-affected ear margins
- Non-affected lumbodorsal area

9.8 Criteria for the diagnosis of canine atopic dermatitis. (*Favrot et al.*, 2010)

Food-responsive dermatosis

Pathogenesis

There is much less known about the pathogenesis of food-responsive dermatosis compared with canine atopic dermatitis; however, histological, clinical and immunological features of food-induced and environmentally induced atopic dermatitis in the dog seem to be very similar.

Clinical approach

History

Food-responsive dermatosis in the dog presents as non-seasonal pruritus or recurrent pyoderma. The disease often mimics atopic dermatitis triggered by environmental allergens. Concurrent gastrointestinal signs are significantly more common in dogs with food-induced atopic dermatitis. No sex predilections have been reported. However, almost half of the dogs with food-induced atopic dermatitis are very young at disease onset (<1 year of age) and dogs >6 years of age at the onset of clinical signs are more than twice as likely to have food-induced rather than environmental atopic dermatitis. Thus, an onset of clinical signs in a very young or an older dog should prioritize a work-up for a food-responsive dermatosis, although all dogs with atopic dermatitis should ideally undergo a diet trial. Some studies have suggested a predilection for Labrador Retrievers and West Highland White Terriers. Breed specificities are likely to vary with the local genetic pool. The response to glucocorticoid therapy can be variable. Gastrointestinal signs are often mild and may not be included in the information volunteered by the owner, particularly flatulence or frequent defecation (>3 times daily). Intermittent vomiting, diarrhoea and borborygmus (rumbling bowel sounds) may occur.

Physical examination

Food-responsive dermatosis can present with very similar clinical signs to canine atopic dermatitis due to environmental allergens. However, the author has seen cases

presenting with recurrent pyoderma, recurrent bacterial folliculitis (Figure 9.9) and urticaria, as well as a presentation similar to flea allergy dermatitis.

Diagnostic tests

Serum testing for food-specific antibodies and intradermal testing with food antigens are not suitable for the diagnosis of a food-responsive dermatosis. Similarly, salivary and hair testing have been shown to be useless. Patch testing with food antigens can identify suitable ingredients for an elimination diet, but numerous false-positive reactions make this test unsuitable for diagnosing a food-responsive dermatosis. The only reliable way to diagnose a canine food-responsive dermatosis is to feed a limited antigen diet for a minimum of 4–6 weeks. In the majority of cases, improvement should be noted during this time (Figure 9.10). However, sometimes it may

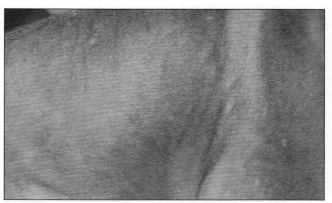

9.9 Multifocal folliculitis on the trunk of a 10-month-old Dogue de Bordeaux with a food-responsive dermatosis.

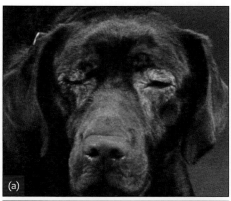

(a)

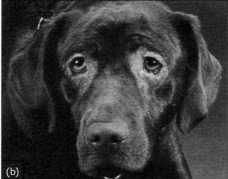

(b)

9.10 (a) A 10-month-old neutered Labrador Retriever bitch with a food-responsive dermatosis. The clinical signs are concentrated on the face. (b) The same dog after 4 weeks on a hypoallergenic diet trial.

be necessary to extend the diet trial to 8–10 weeks to demonstrate significant improvement. In particular, this may be required in those cases that present with recurrent pyoderma. If pyoderma recurs every 4 weeks then a 6–8-week diet trial may be of insufficient length. In addition, if concurrent medication is prescribed to treat secondary infections then the diet trial must be extended for at least 2 weeks more than the expected recurrence of the pyoderma after the course of medication has been completed.

Client compliance is the biggest single issue that results in failure to achieve an adequate diet trial and subsequent diagnosis of a food-responsive dermatosis (Figure 9.11). Explaining the rationale behind diet trials and how to perform one effectively takes time. A handout that reinforces the protocol is a useful addition to the consultation.

Diet selection should be based on a thorough history, which not only includes the main meal of the day but also any additional food sources that may be given (Figure 9.12). The selected diet should be based on a protein to which the animal has had little or no previous exposure; alternatively, a hydrolysed protein diet may be employed. Novel protein diets contain proteins that are not commonly used in regular dog foods, and can vary geographically. Occasionally, a trial with one novel protein diet is not effective, but a response to an alternative diet is seen. One possible reason for this may be the frequent contamination of commercial dog foods with ingredients not listed on the label (Olivry and Mueller, 2018). Another reason may be common antigens in certain diets or existing cross-reactivities; the author usually avoids feeding any poultry (duck, turkey) to dogs with previous exposure to chicken, or any deer, elk or goat to a dog previously fed a beef- or mutton-based diet. Hypersensitivity to additives is theoretically possible but not well documented in the dog.

Hydrolysed diets are a new generation of veterinary diets with an indication for use in animals with gastrointestinal or cutaneous hypersensitivity. The theoretical advantage of these diets is that a novel protein need not be utilized because the dietary protein has been hydrolysed to peptides, which are smaller than those required to provoke an immune response. Although hydrolysed diets have been shown to be beneficial in many dogs with a food-responsive dermatosis, some patients will not improve satisfactorily when fed a hydrolysed protein if they have

had previous exposure to the native source. Hydrolysed diets tend to be less palatable and more expensive than novel protein diets. A lack of response to a food trial using a hydrolysed diet does not rule out the possibility of a food-responsive dermatosis.

Home-cooked diets require a lot of effort to prepare and client compliance is often lower when these diets are employed. The protein source (e.g. fish, rabbit or pork should be novel and readily available, and mixed with a carbohydrate source previously not fed, such as sweet potato, millet or lentils. It should be noted that fish and dairy products may be included in commercially available dog treats and thus may not represent a novel protein source. Home-cooked diets are not nutritionally balanced for long-term feeding and should not be employed in the growing dog.

A food-responsive dermatosis is only confirmed when the dog improves on the diet and relapses on challenge. Improvement may not be complete if the dog has concurrent environmental hypersensitivities. Pruritus typically recurs within the first week of introducing the previously fed foods and often, in the author's experience, within 2–48 hours after challenge.

Treatment

The offending foods can be identified by individual challenge (e.g. chicken, beef, milk and wheat) and a diet free from these allergens selected. The client often elects to maintain the dog on the 'test' diet originally employed. Avoiding known allergens is usually effective in controlling the clinical signs in the long term. However, it is possible that the dog may develop a food-responsive dermatosis to the new diet after months or years, and re-evaluation with a new limited antigen diet will be required.

Although new research is attempting desensitization to foods using immunotherapy, this strategy is currently not adopted in clinical practice.

Key points
• Canine atopic dermatitis can be triggered by environmental or food allergens, or a combination of both
• Additional manifestations of atopy may be seen, such as conjunctivitis and rhinitis
• Dogs with food-responsive dermatosis typically have an early age of onset (<12 months)

• Keep the consistency of the meal the same (i.e. dry, tinned or combination)
• If currently on home-cooked food, switch to an alternative home-cooked source
• Introduce the new food gradually
• Use the new diet for 'treats'
• In a multiple-dog household, put all animals on the same diet

9.11 Tips to improve compliance with diet trials.

• Dog treats
• Dental chews
• Bones
• Flavoured toothpaste
• Food used for tablet administration
• Flavoured tablets
• Table scraps
• Milk
• Gravy
• Treats from neighbours, friends or relatives

9.12 Potential sources of extra food.

References and further reading

Bethlehem S, Bexley J and Mueller RS (2012) Patch testing and allergen-specific serum IgE and IgG antibodies in the diagnosis of canine food-responsive dermatosis. *Veterinary Immunology and Immunopathology* **145**, 582–589

Favrot C, Steffan J, Seewald W *et al.* (2010) A prospective study on the clinical features of chronic canine atopic dermatitis and its diagnosis. *Veterinary Dermatology* **21**, 23–31

Hensel P, Santoro D, Favrot C *et al.* (2015) Canine atopic dermatitis: detailed guidelines for diagnosis and allergen identification. *BMC Veterinary Research* **11**, 19

Jaeger K, Linek M, Power HT *et al.* (2010) Breed and site predispositions of dogs with atopic dermatitis: A comparison of five locations in three continents. *Veterinary Dermatology* **21**, 119–123

Johansen C, Mariani C and Mueller RS (2017) Evaluation of canine adverse food reactions by patch testing with single proteins, single carbohydrates and commercial foods. *Veterinary Dermatology* **28**, 473–480

Marsella R (2013) Hypersensitivity disorders. In: *Muller & Kirk's Small Animal Dermatology, 6th edn*, ed. Miller WH, Griffin CE, and Campbell K, pp. 363–431. WB Saunders, Philadelphia

Mueller RS and Olivry T (2017) Critically appraised topics on adverse food reactions of companion animals (4): can we diagnose adverse food reactions in dogs and cats with *in vivo* or *in vitro* tests? *BMC Veterinary Research* **13**, 275

Mueller RS and Olivry T (2018) Critically appraised topic on adverse food reactions of companion animals (6): prevalence of non-cutaneous manifestations of adverse food reactions in dogs and cats. *BMC Veterinary Research* **14**, 341

Mueller RS and Unterer S (2018) Adverse food reactions: Pathogenesis, clinical signs, diagnosis and alternatives to elimination diets. *The Veterinary Journal* **236**, 89–95

Olivry T and Mueller RS (2018) Critically appraised topic on adverse food reactions of companion animals (5): discrepancies between ingredients and labeling in commercial pet foods. *BMC Veterinary Research* **14**, 24

Olivry T and Mueller RS (2019) Critically appraised topic on adverse food reactions of companion animals (7): signalment and cutaneous manifestations of dogs and cats with adverse food reactions. *BMC Veterinary Research* **15**, 140

Olivry T and Mueller RS (2019) Critically appraised topic on adverse food reactions of companion animals (8): storage mites in commercial pet foods. *BMC Veterinary Research* **15**, 385

Chapter 10

Management of pruritus and atopic dermatitis

Patrick Hensel

Pruritus is a common clinical sign for many skin conditions, including atopic dermatitis, and often has a detrimental impact on the patient's quality of life. It is critical that the cause of the pruritus is identified and eliminated to improve the clinical signs and reduce the need for anti-inflammatory therapy. It should be noted that pruritus is not always associated with an allergic reaction, although many pruritic patients are ultimately diagnosed with some form of allergy. The causes of pruritus are additive and multifactorial and can be aggravated by secondary infections.

Flare factors

Most allergy patients require lifelong care, which is best achieved with an individualized multimodal treatment plan to control acute flares as well as chronic atopic dermatitis. Fleas, food and environmental allergens (e.g. dust mites, pollens), as well as secondary skin and ear infections, are considered to be the major flare factors (Figure 10.1).

Fleas

Pets should be regularly screened for fleas and flea faeces. Repeated exposure to flea bites can increase flea saliva hypersensitivity in atopic animals. Where flea infestation is endemic, atopic patients should be treated with preventatives year-round. The efficacy of topical flea preventatives can be limited by frequent baths with medicated shampoos. As a consequence, flea preventatives may need to be applied more frequently if used topically or, as an alternative, oral insecticides such as isoxazolines may be used.

Food

Acute flares to foods occur most commonly if an animal ingests a food component to which it has been sensitized. Even if a food-responsive dermatosis (also known as food allergy or adverse food reaction) has been ruled out previously, atopic patients can develop new hypersensitivities to food ingredients, resulting in a sudden increase in clinical signs. Another elimination and provocation diet trial may therefore be necessary if a new food-responsive dermatosis is suspected.

Environmental allergens

Seasonal environmental allergens (such as pollen) and non-seasonal allergens (such as dust mites) often cause acute flares. Typical examples are dogs that develop sudden rashes and pruritus after running or rolling in grass. Checking current pollen counts in the region via weather applications or websites may help identify the offending pollen allergens. Avoiding direct contact with the offending allergen may alleviate clinical signs, but it is often not practical. Where contact with offending allergens cannot be avoided, allergen-specific immunotherapy (ASIT) should be considered.

Secondary infections

The skin and ears of atopic patients often show an overgrowth of staphylococci and *Malassezia* species. This can result in skin infections and aggravate the clinical signs. Skin cytology should be performed to identify or rule out the microorganisms. If the findings confirm a skin infection, antimicrobial shampoos or leave-on lotions/foams containing chlorhexidine, ethyl lactate, triclosan and/or topical antifungals such as miconazole and ketoconazole should be used. In more severe bacterial skin infections, oral antibiotics (e.g. 1st generation cephalosporins) may also be necessary (see Chapter 22).

Prevention of acute flares

These flares can be prevented by a combination of skin hygiene (regular baths with antipruritic and/or antimicrobial shampoos/lotions/moisturizers), flea prevention, restricted diet and, if needed, a short course of topical or oral glucocorticoids.

Flare factor	Action
Fleas and other parasites	• Flea combing • Routine ectoparasite prophylaxis
Food	• Strict diet trial and provocation • Avoid future exposure if confirmed food-responsive dermatosis
Environmental allergens	• Check actual pollen count • Avoid direct contact with offending allergen (e.g. grass) • Regular bathing to remove allergens from hair coat and skin (dogs)
Bacteria and yeast	• Identify with cytology ± bacterial culture • Targeted topical therapy with antimicrobial agents • In cases of widespread infection, use systemic antimicrobial therapy

10.1 Flare factors associated with atopic dermatitis.

Medication with proven efficacy

For years, glucocorticoids and ciclosporin have been used for the symptomatic management of atopic dermatitis and pruritus. However, recent advances in understanding the pathomechanism, and the inflammatory and pruritic mediators involved, has helped improve the management of allergies and has led to the development of new therapeutic interventions (Figure 10.2).

With the growing arsenal of anti-inflammatory and antipruritic drugs, treatment can be tailored to manage both the acute and chronic pruritus associated with atopic dermatitis, thus minimizing the risk of potential side effects. Depending on the severity and degree of the pruritus, and associated skin inflammation, the clinician needs to decide whether a broad (e.g. glucocorticoids, ciclosporin), semi-broad (e.g. oclacitinib) or narrow (e.g. monoclonal antibodies, antihistamines) acting drug should be used. If needed, these drugs can also be combined to enhance the efficacy of treatment.

Glucocorticoids

The effects of glucocorticoids are very complex and include a strong antipruritic effect due to their action on a wide range of cells expressing glucocorticoid receptors. These receptors bind to glucocorticoid response elements in the deoxyribonucleic acid (DNA), which then either upregulate or downregulate DNA transcription. This results in alterations of cellular metabolism, thereby causing inhibition of inflammatory cells (e.g. neutrophils, eosinophils, lymphocytes) and suppression of many inflammatory mediators (e.g. cytokines, adhesion molecules, inflammatory enzymes). Glucocorticoids also have an inhibitory effect on both cellular and humoral immunity. The broad, non-specific anti-inflammatory effect results in a positive treatment response for most pruritic skin conditions. The antipruritic effect is considered to be secondary and due to the reduction in skin inflammation. It should be remembered that drugs with such a broad range of actions are more likely to result in side effects.

Topical glucocorticoids

Glucocorticoid sprays, such as 0.015% triamcinolone solution or 0.0584% hydrocortisone aceponate, can be used for acute and localized flares. They are very efficient in reducing localized inflammation and pruritus. They should be used initially twice daily for 1–2 weeks and then, based on clinical response, reduced to alternate day application. These topical drugs are intended for short-term use only. If used long-term, adverse effects such as scaling, cutaneous atrophy, comedones and superficial follicular cysts may occur. However, using hydrocortisone aceponate or other moderately potent topical glucocorticoids on two consecutive days per week for maintenance treatment can delay recurrence of clinical signs without causing visible cutaneous side effects.

Active ingredient	Dosage	Comments
Topical glucocorticoids		
Hydrocortisone aceponate (0.0584%)	Apply q12–24h	• Use for acute flares and localized lesions • Possible adverse effects include skin atrophy and calcinosis cutis
Triamcinolone acetonide (0.015%)	Apply q12–24h	
Oral glucocorticoids		
Prednisone, prednisolone, methylprednisolone	Dogs: initial dose of 0.5–1 mg/kg orally q24h Cats: initial dose of 2.2 mg/kg orally q24h Taper to lowest dose that controls the clinical signs	• Use for acute flares • Fast-acting • Broad anti-inflammatory effect • Many potential side effects • Use prednisolone in cats
Triamcinolone acetonide	Dogs and cats: 0.11–0.22 mg/kg orally q24h	
Dexamethasone	Dogs: 0.07–0.16 mg/kg orally q24h Cats: 0.125–1 mg/kg orally q24h	
Topical calcineurin inhibitor		
Tacrolimus (0.1%)	Apply q12–24h	• Use for long-term management • Use for localized lesions
Oral calcineurin inhibitor		
Ciclosporin	Dogs: initial dose of 5 mg/kg orally q24h Cats: initial dose of 7 mg/kg orally q24h Taper to lowest dose that controls the clinical signs	• Use for long-term management • Slow onset of efficacy • Most common side effect is gastrointestinal signs
Janus kinase (JAK) inhibitor		
Oclacitinib	Dogs: 0.4–0.6 mg/kg orally q12h for up to 14 days, then q24h Cats: 1 mg/kg orally q12h for up to 28 days, then q24h. Note that optimal dosing has not been determined	• Use for acute flare and long-term management • Fast-acting • Do not use in dogs <1 year of age
Monoclonal antibodies		
Lokivetmab	1–2 mg/kg s.c. q30–60days	• Use for acute flares and long-term management • Do not use in cats • Can be used at any age • Very safe

10.2 Drugs with proven efficacy for the treatment of pruritus and atopic dermatitis.

Oral glucocorticoids

Fast-acting drugs, such as prednisone, prednisolone and methylprednisolone, are effective and recommended for short-term treatment of acute flares. They should be given at 0.5 mg/kg once to twice daily, until clinical remission occurs. If long-term systemic glucocorticoids are required, the dose should be decreased to the safest and lowest dose and frequency (e.g. prednisolone at 0.25 mg/kg q48h) that remains efficacious, shows minimal side effects and provides an acceptable quality of life. Other glucocorticoids that can be used orally include triamcinolone acetonide (not available in the UK) and dexamethasone (see Figure 10.2). Side effects of oral glucocorticoids, such as polyuria, polydipsia, polyphagia and predisposition to urinary tract and skin infections, are common and often proportional to dosage and treatment duration. The long-term use of systemic glucocorticoids can also result in calcinosis cutis (especially in Bulldog breeds), and they also predispose to demodicosis. Due to the risk of side effects and the inability to withdraw the drug once administered, the repeated use of long-acting injectable glucocorticoids is not recommended.

Calcineurin inhibitors

This group of broad-acting inflammatory drugs (e.g. tacrolimus, ciclosporin) act predominantly as T-cell inhibitors. By blocking the nuclear factor of activated T-cells (NFAT) transcription factor, the secretion of cytokines such as interleukin (IL)-2 and interferon-gamma is reduced in T-cells. Besides the direct anti-inflammatory effect, calcineurin inhibitors also have a direct antipruritic effect by inhibiting pruritogenic nerve receptors. However, due to the slow onset of treatment effect, calcineurin inhibitors are not recommended for use during acute flares.

Topical calcineurin inhibitors

Tacrolimus (0.1%) can be used for localized, chronic atopic dermatitis. It should be applied twice daily for at least a week and until the inflammation is under control. The frequency of application can then be reduced as needed. Side effects seems to be rare, but signs of skin irritation or a temporary increase in pruritus may be observed. In humans, a sensation of tingling has been reported; it is possible that veterinary patients that appear irritated by this treatment may be experiencing a similar effect.

Oral calcineurin inhibitors

Ciclosporin is approved for long-term management of canine atopic dermatitis. The recommended initial dose for dogs is 5 mg/kg orally q24h, whereas the recommended starting dose for cats is 7 mg/kg orally q24h. It can take up to 4–6 weeks for the ciclosporin to achieve satisfactory clinical improvement; therefore, it is not suitable for the treatment of acute flares. A faster response to treatment can be achieved if ciclosporin is combined with oral glucocorticoids or oclacitinib during the first 2 weeks. Once the clinical signs are under control, the dose of ciclosporin should be reduced by increasing dosage intervals (e.g. every 2–4 days) and/or by reducing the daily dose by, for example, 50%. Gastrointestinal signs, such as vomiting and diarrhoea/soft stool, are relative common side effects, but usually mild to moderate and transient. The risk of these side effects can also be reduced by giving the ciclosporin with food or splitting the daily dose to twice daily administration.

Janus kinase inhibitor

Oclacitinib is a semi-broad, fast-acting antipruritic and anti-inflammatory oral drug. It can be used for the treatment of acute flares as well as chronic atopic disease. Oclacitinib is a Janus kinase (JAK) inhibitor, which preferably inhibits JAK1 and, to a lesser degree, JAK3, resulting in decreased activity of JAK1-dependent cytokines involved in allergy and inflammation (IL-2, IL-4, IL-6 and IL-13) as well as pruritus (IL-31). The recommended initial dose is 0.4–0.6 mg/kg orally q12h for up to 14 days. Thereafter, the dose should be reduced to once daily for maintenance.

Some dogs exhibit increased pruritus when the dosage is reduced to once daily. This may be overcome by splitting the total daily dose and giving the drug twice daily. This regimen may work better because oclacitinib has a short half-life of 4 hours. Oclacitinib is generally well tolerated, but in rare cases can be associated with mild gastrointestinal side effects (e.g. vomiting, diarrhoea). However, it should not be given to dogs <12 months of age due to an increased risk for activating demodicosis and bacterial pneumonia. Oclacitinib is also well tolerated and seems to be safe for short-term use in cats at 1 or 2 mg/kg q12h for 28 days. It should be remembered that the use of oclacitinib in cats is off-label, long-term studies in allergic cats have not been performed and that owners should give consent before oclacitinib is used in this species.

Regular bloodwork and urinalysis (every 3–6 months) should be performed in dogs on long-term oclacitinib to screen for a reduction in white or red blood cells, hypercholesterolaemia and proteinuria.

Monoclonal antibodies

Lokivetmab is a genetically engineered, caninized monoclonal antibody that targets the strongly pruritogenic canine cytokine IL-31. It binds to IL-31 in the extracellular space so that it cannot bind its cytokine receptor to neurons in the skin and transmit the sensation of pruritus. Lokivetmab is injected subcutaneously at 1–2 mg/kg. In most atopic patients, a significant reduction in pruritus can be observed within 48 hours and the effect lasts for 4–8 weeks. Lokivetmab is typically well tolerated and can be used in dogs of all ages. Side effects are very rare and include an allergic reaction to the drug and gastrointestinal upset. This is a caninized monoclonal antibody and should therefore not be used in cats.

Recombinant interferons

Both recombinant canine interferon-gamma and feline interferon-omega may reduce pruritus and other clinical signs in dogs. These drugs act by binding to their respective receptors and it is suspected that they inhibit type 2 pro-allergic cytokines such as IL-4 and IL-13. Recombinant canine interferon-gamma is given subcutaneously at 5,000–10,000 units/kg three times weekly for 4 weeks, then once weekly for canine atopic dermatitis. Recombinant feline interferon-omega is given orally or subcutaneously at 1–5 million units three times weekly for 4 weeks and then monthly thereafter and can have some beneficial effect in canine atopic dermatitis. The efficacy of recombinant interferons has not currently been determined in feline atopic syndrome.

Treatment options with limited efficacy

The following drugs or treatment options have been used in the past as an alternative for anti-inflammatory, antipruritic or adjunct therapy. However, their efficacy is rather limited and is based on insufficient evidence. They can be used in mild forms of atopic dermatitis or in combination with the drugs mentioned above or essential fatty acids.

Antihistamines

Oral type 1 antihistamines act as histamine H1-receptor antagonists with anti-allergic properties, inhibiting histamine-induced wheal and flare responses. Cetirizine may also have an inhibitory effect on eosinophil, T lymphocyte and monocyte chemotaxis during the late phase of an allergic response. Due to their mode of action, and for sufficient antipruritic effect, oral type 1 antihistamines should preferably be given continuously and proactively before a flare occurs to block the effects of histamine. Antihistamines may also be more effective in dogs with mild pruritus and can be used for sparing purposes in combination with glucocorticoids. Commonly used antihistamines in dogs and cats are summarized in Figure 10.3. Antihistamines are in general safe with minimal side effects, such as sedation. In cats, urinary retention can occur.

Antihistamine	Dosage
Cetirizine	1 mg/kg orally q12–24h
Chlorpheniramine (chlorphenamine)	Dogs: 0.5 mg/kg orally q8–12h Cats: 2–4 mg per cat orally q8–12h
Diphenhydramine	2–4 mg/kg orally q8–12h
Fexofenadine	Dogs: 2–5 mg/kg orally q12–24h Cats: 10–15 mg per cat orally q12–24h
Hydroxyzine	2 mg/kg orally q12h

10.3 Commonly used antihistamines in dogs and cats.

Phosphodiesterase inhibitor

Pentoxifylline has a broad anti-inflammatory effect by increasing the second messenger cyclic adenosine monophosphate (AMP) in immune cells and keratinocytes. This results in a decrease in cytokine production (IL-1, IL-4, IL-12, tumour necrosis factor (TNF)-alpha), decrease in leucocyte responsiveness to IL-1 and TNF-alpha, inhibition of B and T lymphocyte activation, a decrease in natural killer cell activation, inhibition of T-cell adherence to keratinocytes and phosphodiesterase-4 inhibition. Due to the slow onset of efficacy (3–4 weeks), this drug is preferably used in chronic inflammatory skin diseases or as an adjunct treatment with drugs such as glucocorticoids and/or essential fatty acids. Pentoxifylline is given at a high dose of 20 mg/kg orally q8h. Reduction of skin lesions and pruritus seem to be enhanced if pentoxifylline is given with essential fatty acids.

Prostaglandin E1 analogue

Misoprostol has an anti-inflammatory effect by reducing eosinophil chemotaxis and survival and inhibiting histamine release from basophils and mast cells after allergen-specific and non-allergenic stimulation. The drug is slow acting and has a modest anti-inflammatory and antipruritic effect. The recommended dose in dogs is 5 mg/kg orally q24h and should be given for 4–6 weeks to determine efficacy. Side effects, such as vomiting and diarrhoea, are commonly observed.

Neurokinin 1 receptor antagonist

Maropitant inhibits pruritus by blocking the binding of substance P to neurokinin 1 receptors in different tissues. The recommended dose in dogs and cats is 2 mg/kg orally q24h. Drooling and vomiting can be observed as potential side effects.

Gamma-aminobutyric acid analogues

Gabapentin and pregabalin are gamma-aminobutyric acid (GABA) analogues used in the treatment of neuropathic pain. These drugs act by binding to the alpha-2-delta subunit of voltage-dependent calcium channels, mainly at the level of the spinal cord. They also inhibit the inflammation-induced release of substance P. The recommended dose range for gabapentin for cats is 5–15 mg/kg orally q8–12h, and 10–20 mg/kg orally for dogs; whereas, for pregabalin, the dose is 2 mg/kg orally q12h in dogs and cats. The drug should be started at the lower dose range. If no effect is seen after 1–2 weeks, the dose should be gradually increased. The most common side effect is drowsiness.

Essential fatty acids

Oral essential fatty acids (EFAs), such as omega-3 fatty acids (eicosapentanoic acid (EPA) and docosapentanoic acid (DHA)) and omega-6 fatty acids (gamma-linolenic acid), are commonly used as an adjunct treatment in allergic, seborrhoeic skin disease and to aid skin barrier regeneration. EFAs can be used in patients with mild pruritus, as part of combination therapy, as a preventative intervention and as sparing agents for glucocorticoids. Omega-6 fatty acids also improve skin and coat quality by altering the superficial skin lipids. Supplementation with omega-3 fatty acids alters the profile of eicosanoids produced when EFAs are metabolized. Dihomo-gamma-linolenic acid (DGLA) competes with arachidonic acid for the enzymes lipoxygenase and cyclooxygenase, resulting in decreased production of inflammatory leucotrienes and prostaglandins. Omega-3 fatty acids can be found in cold water marine fish oil and the suggested dose is 300 mg (180 mg of EPA and 120 mg of DHA)/4.5 kg orally q24h. Linolenic acid is found in sunflower oil (suggested dose: 1.5 ml/kg orally q24h) and safflower oil (suggested dose: 0.5 ml/kg orally q24h). EFAs are slow acting and must be given for up to 3 months before the effect can be assessed. Side effects are uncommon. Gastrointestinal signs (vomiting, diarrhoea, flatulence) may be seen with high dosages.

Ultra-microsized palmitoylethenolamide

Ultra-microsized palmitoylethenolamide (PEA) is a naturally occurring bioactive lipid compound with anti-inflammatory and antipruritic properties. It acts by down-regulating mast cell degranulation and macrophage and pro-inflammatory T-cell activity. It is a slow-acting dietary supplement given at 10 mg/kg orally q24h and should be administered for at least 30 days to assess its efficacy.

Topical lipid formulations

Skin barrier dysfunction plays a major role in atopic disease and may result from a decrease in ceramides, alterations in filaggrin expression and increased trans-epidermal water loss (TEWL) (see Chapter 1). Topical lipid formulations can help normalize existing stratum corneum lipid barrier defects. Such topical products usually contain a combination of cholesterol, EFAs, phytosphingosine and ceramide complexes. These applications are considered as adjunctive therapy and are applied topically at least once weekly for at least two months.

Skin and coat hygiene and care

Frequent bathing (e.g. once or twice a week) with cleansing shampoos may help reduce skin lesions and pruritus by removing irritants, allergens and microorganisms. 'Hypoallergenic' shampoos contain emollients and moisturizers, such as fatty acids, lipids, phytosphingosine, urea, glycerine, colloidal oatmeal and chitosanide. For patients with an increased risk for recurrent bacterial pyoderma and *Malassezia* dermatitis, regular baths with antimicrobial shampoos containing chlorhexidine, benzoyl peroxide, ethyl lactate, complex sugars, miconazole, ketoconazole and climbazole may be used.

The skin and coat should be well lathered and should remain in contact with the shampoo for at least 10–15 minutes before rinsing it off. While shampoos can be very effective, the residual effect is short and may last only for a few days. However, the effects can be prolonged by combining the shampoo treatments with daily use of leave-on conditioners, lotions, foams or wipes containing the same or similar ingredients. Topical therapy may work well for dogs, but managing cats is often difficult. Cats are generally afraid of water and are likely to lick off any topically applied products (see Chapter 27 for more information on topical treatments).

Treatment recommendations

Figure 10.4 details the goals and treatment recommendations for the management of atopic dermatitis.

Managing acute flares of atopic dermatitis

The main goal in managing an acute relapse of pruritus is to identify potential flare factors (see Figure 10.1). Bacterial and yeast skin and ear infections are a common cause of flares. If the infection is superficial and not too severe, topical antimicrobial therapy should be attempted before considering systemic antimicrobials (see Chapter 22). Another important goal is controlling the pruritus and inflammation, in order to prevent skin damage from self-trauma followed by secondary skin infections. In these cases, fast-acting drugs such as glucocorticoids (e.g. prednisolone) or oclacitinib are most commonly used for a short duration. Lokivetmab can be used as an alternative, especially in dogs younger than 12 months of age, where oclacitinib is not indicated. This may advantageous if the pet owner has difficulties with medicating the animal orally; however, it should be remembered that lokivetmab is a narrow-spectrum treatment directed as controlling pruritus. For localized disease, topical glucocorticoids (e.g. hydrocortisone aceponate) can be applied as well. Topical therapy with hypoallergenic shampoos and leave-on products is an important adjunct intervention and will provide additional relief.

Condition	Management goals	Treatment recommendations
Acute flares of atopic dermatitis	Identify and eliminate flare factors	Flea prevention Treat secondary skin and ear infections Elimination and provocation diet trial to identify triggering foods
	Reduce pruritus and skin lesions	Pharmacological agents: • Glucocorticoids • Oclacitinib • Lokivetmab
	Improve skin and coat quality	Hypoallergenic shampoos Leave-on products (e.g. conditioners, lotions, foams)
Chronic atopic dermatitis	Identify and eliminate flare factors	Flea prevention Treat secondary skin and ear infections Elimination and provocation diet trial to identify triggering foods Allergy testing and allergen-specific immunotherapy
	Reduce pruritus and skin lesions	Pharmacological agents: • Ciclosporin • Oclacitinib • Lokivetmab
	Improve skin and coat quality	Hypoallergenic shampoos Topical lipid-containing products Long-term essential fatty acid supplementation
	Long-term prevention	Antihistamines Regular ear cleaning
Inflammation (a targeted approach)	Phase I (reactive therapy) – induction of clinical sign remission	Oral ± topical glucocorticoids followed by oclacitinib
	Phase II (proactive therapy) – prevention of clinical sign recurrence	Allergen avoidance, allergen-specific immunotherapy, topical glucocorticoids and/or lokivetmab followed by oclacitinib and/or ciclosporin, followed by oral glucocorticoids

10.4 The goals and treatment recommendations for atopic dermatitis.

Managing chronic atopic dermatitis

Controlling and avoiding flare factors is also important in the management of patients with chronic atopic dermatitis. Year-round ectoparasitic prevention is recommended. If a previously well controlled patient shows an increase in clinical signs, then repeating an 8-week elimination and provocation dietary trial should be considered as a new food-responsive dermatitis may have developed. As with acute flares, patients with chronic atopic dermatitis are predisposed to secondary bacterial and *Malassezia* skin and ear infections. As a preventative measure, routine ear cleaning should be performed. Identifying the inciting environmental allergens (e.g. pollen, dust mites) and treatment with ASIT should always be considered in chronic atopic dermatitis, especially in young and adolescent animals. ASIT has a minimal risk of side effects, the potential for reducing the frequency of infections and the potential to reduce the need for symptomatic therapy with anti-inflammatory drugs (see Chapter 11).

Topical glucocorticoids can be used for localized chronic atopic dermatitis, but they should be applied intermittently (every 3–4 days) to prevent skin atrophy. Tacrolimus can be used as an alternative, but may be cost-prohibitive.

Oral glucocorticoids, ciclosporin, oclacitinib and lokivetmab are effective for the management of chronic canine atopic dermatitis; however, due to the potential long-term side effects associated with glucocorticoids, they should not be the first choice treatment.

The benefits of ciclosporin include its strong antipruritic and anti-inflammatory effects. The dose of ciclosporin can often be reduced to every 2–4 days once the atopic dermatitis is under control. Oclacitinib is a well-tolerated long-term treatment, although monitoring via routine bloodwork is recommended. Due to its short duration of action, daily administration is required in most patients.

Another, even safer, option is lokivetmab, administered subcutaneously, which is often more convenient for the owner. This can be repeated as needed, and with repeat injections the duration of activity may be extended.

Bathing regularly with hypoallergenic shampoos and topical application of lipid-containing products as an adjunct measure helps stabilize the skin, resulting in reduced skin lesions, pruritus and microbial colonization. Long-term oral supplementation with EFAs is recommended. Besides the beneficial effect on the skin and coat quality, EFAs can have a sparing or synergistic effect with anti-inflammatory drugs. Antihistamines, although not considered very effective, can be beneficial if used as a preventative, adjunct and drug-sparing strategy before the allergy season starts.

Managing inflammation: a targeted approach

Atopic dermatitis is more likely to be a syndrome, which can manifest with a wide range of clinical signs. As a result, an atopic patient may suffer from acute flares (e.g. erythematous macules/patches) as well as chronic skin lesions (e.g. plaques, lichenification, hyperpigmentation)

concurrently at different body sites. This should be taken into account when making a decision regarding treatment; whether a drug should be used for an acute flare or chronic atopic dermatitis is based on the speed of efficacy and not whether they have a broad- or narrow-acting effect. It should be borne in mind that broad-acting drugs will probably work in most patients, but they will also be more likely to cause side effects.

Inflammation targeted therapy is divided into two phases:

- Phase I – reactive therapy
- Phase II – proactive therapy.

The goal of Phase I therapy is to induce clinical remission. In this phase, the skin inflammation is usually prominent and fast- and broad-acting drugs such as oral short-acting glucocorticoids (e.g. prednisolone) should be used. When the inflammation has subsided, the treatment should be changed to oclacitinib. Once the clinical signs have been under control for several weeks, a transition to Phase II therapy is recommended. The goal of Phase II therapy is to prevent recurrence of clinical signs. Proactive strategies include allergen-specific immunotherapy, topical glucocorticoids and lokivetmab.

If, during an early stage of an acute flare, pruritus is noticed, then drugs such as lokivetmab or topical glucocorticoids (e.g. hydrocortisone aceponate applied topically on two consecutive days per week) should initially be used. If the flare cannot be controlled, then a change to broad-acting drugs such as oclacitinib or ciclosporin should be considered.

Key points

- Proactive strategies, such as flea prevention, regular topical skin hygiene and allergen-specific immunotherapy, are key to successful management
- When choosing antipruritic pharmacotherapy, consideration should be given to the speed of action and potential side effects of the drug employed and management can evolve over time
- For most animals, multimodal therapy is required, and it should be tailored to the animal's individual needs

---

References and further reading

Forsythe P and Jackson HA (2020) New therapies for atopic dermatitis. *In Practice* **42**, 82–90

Hensel P, Santoro D, Favrot C *et al.* (2015) Canine atopic dermatitis: detailed guidelines for diagnosis and allergen identification. *BMC Veterinary Research* **11**, 196

Koch SN, Torres SM, Plumb DC (2012) *Canine and Feline Dermatology Drug Handbook, 1st edn.* Wiley-Blackwell, Ames

Olivry T, DeBoer DJ, Favrot C *et al.* (2015) Treatment of canine atopic dermatitis: 2015 updated guidelines from the International Committee on Allergic Diseases of Animals (ICADA). *BMC Veterinary Research* **11**, 210

Chapter 11

Allergy testing and allergen-specific immunotherapy – a practical approach

Dawn Logas and Patrick Hensel

Allergy testing

Diseases caused by ectoparasites, secondary microbial skin infections and food-responsive dermatoses (also known as food allergies or adverse food reactions) should, in most cases, be ruled out in patients with non-seasonal pruritus before allergy testing is considered. Due to the lack of standardization and the possible risk of false-positive and false-negative test results, it is not recommended to rely on allergy testing for the diagnosis of allergies. Atopic dermatitis is a clinical diagnosis (see Chapters 9 and 10). The main purpose of an allergy test is to confirm the clinical diagnosis of atopic disease and to identify the clinically relevant allergens. These allergens can then be selected for individualized allergen-specific immunotherapy (ASIT) for that patient. Allergy testing may also be considered in cats with eosinophilic granuloma complex and feline asthma, if environmental allergies are suspected to play a role in the disease.

Once a clinical diagnosis of atopic dermatitis has been made, several factors may play a role in deciding whether an allergy test is necessary:

- Severity of the clinical signs
- Clinical signs that persist for more than 3 months per year
- Sub-optimal management with symptomatic therapy, due to side effects of the drugs used or an unsatisfactory response achieved
- Poor owner or animal compliance with drug therapy
- The client is committed to pursuing ASIT.

The two established allergy tests in veterinary medicine are intradermal testing (IDT) and allergen-specific immunoglobulin (Ig)E serology testing (ASIS). Although IDT is considered the preferred diagnostic method among dermatologists, ASIS has several advantages over IDT, including:

- No patient risk (no sedation required)
- Less traumatic (no repeated injection required)
- More convenient (no clipping needed, less time-consuming).

ASIS also seems to be less affected by concurrent anti-inflammatory/antipruritic therapy. However, ASIS only measures circulating allergen-specific IgE, does not take into account other allergic pathways, and often shows positive reactions in non-allergic animals. Multi-positive results to plant pollens are also commonly observed in serology testing, due to cross-reacting carbohydrate determinants (CCDs).

IDT and ASIS are still lacking standardization and it is suspected that false-positive and false-negative test results do occur. It is estimated that between 10 and 30% of dogs and cats with clinically confirmed atopic disease may also have a negative allergy test. The significant number of negative test results may be due to factors such as improper technique, the test concentration of allergens being too low, drug interference, intrinsic host factors, age, incorrect selection of allergens, IDT performed too long after (>60 days) or during the peak allergy season, and the presence of a condition called atopic-like dermatitis. Atopic-like disease is clinically identical to atopic dermatitis, but the IgE response to environmental or other allergens cannot be documented. It is possible that other pathomechanisms, such as lymphocyte-mediated reactions, may play a role. IDT and ASIS are very different test methods, which inevitably leads to poor correlation of test results. Nonetheless, the success rate of ASIT based on ASIS *versus* IDT appears similar. When allergy testing is performed, it is important to be aware of possible cross-reactions between related allergens such as house dust and storage mites as well as various grasses, which may not necessarily be clinically relevant. For this reason, it is important to determine whether the tested patient was really exposed to the allergen(s) to which reactions were seen. The proper interpretation of these test results, in conjunction with the clinical history and clinical presentation, can be complex and time-consuming. Referral to a veterinary dermatologist should therefore be considered.

Intradermal testing

IDT is an indirect measure of cutaneous mast cell reactivity and the interaction of the cells with allergen-specific IgE. The appropriate selection of allergens to test is critical to obtain reliable IDT results. Pollens especially are subject to great geographical variability. Therefore, it is important for veterinary surgeons (veterinarians) performing IDT to identify and test with the allergens present in the patient's regional location. Information about relevant allergens can be obtained via veterinary dermatologists, veterinary and medical schools, allergy laboratories, textbooks, local human allergists, the weather bureau and various national pollen count websites.

From time to time, the overall IDT results should be assessed if using this technique in practice and allergens that do not commonly elicit a reaction may be replaced with other possibly more relevant allergens. Intradermal test concentrations may also need to be adjusted since various different test concentrations have been suggested (Figure 11.1). Allergens are relatively stable once diluted and can be stored in glass vials for up to 8 weeks and in plastic syringes for up to 2 weeks at 4°C. The test solutions should be removed from the refrigerator just prior to IDT and allowed to reach room temperature before use. As mentioned above, the selection of test allergens should be made based on the prevalence of the allergens in a specific geographical region. However, the selection of test allergens is often based on personal preference and experience and can vary significantly among dermatologists even within the same geographical region.

IDT is usually performed under light sedation to prevent stress, which may increase blood cortisol levels, and to minimize discomfort. In dogs, the most commonly used sedatives are: medetomidine (10 µg/kg i.v.), dexmedetomidine (150 µg/m² i.v.), a combination of xylazine hydrochloride (0.25–0.5 mg/kg i.v.) and atropine sulphate or zolazepam (4 mg/kg i.v.). In cats, sedation is usually performed with ketamine (10 mg/kg i.v.), ketamine (5 mg/kg i.v.) and diazepam (0.25 mg/kg i.v.), zolazepam, medetomidine or a general gas anaesthesia. If analgesia is desired, then butorphanol can be added.

Intradermal injections are most commonly performed on the lateral thorax, after the hair has been gently clipped and the injection sites marked (minimum 2 cm apart). Generally, a volume of 0.05–0.1 ml of each test concentration is injected intradermally and evaluated after 15–20 minutes. The reaction at each injection site should be compared between those of the positive (histamine phosphate) and negative (saline with phenol) controls. Histamine is used at 1:10,000 w/v (0.1 mg/ml) in Europe and at 1:100,000 w/v (0.01 mg/ml) in the USA; it should be noted that the more concentrated histamine solution (1:10,000) may yield a more consistent positive skin reaction. The negative control should consist of the solution used to dilute the allergens for IDT; this is generally sterile saline with phenol as preservative. The reaction can be interpreted subjectively and/or objectively. For subjective evaluation, the intensity and/or size of the erythema, turgidity and/or wheal formation should be assessed, whereas for objective evaluation, the mean diameter of the area of erythema or wheal formation should be measured. By convention, an allergen reaction is considered positive when the wheal formed is at least equal to or greater than

halfway between the negative and the positive control reactions. If the subjective evaluation is undertaken, the positive control will assume a conventional grade of 4, whereas the negative control will be graded as 0. A reaction to an allergen is considered positive if it is graded as 2 or greater.

Performing and interpreting IDT in cats can be more challenging. The cat's skin is thinner, which increases the risk of injecting the allergen test solution subcutaneously. Skin reactions in cats are often very subtle and appear and fade quickly, which makes interpretation more difficult. Skin test reactions in cats should be assessed as early as 5 minutes after injection.

Allergen-specific immunoglobulin E serology testing

Several assays, mostly based on solid phase enzyme-linked immunosorbent assays (ELISAs), have been tested for allergen-specific serum IgE in both human and veterinary medicine. These assays are used to detect IgE antibodies specific for a panel of allergens (e.g. pollens, moulds, house dust mites and epidermal extracts) considered relevant for the patient. In the past, monoclonal, mixed monoclonal and polyclonal anti-canine IgE have been used to detect allergen-specific IgE antibodies in the serum. However, due to the higher sensitivity and specificity, monoclonal antibodies are most commonly used nowadays.

An alternative veterinary assay uses a unique recombinant fragment of the extracellular portion of the human high affinity IgE receptor alpha-subunit (FcεRIα); this has a strong affinity for canine IgE and does not bind with IgG. There is also the option of an in-clinic immunodot assay (Allercept©, Heska Corporation), which can be used as a screening test. This contains a mixture of flea, house dust mite and pollen allergens and is designed to be used as an indicator as to whether a full serum allergy panel or intradermal testing should be performed. This screening test has a high probability of predicting positive results; however, since it contains mixed allergens, it does not replace performing a complete allergy test.

Another problem that might be encountered with ASIS is multiple positive results to pollen and other allergens. This has been attributed to CCDs. These are highly antigenic, carbohydrate structures commonly found on plants and insects to which individuals may mount a specific IgE response. Importantly, these are not thought to be clinically relevant and, when present on an allergy test, should be interpreted as a false-positive result. The prevalence of CCDs in dogs and cats appears to range between 25 and 70%. A CCD-blocker has been developed (Heska Corporation), which can be employed when false-positive results are suspected, and this significantly improves the quality of the test results.

Currently, many companies are offering allergen-specific serology testing, but test results often show a significant variation between laboratories, which reflects the different detection systems used, allergen sources and cut off values employed.

Miscellaneous

Many laboratories offer allergen-specific IgE panels for food allergens, despite the fact that there are multiple studies that show that IDT and ASIS are not reliable for the diagnosis of food-responsive dermatosis. For this reason,

Allergen	Recommended dilution for IDT
Histamine	1:100,000 to 1:10,000 w/v
Pollens and moulds	1000–8000 PNU/ml
Individual dust mites: • *Dermatophagoides pteronyssinus* • *Dermatophagoides farinae*, *Tyrophagus putrescentiae*, *Lepidoglyphus destructor* • *Acarus siro*, *Blomia tropicalis*	100–250 PNU/ml 75–250 PNU/ml 50–250 PNU/ml
Epidermal extracts (hair, wool, feathers, dander)	250–1250 PNU/ml
Insects	1000–1750 PNU/ml
Whole flea extract	1:1,000 to 1:500 w/v

11.1 Recommended intradermal testing (IDT) concentrations. PNU = protein nitrogen units; w/v = weight to volume.

such serology tests should not be used. Other forms of allergy testing, such as prick or patch testing, which are well established in human medicine, have either not been validated in veterinary medicine, or, in the case of patch testing, are not practical to use in the clinic.

Various drugs, such as antihistamines, glucocorticoids, progestational compounds, beta 2 adrenergic agonists, bronchodilators and tricyclic antidepressants, can inhibit the release of histamine and possibly other inflammatory mediators, inducing false-negative allergy test results. As a consequence, withdrawal of commonly used anti-inflammatory drugs prior to allergy testing is recommended (Figure 11.2). Ciclosporin, oclacitinib and lokivetmab, on the other hand, do not appear to affect the results of allergy testing.

Drug	Withdrawal time
Antihistamines	7 days
Short-acting oral glucocorticoids	14 days
Long-acting injectable glucocorticoids	At least 28 days
Topical glucocorticoids	14 days

11.2 Withdrawal times for common anti-inflammatory drugs. Withdrawal time may vary due to duration of treatment, dosage and type of drugs and it should be observed for both allergen-specific intradermal testing and IgE serology testing.

Allergen-specific immunotherapy

ASIT is defined as the process of administering allergen extracts to a patient in order to decrease their degree of hypersensitivity and reduce the immunological response to environmental allergens. It is still the only currently available therapy for canine and feline atopic dermatitis that can change the course of the disease, as well as provide a chance of cure. The sections below explain what we know about ASIT and how it can be used in general practice.

Allergens

The allergens used for ASIT are natural extracts of pollens, moulds and insects. In the USA, aqueous extracts with phenol as a preservative are most commonly used for subcutaneous ASIT. In Europe and the UK, alum precipitated extracts are used more often. For sublingual ASIT, the allergens are mixed in a 50% glycerine solution. Some sublingual ASIT contains additives that help the allergens adhere to the mucous membranes longer, although there is little published evidence to support this claim.

Mould and insect extracts may contain high concentrations of proteases. These proteases have been shown to degrade certain grass and tree allergens. Some dermatologists place moulds and insects into a separate vial when using aqueous extracts to minimize this proteolysis. Glycerine inhibits the activity of proteases, so moulds and insects can be mixed with pollens when using glycerinated extracts.

In human medicine, the proteins that are considered the major cause of the allergic symptoms for some of the more common pollens are known. Allergen extracts are then standardized with a known quantity of these proteins. In veterinary medicine, non-standardized allergens are still used to make ASIT, which means the proteins that act as the primary allergens are either not known or not measured. The allergy units most commonly used in veterinary medicine are weight per volume (w/v) and protein nitrogen units (PNUs). Both of these units are based on the total micrograms of both allergenic and non-allergenic protein in the extract.

Allergen selection and administration
Selection
Allergen selection for immunotherapy should not be based solely on the strength of a patient's reaction on an intradermal or serum-based allergy test (although recommendations from many companies are based only on this parameter). Other factors that must be considered include the time of year the patient is affected, the severity of the clinical signs during different seasons, and the characteristics of each patient's indoor and outdoor environment. The clinician must also be familiar with most allergenic plants and their pollination schedules for the local area. These airborne pollens can diffuse over many miles, so it is not just plants in the patient's immediate vicinity that are important but those within at least a 15 mile radius. Much of this information can be found on the internet or is available from companies that supply allergens and perform serum allergy testing.

When selecting pollens for inclusion in ASIT, it is important to cover all seasons in which the patient has clinical signs. If the patient's reaction is worse at certain times of the year, more pollens from the season when the patient is more severely affected should be included. The cross-reactivity of pollens should also be taken into account when considering which allergens to include, particularly if the number of allergens is high. However, it is important to remember this is based on human data. To help determine whether indoor allergens should be included in the vial, it is crucial to have information about the patient's indoor environment. House dust mites are ubiquitous, but favour environments with carpets, rugs and fabric furniture. They also prefer homes in areas of higher humidity with no air conditioning. Moulds also like moisture. They are typically present in older structures, particularly those with basements or cellars, but are also common allergens in the outdoor environment in certain temperate geographical areas.

Administration
ASIT can be administered either by subcutaneous injection or as sublingual allergy drops. Subcutaneous ASIT has been used in veterinary medicine for over 70 years, whilst sublingual ASIT has been available for at least the last 10 years. The optimal number and concentration of each allergen for ASIT, as well as the optimal monthly dose, remains unknown for veterinary patients. Thus, all doses are currently calculated on convention.

Subcutaneous injection: For subcutaneous ASIT, on average 10–15 allergens are included in the vial, although some dermatologists routinely include 30 or more allergens. The typical concentration of a maintenance vaccine is 20,000 PNU/ml, but can be up to 40,000 PNU/ml. Most protocols involve a gradual build up to the maintenance dose, typically over 4–12 weeks. However, rush immunotherapy, in which the maintenance dose is reached in 1 day, is sometimes used. Patients are hospitalized and monitored closely for anaphylaxis during this process.

Adverse reactions are rare, even with rush immunotherapy. Most patients are maintained on 1.0–1.5 ml of ASIT monthly. The entire dose may be given once a month or may be divided into smaller weekly or biweekly doses. The dose and frequency should be tailored to suit the individual patient.

Sublingual drops: There is less information of the recommendations for sublingual ASIT. Some companies that prepare sublingual ASIT do not release the concentration of allergens in the vaccine. In the authors' practice, the total monthly dose of allergens is the same for both sublingual and subcutaneous ASIT. The allergen concentration of the maintenance vaccine is 10,000 PNU/ml and the dose is 0.1 ml daily. Sublingual immunotherapy is typically given twice daily (Figure 11.3). It is absorbed by the oral mucosa and should not be swallowed, thus the co-administration of treats is not advised. Although generally well tolerated, some dogs and cats are not amenable to this form of ASIT.

Effectiveness

Most information on the effectiveness of immunotherapy in dogs comes from retrospective studies of subcutaneous ASIT. In these studies, successful treatment was defined as at least a 50% decrease in pruritus and 50–77% of patients met this criterion (Mueller, 2019). The few double-blinded placebo-controlled studies of subcutaneous ASIT in dogs reported a 44–60% efficacy rate after 9–12 months of treatment. The problem with all these studies is that there is no consistency in the dosage of ASIT, type of allergens used (aqueous or alum) or length of the study. Until further information is available, an estimate of a 60–70% response rate to subcutaneous ASIT in dogs in reasonable. There is even less information available about sublingual immunotherapy in dogs and ASIT in general in cats.

The length of time it will take for ASIT to be effective and how long a patient should continue this treatment is not known for either dogs or cats. This is also true for human patients. On average, for humans, it takes 6–12 months for ASIT to begin working and it may take several years to reach full effectiveness. For veterinary patients, the authors normally tell clients not to expect much

change for the first 3–6 months. ASIT should reach its full effect for most patients by 18 months, although in some canine patients it can take 2–3 years before ASIT is completely effective. The authors currently advise owners to expect sublingual ASIT to perform similarly to subcutaneous ASIT, although there are few studies to support these recommendations (Fischer et al., 2020). The authors also inform owners that this is usually a lifelong treatment.

Adverse reactions

The short-term adverse effects of ASIT are usually dose-related and controllable, but there are a very small number of patients that do not tolerate immunotherapy. These adverse effects are seen with both sublingual and subcutaneous ASIT. The most common short-term adverse effect is increased pruritus. This is typically seen during the induction phase and occurs 1–24 hours after the ASIT dose has been administered. To combat the increased pruritus, the dose administered can be decreased and the time taken to reach the maintenance dose lengthened. The administration of antihistamines prior to the ASIT dose can also help decrease pruritus. However, some patients are never able to tolerate the standard maintenance dose and need to remain at a lower dose to present this adverse effect. This is acceptable if the lower dose is able to control the clinical signs. If the patient is undergoing subcutaneous ASIT and the pruritus continues, switching to sublingual ASIT sometimes helps. Conversely, if a patient being treated with sublingual ASIT has chronic oral/perioral pruritus or facial oedema, subcutaneous ASIT may be a better choice.

Anaphylaxis is very uncommon but may occur with ASIT and fatalities are extremely rare. In the authors' practice, it is recommended that the client observe the patient for at least 1 hour after subcutaneous immunotherapy has been administered or for 15 minutes following sublingual ASIT. In most patient, the first signs of anaphylactic shock are vomiting and diarrhoea; if these occur, the client should be instructed to bring the patient back to the clinic immediately. It should be noted that even if the patient has an anaphylactic reaction, it does not mean that ASIT cannot continue to be used. If the patient is undergoing subcutaneous ASIT, they can be switched to sublingual administration. If the patient is already on sublingual ASIT, then the dose can be decreased by half in the long-term. These patients should be monitored closely. In the authors' practice, these patients are pre-medicated with antihistamines and have corticosteroids available at home for emergencies.

The long-term safety profile for ASIT is good and there appears to be no deleterious effects on the liver, kidneys or immune system.

Talking to clients

When discussing ASIT with clients, it is imperative that they understand atopic dermatitis is a chronic disease that, in most cases, will require lifelong therapy. In addition, it is important owners are advised that many patients cannot be maintained with just one therapy, including immunotherapy. The goal is to have the patient on the safest and least expensive long-term treatment possible. The long-term cost of ASIT is usually less than that of any of the currently available drugs for the symptomatic treatment of atopic dermatitis, with the exception of corticosteroids.

In the case of ASIT, it is important to set realistic expectations. ASIT may not completely control the clinical

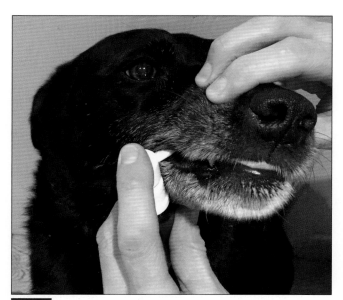

11.3 Administration of sublingual immunotherapy to a dog.

signs, but might effectively decrease the reliance on other medications to manage the associated pruritus and secondary infections. Clients must understand that ASIT does not take effect immediately; it normally takes a minimum of 3–6 months to start seeing an improvement with ASIT, thus it is necessary to keep the patient on symptomatic therapy during this time to stay comfortable. Clients should be given particular goals or endpoints to reach during therapy. Withdrawing symptomatic therapy after a patient has been on ASIT for 2–3 months should be considered. If the patient flares, symptomatic therapy can be restarted and the test tried again following another 2–3 months' treatment. If after 18 months the client feels that ASIT has not made any difference to the patient's quality of life, the treatment should be withdrawn to see if any of the clinical signs worsen. It may be helpful to have handouts for clients to take home that details most of this information (Figures 11.4 and 11.5).

- Allergen-specific immunotherapy (ASIT/allergy vaccine) is beneficial for about 70% of our allergic patients. This is the best long-term treatment option available for allergic patients.
- Improvement is usually seen 3–6 months after starting the treatment; however, some patients may take as long as 12 months to respond.
- In most cases, hyposensitization is a **lifelong therapy**. In patients that have stopped the treatment early, there is a greater than 50% incidence of relapse. For this reason, we usually recommend decreasing the frequency of the therapy instead of stopping completely.
- Some pets may need other therapies in conjunction with hyposensitization, especially during the first year.
- The vials should be kept refrigerated. Do NOT freeze.
- A new needle and syringe should be used with each injection. Injections should be given underneath the skin (subcutaneously). Dispose of used syringes in a sharps container. Return full containers to the veterinary clinic for proper disposal.
- Your pet should not receive a major meal near the time of the injection, but a snack or treat after the injection is recommended.
- Observe your dog for 1–2 hours after the injection, especially during the initial phase of the protocol. Severe reactions are very rare. If your pet vomits, has diarrhoea, develops hives or facial swelling, becomes ataxic (drunken gait), has laboured breathing or collapses, veterinary help should be sought immediately.
- If your pet becomes itchy or has a flare up after the injections, please call us. We will adjust the hyposensitization dose as necessary.
- Please call us with a progress report every 3 months and schedule a clinic visit for your pet every 3–6 months during the first year, so that we may evaluate your pet's progress.
- Please do not hesitate to call us with any questions.
- This treatment is custom-made for your pet and may take 7–10 business days to process, so please call for a refill before you give your last injection.

11.4 Owner instructions for the administration of subcutaneous immunotherapy.

- Sublingual ASIT (allergy drops) is successful for about 70% of our allergic patients and is one of the best long-term treatment options available for allergic patients.
- Improvement is usually seen 3–6 months after starting the drops. However, some patients may take as long as 12 months to respond.
- In most cases, allergy drops are a **lifelong therapy**.
- In some cases, pets may need other therapies in conjunction with the drops, especially during the first year.
- The vials should be kept refrigerated. Do NOT freeze.
- Your pet should not receive anything orally (food, treats or water) for 10 minutes after administering the drops, so they can absorb into the mouth's mucous membranes. The drops have a sweet taste and should not be offensive to your pet.
- Observe your pet for 15–20 minutes after administering the drops, especially during the initial phase of the protocol. Severe reactions are extremely rare. If your pet vomits, has diarrhoea, develops hives or facial swelling, becomes ataxic (drunken gait), has laboured breathing or collapses, veterinary help should be sought immediately.
- If your pet becomes itchy or has a flare up after the receiving the drops, please call us. We will adjust the dosing schedule as necessary.
- Please call us with a progress report every 3 months and schedule a clinic visit for your pet every 3–6 months during the first year, so that we may evaluate your pet's progress.
- Please do not hesitate to call us with any questions.
- The SASI (allergy drops) are custom-made for your pet and can take up to 10 days to prepare so please call for a refill before you run out.

11.5 Owner instructions for the administration of sublingual allergen-specific immunotherapy (ASIT).

Key points

- Allergy testing is indicated after commitment from the client to pursue ASIT for their pet
- Test results should be interpreted in the context of the patient's exposure and should take into consideration potential allergen cross-reactions
- ASIT is a safe and often effective long-term treatment and the only therapy which can change the course of the disease

References and further reading

Fischer NM, Rostaher A and Favrot C (2020) A comparative study of subcutaneous, intralymphatic and sublingual immunotherapy for the long-term control of dogs with nonseasonal atopic dermatitis. *Veterinary Dermatology* **31**, 365–e96

Gram D (2014) Greer allergy immunotherapy compendium. https://www.stagrallergy.com/resources/

Hensel P, Santoro D, Favrot C et al. (2015) Canine atopic dermatitis: detailed guidelines for diagnosis and allergen identification. *BMC Veterinary Research* **11**, 196

Miller WH, Griffin CE and Campbell LC (2013) In: *Muller and Kirk's Small Animal Dermatology, 7th edn.* pp. 373–380 and 390–391, Elsevier Saunders, St. Louis

Mueller RS (2019) Update on allergen immunotherapy. *Veterinary Clinics of North America: Small Animal Practice* **49**, 1–7

Mueller RS, Jensen-Jarolim E, Roth-Walter F et al. (2018) Allergen immunotherapy in people, dogs, cats and horses–differences, similarities and research needs. *Allergy* **73**, 1989–1999

Chapter 12

An approach to scaling

Karen L. Campbell

Excessive scaling is common in dogs and occasionally seen in cats. Scales are composed of exfoliated corneocytes that accumulate on the surface of the skin and within the hair coat as flakes ('dandruff') or extrude from the hair follicles as keratinous plugs (follicular casts). Normal epidermal homeostasis requires finely tuned regulation of keratinocyte growth (epidermopoiesis) and differentiation (keratinization), which leads to the formation of surface corneocytes that then desquamate. Disruption of epidermal homeostasis often results in disordered keratinization and scale formation. Scaling disorders are classified as primary when excess scale formation is a result of genetic abnormalities and secondary when another disease process secondarily affects epidermal proliferation, keratinization, cornification or desquamation.

Seborrhoea is a non-specific term used to describe the clinical signs of excessive scaling: dry scaling (seborrhoea sicca; Figure 12.1ab), greasiness (seborrhoea oleosa; Figure 12.1c) and crusting (seborrhoeic dermatitis; Figure 12.1d). Excessive scaling ('dandruff') is a common presenting complaint in dogs, but is not as common in cats, perhaps owing to their propensity for more meticulous self-grooming. The hair coat may be dry and lusterless with follicular casts (Figure 12.1e); in these cases the scale derived from the upper hair follicle becomes adherent to the hairs. In some animals, patches of greasy, malodorous skin may be present associated with secondary skin infections. It should be noted that secondary skin infections are common due to the impaired integrity of the skin barrier associated with most disorders. Other clinical signs of keratinization disorders include acne, alopecia, calluses, nasal hyperkeratosis, footpad hyperkeratosis, ear margin dermatosis, ceruminous otitis externa and tail gland hyperplasia.

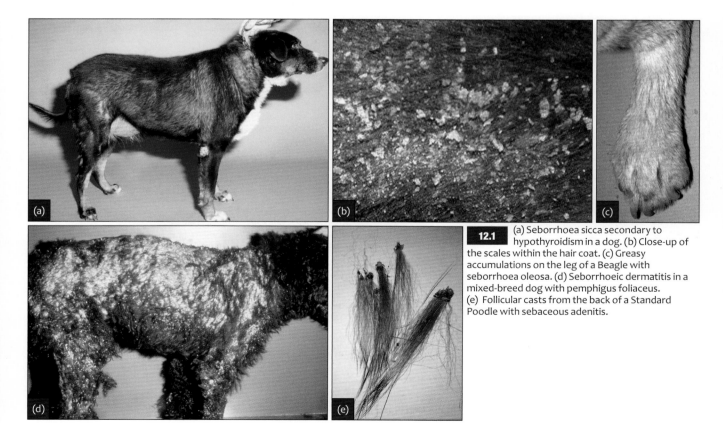

12.1 (a) Seborrhoea sicca secondary to hypothyroidism in a dog. (b) Close-up of the scales within the hair coat. (c) Greasy accumulations on the leg of a Beagle with seborrhoea oleosa. (d) Seborrhoeic dermatitis in a mixed-breed dog with pemphigus foliaceus. (e) Follicular casts from the back of a Standard Poodle with sebaceous adenitis.

Differential diagnosis

Primary keratinization disorders are hereditary and therefore many are associated with certain breeds of dogs and cats (Figure 12.2). In these disorders, excessive amounts of scale result from a defect in the processes of keratinization, cornification or sebaceous gland activity. It is important to be familiar with the clinical presentation of these disorders and their respective breed predispositions to recognize and diagnose the conditions, and to advise owners on the hereditary nature of these diseases (affected animals should be neutered). The diagnosis of primary keratinization disorders is based on early age of onset, knowledge of breed predisposition, history and physical examination findings, genetic testing (when available), ruling out secondary causes of seborrhoea and skin biopsy (dermatohistopathology).

Almost any skin disease can affect keratinization, resulting in secondary scaling (Figure 12.16). The potential causes should be prioritized on the basis of the animal's signalment, history, clinical signs, distribution of lesions and other physical examination findings.

Disorder	Breeds predisposed	Comments
Dogs		
Acrodermatitis of Bull Terriers (Figure 12.3)	Bull Terrier, Miniature Bull Terrier	Autosomal recessive metabolic disease with defects in zinc and/or copper absorption and metabolism. Affected dogs have progressive dermatitis with erythematous, exfoliative lesions on distal extremities, mucocutaneous junctions, muzzle and pinnae; footpads are hyperkeratotic with fissures, dystrophic claws and splayed toes. Chronic diarrhoea, bronchopneumonia and behavioural abnormalities are also common. Mean survival is 7 months
Canine acne	Short-coated breeds with bristly hair coats: Boxer, Dobermann, English Bulldog, German Shorthaired Pointer, Great Dane, Mastiff, Weimaraner,	Age of onset usually <6 months. Lesions on chin and lower lip consist of follicular papules, pustules, nodules and in some cases fistulas; occasionally comedones also present
Canine ear margin seborrhoea (Figure 12.4)	Dachshund, dogs with pendulous ears	Adherent keratinous deposits on medial and lateral margins of pinnae, partial alopecia and occasionally a seborrhoeic odour
Canine primary idiopathic seborrhoea	Basset Hound, Cavalier King Charles Spaniel, Chinese Shar Pei, Cocker Spaniel, Dachshund, Dobermann, English Springer Spaniel, German Shepherd Dog, Irish Setter, Labrador Retriever, Miniature Schnauzer, West Highland White Terrier	Early age of onset is a clue for primary seborrhoea; lesions increase in severity with age. Rule out secondary causes of seborrhoea (diagnose following exclusion of other causes)
Congenital follicular parakeratosis	Labrador Retriever, Rottweiler, Siberian Husky	Generalized exfoliative dermatitis with thick keratinous follicular casts, secondary bacterial and yeast skin infections. Lesions on muzzle and pinnae may be present at birth and rapidly increase in severity
Dermatomyositis	Collies (Rough and Smooth), Shetland Sheepdog	Dermatomyositis (DM) is an immune-mediated disease of the skin and muscle with development influenced by both genetic and environmental factors. Skin lesions usually develop in young dogs; however, sometimes they do not occur until later in life. Scaling, crusting and hair loss most commonly affect the face, ears, feet, legs and the tip of the tail
Epidermal dysplasia (Figure 12.5)	West Highland White Terrier	May be a hereditary exaggerated response to *Malassezia* infection or hypersensitivity. Dogs usually have atopic dermatitis. Clinical signs often develop by 6--12 months of age and include greasy hair coat, severe pruritus, erythema, alopecia, scaling, crusting, lichenification and hyperpigmentation of the face, feet, limbs and ventrum. Ceruminous otitis externa is also common. Large numbers of *Malassezia* are usually found on skin cytology
Epidermolytic ichthyosis (Figure 12.6)	Labrador Retriever, Norfolk Terrier, Rhodesian Ridgeback	Genetic defects in keratin synthesis result in an abnormal cytoskeleton and lysis of keratinocytes. Clinical signs may include areas of erosions and cobblestone-like, hyperpigmented skin in other areas
Exfoliative cutaneous lupus erythematosus	German Shorthaired Pointer	Age of onset is 5–7 months, lesions begin on head and back and often generalize. Dogs have other clinical signs. This is likely a form of hereditary lupus
Familial footpad hyperkeratosis (digital hyperkeratosis) (Figure 12.7)	Dogue de Bordeaux, Golden Retriever, Irish Terrier, Kerry Blue Terrier, Kromfohrländer, Labrador Retriever mixed-breed dogs	Severe keratinous proliferations on surface of all footpads, some may be horn-like. Lameness is common. Lesions develop in puppies
Hereditary nasal parakeratosis	Labrador Retriever	Lesions appear in young dogs (<1 year); develop dry, adherent keratinous debris on nasal planum; crusts on nose may be grey or brown
Lichenoid psoriasiform dermatosis	English Springer Spaniel	May be a hereditary exaggerated response to staphylococcal skin infections. Multiple erythematous hyperkeratotic papules and plaques develop on the inner pinnae and on the skin of the ventral abdomen, inguinal area and prepuce (males)

12.2 Primary scaling disorders. (continues) ▶

Disorder	Breeds predisposed	Comments
Non-epidermolytic ichthyosis (Figures 12.8 and 12.9)	American Bulldog, Australian Terrier, Boston Terrier, Cairn Terrier, Collie, Dobermann, Golden Retriever, Irish Setter, Labrador Retriever, Manchester Terrier, Norfolk Terrier, Parson Russell Terrier, Pit Bull Terrier, Soft Coated Wheaten Terrier, West Highland White Terrier, Yorkshire Terrier	Many causes have been reported, including defects in transglutaminase I expression and activity, defects in intercellular lipids and defects in the cornified envelope. Clinical signs may include tightly adherent scales, keratin debris adherent to hairs and a sparse hair coat. Variably severity and distribution. Genetic tests available for some breeds (see text)
Schnauzer comedone syndrome	Miniature Schnauzer	Comedones develop in a band along dorsal midline, hairs may appear darker and more erect, crusted papules and distended follicular ostia may be seen
Vitamin A-responsive dermatosis	Cocker Spaniel (most common breed affected), Labrador Retriever, Miniature Schnauzer	Affects adult dogs (later age of onset than most primary disorders of keratinization). Clinical signs include follicular papules, follicular casts and multifocal erythematous alopecic plaques, most prominent on the ventral and lateral chest and abdomen. Ceruminous otitis and a rancid odour are also common
Zinc-responsive dermatosis: syndrome I (Figure 12.10)	Alaskan Malamute, Samoyed, Siberian Husky	May have inherited impaired zinc absorption or metabolism. Clinical signs develop between 1 and 3 years of age and include erythema, alopecia, scales and thick adherent crusts involving mucocutaneous junctions and pressure points
Zinc-responsive dermatosis: syndrome II	Seen in rapidly-growing large-breed puppies	Clinical signs include thick, well-demarcated plaques and crusts in the periocular, perioral and genital regions
Dogs and cats		
Nasodigital hyperkeratosis (Figure 12.11)	Basset Hound, Beagle, Cocker Spaniel Bengal cat	Increases in severity with age (late middle-aged to older dogs), lesions may involve either the nasal planum or footpads or both. Prominent, dry, adherent keratinous accumulations may accentuate normal cobblestone pattern or may develop into keratinous proliferations on nose and around the margins of footpads
Sebaceous adenitis (Figures 12.12 and 12.13)	Akita (common), Beagle, Boxer, Chow Chow, Collie, Dachshund, German Shepherd Dog, Havanese, Lhasa Apso, Miniature Pinscher, Old English Sheepdog, Plott Hound, Samoyed (common), Springer Spaniel, Standard Poodle (common), Toy Poodle, Vizsla (common), mixed-breed dogs Cats (rare)	Autosomal recessive inheritance proposed in the Standard Poodle and Akita. Clinical signs include adherent scales, follicular casts and poor hair coat. Lesions most severe on dorsal trunk, temporal region, face and pinnae. Occasional 'rat-tail'. Rarely see focal coalescing firm nodules, annular plaques or facial swelling
Cats		
Feline acne (Figure 12.14)	All breeds	May be cyclic in association with telogen phase of hair cycle; comedones, papules and pustules develop on the chin and occasionally on the lips; dark flakes of keratinous debris may be present. Variable erythema and oedema, occasional nodules, pustules or fistulas
Feline idiopathic facial dermatitis (Figure 12.15)	Persian (including Himalayan)	Thick black exudate and crusts around eyes, mouth and chin. Some also have black waxy debris in ear canals. May be pruritic, often develop secondary bacterial and yeast infections
Feline primary idiopathic seborrhoea	Persian (including Himalayan)	Kittens may have a dirty appearance apparent by 2–3 days of age. Hairs appear curly and are pasted together by keratoseborrhoeic material with a rancid odour. Ceruminous otitis externa is common

12.2 (continued) Primary scaling disorders.

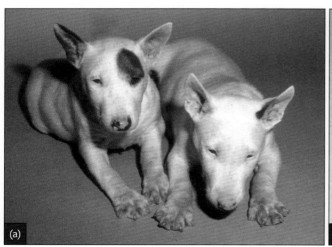
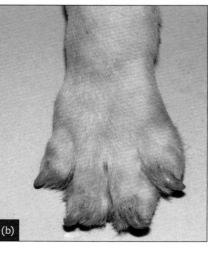

12.3 (a) Bull Terrier puppies with lethal acrodermatitis. (b) Splayed toes of an affected Bull Terrier puppy.

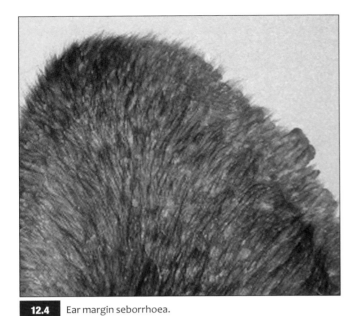

12.4 Ear margin seborrhoea.

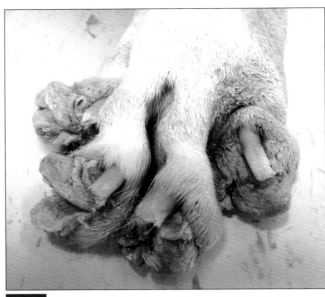

12.7 Severe footpad hyperkeratosis in a mixed-breed dog.

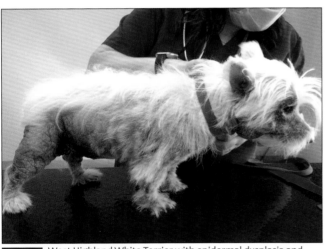

12.5 West Highland White Terrier with epidermal dysplasia and *Malassezia* dermatitis.

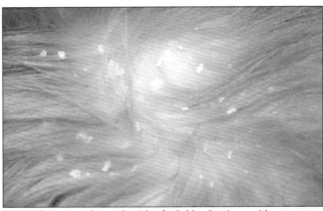

12.8 Large scales on the side of a Golden Retriever with non-epidermolytic ichthyosis.

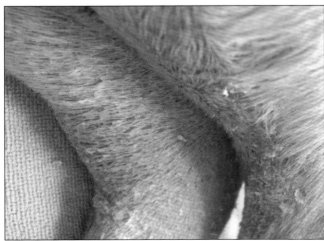

12.6 Scales on the rear legs of a mixed-breed dog with epidermolytic ichthyosis.

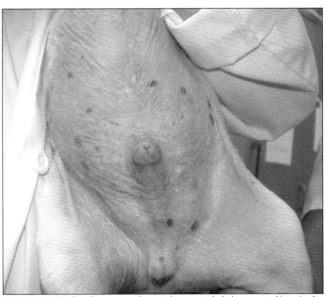

12.9 Tightly adherent scales on the ventral abdomen and inguinal region of a 10-week-old American Bulldog with non-epidermolytic ichthyosis.

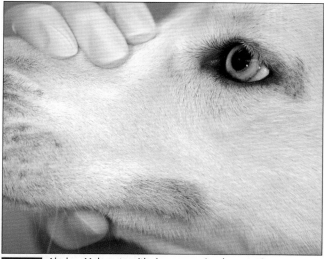

12.10 Alaskan Malamute with zinc-responsive dermatosis: syndrome I.

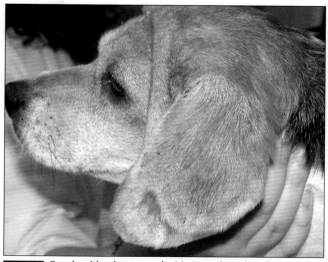

12.13 Beagle with sebaceous adenitis. Note the polycyclic pattern of alopecia on the ear pinna.

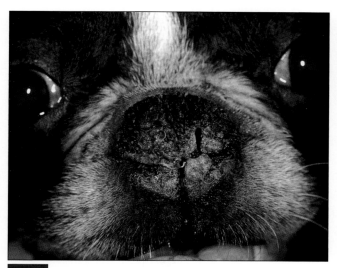

12.11 Nasal hyperkeratosis in a Boston Terrier.

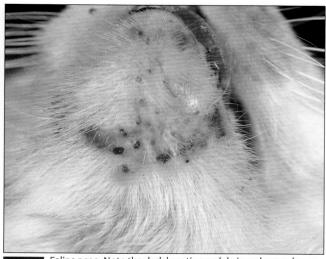

12.14 Feline acne. Note the dark keratinous debris and comedones on the chin.

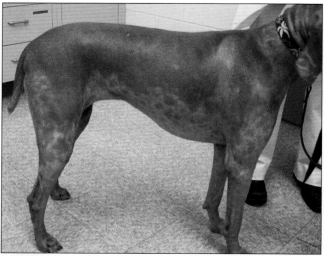

12.12 Vizsla with sebaceous adenitis. Note the polycyclic pattern of alopecia.

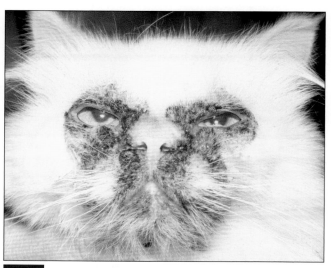

12.15 Idiopathic facial dermatitis in a 1-year-old Persian.

Parasites

- Fleas
- *Demodex*
- *Sarcoptes*
- *Notoedres*
- *Cheyletiella*
- *Otodectes*
- Lice

Allergies

- Flea allergy dermatitis
- Atopic dermatitis
- Food-responsive dermatosis
  - Also known as a food allergy or adverse food reaction
- Contact hypersensitivity
- Adverse drug reactions

Infection

- Bacteria
- *Malassezia*
- Dermatophytes
- *Leishmania*
- Viruses
  - Feline immunodeficiency virus
  - Feline leukaemia virus
  - Canine distemper

Nutritional

- Fatty acid deficiency (rare)
- Protein deficiency (rare)
- Zinc deficiency
- Dietary imbalances

Endocrinopathy

- Hypothyroidism
- Hyperadrenocorticism
- Sex hormone imbalances
- Diabetes mellitus
- Growth hormone-responsive dermatosis

Metabolic disorders

- Superficial necrolytic dermatitis
  - Hepatocutaneous syndrome
- Malabsorption/maldigestion
- Liver disease

Hair follicle disorders

- Black hair follicle dysplasia
- Colour dilution alopecia
- Follicular dysplasia
  - Alopecia X
- Pattern baldness

Immune-mediated disorders

- Pemphigus foliaceus
- Cutaneous lupus erythematosus
- Systemic lupus erythematosus
- Cutaneous drug reactions

Neoplastic diseases

- Epitheliotrophic lymphoma

Paraneoplastic disorders

- Thymoma-associated exfoliative dermatosis (Figure 12.17)

Environmental disorders

- Low humidity
- Degreasing shampoos
- Contact irritants

12.16 Secondary scaling disorders.

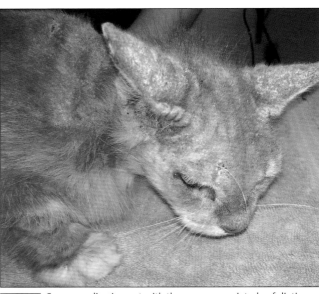

12.17 Severe scaling in a cat with thymoma-associated exfoliative dermatosis.

Clinical approach

History

The history may provide important clues. Pruritus is associated with many secondary causes of scaling (e.g. allergies, parasites). Dogs with primary keratinization disorders may also be pruritic; however, the pruritus is usually associated with secondary skin infections and abates when the infections are treated. Primary keratinization disorders are non-seasonal while some secondary causes of scaling (e.g. fleas, pollen allergies) are seasonal. Other clues in the history may include polyuria, polydipsia and polyphagia with hyperadrenocorticism, or heat-seeking and lethargy with hypothyroidism.

Signalment

Signalment can also be helpful in prioritizing differential diagnoses. Breed predispositions are recognized for the majority of primary keratinization disorders, as well as for many of the secondary causes of scaling (e.g. atopic dermatitis, hypothyroidism and hyperadrenocorticism). The majority of primary keratinization disorders are evident before 1 year of age, whilst clinical signs of atopic dermatitis generally appear between 1 and 3 years of age, and endocrinopathies are most common in middle-aged to older animals.

Lesion distribution

Certain lesion distributions are highly suggestive of various primary and secondary keratinization disorders.

- Examples of site-specific primary keratinization disorders include acne, ear margin dermatosis and nasodigital hyperkeratosis.
- Examples of secondary causes of scaling with typical lesion distributions include flea allergy (tail base, dorsal trunk, hind legs) and scabies (elbows, pinnae, ventral abdomen).

Physical examination

Physical examination findings are most helpful in prioritizing certain secondary causes of scaling.

- Fleas or other parasites may be evident, or the distribution of pruritus and scaling may be highly suggestive.
- Broken hairs are suggestive of pruritus or dermatophyte infections.
- Hairs that epilate easily may be suggestive of endocrinopathies, staphylococcal folliculitis and demodicosis.
- Follicular casts are associated with disorders affecting the hair follicle and adenexae, such as sebaceous adenitis, vitamin A-responsive dermatoses and primary seborrhoea.
- Generalized scaling may be associated with a specific systemic disease, such as thymoma in cats, and more localized scaling may be seen with superficial necrolytic dermatitis (hepatocutaneous syndrome) in dogs and rarely cats.
- Non-cutaneous signs, such as lethargy, muscle wasting and hepatomegaly, support the suggestion of an endocrine disease.

Diagnostic tests

Animals with scaling should be evaluated for parasites using skin scrapings, trichograms or scale examination (see Chapters 3 and 7) and cytology should be performed to assess for secondary infection (see Chapters 3 and 4).

Laboratory tests

Routine haematology and biochemistry are generally normal in animals with primary keratinization defects; however, they may reflect the underlying cause in secondary keratinization disorders. Skin biopsy can be helpful in differentiating primary and secondary keratinization disorders. Epidermal abnormalities may include: increased mitotic activity in basal keratinocytes, dyskeratosis, epidermal hyperplasia, orthokeratotic and/or parakeratotic hyperkeratosis, hyperpigmentation and pigmentary clumping. Other findings may include dystrophic hairs, follicular dilatation and follicular keratosis. Ideally, secondary skin infections should be treated prior to obtaining biopsy samples.

Genetic tests are available for some primary keratinization disorders. Genetic testing may be performed on blood samples from a dog or cat of any age. Buccal or cheek swabs can also be used to obtain cells for deoxyribonucleic acid (DNA) testing; however, this method of sample collection should not be used until the dog or cat is at least 6 weeks old and has been weaned. Clinicians should check with local laboratories regarding the availability of these tests in their area. Genetic tests are available for the following genodermatoses (inherited disorders that present with multisystem involvement) at the time of publication:

- **Epidermolytic hyperkeratosis (rare)** – this disorder results in generalized scaling with hyperpigmentation and epidermal fragility in Norfolk Terriers. Genetic tests are available to detect the base change in the *KRT10* gene. Affected dogs are homozygous for a single base GT→TT change in the consensus donor splice site on intron 5 in *KRT10* (Credille *et al.*, 2005)
- **Exfoliative cutaneous lupus erythematosus (rare)** – this autosomal recessive disorder is a form of lupus that affects German Shorthaired Pointers and Hungarian Vizslas. Affected dogs present with generalized scaling, in addition to other clinical signs (see Chapter 28). Gene sequencing has identified a putative mutation, *A779S* (*2336GT*) on exon 14 of the signal-induced proliferation-associated protein 1 gene (*SIPA1*), located in chromosome 18 (Wang *et al.*, 2011)
- **Familial footpad hyperkeratosis** – also known as hereditary footpad hyperkeratosis and digital hyperkeratosis. Several breeds of dog are affected by this monogenic autosomal recessive disorder characterized by palmoplantar hyperkeratosis. A missense variant (c.155G>C) in the *FAM83G* gene was found in affected Kromfohrländers and Irish Terriers (Drögemüller *et al.*, 2014). Another disease resulting in hyperkeratosis of the footpads is caused by an autosomal recessive mutation in the gene coding for keratin 16 and affects Dogues de Bordeaux
- **Hereditary nasal parakeratosis** – this autosomal recessive disorder is seen in Labrador Retrievers and is associated with a mutation of the T and G nucleotides in the *SUV39H2* gene, which causes dryness of the nose, leading to excessive nasal crusting and the development of painful cracks around the tip of the nose
- **Ichthyosis-AB (American Bulldog type)** – this disorder is characterized by generalized scaling and affected dogs are predisposed to secondary *Malassezia* infections. The genetic test detects a single mutation in the *NIPAL 4* gene associated with ichthyosis in American Bulldogs. A study of 800 American Bulldogs from North America, Australia and Europe showed that 34.3% of the dogs tested were carriers of the mutated *NIPAL 4* gene
- **Ichthyosis-A (Golden Retriever type)** – this is a common autosomal recessive disease in Golden Retrievers due to a variant of the *PNPLA1* gene. Affected dogs present with variable amounts of generalized scale, which readily exfoliates. In a study of 48 breeding dogs, 31% were homozygous for the mutation and 48% were heterozygous, although only 3 of the 48 dogs had clinical signs of ichthyosis (Graziano *et al.*, 2018). It is possible that other genes and/or environmental factors are also involved in the development of ichthyosis in Golden Retrievers
- **Lethal acrodermatitis** – in addition to multifocal crusting, footpad hyperkeratosis and paronychia, affected dogs with this disorder have multisystemic signs and retarded growth. Genetic testing is now available to identify the *MKLN1* splicing defect that results in lethal acrodermatitis in Bull Terriers and Miniature Bull Terriers (Bauer *et al.*, 2018). *MKLN1* encodes the widely expressed intracellular protein muskelin 1. Muskelin 1 has diverse functions in cell adhesion, morphology, spreading and intracellular transport processes. Disease develops in dogs that are homozygous for the splicing defect. The disorder has a poor prognosis for survival
- **Sebaceous adenitis (the genetic basis is unknown)** – breed predilections include the Akita, English Springer Spaniel, Havanese, Samoyed, Standard Poodle and Vizsla. However, sebaceous adenitis has also been reported in over 50 breeds of dog, as well as in cats, rabbits, horses and humans. Destruction of the sebaceous glands leads to scaling and hair loss, which often starts on the dorsal trunk, face, ears and/or tail. Hairs may regrow straighter than normal for the breed and in a different colour. Scales adhering to hairs form follicular casts.

Treatment

For primary keratinization disorders, a combination of topical and systemic medications may be helpful in minimizing excessive scaling and other clinical manifestations. Topical therapies may be indicated daily or every other day initially, with later tapering to use as required to maintain control of the condition. Keeping the hair coat trimmed short may be helpful in increasing the efficacy of topical medications. For secondary keratinization disorders, the focus should be on treating the underlying disease. Bacterial or *Malassezia* skin infections should be treated preferably with topical antiseptics or antimicrobial agents (see Chapters 22 and 26).

Topical therapy

Topical medications (see also Chapter 27) are very useful for managing a wide variety of keratinization disorders. Topical agents may have keratolytic, keratoplastic, degreasing, moisturizing, antibacterial, antifungal, antiparasitic, antipruritic and/or anti-inflammatory properties.

- Keratolytic agents help to remove excessive scales by decreasing keratinocyte cohesion. Keratolytic shampoos include sulphur, salicylic acid, tar, selenium sulphide and benzoyl peroxide. Other agents with keratolytic action include propylene glycol and urea.
- Keratoplastic agents help to normalize keratinization. Examples include sulphur, salicylic acid, tar, selenium sulphide, alpha-hydroxy acids and retinoids such as tretinoin (retinoic acid). Tar is toxic to cats so should only be used in dogs; however, it should be noted that there are concerns regarding carcinogenicity.
- Moisturizing agents include emollients and humectants. Emollients are agents that soften, lubricate or soothe the skin. Occlusive emollients also decrease transepidermal water loss. Examples include fatty acids, oils, hydrocarbons and waxes. Humectants are hygroscopic agents that work by being incorporated into the stratum corneum and binding water. Examples include propylene glycol, glycerine, colloidal oatmeal, urea, sodium lactate, carboxylic acid and lactic acid.
- Ceramides are lipids composed of sphingosines and fatty acids. Ceramides synthesized by keratinocytes have important skin barrier functions, including prevention of epidermal water loss, antimicrobial activity and regulating epidermal cell turnover. Topical products that contain ceramides and/or phytosphingosine may help to repair the abnormal skin barrier associated with primary and secondary keratinization disorders, including canine atopic dermatitis (see Chapter 10).
- Degreasing agents solubilize surface lipids so that they can be removed during bathing. Examples of products useful in treating animals with seborrhoea oleosa include detergents, benzoyl peroxide and selenium sulphide.
- Retinoids, including vitamin A and its synthetic derivatives, regulate the growth, proliferation and differentiation of epithelial cells. Tretinoin (retinoic acid) is useful as a topical medication for treating localized keratinization disorders. Other synthetic retinoids available as topical formulations include adapalene and tazarotene; these agents are more potent and less irritating to the skin. It should be noted that these products are not licensed for use in animals.

Systemic therapy

Systemic therapy should be directed at the correction of any underlying or co-existing diseases. Good nutrition is important for the health of the skin and hair coat, therefore a high quality diet supplemented with essential fatty acids ± zinc should be recommended. Additional systemic treatments should be given as indicated for the specific condition being treated.

- Vitamin A at 800–1000 IU/kg orally q24h is effective in treating dogs with vitamin A-responsive dermatosis. Side effects can include keratoconjunctivitis sicca, skin rashes, vomiting, diarrhoea, joint stiffness, skeletal abnormalities, hepatitis, hypertriglyceridaemia and hypercholesterolaemia. These side effects are uncommon in adult dogs. Monitoring of tear production and biochemical profiles every 3–6 months is recommended. Synthetic retinoids have been used for these conditions, but are subject to prescribing restrictions in some countries.
- Calcitrol (vitamin D) at 10 mg/kg orally q24h may be helpful in some cases of refractory primary seborrhoea. Serum calcium levels should be monitored weekly.

Key points

- Crusting and scaling are secondary to an underlying primary disease in the majority of cases. Ectoparasites and secondary infections are common
- Primary genetically inherited diseases are uncommon, but genetic testing is becoming increasingly available for identification of these cases
- Management should be tailored to the individual case and often involves topical treatment, specific management of the primary disease and dietary modification

References and further reading

Bauer A, Jagannathan V, Hogler S *et al.* (2018) MKLN1 splicing defect in dogs with lethal acrodermatitis. *PLoS Genetics* **14**, e1007264; doi: 10.1371/journal.pgen

Casal ML, Want P, Mauldin EA *et al.* (2017) A defect in NIPAL4 is associated with autosomal recessive congenital ichthyosis in American Bulldogs. *PLoS One* **12**, e0170708

Credille KM, Barnhart KF, Minor JS *et al.* (2005) Mild recessive epidermolytic hyperkeratosis associated with a novel keratin 10 donor splice-site mutation in a family of Norfolk Terrier dogs. *British Journal of Dermatology* **153**, 51–58

Drögemüller M, Jagannathan V, Becker D *et al.* (2014) A mutation in the FAM83G gene in dogs with hereditary footpad hyperkeratosis (HFH). *PLoS Genetics* **10**, e1004370

Evans JM, Noorai RE and Tsai KL *et al.* (2017) Beyond the MHC: A canine model of dermatomyositis shows a complex pattern of genetic risk involving novel loci. *Plos Genetics* **13**, e1006604

Graziano L, Vasconi M and Cornegliani L (2018) Prevalence of PNPLA1 gene mutation in 48 breeding Golden Retriever dogs. *Veterinary Sciences* **5**, 48

Gross TL, Ihrke PJ, Walder EJ and Affolter VK (2005) Diseases with abnormal cornification. In: *Skin Diseases of the Dog and Cat: Clinical and Histologic Diagnosis, 2nd edn*, ed. TL Gross *et al.*, pp. 161–198. Blackwell Science, Oxford

Mauldin EA, Credille KM, Dunstan RW *et al.* (2008) The clinical and morphologic features of non-epidermolytic ichthyosis in the Golden Retriever. *Veterinary Pathology* **45**, 174–180

Medleau L and Hnilica KA (2006) Keratinization and seborrheic disorders. In: *Small Animal Dermatology: A Color Atlas and Therapeutic Guide, 2nd edn*, ed. L Medleau and KA Hnilica, pp. 295–326. WB Saunders, Philadelphia

Messinger L (2002) Canine keratinization disorders. In: *The 5-Minute Veterinary Consult Clinical Companion: Small Animal Dermatology*, ed. KH Rhodes, pp. 532–541. Lippincott Williams & Wilkins, Philadelphia

Miller WH, Griffin CE and Campbell KL (2013) Keratinization defects. In: *Muller and Kirk's Small Animal Dermatology, 7th edn*, pp. 630–646. Elsevier, St. Louis

Paterson S (2008) Keratinisation defects. In: *Manual of Skin Diseases of the Dog and Cat, 2nd edn*, ed. S Paterson, pp. 277–291. Blackwell Publishing, West Sussex

Wang P, Zangerl B, Werner P *et al.* (2011) Familial cutaneous lupus erythematosus (CLE) in the German Shorthaired Pointer maps to CFA18, a canine orthologue to human CLE. *Immunogenetics* **63**, 197–207

Wartewig S and Neubrt RHH (2007) Properties of ceramides and their impact on the stratum corneum structure: a review. *Skin Pharmacology and Physiology* **20**, 220–229

Werner HA and Messinger L (2002) Exfoliative dermatoses. In: *The 5-Minute Veterinary Consult Clinical Companion: Small Animal Dermatology*, ed. KH Rhodes, pp. 74–84. Lippincott Williams & Wilkins, Philadelphia

Chapter 13

An approach to papules and pustules

Rosanna Marsella

Papular and pustular eruptions are extremely common in veterinary dermatology. Papules are small solid elevations of the skin. Papules are erythematous and typically due to the infiltration of inflammatory cells. Pustules are small skin elevations filled with pus. Pustules start as papules and then progress to epidermal collarettes (which are secondary lesions). Pustules are transient and may not be visible in all cases.

Differential diagnosis

Papules and pustules are both primary lesions, which may or may not be centred around the hair follicles. For this reason, when considering the differential diagnoses of these lesions, it is common to divide them into two main categories: follicular and non-follicular diseases (Figure 13.1). However, it can be difficult to determine whether pustules have a follicular orientation without the aid of magnification; as a general rule, if the pustules appear large and span multiple follicles, they are not follicular in nature. A classic example of a pustular disease that spans multiple follicles is impetigo (Figure 13.2). When determining the differential diagnoses, it is also crucial to consider the distribution of the lesions (see below), how commonly the disease occurs and whether pruritus is present (e.g. both sarcoptic mange and flea allergy dermatitis are typically very pruritic). However, it should be borne in mind that diseases that would not necessarily be pruritic, may be associated with pruritus following secondary skin infection. *Demodex* and staphylococcal infection are more common causes of folliculitis in dogs than dermatophytes and therefore should be considered in all canine cases of pustular and papular skin disease. In contrast, dermatophytosis is more commonly seen in cats.

Follicular
• Demodicosis
• Dermatophytes
• *Staphylococcus*

Non-follicular
• Flea bites or other insect bite hypersensitivities
• *Sarcoptes*
• Hookworm dermatitis
• Contact allergy

13.1 Differential diagnoses for follicular and non-follicular diseases presenting with papules and pustules. (continues) ▶

Non-follicular *continued*
• *Malassezia* dermatitis
• Atopic dermatitis (very small papules are sometimes present in dogs allergic to house dust mites)
• Food-responsive dermatosis (also known as food allergy or adverse food reaction)
• Impetigo
• Chin acne
• Pemphigus complex (foliaceus and erythematosus)
• Systemic lupus erythematosus
• Canine familial dermatomyositis
• Subcorneal pustular dermatitis
• Sterile eosinophilic pustular dermatitis
• Idiopathic linear pustular acantholytic dermatosis
• Drug eruptions
• Juvenile cellulitis
• Mast cell tumours
• Calcinosis cutis (dogs)
• *Leishmania*
• Miliary dermatitis (cats)
∘ Underlying causes include:
– Bacterial, yeast and viral infections
– Ectoparasites (e.g. fleas, lice, *Cheyletiella*, *Notoedres*)
– Allergy (e.g. fleas, atopic dermatitis, food, contact)
– Cutaneous lymphoma
– Immune-mediated (e.g. pemphigus)
– Manifestations of internal disease (e.g. hyperthyroidism)

13.1 (continued) Differential diagnoses for follicular and non-follicular diseases presenting with papules and pustules.

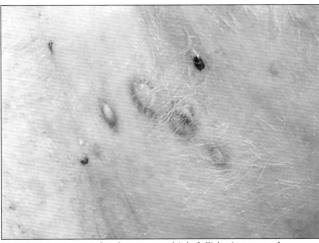

13.2 Large pustules that span multiple follicles in a case of impetigo.

Clinical approach

Physical examination

It is important that clinicians are familiar with the lesion distribution of various diseases in order to aid identification. For example:

- The classic distribution of lesions seen in cases of sarcoptic mange includes the ventral abdomen, the margins of the pinnae, the elbows and the hocks (Figure 13.3)
- Typical lesion distribution in dogs with a flea allergy is the rump, hind legs and tail; it is classically a disease that affects the body from the waist caudally. Interestingly, many dogs exposed to fleas have bites in the umbilical area
- The lesion distribution in cats with a flea allergy manifests as one of four reactive patterns (see Chapters 23 and 24), mainly affecting the head and neck, although a more dorsal distribution may be seen with multifocal papules or the development of miliary dermatitis
- The lesions associated with pemphigus foliaceus often begin on the face and can have a 'butterfly' appearance, affecting the periocular areas, the bridge of the nose and the whole surface of the pinnae (Figure 13.4).

In addition, it is important to note whether or not the lesions all appear at the same stage of development. For example, with superficial pyoderma in dogs, it is common to see erythematous and hyperpigmented macules, collarettes and papules in the same patient (Figure 13.5). These

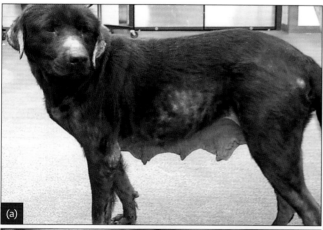

(a)

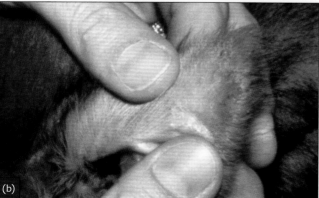

(b)

13.3 Lesion distribution associated with sarcoptic mange in the dog. (a) Typical lesion distribution includes the ventral abdomen, the margins of the pinnae, elbows and hocks. (b) Crusting and lesions on the margins of the pinna.

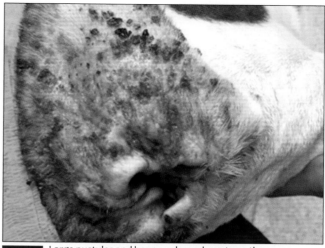

13.4 Large pustules and honey-coloured crusts on the concave surface of the pinna of a patient with pemphigus.

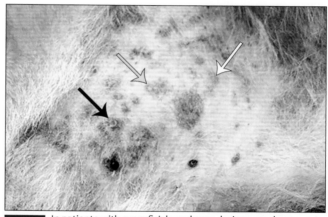

13.5 In patients with superficial pyoderma, lesions may be seen at various stages of development. Note that erythematous macules (yellow arrow), papules (white arrow) and collarettes (black arrow) are visible in this case.

lesions are all different stages of the same process. The inguinal area is a good site to observe these lesions due to the paucity of the hair coat. In contrast, if an animal has a contact allergy, the insult occurs at a single point in time and the lesions will all be at the same stage of development (Figure 13.6).

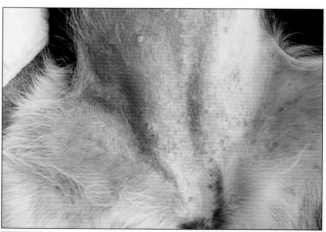

13.6 Severe erythema and papular eruption in the inguinal area of a dog with a contact allergy to grass.

Diagnostic tests

Secondary skin infections are very common and can complicate the clinical picture both in terms of lesions and the presence of pruritus. Thus, if an infection is identified, it should be addressed first and the patient re-evaluated once the infection is under control. At this point, it is much easier to identify the underlying disease process and determine whether it is associated with pruritus. In the past, it was commonplace to treat these infections with a empirically prescribed systemic antibiotic and to re-revaluate the patient after 3–4 weeks' treatment. However, with the increase in antibiotic-resistant bacteria, topical therapy may be preferred. This course of action may also apply to secondary *Malassezia* infections. The reader is referred to Chapters 21, 22 and 26 for a full discussion of treatment for superficial skin infections.

If the pruritus persists once the secondary skin infection has been addressed, and is associated with a papular eruption, then it is important to consider parasitic diseases and allergies. Parasitic diseases usually have a sudden onset, rather than the indolent course associated with atopic dermatitis or a food-responsive dermatosis. If parasites are not found on the physical examination, then a therapeutic trial with a parasiticide (e.g. an isoxazoline) may be justified and, in the case of fleas, aggressive environment treatment should also be undertaken.

If the history of the patient reveals a non-seasonal pruritus that waxes and wanes, then differential diagnoses such as a food-responsive dermatosis, contact allergy to non-seasonal triggers and atopic dermatitis triggered by non-seasonal allergens, such as dust mites, should be considered. The reader is referred to Chapters 9 and 10 for a detailed discussion about the approach to these cases.

The diagnostic approach to dogs and cats with papular and pustular skin disease is summarized in Figure 13.7.

Deep skin scrapings

For dogs presenting with papules and/or pustules, the recommended clinical approach is to begin with deep skin scrapings (to look for evidence of *Demodex*) and cytology (see below). If the deep skin scrapings are negative, in most instances, demodicosis can be ruled out. Exceptions are cases where the skin is fibrotic or in breeds, such as the Shar Pei, where it can be difficult to extrude the mites and a biopsy may need to be performed to rule out the disease. Many clinicians employ hair plucking (trichograms) or squeezing the skin and applying adhesive tape as alternative methods for collecting samples from sensitive areas of skin where deep skin scrapings may be challenging or painful.

Cytology

Cytology should be performed to identify:

- The type of inflammatory cells present
- The presence of bacteria and yeasts
- The presence of acantholytic keratinocytes.

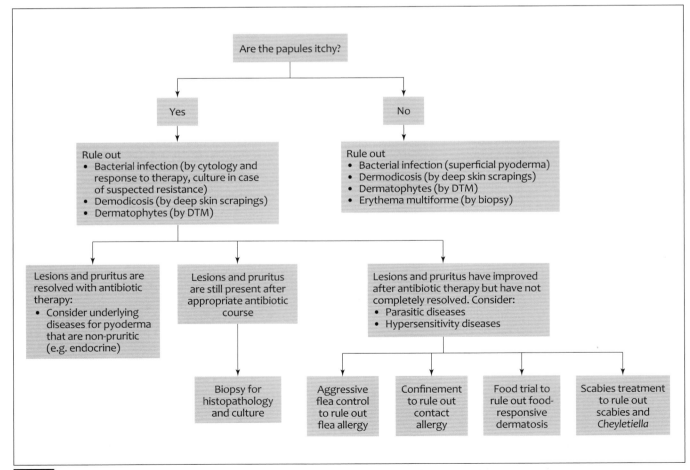

13.7 Diagnostic approach to a case presented with papular eruptions. DTM = dermatophyte test medium.

It is important to emphasize that the cytological findings should always be interpreted in light of the clinical signs (see Chapters 3 and 4). For example, identifying the presence of acantholytic keratinocytes does not always support a diagnosis of pemphigus foliaceus; they may be seen with other diseases in which there is severe inflammation and disruption of the epidermis, such as superficial pyoderma, dermatophytosis and severe contact allergy.

Dermatophyte culture

Dermatophytosis is commonly seen in cats and should be ruled out by performing a fungal culture (i.e. plucking hairs and placing them on a dermatophyte test medium plate). Dermatophyte culture may not be necessary for all canine cases.

Biopsy

Less commonly, papules and pustules may be associated with an immune-mediated or autoimmune disease, unusual infection or neoplasia, and collecting biopsy samples for histopathology and culture should be considered. Biopsy samples should be taken from a primary lesion wherever possible and should be obtained prior to the initiation of immunomodulation (see Chapters 3 and 5).

Key points

- It is helpful to determine on clinical examination whether papules and pustules have a follicular orientation
- Lesion distribution on the body is also helpful in generating a differential diagnosis
- Papules and pustules are often associated with pyoderma, and this should be treated before any further evaluation is made

References and further reading

Fadok VA and Irwin K (2019) Sodium hypochlorite/salicylic acid shampoo for treatment of canine staphylococcal pyoderma. *Journal of the American Animal Hospital Association* **55**, 117–123

Kano R, Aramaki C, Murayama N *et al.* (2019) High multi-azole-resistant *Malassezia* pachydermatis clinical isolates from canine *Malassezia* dermatitis. *Medical Mycology* **58**, 197–200

Loeffler A and Lloyd DH (2018) What has changed in canine pyoderma? A narrative review. *Veterinary Journal* **35**, 73–82

Morris DO, Loeffler A, Davis MF *et al.* (2017) Recommendations for approaches to meticillin-resistant staphylococcal infections of small animals: diagnosis, therapeutic considerations and preventative measures.: Clinical Consensus Guidelines of the World Association for Veterinary Dermatology. *Veterinary Dermatology* **28**, 304–e69

Ramos SJ, Woodward M, Hoppers SM *et al.* (2019) Residual antibacterial activity of canine hair treated with five mousse products against *Staphylococcus pseudintermedius in vitro*. *Veterinary Dermatology* **30**, 183–e57

Sjöström Y, Mellor P and Bergvall K (2018) A novel non-azole topical treatment reduces *Malassezia* numbers and associated dermatitis: a short term prospective, randomized, blinded and placebo-controlled trial in naturally infected dogs. *Veterinary Dermatology* **29**, 14–e7

Chapter 14

An approach to erosions and ulcerations

Manolis N. Saridomichelakis

An erosion is a circumscribed depressed lesion that represents a defect of the epidermis that does not penetrate the basement membrane. Erosions do not bleed and heal without scarring (Figure 14.1a). They are typically the result of self-trauma. An ulcer is a deeper defect that extends into the dermis after disruption of the basement membrane. These lesions are frequently covered by crusts, bleed easily and, at least when they involve deep dermis, heal with scar formation (Figure 14.1b).

Ideally, the differentiation between erosions and ulcers should be based on histopathology, because it may be impossible to differentiate deeper erosions from shallow ulcers during clinical examination (Figure 14.1c). Nevertheless, this distinction may not be particularly helpful in the diagnostic process because the canine and feline

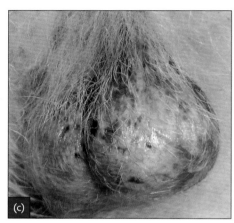

14.1
(continued)
(c) Erosions or superficial ulcers on the scrotum of a 4-year-old male Akita with irritant contact dermatitis.

epidermis is thin and therefore erosions frequently evolve into ulcers, especially if they become infected or self-traumatized. Thus, erosions and ulcers are discussed collectively for the remainder of this chapter, although more severe or deeper pathological processes are generally responsible for ulcer formation.

Pathophysiology

Erosions and ulcers are common lesions that may occur as a result of various external and internal factors that affect the epidermis, dermoepidermal junction and dermis.

- **External factors:** mechanical trauma; ultraviolet light skin damage; pressure; and chemical, electrical, thermal or toxic damage. External factors are the most common cause, especially when self-trauma secondary to pruritic skin diseases is considered (see Chapter 6).
- **Internal factors:** severe inflammation; degeneration, necrosis and apoptosis of keratinocytes; vesicular, pustular (see Chapters 13 and 28) and bullous diseases; detachment of epidermal layers caused by maceration; widening of fissures; disruption of blood supply (ischaemia); absence, destruction or catabolism of specific structural and adhesion molecules; transcutaneous elimination of minerals; and neoplastic invasion (see Chapter 34).
- In some cases, both **external and internal factors** are involved (e.g. external pressure and resultant ischaemia causing pressure sores).

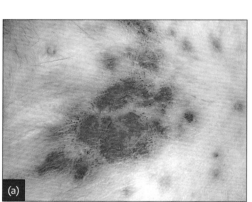

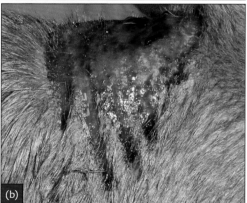

14.1 (a) Erosions on the ventral abdomen of a 12.5-year-old neutered female Domestic Shorthaired cat with eosinophilic plaques caused by allergic dermatitis. (b) Ulcer on the dorsal trunk of a 3-year-old male crossbreed dog with a chemical burn. (continues) ▶

Failure of skin barrier function in erosive and ulcerative diseases results in the loss of fluid, protein and electrolytes and in tissue colonization by opportunistic bacteria. Widespread ulceration may become life-threatening as a result of dehydration, hypoproteinaemia and septicaemia and, therefore, rapid diagnostic investigation and institution of specific and palliative treatment is warranted.

Differential diagnosis

A heterogeneous group that includes a large number of diseases (Figure 14.2) may manifest with erosions and/or ulcers, which can be accompanied by other primary or secondary skin lesions. There is no further discussion on erosions and ulcers caused by self-trauma (Figure 14.6) here; readers are referred to Chapter 6 for a more complete discussion.

Bacterial (see Chapters 21 and 30)

- Surface (e.g. intertrigo, pyotraumatic dermatitis)
- Superficial (e.g. mucocutaneous pyoderma, superficial exfoliative (spreading) pyoderma)
- Deep (e.g. German Shepherd Dog pyoderma, post-grooming furunculosis (Figure 14.3), cellulitis)
- Due to specific organisms (e.g. mycobacterial, actinomycosis, nocardiosis)

Fungal and others (see Chapters 25 and 30)

- Dermatophytosis (e.g. kerion, pseudomycetoma)
- Candidiasis
- Subcutaneous mycoses (e.g. sporotrichosis)
- Systemic mycoses (blastomycosis, coccidiomycosis, cryptococcosis, histoplasmosis)
- Prototheocosis
- Pythiosis

Protozoal (see Chapter 30)

- Canine (Figure 14.4) and feline leishmaniosis

Viral

- Feline leukaemia virus infection (giant cell dermatosis)
- Feline cowpox virus infection
- Feline herpesvirus infection
- Feline calicivirus infection

Parasitic (see Chapter 7)

- Cutaneous microfilariosis (Figure 14.5)
- Arthropod bites (ticks, spiders)
- Insect stings or bites (flies, mosquitoes)
- Myiasis

Allergic (see Chapter 23)

- Feline mosquito bite hypersensitivity

Autoimmune and immune-mediated (see Chapter 28)

- Pemphigus (e.g. foliaceus, vulgaris, paraneoplastic)
- Subepidermal bullous dermatoses (e.g. mucus membrane pemphigoid, bullous pemphigoid, epidermolysis bullosa acquisita)
- Lupus erythematosus (cutaneous and systemic)
- Vascular insufficiency or vasculitis
- Adverse drug reactions
- Erythema multiforme, Stevens-Johnson syndrome, toxic epidermal necrolysis
- Canine uveodermatological syndrome

Metabolic and toxic (see Chapter 31)

- Superficial necrolytic dermatitis (hepatocutaneous syndrome)
- Feline acquired skin fragility syndrome

Congenital and hereditary

- Facial dermatitis of Persian and Himalayan cats
- Epidermolysis bullosa

14.2 Aetiological classification of skin diseases that may present with erosions and/or ulcers. (continues) ▶

Congenital and hereditary continued

- Ehlers-Danlos syndrome
- Canine dermatomyositis
- Acrodermatitis of Bull Terriers

Environmental (see Chapter 32)

- Actinic dermatoses
- Irritant contact dermatitis
- Burns (e.g. chemical, electric, thermal)
- Frostbite
- Snake bites
- Foreign bodies
- Trauma, pressure sores

Nutritional (see Chapter 31)

- Zinc-responsive dermatosis
- Generic dog food dermatosis

Neoplastic and non-neoplastic tumours (see Chapter 34)

- Squamous cell carcinoma
- Mast cell tumour
- Cutaneous lymphoma
- Histiocytic neoplasms, reactive histiocytosis
- Cutaneous metastases of lung carcinomas
- Calcinosis cutis/calcinosis circumscripta

Self-trauma in pruritic (see Chapter 6), behavioural and neurological disorders

Unknown or multiple aetiology (see Chapters 23 and 33)

- Feline plasma cell pododermatitis
- Feline indolent ulcer, feline eosinophilic plaque, feline and canine eosinophilic granuloma
- Panniculitis
- Canine juvenile cellulitis
- Canine perianal fistulae
- Canine eosinophilic furunculosis of the face

14.2 (continued) Aetiological classification of skin diseases that may present with erosions and/or ulcers.

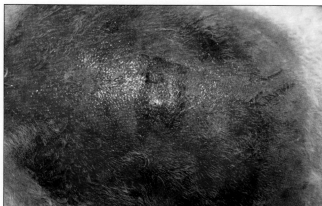

14.3 Erosions and ulcers on the rump of a 13-year-old neutered Poodle bitch with post-grooming furunculosis.

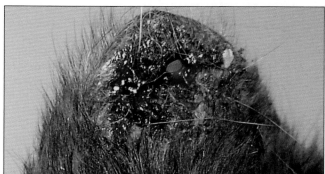

14.4 Ulcer of the tip of the ear pinna of a 7-year-old male German Shepherd Dog with leishmaniosis.

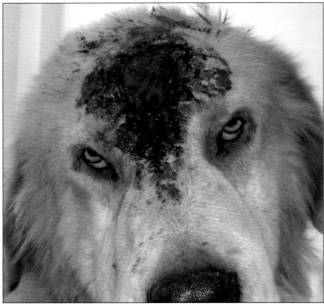

14.5 Ulcer on the forehead of a 6-year-old male dog with cutaneous dirofilariosis caused by *Dirofilaria immitis*.

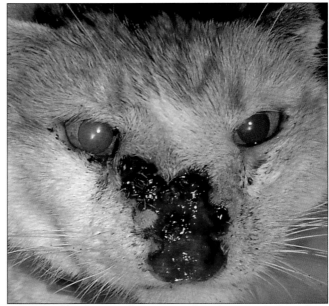

14.7 Ulcerative type of squamous cell carcinoma on the face of a 15-year-old female Domestic Shorthaired cat.

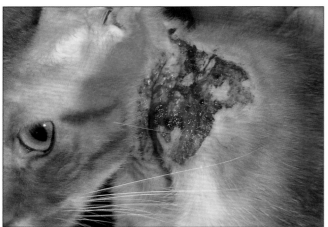

14.6 Self-induced erosions and ulcers on the neck of a 3-year-old male Domestic Shorthaired cat with a food-responsive dermatosis (also known as food allergy or adverse food reaction).

Clinical approach

Erosions and ulcers are generally considered to be secondary skin lesions, although in a few cases they can be the primary manifestation of the disease pathology (e.g. in the ulcerative type of squamous cell carcinoma; Figure 14.7). When more diagnostic primary skin lesions are present (e.g. erythematous or haemorrhagic macules, papules, plaques, pustules, bullae, nodules, tumours), it is usually more rewarding to follow the clinical approach described in the relevant chapters. However, owing to the transient nature of many primary lesions, they can be absent at the time of consultation; therefore, erosions/ulcers, along with hypotrichosis, alopecia, erythema, scales and crusts may be the only lesions left. In these cases, the diagnostic approach is based on the history, signalment, general and dermatological physical examination findings, and the laboratory test results.

History

The living conditions of the dog or cat are particularly important in the diagnostic investigation of erosive and ulcerative skin diseases. Animals that live outdoors are more prone to environmental (e.g. actinic dermatoses, chemical burns, frostbite, snake bites, foreign bodies and trauma), some fungal (e.g. sporotrichosis, blastomycosis, coccidioidomycosis, cryptococcosis) and parasite-induced (e.g. canine eosinophilic furunculosis of the face, feline mosquito bite hypersensitivity) diseases. Cats residing in rural areas are at increased risk for mycobacterial and cowpox virus infections. Other contagious diseases (e.g. dermatophytosis and feline leukaemia virus, herpesvirus and calicivirus infections) are encountered more frequently in animals that live in close proximity with others. Sun exposure not only provokes erosive and ulcerative skin diseases, such as actinic dermatoses and squamous cell carcinoma, but also aggravates many others (e.g. pemphigus foliaceus, lupus erythematosus, canine dermatomyositis). In addition, the travel history of the animal may be particularly important in raising the suspicion of certain regional diseases, such as subcutaneous and systemic mycoses, leishmaniosis and cutaneous microfilariosis.

The onset of lesions may be gradual or abrupt, and may be associated with certain circumstances (e.g. spider bites, insect stings or bites, drug administration including vaccination, environmental insults such as trauma, fractures, burns and exposure to extreme cold). In particular, some erosive and ulcerative skin diseases may appear as a result of idiosyncratic adverse drug reactions (e.g. pemphigus, lupus erythematosus-like dermatosis, vasculitis, Stevens–Johnson syndrome, toxic epidermal necrolysis, panniculitis) or be due to the effects of medication on the immune system and metabolism (e.g. candidiasis, cryptococcosis, feline herpesvirus infection, and feline acquired skin fragility syndrome after the administration of glucocorticoids or progestogens). Finally, owners should be asked specifically about the presence of systemic clinical signs that may have appeared before or after the occurrence of skin lesions (see below).

Signalment

Some breeds are predisposed to specific erosive and ulcerative skin diseases; for example, injection (usually vaccine) site reactions like vasculitis are more common in small-breed dogs, such as the Lhasa Apso, Maltese, Pekingese, Pomeranian, Poodle and Yorkshire Terrier, whereas actinomycosis, nocardiosis and some mycoses are more frequently seen in large-breed dogs.

Strong sex predispositions have not been recognized for most of these diseases: a male predisposition for German Shepherd Dog pyoderma and subcutaneous/systemic mycoses may be an important exception.

The age of the animal is very helpful in prioritizing the differential diagnosis; for example, congenital and hereditary skin diseases and canine juvenile cellulitis occur at a young age, German Shepherd Dog pyoderma and perianal fistulae are seen in middle-aged dogs, and cutaneous neoplasms are more common in older dogs and cats.

General physical examination

Dogs and cats with widespread erosions, especially those with deep ulcers, commonly present with systemic clinical signs such as depression, lethargy, anorexia, fever and peripheral lymphadenomegaly, as a result of dehydration, hypoproteinaemia, electrolyte imbalances, secondary pyoderma and septicaemia. Furthermore, pain and lameness can accompany ulcerative skin diseases, especially when the lower limbs are involved.

On the other hand, systemic clinical manifestations may occur because many skin diseases that cause erosions and ulcers can also affect the internal organs and/or because such diseases represent cutaneous manifestations of a systemic pathology (for example vasculitis due to bacterial septicaemia, various systemic infections and neoplasia; and feline acquired skin fragility syndrome due to hyper-adrenocorticism, diabetes mellitus or hepatic lipidosis). Recognition of these cutaneous manifestations is important to direct further diagnostic investigation.

Dermatological examination

Gloves should be worn when examining dogs and cats with erosive and ulcerative skin diseases because some of them are zoonotic (e.g. sporotrichosis, feline cowpox virus infection). A thorough search for primary lesions is necessary (see above) and it is also important to examine the animal meticulously for altered skin pigmentation, especially hypopigmentation (see Chapter 16).

When erosions or ulcers are present, the following features should be noted:

- Their shape and delineation
- The appearance of the base
- The borders of the lesion and the surrounding skin
- The presence and type of discharge
- The distribution on the body surface and visible mucous membranes.

The shape of the lesions depends on the underlying pathogenic mechanism. For example, they are frequently linear when caused by self-trauma, punched out when due to disruption of the blood supply, and circular when they follow rupture of pustules, vesicles or bullae. In the latter case, they also appear well delineated, in contrast to erosions and ulcers caused by necrosis of the skin, which are usually not well demarcated. The base of the ulcers may be smooth, ragged or necrotic, and their edge undermined or thickened, smooth, rolled or jagged and necrotic. The surrounding skin may present a variety of skin lesions or can be macroscopically normal; a positive Nickolsky sign (extension of the erosion or ulcer by applying digital pressure to the adjacent skin) indicates poor epidermal or dermoepidermal cohesion.

When discharge is present on the base of the lesion, it is usually purulent or haemorrhagic and when dried it leads to crust formation. The distribution of the lesions is quite variable, depending on the cause. It is particularly important to look closely at the visible mucous membranes (oral, conjunctival, genital), mucocutaneous junctions (lips, nostrils, eyelids, prepuce, vulva, anus), nasal planum, ear pinnae and footpads, because many erosive and ulcerative skin diseases affect these areas preferentially (Figures 14.8 and 14.9).

Disease	Mucous membranes	Mucocutaneous junctions	Nasal planum	Ear pinnae	Footpads
Actinic dermatoses		+	+	+	
Adverse drug reactions	+	+	+	+	+
Canine dermatomyositis	+	+	+	+	+
Canine juvenile cellulitis		+		+	
Canine leishmaniosis	+	+	+	+	+
Canine uveodermatological syndrome	+	+	+	+	+
Cryptococcosis	+	+	+	+	+
Cutaneous lymphoma	+	+	+	+	+
Erythema multiforme, Stevens-Johnson syndrome, toxic epidermal necrolysis	+	+	+	+	+
Feline calicivirus infection	+	+	+	+	+
Feline cowpox virus infection	+				+
Feline herpesvirus infection	+	+	+		+
Feline indolent ulcer, feline eosinophilic plaque, feline and canine eosinophilic granuloma	+	+		+	+
Feline mosquito bite hypersensitivity		+	+	+	+

14.8 Distribution of erosive and ulcerative skin diseases. (continues) ▶

Disease	Mucous membranes	Mucocutaneous junctions	Nasal planum	Ear pinnae	Footpads
Feline plasma cell pododermatitis	+				+
Fly bite dermatitis				+	
Frostbite				+	
Hereditary epidermolysis bullosa	+	+		+	+
Intertrigo		+			
Irritant contact dermatitis	+	+	+	+	+
Lupus erythematosus	+	+	+	+	+
Mucocutaneous pyoderma		+	+		
Myiasis		+			
Pemphigus complex	+	+	+	+	+
Squamous cell carcinoma	+	+	+	+	
Subepidermal bullous dermatoses	+	+	+	+	+
Superficial necrolytic dermatitis	+	+	+	+	+
Vascular insufficiency	+	+	+	+	+
Zinc-responsive dermatosis, generic dog food dermatosis		+	+	+	+

14.8 (continued) Distribution of erosive and ulcerative skin diseases.

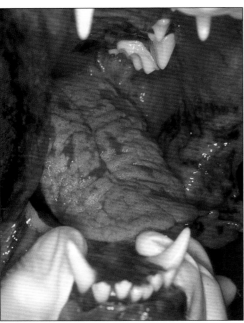

14.9 Ulcerations on the tongue of a dog with erythema multiforme.

Diagnostic tests

Various diagnostic tests may be employed in an effort to reach a final diagnosis in a dog or cat with erosions and ulcers. Selection of the appropriate tests depends upon the most probable differential diagnoses based on the signalment, history and the results of general physical and dermatological examinations.

Cytology

Cytology (see Chapter 4) may be helpful diagnostically and this is more often the case with erosive than ulcerative skin diseases. Impression smears can be obtained from the surface of the lesions, the under surface of the overlying crusts and the incision surface of biopsy specimens. When the surface is dry, it can be gently freshened with a scalpel blade. When a nodule with an eroded or ulcerated surface is encountered, it is recommended first to scrub the surface thoroughly and, after it dries, to squeeze the lesion in order to extrude fresh exudate. Organisms (bacteria, fungi, *Leishmania* amastigotes), inflammatory cells, acantholytic keratinocytes, viral inclusions within keratinocytes (feline cowpox) and neoplastic cells may be found in these preparations.

The significance of surface bacteria as a primary cause of the skin disease is often questionable. Erosions and ulcers are frequently contaminated by opportunistic organisms from the environment or, as a result of licking, from the oral cavity (e.g. *Simonsiella* spp.). However, when phagocytosed cocci or rods are present, the lesions are considered to be infected and prompt topical and perhaps systemic antibacterial treatment should be instituted. Special stains may be required to demonstrate specific organisms (e.g. mycobacteria, *Actinomyces* spp., *Nocardia* spp.).

Neutrophils are the most common inflammatory cell type and may be normal or degenerated. Ulcers, irrespective of their cause, are accompanied by an inflammatory cell infiltrate that is usually dominated by neutrophils. However, degenerative changes of these cells are further evidence in favour of the pathogenic role of the bacterial organisms. Additional inflammatory cell types include macrophages (i.e. pyogranulomatous or granulomatous inflammation) that may contain lipids (panniculitis), eosinophils (e.g. some subcutaneous mycoses, insect stings or bites, canine eosinophilic furunculosis of the face, feline eosinophilic granuloma complex), lymphocytes, plasma cells (e.g. feline plasma cell pododermatitis) and mast cells. Acantholytic keratinocytes, especially when seen in large numbers and/or arranged in clusters, are most commonly associated with pemphigus foliaceous (see Chapters 4 and 28).

Neoplastic cells are usually hard to find in impression smears from the ulcerated surface of skin neoplasms (Figure 14.10). In these cases, fine-needle biopsy (with or without aspiration) of the underlying tumour is indicated to obtain a representative sample. The same is true when dealing with eroded or ulcerated nodules; this sampling technique may also be rewarding when used to sample the raised edge of deep ulcers.

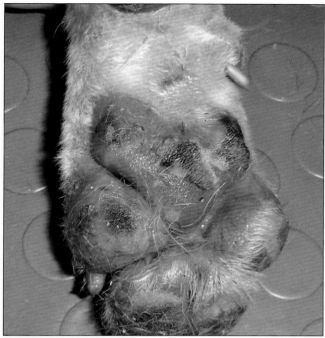

14.10 Erosions on the footpads of a 5.5-year-old neutered Boxer bitch with epitheliotrophic lymphoma.

Culture and sensitivity

Bacterial culture and antimicrobial sensitivity testing are indicated when bacteria are suspected to contribute to the disease pathology, either as a primary cause (*Nocardia*, *Actinomyces*, mycobacterial disease) or as a secondary invader. In both cases, it is advisable to avoid surface sampling and to obtain tissue biopsy samples after aseptic preparation of the skin surface (see above). Samples should be sent to an appropriate laboratory, which should be notified if specific pathogens are suspected. Whenever bacterial pyoderma is confirmed, a thorough search for underlying diseases, such as canine demodicosis (Figure 14.11), is always indicated (see Chapter 21).

Dermatophyte testing

Testing for dermatophytosis, including Wood's lamp examination, microscopy of hair and crusts, polymerase chain reaction (PCR) and fungal culture (see Chapter 25),

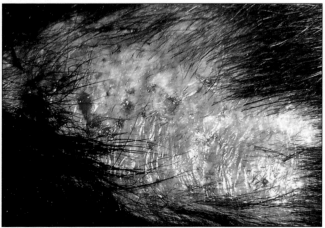

14.11 Erosions and ulcers on the dorsal trunk of a 6-month-old Greek Hound bitch with deep bacterial pyoderma secondary to juvenile-onset generalized demodicosis.

is indicated when ringworm kerion or pseudomycetoma is suspected. It is important to remember that:

- The exudate present on the surface of erosions and ulcers may result in false fluorescence under Wood's lamp examination
- Histopathology may be necessary for a final diagnosis, especially for culture-negative cases of dermatophyte kerion and pseudomycetoma.

Surface sampling for fungal culture is also indicated when candidiasis is included in the list of differential diagnoses. However, if subcutaneous and systemic mycoses or protothecosis are suspected, tissue biopsy samples should be submitted and the laboratory should be notified about the suspected organism involved. Special caution is warranted in the case of systemic mycoses, blastomycosis, coccidioidomycosis and histoplasmosis because the mycelial forms of these organisms pose a great danger to laboratory personnel.

Biopsy and histopathology

Cutaneous histopathology is perhaps the most rewarding examination for erosive and ulcerative skin diseases and in many cases will give a definitive diagnosis (e.g. autoimmune and immune-mediated, congenital and hereditary, nutritional, neoplastic diseases). However, this is highly dependent on the samples collected and important consideration should be given to the age of the lesion, site selection, technique and the number of biopsy specimens that are obtained.

Optimally, samples should be obtained from early lesions. In addition, biopsy is always indicated early in the diagnostic investigation when cutaneous and mucous membrane involvement is widespread and/or accompanied by systemic clinical signs. On the other hand, mucocutaneous pyoderma can mimic, both clinically and histopathologically, some autoimmune diseases (such as cutaneous lupus erythematosus) and secondary bacterial infection may mask the characteristic histological lesions of the primary skin disease. In these cases, it is preferable (though not always feasible) to postpone skin biopsy until the bacterial infection has been resolved by appropriate antimicrobial treatment administered for at least 3–4 weeks. On the contrary, anti-inflammatory and immunosuppressive treatment should be avoided prior to biopsy.

Site selection is very important in order to maximize the chances for an informative result. Whenever possible primary lesions should be sampled; ulcers and erosions are secondary lesions and less likely to provide diagnostic clues. Biopsy of the base of ulcers should be avoided because, irrespective of the cause, the samples may show only a non-specific neutrophilic inflammation, which is non-diagnostic. The most informative specimens are usually obtained across the edge of the lesions and, sometimes, from the adjacent skin. For these reasons, skin biopsy may be accomplished in three ways:

- By taking separate punch biopsy samples from the edge of the ulcer and the adjacent skin and submitting them in different vials
- In the case of small ulcers, by excising them totally along with a rim of adjacent skin
- By taking, with a scalpel blade, elliptical excisional biopsy specimens with the long axis of the sample perpendicular to the edge of the ulcer (Figure 14.12).

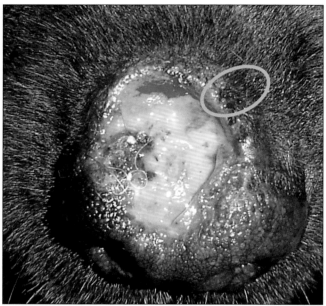

14.12 Proper orientation of wedge biopsy from the edge of an ulcer and adjacent skin. Blue ellipsis represents the incision line.

The last is the most practical option and has the additional advantage that, owing to its shape, the specimen will be trimmed in the proper direction, thus enabling the pathologist to examine consecutively, first the adjacent skin, then the border of the lesion, and finally its base. Excisional biopsy samples are also preferred for erosive diseases, although punch biopsy specimens can be adequate when diffuse erosions are sampled. Finally, it is very important to obtain and submit multiple samples from lesions with a different appearance or from lesions located on different areas of the body and from mucous membranes. Good communication between the clinician and the pathologist is mandatory, especially when a straightforward pathological diagnosis is not possible and additional examinations, including special stains, immunohistochemistry, immunofluorescence and PCR, are needed (see Chapter 5). Further laboratory tests may be indicated to reach a final diagnosis and to evaluate the general health of the animal.

Key points

- Erosions and ulcerations are often the result of self-trauma due to pruritus
- Well demarcated lesions; however, may be primary and the result of an immune-mediated process
- Histopathology can be rewarding in erosive/ulcerative diseases, if biopsy samples are obtained from multiple early lesions

---

References and further reading

Gross TL, Ihrke PJ, Walder EJ and Affolter VK (2005) *Skin Diseases of the Dog and Cat: Clinical and Histopathologic Diagnosis, 2nd edn*. Blackwell Publishing, Oxford

Hill PB (2002) *Small Animal Dermatology: a Practical Guide to the Diagnosis and Management of Skin Diseases in Dogs and Cats*. Butterworth Heinemann–Elsevier Science Ltd, Edinburgh

Miller WH, Griffin CE and Campbell KL (2013) *Muller and Kirk's Small Animal Dermatology, 7th edn*. Elsevier, St Louis

Chapter 15

An approach to nodules and draining sinus tracts

David H. Shearer and Jane M. Dobson

Nodules and sinus tracts are common signs in small animal dermatology and are the manifestation of a diverse group of underlying pathological processes, some of which may be common, as in a cat bite abscess, or rare, as in the case of some mycoses or bacterial infections.

Nodules are solid, cystic or oedematous elevations of the skin that may extend into the subcutis, panniculus and/or muscle. Microscopically, they are made up of accumulations of cells and fluid within the epidermis, dermis and hypodermis. These cells may be neoplastic, inflammatory/reactive or both. Disruption of the epidermis over nodules occurs frequently as a result of inflammation or ischaemia. The clinical features associated with the necrosis and inflammation are sinus tracts and/or ulceration.

A sinus tract represents an attempt at rejection and removal of various types of material from the dermis and subcutis. The material can enter the skin by penetration, via the hair follicles, by systemic routes or may be formed within the skin and subcutis.

Differential diagnosis

Nodules may be classified as:

- Inflammatory
  - Infectious
  - Non-infectious
- Non-inflammatory
- Neoplastic.

Inflammatory nodular lesions
Infectious and parasitic causes

Nodules comprised of inflammatory cells, with sinus tract formation (e.g. abscesses) or without may be the sequel of a folliculitis, furunculosis or panniculitis, depending on the focus of the inflammatory response. A variety of organisms can cause infectious nodules, including mycobacteria, *Actinomyces/Nocardia*, *Staphylococcus*, *Leishmania* and various fungi (Figure 15.1).

Abscesses:
Clinical presentation: Abscesses are common in cats and seen occasionally in dogs. The lesions are usually single, occasionally multiple, subcutaneous, painful nodules with or without ulceration and discharging sinus formation. Abscesses are usually caused by penetrating injury and infection (bite, claw injury, foreign body).

Bacterial
- Furunculosis secondary to staphylococcal folliculitis and/or *Demodex*
- *Actinomyces/Nocardia* infections
- Cutaneous mycobacterial infections
- Post-traumatic and foreign body abscesses
- Feline mycoplasma-induced abscesses
- Cutaneous bacterial granuloma
- Focal adnexal dysplasia (usually the result of chronic focal folliculitis/furunculosis)

Fungal
- Subcutaneous dermatophytic granuloma
- Sporotrichosis
- Opportunistic subcutaneous fungal infections:
  - Eumycetoma
  - Phaeohyphomycosis
  - Zygomycosis
  - Hyalohyphomycosis
- Cutaneous involvement with systemic mycoses:
  - Cryptococcosis
  - Coccidioidomycosis
  - Blastomycosis
  - Histoplasmosis
- Pythiosis

Algal
- Protothecosis
- Disseminated infections with Protista

Parasitic
- Leishmaniosis
- Rhabditic dermatitis

15.1 Infectious and parasitic causes of inflammatory nodular lesions.

Diagnosis: The diagnosis is usually based on clinical examination and surgical exploration.

Prognosis: The prognosis following appropriate treatment is usually good; however, in immunosuppressed individuals the causative organism may spread to involve internal organs.

Treatment: Drainage and systemic antibiotics for 5 days is usually effective. In poorly responsive cases, samples should be collected for microbiological culture and sensitivity testing.

Panniculitis:
Clinical presentation: Panniculitis is the term used to refer to inflammation of the subcutaneous adipose tissue. It is not a specific disease. Focal panniculitis can occur as a bystander effect in follicular disease (especially if furunculosis

has developed) or it can be a process that specifically involves the adipose tissue. The lesions present as single or multiple, discrete or diffuse, subcutaneous nodules, with or without ulceration and discharging sinus formation. The lesions may be painful.

Diagnosis: A variety of causes have been reported in dogs and cats, including:

- Infectious (bacterial, mycobacterial, fungal)
- Parasitic (arthropod bites)
- Immune-mediated (lupus erythematosus, drug reaction, vasculitis, sterile panniculitis in dogs)
- Physicochemical (mechanical trauma, foreign material)
- Pancreatitis/pancreatic neoplasia
- Nutritional (vitamin E deficiency)
- Idiopathic.

The diagnosis is based on ruling out these potential causes through appropriate diagnostic techniques. Multiple deep biopsy samples and histopathology with additional tissue culture are essential to confirm panniculitis and establish whether or not there is an infectious cause. A sterile idiopathic nodular dermatitis is diagnosed on the basis of histological and microbiological results.

It is important to remember that some causative organisms require special culture media and may be present in very small numbers. This is the case for canine sporotrichosis, which can be challenging to diagnose, as well some atypical mycobacterial infections. For this reason, clinicians need to consider the test results alongside the history of development of the lesions and lesion distribution. The laboratory should be notified if unusual agents are suspected, as special culture media and conditions are often required. For some diseases, it is not uncommon to have to repeat the tests several times to identify the infectious agent. In the future, further specific causes, especially novel infectious agents, are likely to be identified in cases that are currently diagnosed as sterile idiopathic nodular dermatitis.

Prognosis: The prognosis depends upon the aetiology.

Treatment: The treatment depends upon the aetiology. Single lesions caused by trauma, or at injection sites, can be excised surgically. Animals with multiple sterile lesions usually respond to glucocorticoids: prednisolone at 2 mg/kg orally q24h (dogs) and 4 mg/kg orally q24h (cats).

Non-infectious causes

Nodules are also seen with accumulations of inflammatory cells without the involvement of microorganisms (Figure 15.2). These nodules may occur with or without sinus tract formation. Debris may be released into the dermis from ruptured hair follicles, producing a 'foreign body' response. Other endogenous substances recognized as 'foreign' and targeted by the immune/inflammatory response are fatty acids/lipids released during adipocyte necrosis (e.g. sterile panniculitis) and the products of dermal mineralization (calcinosis cutis).

Neoplastic and non-inflammatory nodular lesions

Neoplasia, both benign and malignant, is one of the major causes of nodule formation in the skin and subcutaneous tissues, and may be seen with or without sinus tract formation. Neoplasms of the skin and subcutis are the

Mast cell degranulation
- Urticaria
- Angiogenic oedema

Degenerated collagen
- Arthropod-bite granuloma
- Eosinophilic granuloma

Fatty acids/lipids
- Sterile nodular panniculitis
- Traumatic panniculitis
- Post-injection panniculitis
- Xanthoma

Calcium
- Calcinosis cutis
- Calcinosis circumscripta

Extravasated blood (haematoma/seroma)
- Vascular disease, vasculitis, thrombosis
- Clotting disorders

Amyloid
- Nodular cutaneous amyloidosis

Idiopathic
- Sterile nodular granuloma and pyogranuloma
- Canine juvenile cellulitis syndrome
- Canine cutaneous histiocytosis
- Nodular dermatofibrosis in German Shepherd Dogs

15.2 Non-infectious causes of inflammatory nodules.

most frequently diagnosed tumours of domesticated animals. The prevalence varies depending on the study, but in dogs and cats they represent between 25% and 58% of all neoplasms seen. More than 25 morphologically distinct cutaneous neoplasms have been described (Figure 15.3; see Chapter 34).

Other non-neoplastic, non-inflammatory conditions may cause nodule formation (Figure 15.4). These include: hyperplastic, dysplastic or developmental accumulations (e.g. hamartomas) of cells; excesses of non-cellular tissue components, such as collagen; and benign cystic structures. Calcinosis circumscripta is also an example of a non-inflammatory and non-neoplastic nodular disease.

Tumours of epithelial origin

Epidermal cells:
- Squamous papilloma/papillomatosis
- Squamous cell carcinoma
- Multicentric squamous cell carcinoma *in situ* (Bowen's syndrome)
- Basal cell tumour (including the rarer basal cell carcinoma)
- Keratoacanthoma/intracutaneous cornifying epithelioma

Follicular hair matrix/follicular epithelial components:
- Trichoepithelioma
- Pilomatrixoma

Sebaceous/hepatoid gland cells/apocrine/ceruminous:
- Adenoma/adenocarcinoma

Tumours of melanocyte origin

Melanoma:
- Benign dermal
- Malignant

Tumours of round cell origin

Mast cell tumour
Plasmacytoma
Lymphoma:
- Epitheliotrophic
- Non-epitheliotrophic
- Angiotropic lymphoma (lymphomatoid granulomatosus)

15.3 Neoplastic causes of nodular lesions. (continues) ▶

Tumours of round cell origin *continued*

Histiocytoma (canine cutaneous):
- Histiocytic sarcoma – localized
- Histiocytic sarcoma – disseminated (malignant histiocytosis)

Transmissible venereal tumour

Tumours of mesenchymal origin

Spindle cell sarcoma:
- Perivascular wall tumour (haemangiopericytoma)
- Schwannoma (peripheral nerve sheath tumour)
- Fibrosarcoma (fibroblast origin)
- Myxosarcoma

Blood and lymphatic vessels:
- Haemangioma/haemangiosarcoma
- Lymphangioma/lymphangiosarcoma

Adipose tissue:
- Lipoma/liposarcoma
- Fibrolipoma
- Infiltrative lipoma

Fibrous tissue:
- Fibroma/fibrosarcoma

Miscellaneous/other:
- Fibropapilloma (feline sarcoid)
- Benign fibrous histiocytoma
- Leiomyosarcoma
- Dermatofibroma
- Nodular dermatofibrosis

Metastatic neoplasms

Many (carcinomas)

15.3 (continued) Neoplastic causes of nodular lesions.

- Benign nodular sebaceous hyperplasia (Figure 15.5)
- Skin tag (skin polyp, acrochondron)
- Naevi/hamartomas:
  - Collagenous
  - Vascular
  - Follicular
  - Sebaceous
- Fibroadnexal dysplasia
- Dermoid cyst/dermoid sinus
- Follicular cyst/epidermoid cyst/epidermal inclusion cyst
- Lipomatosis
- Nodular dermatofibrosis
- Apocrine cystomatosis

15.4 Non-neoplastic, non-inflammatory causes of nodular lesions.

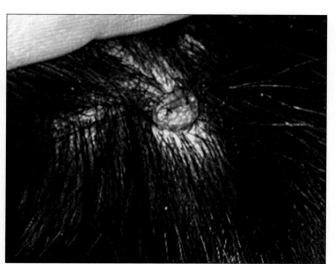

15.5 Nodular sebaceous hyperplasia: one of several lesions in the skin of this elderly dog.

Clinical approach

History and clinical examination

The clinical history, age, breed and sex of the patient, the distribution, duration and rate of progression of the lesion(s) and the associated clinical signs (e.g. pruritic or non-pruritic) are important in establishing likely differential diagnoses. Older animals are more likely to develop cutaneous neoplasia, whereas infectious inflammatory lesions can occur at any age. The gross appearance (erythema, alopecia, ulceration) and texture (soft, fluctuant, firm, fixed) of lesion(s) on clinical examination may also give clues to the aetiology. Although infectious inflammatory lesions often produce erythema and pain, many neoplastic lesions (e.g. mast cell tumours) can also induce a local paraneoplastic inflammatory response. Some infectious inflammatory lesions also include a foreign body reaction to material released into the dermis or subcutis; one common example is keratin and hair released from ruptured hair follicles in a deep pyoderma. The authors also see apparently inflammatory lesions that progress to neoplasia (e.g. feline injection-associated sarcomas appear to develop at the site of an inflammatory reaction, lymphoma can also be a sequel to inflammation in some organs). If apparently infectious inflammatory lesions fail to respond to initial rational therapy, then further investigations are required.

Diagnostic tests

Skin scraping and hair pluck examination

It is important not to forget to perform the basic tests such as scrapings/hair plucking for the identification of *Demodex* spp. or dermatophytes, which can present clinically as discharging sinuses and nodules once furunculosis has developed.

Cytology

Cytology is a useful screening tool for obtaining rapid diagnostic information but the technique requires some practice. It is most useful when performed in the practice before carrying out more invasive techniques; indeed, for most skin nodules in cats and dogs an aspirate should be attempted (fine-needle aspiration biopsy, FNAB) prior to biopsy or excision. One limitation is the false-negative sample, such as one from an inflamed neoplasm that contains none of the neoplastic cells, or samples from cases of infectious diseases (e.g. atypical mycobacteria infections) in which only very few organisms are present in the tissue, warranting wedge biopsy. Inflammation is a common feature within neoplastic lesions; therefore, samples may contain a heterogeneous population that includes atypical neoplastic cells as well as mixed inflammatory cells. One downside of FNAB is that it may induce inflammation within the lesion and occasionally make histopathology more difficult.

Material for cytology may be collected by:

- Fine-needle aspiration (FNA), especially useful for nodules and lymph nodes
- Impression from the lesion (especially a freshly cut surface or exudates) or a scraping
- Smears or touch impressions of sinus tract contents.

One advantage of cytology is that minimal restraint of the patient is required for these procedures. If the specimen is acellular, the lesion can be re-aspirated or a biopsy performed to obtain samples for culture and histopathology. It is easy to miss the lesion on aspiration and obtain adipocytes that wash off during fixation and staining, leaving a blank slide. The same is true with aspirates from lipomas.

Microbial culture and identification

The cytology result may indicate whether the lesion is likely to be inflammatory rather than neoplastic; however, the sample can contain both types of lesion, e.g. fine-needle aspirates from histiocytomas usually contain proliferating Langerhans' cells and lymphocytes, while those from mast cell tumours often contain eosinophils and fibroblasts as well as neoplastic mast cells. If inflammatory cells and organisms are seen, collection of material for microbiology or other techniques may be indicated. In general, a representative tissue sample, such as from a wedge incision biopsy or punch biopsy, is the most rewarding type of material for microbiology. However, if tissue grains or granules are present within a mass or a sinus tract, they may be packed with organisms and some material should be collected for culture as well as cytology, which may give an immediate indication of an infectious agent (e.g. *Actinomyces*).

Cultures from swabs of nodules rarely identify the causative agent and superficial samples commonly collect secondary colonizers, particularly where the lesions are ulcerated. It is important to consider which organisms are likely to be involved, based on the clinical features and cytology results, so that the correct culture conditions can be used and potential safety hazards assessed. The differential diagnoses should be stated clearly on the microbiology submission form so that the laboratory will perform the appropriate type(s) of culture from the submitted specimen(s). Ideally, the laboratory should be told whether anaerobic and aerobic bacterial culture, fungal culture or much more specialized mycobacterial culture is required. Subsampling and transport to a reference laboratory may be required for particular organisms (e.g. for the culture and identification of mycobacteria). Apart from swabs in transport media, solid tissue samples can be submitted in sterile universal containers (a drop of sterile saline placed in the container will help to prevent them drying out, but this is not necessary if delivery to the laboratory is rapid; if in doubt the laboratory should be contacted and asked how they like to receive the samples).

If an infectious agent is not immediately suspected or cannot be identified, multiple representative skin biopsy samples should be submitted for histopathology. Before placing all the samples in formalin, several biopsy specimens should be chilled or frozen for future microbiological diagnosis or polymerase chain reaction (PCR). Histopathology samples should be accompanied by a list of differential diagnoses and requests for special staining to rule out difficult microbial infections; most pathologists will perform these if the histological pattern raises the possibility of an infectious cause. Some organisms, such as some forms of mycobacteria, are not easy to culture or may take some months to grow *in vitro*. Mycobacteria can also be very difficult to find in histological sections.

Polymerase chain reaction for microbes

PCR is now used for the detection of microbial deoxyribonucleic acid (DNA) in tissue samples. Examples include arthropod-borne infections (e.g. *Borrelia*), bacteria, fungi and mycobacteria. Although it can be attempted on formalin-fixed tissue, false-negative results are a problem with some organisms (e.g. mycobacteria) and fresh tissue is recommended. Stored fresh frozen tissue can be used for mycobacterial PCR in the cat after a histopathological diagnosis of likely mycobacterial disease. Freezing some fresh tissue collected when taking biopsy samples for histopathology is recommended for all cutaneous and subcutaneous masses in the cat.

PCR is being used to study the cutaneous microbiome and is likely to become the gold standard for diagnosis of some infectious diseases in the future. A drawback with PCR is its sensitivity and that it may provide a false-positive result; it must be interpreted in light of the histopathological and clinical information. A good example of this problem is quiescent feline herpesvirus, which can be detected in a carrier cat's skin biopsy samples, but is not necessarily involved in the disease process.

Fluorescent *in situ* hybridization for microbes

This is a molecular technique, which is now being used routinely to identify the presence of specific sequences of microbial DNA or ribonucleic acid (RNA) in tissue sections. Along with the histopathology, this can indicate the cause of a disease.

Blood tests in nodular skin disease

Serology is important in the diagnosis of a number of infectious diseases, such as leishmaniosis. An interferon gamma release assay (IGRA) is a blood test that has been adapted for use in cats. The IGRA can indicate a likely causal species in cases of infection with *Mycobacterium bovis* or *M. microti*, and can be suggestive of *M. avium-intracellulare complex* (MAC) infection. Ziehl–Neelsen-positive organisms identified histopathologically with a negative IGRA test indicate infection with a non-tuberculous mycobacterial (but not MAC) organism.

Skin biopsy and histopathology

General considerations: There are no general contraindications for skin biopsy. Sedation and local anaesthesia are sufficient for most techniques other than total surgical excision of large nodules. Potential bleeding disorders should be evaluated prior to biopsy, including punch biopsy, if there is any clinical evidence to suggest that abnormal haemostasis is likely. The theory that performing a biopsy hastens the growth or dissemination of malignant neoplasms is largely unfounded, but the soft tissue tract through which the biopsy specimen is collected should be removed in its entirety at subsequent excision of the tumour, because tumour cells may be spread locally on instruments or through haemorrhage. The growth of neoplasia is determined by the innate ability of the malignant cells to avoid self-death, support their own replication by angiogenesis and spread through the circulation, and by the inability of the host defence mechanisms to prevent establishment of tumour foci in tissues distant from their original site.

Biopsy technique: For inflammatory lesions, multiple deep punch biopsy samples may be taken. However, the best sample for histopathology is from an elliptical incision biopsy that includes the margin of the nodule. If this is excisional, the whole nodule should be positioned in the centre of the ellipse. For most solitary cutaneous nodules in cats and dogs, it is advisable to collect and cytologically examine a fine-needle aspirate prior to excisional biopsy, to ensure that the lesion is not a mast cell tumour or other locally invasive tumour that might require a wide margin of excision. Using the elliptical biopsy technique, the sample is cut in half along the long axis, thus providing an excellent margin in which to evaluate the invasiveness of the lesion. It is important that the biopsy sample is removed *en bloc* to ensure that there is representative deeper tissue available for evaluation. The surgical margins can be marked using histological inks or sutures to indicate particular points of interest to the laboratory. Most laboratories will provide the histopathologist with multiple sections in two vertical planes at 90 degrees to one another. The pathologist will evaluate the margins of these sections and provide an indication as to whether or not a tumour-free margin has been achieved. In well circumscribed tumours, this will provide a good indication of the surgical margins. In more invasive tumours, it is possible to have tumour-free margins in the sections produced and examined, and these are usually reliable indicators of complete excision. It is important to note that, occasionally, the histological sections are not representative and the tumour cells are at the surgical margin elsewhere.

Biopsy of the local lymph node: Correctly staging a tumour for oncological management requires evaluation of the draining lymph node(s). Enlarged soft nodes may be seen with inflammatory nodules as a result of antigenic stimulation, lymphatic spread of infectious foci, or an inflammatory reaction to neoplasia. All enlarged lymph nodes should be aspirated for cytology. If a firm lymph node is negative for neoplasia on FNA, a biopsy should be performed under general anaesthesia. Infiltration with local anaesthetic can destroy lymph node architecture. Although the sample provided by a Tru-cut needle may be sufficient, excisional biopsy of the affected lymph node provides the best information, particularly in cats.

Immunohistochemistry

Organisms and cell types within lesions can, in some cases, be identified on the basis of the presence of cell surface molecules (markers) using immunohistochemistry (IHC). This technique employs binding labelled immunoglobulins directed at the cell surface molecules. Although many antibodies work with formalin-fixed tissues, most work best on fresh frozen specimens. IHC is being increasingly used for routine tumour phenotyping in veterinary pathology.

IHC can be used to identify organisms and the phenotype of the cells within neoplasms. Tumour identification depends upon the expression of phenotype-specific molecules by the tumour cells. Given that tumours may share surface molecules, it is usual to employ a panel of reagents against a variety of markers (Figure 15.6); the

Cell type	Panel of stains employed
Melanocytes	MelanA PNL2 S100
Keratinocytes	Cytokeratin
Lymphocytes	CD79a (B-cells) CD3 (T-cells) CD45 (all leucocytes)
Histiocytes	Lysozyme Fascin Mac387/CD18
Plasma cells	MUM1
Mast cells	c-Kit Mast cell tryptase
Endothelium	Factor VIII

15.6 Commonly used immunohistochemistry stains for tissue types in skin tumours.

'profile' of positive markers obtained leads to the identification of the phenotype. It is important to note that anaplastic tumours, whose histogenesis and phenotype cannot be identified by microscopy, can also lose their expression of characteristic markers. Hence, anaplastic tumours, for which IHC would help phenotyping, can have equivocal staining. In this circumstance, the results of IHC may add little or nothing to the microscopic examination and interpretation by a pathologist.

Proliferation markers for tumours

Proliferation markers such as Ki67 and AgNOR are now being used routinely for differentiating histologically low or intermediate grade mast cell tumours from high grade tumours. Ki67 is a large nuclear protein that is expressed exclusively by cells in all phases of the cell cycle except G0 and, therefore, if a cell is expressing Ki67, it is replicating. It is an independent prognostic factor in many human tumours and has been shown to be an independent prognostic factor in canine mast cell tumours (Scase *et al.*, 2006).

Tumour clonality by PCR for antigen receptor rearrangement

In canine and feline lymphoma cases, clonality by PCR for antigen receptor rearrangement (PARR) is now routinely performed on formalin-fixed tissue to support the diagnosis of lymphoma. Lymphoid cells normally contain DNA antigen binding regions (encoded by specific DNA sequences) that are unique. Clonality testing (PARR) uses PCR to detect and amplify antigen receptor genes in order to establish whether populations of lymphoid cells are clonal (with the same receptor rearrangement) or polyclonal.

> ### Key points
> - Infectious agents should always be considered in the case of inflammatory nodules; these may be unusual or present in very small numbers
> - Tissue biopsy provides the optimal sample for microbial culture from nodules and draining tracts
> - Freezing fresh tissue for further PCR testing is advantageous if an unusual infection is suspected

References and further reading

Goldschmidt MH and Shofer FS (1992) *Skin Tumours of the Dog and Cat.* Pergamon Press, Oxford

Gross TL, Ihrke PJ and Walder EJ (1992) *Veterinary Dermatopathology. A Macroscopic and Microscopic Evaluation of Canine and Feline Skin Disease.* Mosby-Year Book, St Louis

McEntree MC and Page RL (2001) Feline vaccine-associated sarcomas. *Journal of Veterinary Internal Medicine* **15**, 176–182

Scase TJ, Edwards D, Miller J *et al*. (2006) Canine mast cell tumors: correlation of apoptosis and proliferation markers with prognosis. *Journal of Veterinary Internal Medicine* **20**, 151–158

Scott DW, Miller WH and Griffin CE (2001) *Muller & Kirk's Small Animal Dermatology, 6th edn.* WB Saunders, Philadelphia

Yager JA and Wilcock BP (1994) *Colour Atlas and Text of Surgical Pathology of the Dog and Cat.* Mosby-Year Book Europe Limited, London

Chapter 16

An approach to disorders of pigmentation

Zeineb Alhaidari

In veterinary dermatology, disorders of pigmentation are disorders of melanogenic pigmentation; the role of other factors that contribute to pigmentation in hairless skin, such as haemoglobin or carotenes, is anecdotal.

Melanin pigments are synthesized in specialized cells, the melanocytes, which are present in the hair follicle and epidermal basal layer. Melanocytes are dendritic cells that send connections to a determined number of neighbouring keratinocytes, to form a pigmentary functional unit. In the human epidermis, every melanocyte is associated with 36 keratinocytes, whilst the bulbar melanocyte is associated with only four cortical keratinocytes. These follicular melanocytes have specific properties. They are taller than epidermal melanocytes and synthesize larger melanosomes, which are distributed individually to the cortical cells. They are characterized by cyclic activity, synthesizing melanin during the anagen phase and entering apoptosis during the catagen phase, to be replaced at the next cycle by non-differentiated cells that reside in the permanent upper part of the outer root sheath.

The precursors of melanocytes, melanoblasts, originate in the neural crest. After migration to their final location in the skin, eyes, inner ears and leptomeninges, these precursor cells proliferate and differentiate into melanin-producing melanocytes. These cells are characterized by the highly organized membrane-bound organelles called melanosomes in which melanin biosynthesis takes place. Melanin synthesis is dependent on the production of competent melanogenic enzymes. Tyrosinase is the critical and rate-limiting enzyme in melanin production.

Once established, the melanocyte, a fragile cell almost devoid of proliferation potential, is unable to produce growth factors and is dependent on the neighbouring keratinocytes and fibroblasts to survive. Ultraviolet (UV) light is the most potent stimulus for melanogenesis. It has both direct and indirect effects on melanocytes, resulting in an increased number of dendrocytes and increased synthesis of both melanosomes and tyrosinase. The result of these effects may be seen as tanning in alopecic dogs (Figure 16.1).

Disorders of pigmentation occur when any of these distinct and specific mechanisms is disturbed. They are, therefore, common clinical problems. Pigmentation disorders not only have a cosmetic importance, but sometimes a medical or zootechnical significance because they can reflect systemic diseases or genodermatoses. Compiling the list of differential diagnoses requires a methodical approach based on the three classical major steps of every dermatological examination: history, physical examination and diagnostic tests.

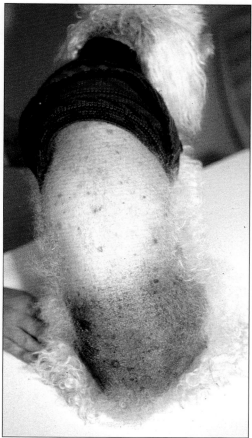

16.1 Tanning observed in an alopecic white Poodle incompletely protected from the sun by a coat.

Hypopigmentation disorders

Differential diagnosis

The differential diagnoses for hypopigmentation disorders are listed in Figure 16.2.

Clinical approach

Figure 16.3 summarizes the clinical approach to hypopigmentation disorders.

Extensive lesions	
Inherited	Piebaldism Waardenburg syndrome Oculocutaneous albinisms Chediak–Higashi syndrome
Acquired	Nutritional imbalances: • Copper deficiency • Zinc deficiency • Severe protein deficiencies (rare)
Circumscribed lesions	
Acquired	Traumatic: • Physical trauma (X-rays, burns, cold, mechanical) • Chemical trauma • Surgical scars Immune-mediated: • Vitiligo • Uveodermatological syndrome Post-inflammatory: • Lupus • Bullous autoimmune dermatoses • Contact dermatitis • Any inflammatory dermatitis Infectious: • Leishmaniosis (humans and dogs) Idiopathic: • Idiopathic nasal hypopigmentation (not a disease) • Periocular depigmentation of the Siamese cat

16.2 Differential diagnoses for hypopigmentation disorders.

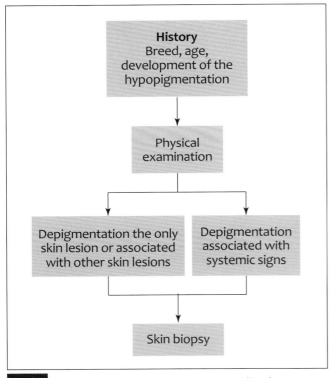

16.3 Diagnostic approach to hypopigmentation disorders.

History and signalment

Breed disposition: Certain breeds are recognized as being most at risk for circumscribed hypomelanoses.

- Vitiligo: this is most prevalent in the Belgian Shepherd, Rottweiler, Dobermann, Rough Collie, Newfoundland, German Shorthaired Pointer, German Shepherd Dog and Old English Sheepdog, and in the Siamese cat.

- Uveodermatological syndrome: this is reported mainly in northern breeds of dog such as the Siberian Husky, Akita Inu and Samoyed.
- Cutaneous lupus: this predominantly affects the Rough Collie, Shetland Sheepdog and the German Shepherd Dog.
- Dermatomyositis: this is described mainly in the Rough Collie, Shetland Sheepdog and Beauceron Shepherd Dog.
- Acquired nasal idiopathic hypopigmentation: this condition is observed more frequently in the Labrador Retriever, Siberian Husky, Samoyed, Poodle and German Shepherd Dog.

Age of onset: The age of onset of hypomelanosis is of major diagnostic importance. If the lesions are present at birth or appear early in life, they are indicators of geno-dermatoses, such as Waardenburg syndrome (Figure 16.4), albinism (see below) or dermatomyositis. The development of achromic macules on the mucocutaneous junctions in young adults points towards vitiligo or lupus. Development of depigmentation in middle-aged animals may be suggestive of an autoimmune disease, while in older animals it may be more suggestive of a neoplastic disease, such as cutaneous lymphoma.

Development of the condition: The development of hypopigmentation should be documented carefully. The circumstances of its onset should be considered. Any trauma can potentially induce spongiosis, which interferes with the distribution of melanosomes to adjacent keratinocytes. It can even result in the death of melanocytes, with subsequent irreversible amelanosis. Any preceding drug administration should be reported.

The location of the initial lesion is of great importance, particularly if dealing with nasal depigmentation:

- Achromic macules that appear at the junction of the nasal planum with hairy skin can be associated with mucocutaneous pyoderma, autoimmune skin disease or, in the older dog, epitheliotrophic lymphoma
- The rostral nares are often a primary site for contact dermatitis
- If the depigmentation is unilateral, typically located on the floor of the nares, and associated with a purulent discharge, nasal aspergillosis should be considered.

Seasonality of depigmentation is an indicator for some cases of lupus and pemphigus erythematosus because the lesions in these diseases are photo-aggravated. These disorders are generally associated with other clinical signs such as crusting, erosions or ulceration.

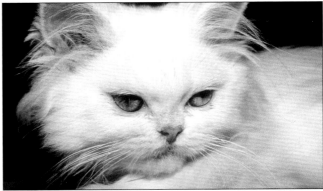

16.4 Waardenburg syndrome in a white Persian kitten, which presented with complete deafness and heterochromic irides.

General physical examination

Hypomelanoses are sometimes associated with multisystemic diseases:

- The joints and other body systems are involved in both systemic lupus erythematosus (SLE) and leishmaniosis
- Ocular involvement is reported in leishmaniosis, systemic mycoses (such as cryptococcosis) and uveodermatological syndrome
- Blood cells are affected in SLE or canine cyclic haemopoiesis (a rare genodermatosis described in the collie).

Dermatological examination

A thorough dermatological examination must be carried out to ascertain whether depigmentation is the only cutaneous lesion present. If this is the case, and if the lesions arelimited to the nose, the persistence of nasal markings suggests a non-inflammatory dermatosis, such as acquired idiopathic nasal hypopigmentation (Figure 16.5) or vitiligo. However, sunlight can induce an actinic dermatitis in any unpigmented, initially non-inflamed lesion with subsequent disappearance of nasal markings.

When depigmentation is associated with other skin lesions, the type of lesion may point towards a possible diagnosis:

- Scales: leishmaniosis should be considered
- Pustules, vesicles, crusts and ulcers: autoimmune disease should be considered
- Nodules: infectious diseases such as systemic mycoses and tumours should be considered.

Diagnostic tests

Skin biopsy: This is the fundamental diagnostic test when dealing with hypopigmentation. The biopsy specimens should be taken from the centre of the lesions, but

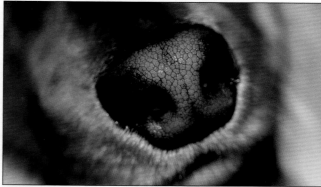

16.5 Persistence of nasal markings in a case of idiopathic acquired nasal hypopigmentation.

should also include the margins, especially if the lesions are extending.

- The absence of both an inflammatory infiltrate and melanocytes points towards post-inflammatory depigmentation or vitiligo.
- If melanocytes are present and there is no inflammatory infiltrate, acquired idiopathic nasal hypopigmentation should be suspected (however, the diagnosis remains a clinical one).
- Lymphocytic lichenoid (interface) infiltrates (band of inflammatory cells in the superficial dermis) are of interest in cutaneous lupus, epitheliotrophic lymphoma and uveodermatological syndrome, where a granulomatous lichenoid infiltrate is pathognomonic of the uveodermatological syndrome
- When dealing with granulomatous or pyogranulomatous nodular to diffuse infiltrates, special stains should be used to try to demonstrate infectious agents such as *Leishmania*, mycobacteria or fungal organisms.

Vitiligo

Vitiligo is a circumscribed melanocytopenic amelanosis that results from the selective destruction of melanocytes.

Pathogenesis

Vitiligo is an autoimmune disease in which cutaneous melanocytes are destroyed by CD8+ T-cells. Exogenous and endogenous stimuli promote oxidative stress leading to excessive reactive oxygen species (ROS), which are responsible for the production of damage-associated molecular patterns (DAMPs) and the release of melanosomal antigens that activate innate immunity through dendritic cells, leading finally to the recruitment of CD8+ T-cells that destroy the melanocytes. By the production of tumour necrosis factor (TNF)-alpha and interferon-gamma, oxidative stress enhances the secretion of interleukin (IL)-6 and IL-8, increasing the recruitment of CD8+ T-cells, thus amplifying the inflammatory network. There is also a lower T regulatory response and a higher dendritic cell induced Th 17 response, supporting a Th 17 mediated autoimmunity via the activation of dendritic cells.

Predisposing factors

Various breeds are predisposed (see above).

Clinical presentation

Vitiligo is characterized by the development of achromic macules on facial mucocutaneous junctions in young animals (Figure 16.6). With time, these macules spread progressively and symmetrically, and could extend to the footpads, nails and hair without other accompanying skin pathology.

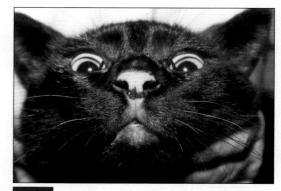

16.6 Vitiligo in a young Siamese crossbreed cat.

▶

Vitiligo *continued*

Diagnosis

Biopsy samples from depigmenting lesions demonstrate an active process with a discrete superficial perivascular lymphocytic inflammatory infiltrate. Established lesions are characterized by the absence of melanocytes and the absence of inflammatory infiltrate.

Treatment

Classically, there is no treatment that provides reliable results and the development of the condition is unpredictable. In some early cases, glucocorticoids are useful and may give a satisfying re-pigmentation. In one study L-phenylalanine treatment for 6 months resulted in clinical improvement (Guaguère and Mueller, 2008). Currently, therapies that disrupt the inflammatory pathway, targeting interferon-gamma, interferon-gamma receptor or downstream signals, such as the Janus kinase (JAK)-signal transducer and activator of transcription (STAT) pathway, are under investigation. As a consequence, the JAK kinase inhibitors could be a promising therapy.

Uveodermatological syndrome

Uveodermatological syndrome has been described mainly in Akitas, Samoyeds and Siberian Huskies (Figure 16.7), but it has been reported in other breeds as well. It resembles the Vogt-Koyanagi-Harada syndrome in humans, in which a combination of neurological symptoms (meningitis) with ophthalmological signs (uveitis) and cutaneous manifestations (alopecia and depigmentation) is seen. In the dog, neurological manifestations are rare and may only be found on post-mortem examination (Denerolle *et al.*, 2000). Males are affected twice as often as females.

Pathogenesis

This condition is caused by an immune-mediated reaction directed against melanocytes. In humans, it has been demonstrated that the proteins of the tyrosinase family are the target for the autoimmune T-cells. In both humans and dogs, anti-retinal antibodies have been detected but could be produced in response to the retinal damage.

Clinical presentation

Dogs classically present with severe uveitis, which may precede or follow depigmentation of the facial mucocutaneous junctions, extending sometimes to the hair (poliosis), other mucocutaneous junctions or the footpads. The cutaneous lesions can progress to erosions and ulcers. Since progression of the ocular lesions can lead to blindness, it is imperative that this is identified and treated promptly.

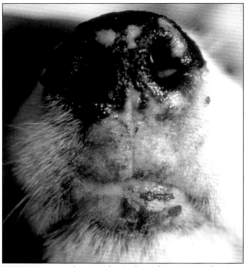

16.7 Uveodermatological syndrome in a Siberian Husky, with partial depigmentation of the nose, muzzle and lips.

Diagnosis

Skin histology is diagnostic and the lesions are characterized by a granulomatous to pyogranulomatous lichenoid infiltrate with pigmentary incontinence. Histopathological findings in the eye demonstrate a granulomatous panuveitis and retinitis.

Treatment

Treatment involves a combination of oral immunosuppressive doses of corticosteroids and/or cytotoxic drugs, with topical corticosteroids and cycloplegics. The ophthalmological prognosis is poor unless treatment is instituted early; whilst the skin lesions generally re-pigment fairly easily, relapses are usually seen if the treatment is not maintained.

Epitheliotrophic lymphoma

An important consideration for depigmentation in the older dog is epitheliotrophic lymphoma (see Chapter 34). This often presents in the early stages with depigmentation and loss of normal skin architecture of the nasal planum and mucocutaneous junctions.

Albinism

The different forms of albinism result from disorders of melanocyte functions and are characterized by homogeneously reduced pigmentation that is usually due to deficient melanin biosynthesis. The defect can be restricted to melanosomes, as in oculocutaneous albinisms (OCAs), or can affect organelles that have a similar origin, such as lysosomes or platelets. Reduction of melanin in the eyes results in reduced visual acuity, caused by foveal hypoplasia and misrouting of the optic nerve fibres.

Oculocutaneous albinisms

OCAs are caused by either a complete lack or a reduction of melanin biosynthesis in the melanocytes. The most common mutations are associated with no residual enzyme activity and are called tyrosinase negative OCA (OCA1A). These mutations lead to the most obvious phenotype: white hairs and skin, translucent irides, severe photophobia and nystagmus. The milder forms (OCA1B, OCA2, OCA3 and OCA4, recognized in humans) have been associated with variable amounts of pigmentation. In humans, OCA6 and OCA7 demonstrate the classic visual symptoms but without an obvious change in the pigmentation patterns. All types are inherited as autosomal recessive disorders. OCA1 is caused by mutation in the tyrosinase gene (TYR), tyrosinase being the copper-containing enzyme catalyzing the first two steps in the melanin biosynthesis pathway. In humans, 303 mutations in tyrosinase are known.

Type 1 temperature-sensitive oculocutaneous albinism (OCA1-TS) is associated with unusual enzyme activity. A mutation in tyrosinase interferes with its thermostability; the enzyme is inhibited in warmer areas of the body and activated in cooler areas, such as the extremities. This form of OCA has been reported in humans and is the result of genetic selection in Siamese and Himalayan cats, mice and rabbits.

Other partial albinism disorders

The Chediak Higashi syndrome is a rare autosomal recessive disorder caused by the mutation of a lysosomal trafficking regulator protein that leads to a decrease in phagocytosis, resulting in recurrent pyogenic infection, peripheral neuropathy and partial albinism. The Chediak Higashi syndrome has been described in several species, including humans, Persian cats, Aleutian minks, beige mice, blue and silver foxes, Hereford cattle and killer whales.

Hyperpigmentation disorders

Differential diagnosis

The differential diagnoses for hyperpigmentation disorders are listed in Figure 16.8.

Clinical approach

Figure 16.9 summarizes the clinical approach to hyperpigmentation disorders.

Focal lesions		
Inherited	Lentigo Naevus	
Acquired	Demodicosis Dermatophytosis Pyoderma Trauma Neoplasia	
Multifocal lesions		
Inherited	Lentigines Naevus	
Acquired	Demodicosis Dermatophytosis Pyoderma Multicentric pigmented tumours	
Diffuse lesions		
Acquired	Demodicosis *Malassezia* dermatitis Endocrinopathies (hypothyroidism, hyperadrenocorticism, hyperoestrogenism) Recurrent flank alopecia Alopecia X Ultraviolet light on alopecic dogs	

16.8 Differential diagnoses for hyperpigmentation disorders.

History and signalment

Breed disposition: Lentigo (see below) is a congenital hypermelanosis. Demodicosis and most endocrinopathies are highly prevalent in certain breeds (see Chapter 18).

Age of onset: Young animals are prone to infectious disorders, either parasitic or bacterial. Older animals are prone to endocrinopathies and neoplastic diseases.

Development of the condition: The circumstances of the onset and development of the hyperpigmentation should be detailed. Any inflammatory condition can result in post-inflammatory hyperpigmentation.

Physical examination

The distribution of the lesions is important:

- A focal lesion may be caused by trauma, demodicosis, dermatophytosis or neoplasia
- Multifocal lesions (Figure 16.10) may be associated with pyoderma, demodicosis or dermatophytosis
- Diffuse hyperpigmentation (Figure 16.11) may be caused by demodicosis or an endocrinopathy. In both cases, it is typically the result of comedone formation and/or a diffuse increase in pigment. Endocrinopathies are frequently associated with systemic signs such as lethargy and obesity in hypothyroidism, and with polyuria/polydipsia in hyperadrenocorticism.

Diagnostic tests

Basic tests: These should be prioritized when dealing with hyperpigmentation.

- Deep skin scrapings are mandatory in all cases of hyperpigmentation to rule out demodicosis.

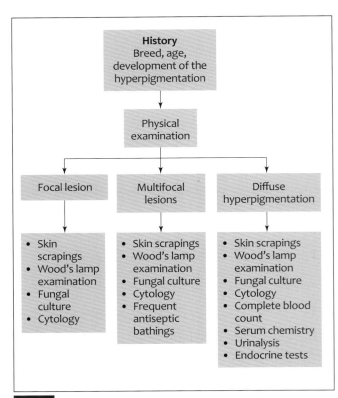

History
Breed, age, development of the hyperpigmentation

↓

Physical examination

→ Focal lesion
→ Multifocal lesions
→ Diffuse hyperpigmentation

Focal lesion:
- Skin scrapings
- Wood's lamp examination
- Fungal culture
- Cytology

Multifocal lesions:
- Skin scrapings
- Wood's lamp examination
- Fungal culture
- Cytology
- Frequent antiseptic bathings

Diffuse hyperpigmentation:
- Skin scrapings
- Wood's lamp examination
- Fungal culture
- Cytology
- Complete blood count
- Serum chemistry
- Urinalysis
- Endocrine tests

16.9 Diagnostic approach to hyperpigmentation disorders.

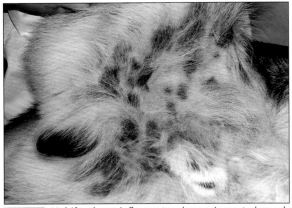

16.10 Multifocal post-inflammatory hyperpigmented macules in a case of bacterial folliculitis.

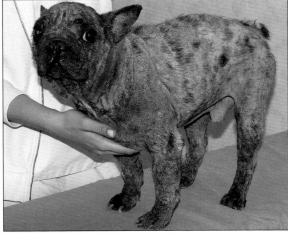

16.11 Diffuse hyperpigmentation in a case of generalized demodicosis in a French Bulldog.

- Wood's lamp examination and fungal culture are recommended.
- Cytology should be used in every case to check for the presence of *Malassezia* and bacteria.

Haematology, serum chemistry profile and urinalysis may support a possible hormonal imbalance. In such cases, specific endocrine tests are indicated.

Biopsy: This is usually not very rewarding when dealing with hypermelanoses, although some conditions may be diagnosed histologically, such as recurrent flank alopecia or neoplasia. A biopsy should be performed if these conditions are strongly suspected.

Lentigo

Clinically, the term lentigo describes a black macule that results from an increased number of basal melanocytes and an increased basal melanin load. Lentigo may present as either single or multiple lesions (lentigines) (Figure 16.12). It is the only recognized congenital form of hypermelanosis in animals. Ginger cats frequently present with multiple lentigines affecting the facial mucocutaneous junctions, which increase progressively in number and size with age and eventually coalesce.

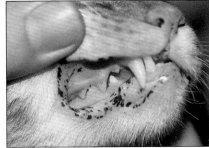

16.12 Three-year-old Domestic Shorthaired ginger cat with lentigo simplex.

Key points

- Any progressive depigmentation should be investigated as it may potentially be associated with significant clinical disease
- Hyperpigmentation is often post-inflammatory and will resolve if the underlying condition is treated
- Depigmentation of the nasal planum and mucocutaneous junctions in the older dog may be an early sign of epitheliotrophic lymphoma

References and further reading

Balu K and Puhorit R (2014) Mutational analysis of oculocutaneous albinism: a compact review. *BioMed Research International*. Article ID 905472

Denerolle P, Tessier M and Molon-Noblon S (2000) Nerve lesions in a Siberian Husky suffering from a uveodermatological syndrome. *Pratique Médicale et Chirurgicale de l' Animal de Compagnie* **35**, 273–278

Guaguère E and Muller A (2008) Efficacy of L-phenylalanine in the treatment of canine vitiligo: a preliminary report of 4 cases. *Veterinary Dermatology* **19**, 75

Rashighi M and Harris JE (2017) Vitiligo pathogenesis and emerging treatments. *Dermatologic Clinics* **35**, 257–265

Tham HL, Linder KE and Olivry T (2019) Autoimmune diseases affecting skin melanocytes in dogs, cats and horses: vitiligo and the uveodermatological syndrome: a comprehensive review. *BMC Veterinary Research* **15**, 251–268

Yamaki K, Gocho K, Hayakawa K *et al.* (2000) Tyrosinase family proteins are antigens specific to Vogt-Koyanagi-Harada disease. *The Journal of Immunology* **165**, 7323–7329

Chapter 17

An approach to focal and multifocal alopecia

Dunbar Gram and Megan Boyd

The term alopecia refers to the lack of hair on a normally haired area of skin. Alopecia is a common clinical finding and can be either primary (due to a disease affecting the hair follicle, disruption in nutrition to the hair follicle or a systemic disease affecting the hair cycle; Figure 17.1) or secondary (due to self-trauma as a result of a pruritic disease; Figure 17.2). Alopecia can also be focal (one small area), multifocal (multiple areas on the body) or generalized (affecting large areas on the body, such as the trunk).

There is a wide range of conditions that result in alopecia, and understanding the underlying pathophysiological processes will enable practitioners to develop a focused differential diagnosis list and diagnostic plan. This will allow unnecessary and potentially invasive diagnostic procedures to be avoided. The diagnostic work-up for pruritic and non-pruritic cases may differ, so it is important to determine

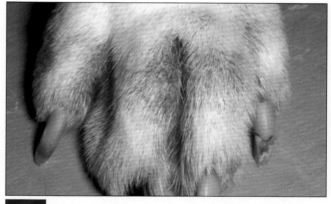

17.2 Patchy self-induced alopecia on the paw of an atopic dog.

from the history and clinical signs whether alopecia or pruritus was the initial presenting sign. However, it should be remembered that pruritus may occur concurrently with a non-pruritic disease when a secondary infection is present.

History and physical examination

The history should include the age of the animal when the clinical signs first occurred and the speed of onset. The presence or absence of other clinical signs should also be noted. In some cases, there may be an association with drugs such as vaccines or spot-on therapies and this should be recorded in the history. The signalment of the animal should be noted as some forms of alopecia have a breed or gender predisposition (e.g. sebaceous adenitis and X-linked hypohidrotic ectodermal dysplasia). The coat colour of the animal should be noted as there are conditions, such as colour dilution alopecia, that affect particular hair coat colours.

The distribution of the alopecia should be noted during the physical examination. Spontaneous alopecia tends to be well demarcated. The physical examination also may reveal findings that indicate pruritus, including excoriations, poorly demarcated alopecia, a barbered hair coat, hairs trapped within the gingival line of the incisor or canine teeth, a positive pinnal-pedal reflex and even attrition of the incisor teeth. The presence of follicular casts indicates a follicular disease.

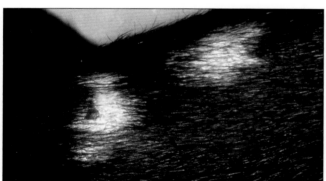

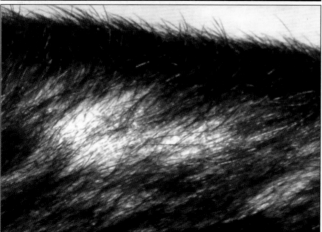

17.1 Multifocal areas of non-pruritic alopecia in an adolescent mixed-breed dog.

Diagnostic tests

Routine dermatological tests are invaluable in determining the cause of alopecia. The minimum database for cases of alopecia should include skin cytology, deep skin scrapes (or hair plucks), trichography, Wood's lamp examination and dermatophyte culture/polymerase chain reaction (PCR) (Figure 17.3). Ancillary tests, including bacterial culture, bloodwork, endocrine tests (both screening and confirmatory) and dermatohistopathology should be selected on a case-by-case basis (Figures 17.4 and 17.5).

Diagnostic test	Findings	Interpretation
Trichography	Anagen *versus* telogen hairs	A mixture of anagen and telogen hairs is normal (dependent on hair coat type) Predominantly telogen hairs is consistent with endocrine disease
	Fractured hair shafts	Alopecia secondary to pruritus
	Demodex mites/eggs	Demodicosis
	Dermatophyte hyphae and arthrospores	Dermatophytosis
	Fractured shafts associated with clumps of melanin	Colour dilution alopecia
Deep skin scrapings	*Demodex* mites/eggs	Demodicosis
Skin surface cytology	Presence of bacteria or *Malassezia*	Significant numbers associated with clinical signs suggest a secondary infection
Wood's lamp	Apple green fluorescence of hair shafts	Supports the presence of *Microsporum* spp. Culture/polymerase chain reaction (PCR) indicated to confirm

17.3 Minimum database of diagnostic tests for cases of alopecia.

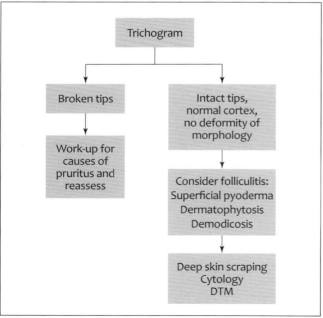

17.4 General approach to alopecia. DTM = dermatophyte test medium.

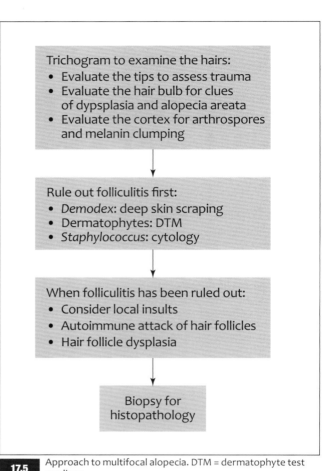

17.5 Approach to multifocal alopecia. DTM = dermatophyte test medium.

Differential diagnosis

Folliculitis and furunculosis

Folliculitis refers to inflammation within the hair follicle, which ultimately results in loss of the hair shaft. Folliculitis is the most common cause of focal and multifocal alopecia; the presence of pruritus can be variable. Furunculosis may develop if the integrity of the hair follicle is breached, resulting in inflammation within and involving the surrounding area of the hair follicle. Extensive furunculosis is painful.

In addition to alopecia, primary lesions may include papules, pustules and furuncles. Causes of folliculitis include bacterial pyoderma, demodicosis (Figure 17.6) and dermatophytosis. It should be noted that these conditions can occur concurrently and may be clinically indistinguishable in the dog. Dermatophytosis is more common in the cat. The potentially contagious and zoonotic nature of dermatophytosis means that careful consideration should be given to diagnostic testing, even when the diagnosis is considered less likely.

Demodicosis and bacterial folliculitis should form part of the initial differential diagnosis list in dogs and should be checked for at subsequent consultations if alopecia is present. This is particularly important in atopic patients if anti-inflammatory drugs are being administered to control the pruritus. The author has been referred many patients with undiagnosed demodicosis and/or pyoderma that were previously well controlled atopic patients receiving long-term medical therapy for pruritus.

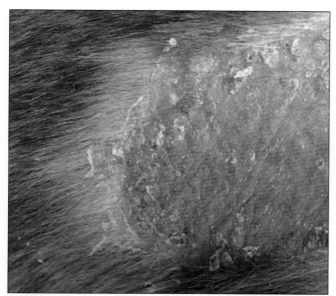

17.6 Well demarcated alopecia due to bacterial pyoderma and demodicosis. The patient had been receiving antipruritic and anti-inflammatory drugs for allergic dermatitis.
(Courtesy of the University of Florida)

Protozoal folliculitis

Leishmaniosis is an important differential diagnosis to consider in patients with alopecia that are living in, or have a history of travel from, an endemic country (Figure 17.7). The protozoan is transmitted during a blood meal from a sand fly and the development of clinical disease is dictated by the immune response of the patient. Systemic and cutaneous signs are markedly variable, although granulomatous perifolliculitis is a common inflammatory pattern (see Chapter 30).

Ischaemia

Ischaemic damage to the hair follicle can occur as a sequela to vascular compromise (see Chapter 28). In addition to alopecia, lesions created by tissue hypoxia include scale, cicatrix and comedones. There are multiple potential causes. A region of focal alopecia at the site of an injection given within the last 6 months is suggestive of a drug reaction (Figure 17.8); this can be confirmed by histopathology. However, it should be remembered that ischaemic damage due to a drug reaction may become more generalized and affect regions of the body where circulation can be readily compromised (e.g. the pinnal apices, central paw pads, tail tip and bony prominences).

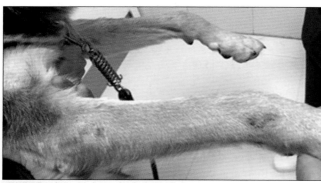

17.7 Alopecia due to leishmaniosis.
(Courtesy of Maite Verde, Zaragoza University)

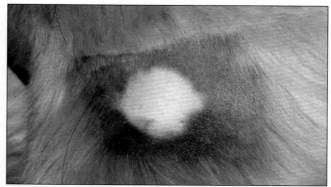

17.8 Localized vaccination reaction, resulting in focal alopecia and depigmentation. (Note that the area has been shaved for better visualization)

Dermatomyositis is a disorder involving the vascular supply to the skin and musculature. It is typically seen in young Rough Collies and Shetland Sheepdogs. Primary lesions are erosive to ulcerative, but cicatricial alopecia develops over the face, limbs and extremities (Figure 17.9). In cases where the musculature is involved, problems with chewing and locomotion may develop and muscular atrophy ensues. Both hereditary and non-hereditary cases of dermatomyositis have been described and there appears to be a complex association with genetic mutations and environmental factors.

The diagnosis of ischaemic disorders can be confirmed with histopathology.

Trauma and toxins

Trauma or toxin related causes of alopecia include direct irritant reactions from topical drugs (e.g. flea control products), subcutaneous injections (Figure 17.10), acute or chronic heat exposure, traction alopecia from tightly bound hair in a hair tie and compression alopecia, often from constant bumping against the roof of a kennel. The history and location of the alopecia often identifies the cause. Cytology should be performed to check for evidence of secondary infections and histopathology may help to confirm the disease process.

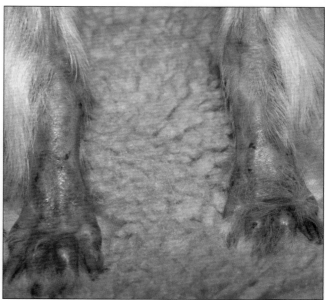

17.9 Cicatricial alopecia on the forelimbs of a Shetland Sheepdog with dermatomyositis.

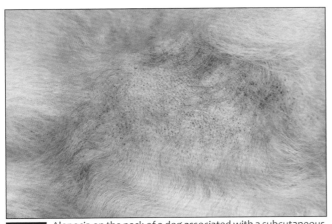

17.10 Alopecia on the neck of a dog associated with a subcutaneous injection.
(Courtesy of the University of Florida)

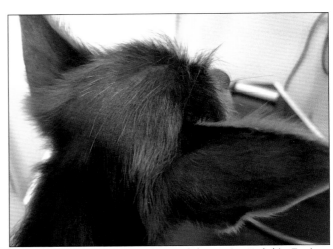

17.12 Black hair follicle dysplasia and alopecia in a Yorkshire Terrier. Note that the alopecia only affects the dark hairs.

Congenital or hereditary alopecia

Congenital or hereditary alopecia occurs early in life. There may be a familial history of the disease or, at the very least, a breed disposition. Many dogs and cats have been bred to manifest absent or sparse hair coats, including the Xoloitzcuintle (Mexican hairless dog) and the Sphynx cat. These breeds may have microscopic hairs or dysplastic hair follicles, leading to comedone formation, milia and seborrhoea considered normal for the patient. Supportive topical treatment is often required to prevent secondary infection.

Animals with a mild form may not have complete alopecia but rather demonstrate hypotrichosis. In some cases, genetic mutations can lead to multifocal alopecia; for example, canine X-linked hypohidrotic ectodermal alopecia (Figure 17.11), where the alopecia is associated with an absence of apocrine and sebaceous glands, as well as altered dentition.

Colour dilution alopecia

Colour dilution alopecia occurs in dog breeds where a breeding selection for a diluted coat colour (such as blue and fawn) has been made. A similar disorder which affects only the black hairs in a coat (black hair follicular dysplasia) is also seen (Figure 17.12). In these cases, a genetic mutation in melanophilin, responsible for the distribution of melanosomes, has been identified. The result is an accumulation of macromelanosomes in the hair shaft, which are thought to lead to weakness and fracture of the hair.

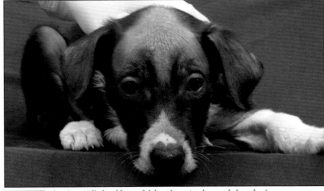

17.11 Canine X-linked hypohidrotic ectodermal dysplasia.
(Courtesy of Hilary Jackson)

This can be demonstrated on trichography and confirmed by dermatohistopathology. Affected animals present with sparse hair coats (hypotrichosis) and are predisposed to secondary infections. There is no effective treatment, but routine antimicrobial shampoos and gentle grooming of the hair coat are recommended.

Autoimmune alopecia

Alopecia areata is a rare disease that affects both dogs and cats. Cases present with well-demarcated areas of alopecia, often on the head or face but other regions of the body may also be involved. The pathogenesis for alopecia areata has not been completely determined, but auto-antibodies have been demonstrated directed at follicular proteins in the region of the hair bulb. The diagnosis is made based on histology characterized by peribulbar lymphocytic inflammation. There is not consistently effective treatment for this condition; glucocorticoids and calcineurin inhibitors have been tried with variable success.

Neoplasia

Alopecia can develop as a result of any invasive neoplasm. Multifocal patchy alopecia, often associated with variable scale and pruritus, can be a feature of epitheliotrophic lymphoma (see Chapter 34).

Key points

- The three most important causes of folliculitis resulting in multifocal alopecia are:
  - *Demodex*
  - Dermatophytes
  - *Staphylococcus*
- Deep skin scrapings and cytology should be performed for all dogs with alopecia
- Although some diseases may be considered non-pruritic (e.g. *Demodex*), pruritus can occur when secondary infections are present, therefore it is important not to assume that any patient that scratches has an allergy
- If common causes of folliculitis have been ruled out, then skin biopsy to identify less common disorders may be indicated

Chapter 18

An approach to canine symmetrical alopecia and management

Manon Paradis

The causes of alopecia in dogs are numerous and include infections, self-inflicted hair loss, endocrinopathies and follicular dysplasias. This chapter is restricted to cases of non-pruritic canine symmetrical alopecia. Hair growth is influenced by, amongst other factors, gonadal, adrenal, thyroid, pituitary and pineal hormones. Excesses, deficiencies and hormonal imbalances have been implicated in a myriad of clinical syndromes in dogs. In some endocrinopathies (e.g. hypothyroidism, hyperadrenocorticism, hyperoestrogenism and pituitary dwarfism), the hormonal mechanisms are understood and these disorders are relatively well characterized clinically. Many other alopecic disorders may resemble endocrinopathies clinically (e.g. canine recurrent (seasonal) flank alopecia, alopecia X, colour dilution alopecia and other follicular dysplasias) but, in many instances, the final diagnosis can be more difficult to establish.

Clinical approach

Figure 18.1 shows an approach to the evaluation of canine alopecia.

History and signalment

A complete history should be taken and a general physical examination conducted in order to detect any abnormalities present in other organs. A history of polyuria/polydipsia (PU/PD), the presence of a pendulous abdomen or abnormal genitalia (testicular asymmetry or cryptorchidism, vulvar enlargement) may greatly influence the selection of further tests.

The history and dermatological examination should allow the clinician to rule in or out the presence of pruritus. If present, it should be investigated first (see Chapter 6). If pruritus is absent or minimal, then it is necessary to determine whether the pattern of hair loss is focal, symmetrical or diffuse. It is important to look for the presence of inflammation and/or any primary lesions, such as papules or pustules. If such skin lesions are present, skin scrapings, skin cytology and/or dermatophyte culture should be performed. If pruritus, inflammation or any other primary lesions are absent, the next most pertinent diagnostic procedure to perform is influenced by the age of onset, breed and reproductive status. To help compile a list of differential diagnoses, the following considerations should be made:

- The dog's age at the time of onset of alopecia
- The rate of development of the alopecia
- Spontaneous resolution or progression of the disease
- The presence of a cyclical pattern.

Age and time of onset

The onset of alopecia should always be related to the dog's age and any physiological and/or pathological event, management change or treatment. Alopecia sometimes occurs several weeks after physiological events, such as pregnancy and lactation, or pathological events, such as severe systemic disease, shock or surgery (e.g. telogen effluvium). Failure of hair regrowth after clipping is suggestive of hypothyroidism, hyperadrenocorticism or alopecia X. Many disorders have an age at onset that is quite predictable:

- Congenital alopecia is present at birth
- Demodicosis usually occurs before 1 year of age
- Hypothyroidism typically develops after 3 years of age
- Hyperadrenocorticism occurs generally in middle-aged to old dogs.

Spontaneous remission

Spontaneous remission usually occurs in canine recurrent flank alopecia, anagen and telogen defluxion and post-clipping alopecia, disorders that are unrelated to endocrine imbalance. Spontaneous remission can also be seen with dermatophytosis and demodicosis. However, in these cases, some inflammation and scaling is usually present at the time of active lesions.

Breed predisposition

Certain breeds are predisposed to alopecic conditions, such as hypothyroidism, alopecia X, pattern alopecia and canine recurrent flank alopecia. Figure 18.2 lists the breed predisposition to diseases that present with symmetrical alopecia.

Coat colour

Coat colour may provide useful diagnostic information in pigment-related alopecia, such as black hair follicular dysplasia, colour dilution alopecia and follicular lipidosis. Careful evaluation of the coat may be required, as some dilute colours are subtle.

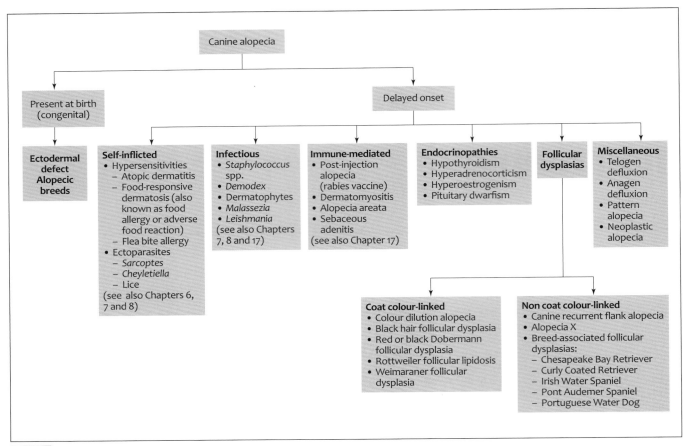

18.1 Evaluation of canine alopecia.

Condition	Predisposed breeds
Alopecia X	Alaskan Malamute, Chow Chow, Keeshond, Miniature Poodle, Pomeranian, Samoyed, Schipperke, Siberian Husky
Breed-specific follicular dysplasia	Chesapeake Bay Retriever, Curly Coated Retriever, Dobermann, Irish Water Spaniel, Pont Audemer Spaniel, Portuguese Water Dog
Canine recurrent flank alopecia (CRFA)	Airedale, Bearded Collie, Boxer, Bouvier des Flandres, English and French Bulldogs, Golden and Labrador Retrievers, Griffon Korthal, Schnauzer
Colour dilution alopecia (CDA)	Bernese Mountain Dog, Chihuahua, Chow Chow, Dachshund, Dobermann, Great Dane, Italian Greyhound, Labrador Retriever (silver), Large Munsterlander, Miniature Pinscher, Newfoundland, Poodle, Saluki, Shetland Sheepdog, Schipperke, Silky Terrier, Staffordshire Bull Terrier, Whippet, Yorkshire Terrier
Hyperadrenocorticsm	Boston Terrier, Boxer, Miniature Poodle
Hypothyroidism	American Pitt Bull Terrier, Beagle, Boxer, Cocker Spaniel, Dalmatian, English Setter, German Wirehaired Pointer, Giant Schnauzer, Golden Retriever, Maltese, Old English Sheepdog, Rhodesian Ridgeback, Shetland Sheepdog
Pattern alopecia	Boston Terrier, Boxer, Chihuahua, Dachshund, Greyhound, Miniature Pinscher, Whippet
Sebaceous adenitis	Akita Inu, Border Collie, Chow Chow, English Springer Spaniel, German Shepherd Dog, Havanese, Samoyed, Standard Poodle, Vizsla

18.2 Breeds predisposed to diseases that present with symmetrical alopecia (all of these conditions can also be seen in crossbreed dogs).

Sexual status

Hyperoestrogenism caused by a Sertoli cell tumour, or ovarian cysts or tumours may also lead to alopecia. Lack of the oestrous cycle in bitches may be seen with hypothyroidism or hyperadrenocorticism.

Diagnostic tests

If the history and signalment fail to produce a definitive diagnosis, further tests are necessary. These should be selected according to the index of suspicion (Figure 18.3). Haematology, biochemistry and urinalysis may be useful to evaluate the general health status of adult dogs with an alopecic condition, or if a systemic disease that may lead to alopecia is suspected. Hormone tests should be carried out if the clinical signs and results of blood tests and urinalysis suggest an endocrinopathy.

Skin biopsy may be the initial and only diagnostic procedure performed if sebaceous adenitis is strongly suspected.

Condition	Underlying pathology	Age of onset	Cutaneous signs apart from alopecia	Systemic signs	Laboratory findings	Diagnostic tests	Therapy
Alopecia X	Unknown	Adult	Hyperpigmentation, hair regrowth at the biopsy site	None	None	Rule out other causes, skin biopsy (large number of flame follicles suggestive)	Neutering, melatonin, benign neglect, deslorelin, dutasteride, trilostane, mitotane
Anagen defluxion	Cessation of mitotic activity in rapidly dividing hair matrix cells	Variable	None	Related to severe systemic disease or to cytotoxic therapy	Related to underlying pathology	Trichogram	Withdraw offending drug
Breed-specific follicular dysplasia	Unknown	Variable	Secondary pyoderma	None	None	Trichogram, skin biopsy	None
Canine recurrent flank alopecia	Unknown	Adult	None	None	None	Skin biopsy may be helpful	Melatonin or benign neglect
Colour dilution alopecia	Abnormality of melanization	<1 year	Comedones, secondary pyoderma	None	None	Trichogram, skin biopsy	None
Congenital alopecia	Ectodermal defect	At birth	None	Anomalies of dentition	None	Skin biopsy	None
Hyperadrenocorticism	Pituitary or adrenal neoplasia	Adult/old	Atrophic skin, calcinosis cutis, comedones, prominent cutaneous blood vessels	PU/PD, polyphagia, panting, pot-belly muscle atrophy, lethargy, testicular atrophy, abnormal oestrus	↑ Cholesterol, ↑ triglycerides, ↑ ALP, moderate ↑ other liver enzymes, stress leucogram, dilute urine	Abnormal cortisol response to ACTH stimulation test, LDDST and HDDST, ↑ urinary C:C ratio, ultrasonography	Surgical: adrenalectomy Medical: mitotane, trilostane
Hyperoestrogenism	Functional gonadal neoplasia or ovarian cyst, exogenous oestrogen	Adult	Hyperpigmentation, enlarged vulva, linear preputial dermatosis, gynecomastia	Abnormal oestrus, abnormal sexual behaviour	Bone marrow suppression	Ultrasonography, radiography, histopathology (gonads)	Surgical neutering, stop exogenous source of oestrogen
Hypothyroidism	Lymphocytic thyroiditis	Middle age	Dull hair coat, scaling, myxoedema,	Lethargy, obesity	↑ Cholesterol, non-regenerative anaemia	↓ Total T4, ↑ TSH	Levothyroxine
Pattern alopecia	Unknown	<1 year	None	None	None	Skin biopsy	Melatonin
Pituitary dwarfism	Abnormal pituitary gland development. Autosomal recessive inherited (German Shepherd Dog)	<1 year	Hyperpigmentation, secondary pyoderma	Proportionate dwarfism, ± hypothyroidism, hypogonadism	None	Growth hormone response test ± total T4, free T4	Growth hormone, progestin, ± levothyroxine, antibacterial shampoos, systemic antibiotics
Sebaceous adenitis	Unknown	Variable	Scaling, follicular casts	None	None	Skin biopsy, trichogram,	Ciclosporin, retinoids (vitamin A), keratolytic, moisturisers
Telogen effluvium	Synchronous arrest of the hair cycle	Variable	None	Only if systemic disease or physiological stress is present	None	Trichogram, skin biopsy	None, rapid resolution

18.3 Characteristics and treatment in canine symmetrical alopecia. ACTH = adrenocorticotropic hormone; ALP = alkaline phosphatase; C:C = cortisol:creatinine ratio; HDDST = high-dose dexamethasone suppression test; LDDST = low-dose dexamethasone suppression test; PU/PD = polyuria/polydipsia; T4 = thyroxine; TSH = thyroid-stimulating hormone.

Congenital alopecia

The partial or total absence of hair at birth is a rare condition. Congenital alopecia is often associated with abnormalities in other ectodermal-derived cutaneous appendages (e.g. epitrichial and atrichial glands, claws) and teeth. The condition has been reported occasionally in various breeds (see Chapter 17). In addition, it is a characteristic of some breeds selected for a hairless phenotype, such as the Mexican Hairless Dog (Xoloitzcuintle), the Peruvian Hairless Dog (Peruvian Inca Orchid; Figure 18.4a) and the Chinese Crested Dog (Figure 18.4b). This ectodermal dysplasia (associated with abnormal dentition), due to a mutation in the FOX13 gene, is inherited as a monogenic autosomal semidominant trait in these three breeds (Drögemüller et al., 2008). Heterozygous dogs are hairless and homozygous mutants die during embryogenesis. The alopecia seen in the American Hairless Terrier is inherited as an autosomal recessive trait. It is due to a mutation in the SGK3 gene and is not associated with abnormal dentition (Parker et al., 2017).

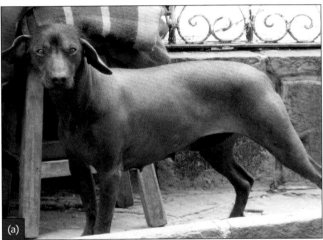

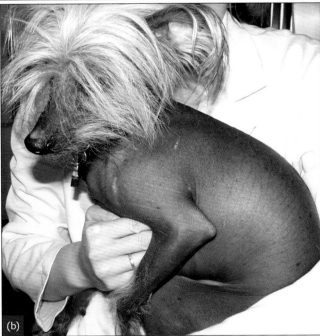

18.4 (a) Peruvian hairless dog. (b) Chinese crested dog.

Endocrinopathies

An endocrine aetiology should be suspected in dogs with a bilateral, non-pruritic, symmetrical alopecia, failure of hair regrowth after clipping, cutaneous hyperpigmentation and the presence of comedones, especially if concurrent systemic clinical signs are present.

Hypothyroidism

Hypothyroidism is a common canine endocrinopathy. However, owing to the polysystemic and often vague clinical signs, and to the lack of a perfect diagnostic test, hypothyroidism is also commonly misdiagnosed in this species.

Pathogenesis

The most common cause of canine thyroid dysfunction is heritable lymphocytic thyroiditis. Thyroid hormones have a myriad of physiological effects and are necessary for normal cell metabolism. They stimulate erythropoiesis and regulate both cholesterol synthesis and its degradation. Thyroid hormones are needed for the initiation of anagen hair follicles, regulation of the cornification process and sebaceous gland secretion. Hypothyroidism occurs most commonly in mid- to large purebreed dogs and usually has an onset of clinical signs between 3 and 6 years of age. Several breeds are reported to be at increased risk of developing hypothyroidism (see Figure 18.2).

Clinical presentation

Hypothyroidism is characterized by a plethora of clinical signs affecting the skin and other organ systems (Figure 18.5):

- Common: dry, dull and brittle hair coat; scaling; lack of hair regrowth after clipping; alopecia and hyperpigmentation on the bridge of the nose, tail and friction areas; generalized hyperpigmentation; weight gain/obesity (without polyphagia); lethargy; mental dullness
- Uncommon: pyoderma; facial myxoedema (tragic look); weakness; exercise intolerance; cold intolerance; truncal alopecia
- Rare: ceruminous otitis; bradycardia; hypothermia; ocular disorders; reproductive disorders; facial paralysis.

None of the clinical signs is pathognomonic for hypothyroidism and their development is generally gradual and insidious. Congenital hypothyroidism is rare and results in disproportionate dwarfism (with epiphyseal dysgenesis), macroglossia, delayed dental eruption and cretinism, in addition to the usual clinical signs. In a clinical context, hypothyroidism is rare in dogs <2 years of age.

Diagnostic tests

Of the numerous diagnostic tests available to evaluate thyroid function, no single test is optimal, and hypothyroidism is sometimes difficult to diagnose with confidence. Each test has advantages and limitations that the veterinary surgeon (veterinarian) should be aware of, and so far none can accurately confirm or rule out hypothyroidism in all cases. Readers are referred to specialist textbooks for more details about the diagnostic tests available.

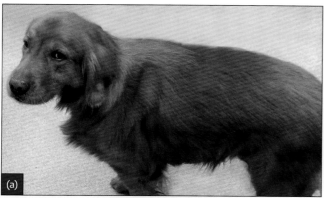

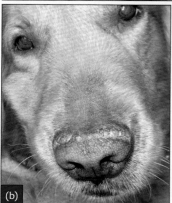

18.5 Hypothyroidism in a Golden Retriever.
(a) Tragic face with myxoedema and poor hair coat. (b) Alopecia and hyperpigmentation of the bridge of the nose.
(c) Alopecia of the tail.

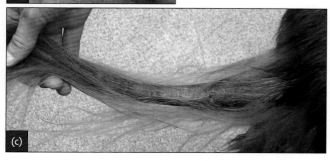

When evaluating thyroid function in a dog, the clinician should:

- Select patients with clinical signs and age (>2 years old) that are compatible with hypothyroidism
- Be aware of the factors (mostly drugs and non-thyroidal illnesses) that can alter the test results
- Postpone thyroid evaluation, if possible, until resolution of the illness or withdrawal of the drug
- Send samples to a laboratory that has validated assays for dogs and has established reference values.

A definitive diagnosis of hypothyroidism can best be made based on a combination of compatible clinical signs and abnormal specific thyroid test results, coupled with successful long-term response to levothyroxine supplementation. Any thyroid function test results (and response to therapy) in dogs should be interpreted carefully, and always with a healthy dose of scepticism. If there is discordance between two tests results (e.g. total thyroxine (TT4) and canine thyroid-stimulating hormone (cTSH)) or if the results are ambiguous, it is preferable to resubmit blood samples a few weeks to a few months later or to perform additional tests, such as free thyroxine (FT4), thyroglobulin auto-antibodies (TgAA) or thyroid-stimulating

hormone (TSH) stimulation test using recombinant human TSH (rhTSH). The measurement of TgAA, along with FT4 and cTSH, has been advocated for screening at-risk animals prior to breeding (Orthopedic Foundation for Animals, North America), with the aim of ultimately eliminating heritable forms of thyroiditis.

Treatment

Lifelong therapy with levothyroxine is required. It is administered orally, at the induction dose of 20 μg/kg q12h (or 0.5 mg/m² q12h). Lethargy can resolve within a few days, but it can take a few months for the hair coat to return to normal. After levothyroxine replacement therapy has been administered for 4–8 weeks, or when all the clinical signs have resolved, a 'post-pill' serum TT4 concentration should be measured 4–6 hours after administration to determine whether an adequate concentration of the hormone is present in the blood. Typically, the author aims for a TT4 level in the high normal range, or slightly above the normal range. The serum cTSH concentration should normalize with appropriate therapy. However, it is not the most useful parameter to measure for the monitoring of adequate dosing because it can detect hypothyroid dogs that are undertreated but cannot distinguish between dogs that are adequately supplemented and those that are oversupplemented.

Thyrotoxicosis (associated with PU/PD, weight loss, panting, nervousness and tachycardia) is rare in dogs, owing to the rapid metabolism and renal/hepatic excretion of thyroid hormones. Nevertheless, in most hypothyroid dogs, treatment can be reduced to once daily administration (20 μg/kg or 0.5 mg/m² orally q24h) after an adequate clinical response is noted, without reduction in efficacy. Owing to the hereditary nature of this disorder, hypothyroid dogs (or dogs with results compatible with lymphocytic thyroiditis) should not be allowed to breed.

Hyperadrenocorticism

Spontaneous and iatrogenic hyperadrenocorticism are common and well recognized disorders in dogs. However, the occurrence of iatrogenic hyperadrenocorticism has declined over recent decades, owing to increased recognition and an improved therapeutic approach to several disorders (e.g. allergies, yeast dermatitis), which were historically poorly controlled by relatively high doses and long-term use of glucocorticoids.

Approximately 85% of dogs with spontaneous hyperadrenocorticism suffer from pituitary-dependent hyperadrenocorticism. The remaining 15% of cases are caused by an adrenocortical neoplasm (adenoma or adenocarcinoma) that secretes excessive amounts of cortisol. Spontaneous hyperadrenocorticism occurs more frequently in middle-aged to older dogs, and some breeds such as the Dachshund, Boxer, Boston Terrier and Miniature Poodle are at increased risk. The onset of clinical signs is insidious and slowly progressive.

Clinical presentation

The clinical signs of hyperadrenocorticism are usually fairly characteristic:

- Common: PU/PD; polyphagia; abdominal enlargement/truncal obesity (caused by hepatomegaly, muscle weakness and/or intra-abdominal fat accumulation) (Figure 18.6a); lethargy; muscle weakness; panting; symmetrical alopecia; skin hyperpigmentation; thin and hypotonic skin (Figure 18.6b); comedones

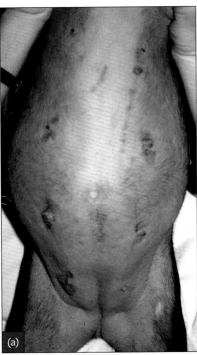

18.6 (a) Pituitary-dependent hyperadrenocorticism in a Boston Terrier, showing alopecia and pot-bellied appearance.
(b) Hyperadrenocorticism in a mixed-breed dog. Note the alopecia and thin abdominal skin showing dermal blood vessels.

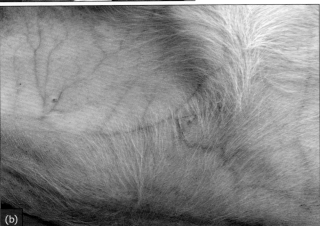

an elevated UCCR. However, most dogs with an elevated UCCR do not have hyperadrenocorticism. If the UCCR is normal, it is most likely that the dog does not have hyperadrenocorticism. If the ratio is elevated, more specific tests, such as the low-dose dexamethasone suppression test (LDDST) or the adrenocorticotropic hormone (ACTH) stimulation test, must be performed to determine whether hyperadrenocorticism is truly present

- LDDST and ACTH stimulation test these have a sensitivity of approximately 90–95% and 85%, respectively. Therefore, the LDDST will be normal in 5–10% of patients and the ACTH stimulation test will be normal in about 15% of patients with hyperadrenocorticism. If the dog has the classical signs and laboratory abnormalities but no non-adrenal gland illness, the diagnosis of hyperadrenocorticism can be made with confidence. However, if non-adrenal gland illness is present, the LDDST has about a 50% false–positive rate and the ACTH stimulation test has about a 15% false–positive rate

If an animal has been receiving any form of steroid, even topically, for weeks to months, either test can be altered owing to feedback effects. The time needed for withdrawal and recovery of the pituitary–adrenal axis depends on the duration of treatment and type of steroid used

Steroid therapy can cause clinical signs of hyperadrenocorticism (iatrogenic) and can also cause atrophy of the adrenal gland cortex. This can be diagnosed by evaluating the lack of response to the ACTH stimulation test.

Tests to differentiate between pituitary- and adrenal-dependent hyperadrenocorticism:

- Ultrasonography should not be used to diagnose hyperadrenocorticism but rather to differentiate pituitary-dependent hyperadrenocorticism from a functional adrenal gland tumour. With a good ultrasound machine, skill and adequate abdominal echogenicity allowing good visualization of the adrenal glands, it may not be necessary to perform diagnostic procedures such as the high-dose dexamethasone suppression test (HDDST) or measurement of endogenous ACTH
- The origin of the hyperadrenocorticism can be determined in about 75% of dogs using the HDDST. If cortisol levels are suppressed, the diagnosis is pituitary-dependent hyperadrenocorticism. If cortisol levels are not suppressed by the HDDST in a dog with confirmed hyperadrenocorticism, then the dog could still have either form, with odds of pituitary-dependent *versus* adrenal-dependent hyperadrenocorticism of 50:50. If there is no suppression, abdominal ultrasonography should be performed or the endogenous ACTH level measured.

- Less common: calcinosis cutis; easy bruising; phlebectasia; coat colour change; non-healing wounds; chronic infections; neurological signs secondary to a pituitary gland tumour; testicular atrophy; anoestrus; clitoral hypertrophy.

Diagnostic tests

No single clinical sign, haematological finding or biochemical change is always present in each case of hyperadrenocorticism and, furthermore, all of the changes can be seen in several other disorders. Therefore, before a diagnosis of hyperadrenocorticism can be established, several screening tests and diagnostic procedures must be performed in order to avoid the misdiagnosis of hyperadrenocorticism and missing concomitant disorders. The diagnostic procedures that can be performed to confirm and localize hyperadrenocorticism are outlined in Figure 18.7.

Tests for hyperadrenocorticism include:

- Urinary cortisol:creatinine ratio (UCCR): this is useful only in ruling out hyperadrenocorticism. Nearly 100% of dogs with spontaneous hyperadrenocorticism have

Treatment

- In cases of iatrogenic hyperadrenocorticism, the patient should be gradually weaned off exogenous glucocorticoids until the hypothalamus–pituitary–adrenal axis is normalized.
- In cases with an adrenal gland neoplasm, unilateral adrenalectomy is the treatment of choice.
- In patients with pituitary-dependent hyperadrenocorticism, several therapeutic options are available, with mitotane and trilostane being used most commonly.

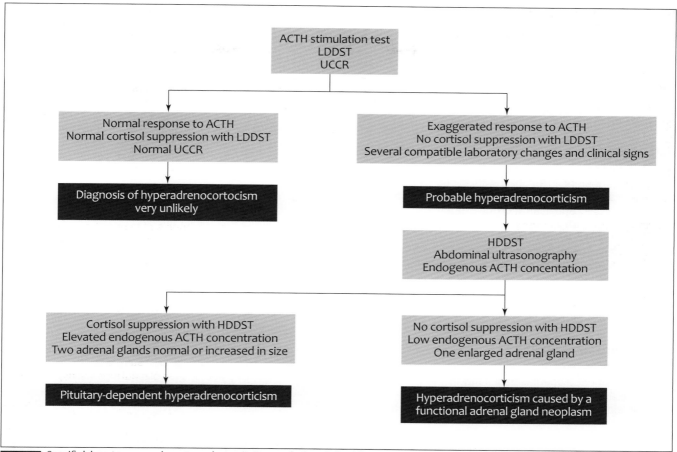

18.7 Specific laboratory procedures to evaluate pituitary and adrenal gland function in suspected cases of canine hyperadrenocorticism. ACTH = adrenocorticotropic hormone; HDDST = high-dose dexamethasone suppression test; LDDST = low-dose dexamethasone suppression test; UCCR = urinary cortisol:creatinine ratio.

Before initiating treatment, the cost, benefits and potential side effects should be discussed in detail with the owner. Irrespective of the treatment chosen, each dog should be monitored carefully, with the treatment adjustment as needed.

Mitotane (Op'-DDD): Mitotane, not currently licensed for dogs in the UK (can be obtained/prescribed per the cascade as a human drug), has been used extensively in the treatment of pituitary-dependent hyperadrenocorticism. Mitotane causes necrosis of the zona fasciculata and zona reticularis, but usually spares the zona glomerulosa of the adrenal gland.

An induction dose of 25–50 mg/kg/day orally (divided q12h and administered with food) is used to effect (5–21 days; average 5–8 days). Daily administration should be stopped if water intake decreases to <60 ml/kg over 24 hours, if partial or total anorexia, lethargy, diarrhoea or vomiting occurs, or if the cortisol concentration measured pre- and post-ACTH stimulation performed on day 8 or 9 of treatment is low or normal. The maintenance dose is approximately 50 mg/kg per week. This dose can be divided and the drug administered q24–48h, if possible.

The side effects related to treatment are due to a decrease in the cortisol level to below that required for physiological needs. The side effects include lethargy, anorexia, weakness, vomiting and diarrhoea. If such side effects are encountered, the administration of mitotane must be stopped and a physiological dose of glucocorticoid (prednisone at 0.25 mg/kg orally q24h) given for a week if needed. Prednisone must be stopped at least 24 hours before measuring cortisol because it cross-reacts in the assay.

Treated dogs need to be re-evaluated periodically. An ACTH stimulation test may need to be performed every 3–6 months because the mitotane dose may need to be increased during the first year of treatment.

Trilostane: The use of trilostane has gained increasing popularity among veterinary surgeons over the last two decades and in many countries it is the only drug that is approved for the treatment of canine hyperadrenocorticism. Trilostane inhibits adrenal steroidogenesis, including the synthesis of cortisol and aldosterone.

An initial dose of 0.5–1 mg/kg orally q12h is currently recommended (Pérez-Alenza, 2017). The dose is adjusted according to the clinical signs and serum cortisol values 2–4 hours post ACTH stimulation.

Trilostane is well tolerated in most dogs but severe adverse effects may occur. Dogs treated with trilostane should be evaluated after 10–15 days of treatment and again after 1 month, 3 months and every 3–6 months thereafter. Most dogs show resolution of PU/PD within 1 month and dermatological clinical signs within 3 months.

Trilostane is the drug of choice for dogs with adrenal-dependent hyperadrenocorticism to prepare them for adrenalectomy and to reduce postoperative complications. Trilostane can also be used in patients with inoperable adrenal gland tumours.

Hyperoestrogenism and other problems related to sex hormones

Excesses, deficiencies and imbalances of sex hormones have been implicated in a myriad of clinical syndromes in dogs that lead to alopecia. However, with the exception of hyperoestrogenism, most previously reported ill-defined dermatoses associated with sex hormones of gonadal origin are probably non-existent.

Pathogenesis

Hyperoestrogenism may occur in males with a functional testicular tumour or in bitches with cystic ovaries, functional ovarian tumours (usually a granulosa cell tumour) or following chronic administration of exogenous oestrogen. Testicular neoplasia is common, especially in cryptorchid dogs, and Sertoli cell tumours are the most common type to cause hyperoestrogenism, leading to endocrine alopecia (seen in about one-third of cases). Metastases occur in fewer than 10% of cases. Clinical signs related to hyperoestrogenism can also occur in dogs in direct contact with, or following licking of, oestrogen creams (e.g. hormone replacement skin products) applied to human skin.

Clinical presentation

Dermatological signs of hyperoestrogenism include bilateral, symmetrical alopecia, beginning in the perineal and genital areas and progressing from the rear to the front of the dog along the ventral trunk and neck, with frequent hyperpigmentation. A preputial linear dermatosis with erythema or hyperpigmentation from the prepuce to the scrotum can be also seen. The affected dog may have symmetrical alopecia, feminization or both. Feminization is characterized by a pendulous prepuce, nipple enlargement and the attraction of other male dogs. In bitches, hyperoestrogenism is manifested clinically by vulvar and nipple enlargement associated with oestrous cycle abnormalities such as prolonged oestrus and nymphomania.

Diagnostic tests

In intact males, diagnosis is often made by clinical examination and palpation of a testicular mass, testicular asymmetry (contralateral testicular atrophy) or cryptorchidism. Abdominal ultrasonography is useful to evaluate intra-abdominal testes, the prostate gland and investigate the presence of metastases. Prostatomegaly (due to oestrogen-induced squamous metaplasia) or oestrogen-induced bone marrow depression (resulting in anaemia, leucopenia or pancytopenia) can occur, and pale mucous membranes and/or petechiae may be seen. In intact bitches, the diagnosis is usually straightforward, especially if oestrus and cutaneous changes are present. Abdominal ultrasonography in bitches may show cystic or neoplastic ovaries or the presence of metastases.

Treatment

Surgical neutering (bilateral castration, ovariohysterectomy) or withdrawal of the exogenous source of oestrogen is the treatment of choice.

Pituitary dwarfism

Pituitary dwarfism is a rare disorder that results from the inadequate secretion of growth hormone with resultant retardation of growth and progressive hair loss. It has been reported most commonly in German Shepherd Dogs (Figure 18.8), in which it has been shown to be inherited as an autosomal recessive trait.

Clinical presentation

Affected dogs appear normal at birth, but growth retardation is usually evident by 2–3 months of age. Proportionate dwarfism and bilaterally symmetrical alopecia and hyperpigmentation become obvious before the dog reaches adulthood. The clinical signs are related to growth hormone deficiency, with or without concurrent thyroid, adrenocortical and gonadal abnormalities.

Treatment

Growth hormone administration has been the treatment of choice for several years; however, it is expensive and exogenous administration can be associated with the development of antibodies and diabetes mellitus. Progestin, which induces the production of growth hormone from the mammary glands, can also been used. Levothyroxine should be used if secondary hypothyroidism is present.

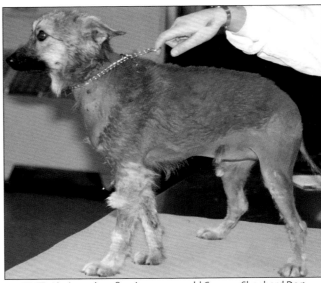

18.8 Pituitary dwarfism in a 1.5-year-old German Shepherd Dog bitch.

Follicular dysplasias

The term follicular dysplasia embraces a group of often ill-defined alopecic disorders that could be linked to coat colour, including:

- Colour dilution alopecia
- Black hair follicular dysplasia
- Canine recurrent flank alopecia
- Alopecia X
- Various breed-associated follicular dysplasias.

Colour dilution alopecia
Pathogenesis

Coat colour dilution in dogs is a specific pigmentation phenotype caused by defective transport of melanosomes, which leads to the accumulation of large clumps of pigment in the hair shaft. More than 20 breeds segregate for dilute coat colour (Welle *et al.*, 2009). It is inherited as an autosomal recessive trait and is often accompanied by alopecia. However, the dilute mutation is not sufficient to result in clinical signs of the disease. The risk of developing colour dilution alopecia seems to be breed-specific; for example, most (if not all) blue Dobermanns develop some degree of alopecia, while most Weimaraners do not (Laffort-Dassot *et al.*, 2002).

Clinical presentation

Affected dogs show a progressive alopecia that affects only the dilute areas between 3 months and 3 years of age (Figure 18.9). Scaling and comedones with secondary bacterial infection are also present in affected areas.

Diagnostic tests

Breed predisposition and the presence of alopecia restricted to the diluted areas should suggest such a condition. The trichogram shows large melanin clumps along the hair shafts, causing distortion and fracture of the hairs. Histological examination of skin specimens from affected areas shows abnormal melanin aggregates in the epidermal and follicular basal cells.

Treatment

Palliative therapy may be attempted with melatonin, retinoids or essential fatty acids to improve the condition of the hair and skin. Secondary pyoderma should be treated with antibacterial shampoos and, in refractory cases, systemic antibiotics. Since the hair of these patients is fragile and prone to break, it is important to select products that are not too harsh or drying, and mild moisturizing formulations are preferable.

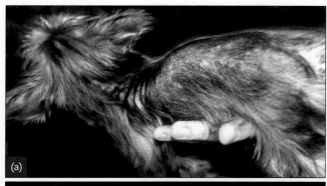

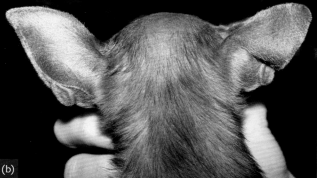

18.9 (a) Yorkshire Terrier with colour dilution alopecia affecting the blue area of the body. (b) Chihuahua showing colour dilution alopecia on the head and ear pinnae, with a normal hair coat in the brown areas.

Canine recurrent flank alopecia

Canine recurrent (seasonal) flank alopecia is characterized by episodes of truncal hair loss, which often occur on a recurrent basis.

Pathogenesis

The cause of canine recurrent flank alopecia is unknown but the seasonal nature and recurrence suggests that photoperiod may be involved (Paradis, 2019c). There is a higher incidence of canine recurrent flank alopecia at higher latitude (around or north of the 45 degree parallel). In Australia and New Zealand, the onset of canine recurrent flank alopecia appears to be the reverse of what is seen in the northern hemisphere (but also during their short photoperiod season), which supports the involvement of light exposure in this disorder. The high incidence in some breeds and the familial character of canine recurrent flank alopecia suggest a genetic influence.

Clinical presentation

Canine recurrent flank alopecia is characterized by a fairly abrupt onset of non-scarring alopecia, usually bilaterally symmetrical, with well demarcated borders and often markedly hyperpigmented alopecic skin (Figure 18.10). The alopecia is usually confined to the thoracolumbar region,

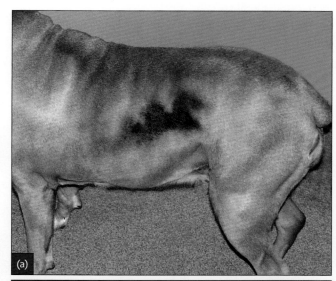

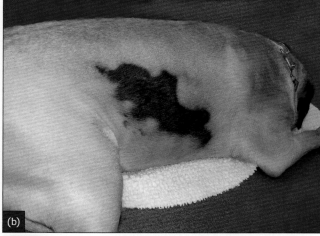

18.10 Canine recurrent flank alopecia in (a) a Boxer and (b) a Mastiff.

but occasionally it is seen in association with alopecia on the dorsum of the nose, base of the ears, base of the tail and perineum.

Spontaneous regrowth of a normal pelage generally occurs within 3–8 months (range: 1–14 months), although some individuals have coat colour changes in areas affected previously (melanotrichia in Boxers; aurotrichia in Miniature Schnauzers). In some cases, hair regrowth may become less complete after several episodes; it may even progress to an end-stage of permanent flank alopecia and marked hyperpigmentation. Up to 20% of canine recurrent flank alopecia cases may have only one isolated episode of flank alopecia during their lifetime; however, most dogs develop recurrent alopecic episodes for years. Some dogs have an occasional year when the alopecia does not recur. The degree of alopecia is variable, with some dogs developing virtually identical hair loss (size and duration) year after year, and other dogs developing larger areas and/or longer episodes of hair loss as years go by.

The mean age at onset of the first episode is approximately 4 years (range: 8 months to 11 years). The majority of dogs have an onset of alopecia between November and March in the northern hemisphere. Dogs of either sex and of any reproductive status can be affected. Several breeds are at higher risk of developing canine recurrent flank alopecia, and Boxers account for approximately half of all cases (see Figure 18.2). The condition appears to be rare or absent in the plush-coated Nordic breeds, German Shepherd Dog and Cocker Spaniel.

Diagnostic tests

In most cases, the diagnosis is based on the history and clinical signs. Histopathological findings (such as 'witch's feet') are suggestive of, but not pathognomonic for, canine recurrent flank alopecia. In dogs presented during their first episode, other causes of alopecia such as endocrinopathies (hypothyroidism, hyperadrenocorticism) and other follicular dysplasias need to be ruled out. Although hypothyroidism does not typically cause an abrupt onset of truncal alopecia, it is important to rule it out because both hypothyroidism and canine recurrent flank alopecia can occur in the same animal (Daminet and Paradis, 2000).

Treatment

The unpredictable course of canine recurrent flank alopecia and the spontaneous regrowth of hair render the evaluation of any therapeutic agent difficult, whether it is used to prevent canine recurrent flank alopecia or to shorten an existing episode of alopecia. Oral melatonin (3–6 mg/dog q8–12h) can be administered before an expected episode of alopecia or shortly after the onset of alopecia (Paradis, 1999, 2019c). The probability of recurrence without treatment is approximately 70% in any given year. Dogs affected with canine recurrent flank alopecia are healthy otherwise, and benign neglect is also a valuable therapeutic approach.

Alopecia X

Alopecia X is the name most veterinary dermatologists are now using to refer to the following diseases:

- Pseudo-hyperadrenocorticism
- Adult-onset growth hormone deficiency
- Growth hormone-responsive alopecia
- Adrenal gland sex hormone imbalance
- Congenital adrenal gland hyperplasia-like syndrome
- Lysodren-responsive dermatosis
- Follicular dysplasia of Nordic breeds (woolly syndrome, coat funk in Malamutes)
- Follicular growth dysfunction of the plush-coated breeds.

More recently, the name 'hair cycle arrest' has been proposed but the author finds this term confusing because it either refers to alopecia X exclusively or to all acquired non-inflammatory alopecic disorders.

Pathogenesis

The aetiology of alopecia X remains obscure. A genetic predisposition to an unidentified hormonal imbalance is plausible, but a defect residing at the hair follicle level is also possible. If the problem is a primary disorder of the hair growth cycle, various stimuli (including different hormones) could draw the hair follicles into the anagen phase.

Clinical presentation

Initially, there is loss of the primary hairs (with retention of secondary hairs) in the frictional areas (around the neck, caudomedial thighs and tail) (Figure 18.11). Gradually, all hair is lost in these regions and eventually the truncal primary hairs are also lost, giving the remaining coat a puppy-like appearance. With time (several months to

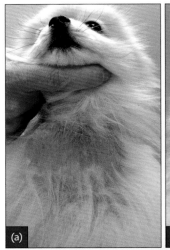
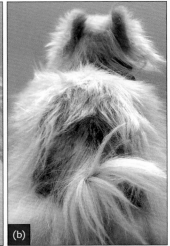
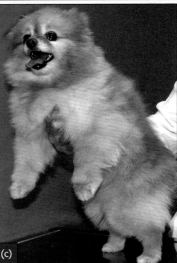

18.11 Pomeranian with alopecia X showing hair loss (a) around the neck and (b) on the rump. (c) The same dog after melatonin treatment.

years), the secondary hairs become sparse and hyper-pigmentation of the exposed skin and/or a colour change in the remaining hair coat may be seen. The head and legs are usually spared. A tendency to regrow hair at the skin biopsy site or at the site of traumatic stimuli (e.g. skin scraping, sunburn, pyoderma) is a common finding in this syndrome.

Alopecia X is seen most commonly in young adults, but it can also develop in older dogs. Dogs of either sex and of any reproductive status can be affected. Breeds more at risk of developing this syndrome are the Nordic breeds and Poodles (see Figure 18.2).

Diagnostic tests

The diagnosis is based on the history, physical examination findings and ruling out other diseases (e.g. hypothyroidism, spontaneous and iatrogenic hyperadrenocorticism, hyperoestrogenism, sebaceous adenitis, telogen effluvium and other follicular dysplasias). Skin biopsy may be useful to rule out sebaceous adenitis. In addition, the presence of a large number of hair follicles with excessive trichilemmal keratinization (flame follicles) is suggestive of alopecia X. A reproductive hormone panel before and following ACTH stimulation has been used in the past; however, a retrospective study has demonstrated that this is not useful in the diagnosis of alopecia X (Frank et al., 2003).

Treatment

Various medical and surgical treatments have been suggested. Castration induces hair growth in up to 70% of cases. Oral melatonin is the treatment of choice in neutered animals. It is given at a rate of 3–6 mg/dog q8–12h for up to 3 months and is effective in up to 40% of cases (Paradis, 1999; Frank et al., 2003) (see Figure 18.11c). Deslorelin is effective in approximately 80% of intact male dogs but appears ineffective in neutered females. Dutasteride, a 5-alpha reductase inhibitor, may be effective in approximately 50% of the cases. Mitotane and trilostane have been used successfully in some dogs but should be used with caution. Benign neglect is a valid option because alopecia X is essentially an aesthetic problem.

Breed-associated follicular dysplasias

Distinct types of follicular dysplasia have been described in the Irish Water Spaniel (Cerundolo et al., 2000), Portuguese Water Dog (Miller and Scott, 1995), Chesapeake Bay Retriever (Cerundolo et al., 2005), Pont Audemer Spaniel (Guaguère et al., 2000) and Curly Coated Retriever (Bond et al., 2016). It is possible that the disorder in the Chesapeake Bay Retriever is the same as that in the Irish Water Spaniel, because the latter was one of several breeds used to create the Chesapeake Bay Retriever.

Clinical presentation

Affected dogs are born with a normal hair coat. Focal or diffuse symmetrical alopecia, usually affecting the dorsum and flanks, develops during adulthood. Some Portuguese Water Dogs (Figure 18.12) and Irish Water Spaniels present with clinical lesions identical to those of canine recurrent flank alopecia with spontaneous remission and recurrence of flank or truncal alopecia.

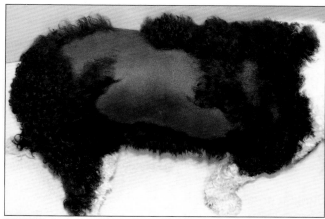

18.12 Portuguese Water Dog with follicular dysplasia affecting the trunk.

Diagnostic tests

The breed predisposition and clinical signs are indicative of this condition. Histology of skin specimens shows varying degrees of follicular hyperkeratosis, melanin clumping and dysplastic hair follicles.

Treatment

These genetically based dermatoses are incurable. Affected dogs are otherwise healthy, with the exception of secondary pyoderma. In some cases, melatonin and essential fatty acid supplementation may improve coat quality and reduce the severity of the alopecia. Secondary pyoderma should be treated with antibacterial shampoos and, in refractory cases, systemic antibiotics.

Miscellaneous conditions

Miscellaneous conditions that result in symmetrical alopecia include:

- Anagen defluxion
- Telogen defluxion
- Pattern alopecia
- Sebaceous adenitis.

Anagen defluxion

This is a rare condition, typically seen in dogs with an anagen predominant hair cycle (e.g. Poodles). It is caused by an abrupt cessation of mitotic activity in rapidly dividing hair matrix cells (anagen hair), usually associated with severe systemic disease or the administration of cytotoxic medications, such as doxorubicin, for which the risk of developing alopecia increases with cumulative dose (Falk et al., 2017).

Clinical presentation

Hair loss, which occurs within days to weeks of drug administration, can be localized to the face or trunk, or can be generalized.

Diagnostic tests

A history of previous treatment with a cytotoxic drug or possible contact with toxic substances is suggestive. The trichogram shows anagen hair bulbs and irregular hair shafts.

Treatment

There is no specific treatment for this condition; spontaneous resolution occurs if the offending drug is withdrawn.

Telogen defluxion

This is an uncommon condition in which the hair follicles go into a premature resting phase. It is associated with stressful events, such as pregnancy, parturition, lactation, severe systemic illness, marked febrile episodes, shock, surgery and various drugs. The cause of hair loss is the synchronous premature progression from the anagen to telogen phase.

Clinical presentation

Patchy to diffuse alopecia can occur within 2–4 months and affects the trunk. Hairs are usually easily epilated.

Diagnostic tests

A history of metabolic stress and excessive epilation are suggestive. The trichogram shows a predominance of telogen hairs.

Treatment

Specific therapy is not required because complete hair regrowth occurs a few months after the cause of the metabolic stress has been resolved.

Pattern alopecia

Canine pattern alopecia is a relatively common disorder that may present with several different syndromes. The two main forms of canine pattern alopecia are the ventral type (the most common syndrome) and the pinnal type.

Pathogenesis

Canine pattern alopecia has been recognized in several short-coated breeds (see Figure 18.2). The aetiology is unknown, but the strong breed and familial predisposition suggests that genetic predisposition is involved. Canine pattern alopecia may be an overshoot reaction to artificial selection pressure favouring the fine, delicate coat sought by breeders. Over recent decades, breeders of smooth-coated Dachshunds have been able to decrease the incidence of the ventral type of canine pattern alopecia significantly by selective breeding, but with the result that the dogs generally have a coarser hair coat (Paradis, 2019b).

Clinical presentation

Canine pattern alopecia affects dogs of either sex and of any reproductive status. A progressive alopecia that remains restricted to the described areas usually starts before 1 year of age.

- Canine pattern alopecia, ventral type: progressive alopecia that develops along the ventral neck, chest and abdomen, the caudomedial aspect of the thighs, the perineum and the postauricular regions (base of the ear pinnae) (Figures 18.13 and 18.14).
- Canine pattern alopecia, pinnal type: progressive alopecia of the convex aspect of the ear pinnae as well as the bridge of the nose in many cases.
- Alopecia and melanoderma of the Yorkshire Terrier: alopecia and hyperpigmentation of the convex aspect of the ear pinnae and the bridge of the nose. This is probably the same disorder as canine pattern alopecia, pinnal type but reported under a different appellation.

Diagnostic tests

The diagnosis is based on the history, dermatological examination and exclusion of other differential diagnoses. The histopathological findings are characterized by miniaturization of the hair follicles.

Treatment

This disorder is strictly aesthetic and no effective treatment has been reported, with the exception of melatonin (see Figure 18.14b). Good results have been observed in several dogs treated with this drug.

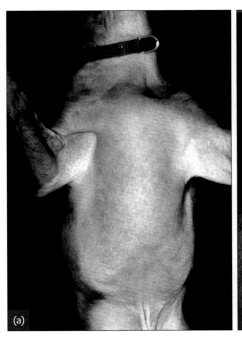 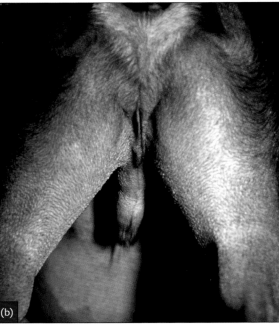

18.13 Miniature Pinscher with pattern alopecia affecting (a) the ventral chest and (b) the caudomedial aspect of the thighs.

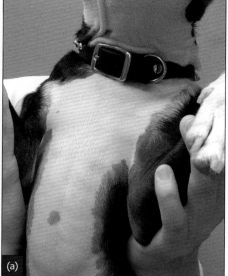
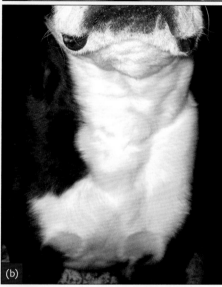

18.14 Boston Terrier with pattern alopecia affecting the ventral chest (a) before and (b) after melatonin administration.

Sebaceous adenitis

Sebaceous adenitis is characterized by a granulomatous inflammation involving the sebaceous glands, with their progressive destruction. The aetiopathogenesis is unknown, but breeds such as the Standard Poodle and Akita are genetically predisposed (see Figure 18.2).

Clinical presentation

Varying degree of alopecia with severe scaling and crusting affecting the head and trunk. The hair coat becomes dull, dry and brittle and is easily epilated. Follicular casts are often present.

Diagnostic tests

The presence of follicular casts in a predisposed breed is suggestive of sebaceous adenitis. Histology of skin specimens shows variable degrees of sebaceous adenitis with complete absence of the glands in the late stage of the condition.

Treatment

Sebaceous adenitis cannot be cured; however, clinical control can be attained with topical and/or systemic therapy. Topical therapy (propylene glycol, oil soak, antiseborrhoeic shampoos) may improve the quality of the coat but the destruction of the sebaceous glands is permanent unless systemic ciclosporin is used (Linek *et al.*, 2005). Oral administration of essential fatty acids or retinoids may be helpful in some cases. Secondary pyoderma should be treated with antibacterial shampoos or systemic antibiotics in severe cases.

Key points

- When evaluating a middle-aged dog with symmetrical truncal alopecia, it is important to rule out endocrine disease. This is rarely a problem in young dogs
- There are a number of breed-related genodermatoses the clinician should be aware of, which present in younger dogs
- A skin biopsy can be helpful and lead to a definitive diagnosis in some diseases, such as sebaceous adenitis, but may only be supportive in other alopecic diseases

---

References and further reading

Behrend EN (2014) Chapter 10, Canine hyperadrenocorticism. In: *Canine and Feline Endocrinology, 4th edn*, eds. EC Feldman, R Nelson, C Reusch and JC Scott-Moncrieff, pp. 377–451. Elsevier Saunders, St. Louis, Missouri

Behrend EN, Kooistra HS, Nelson R *et al.* (2013) Diagnosis of spontaneous canine hyperadrenocorticism: 2012 ACVIM Consensus statement (Small Animal). *Journal of Veterinary Internal Medicine* **27**, 1292–1304

Bond R, Varjonen K, Hendricks A *et al.* (2016) Clinical and pathological features of hair coat abnormalities in Curly Coated Retrievers from UK and Sweden. *Journal of Small Animal Practice* **57**, 659–667

Cerundolo R, Lloyd DH, McNeil P *et al.* (2000) An analysis of factors underlying hypotrichosis and alopecia in Irish Water Spaniels in the United Kingdom. *Veterinary Dermatology* **11**, 107–122

Cerundolo R, Maudlin EA, Goldschmidt MH *et al.* (2005) Adult-onset hair loss in Chesapeake Bay Retrievers: a clinical and histological study. *Veterinary Dermatology* **16**, 39–46

Cerundolo R, Paradis M and Mecklenburg L (2009) Breed specific hair-cycle abnormalities. In: *Hair Loss Disorders in Domestic Animals*, ed. L Mecklenburg *et al.*, pp. 169–175. Wiley-Blackwell, Iowa

Daminet S and Paradis M (2000) Evaluation of thyroid function in dogs suffering from recurrent flank alopecia. *Canadian Veterinary Journal* **41**, 699–703

Drögemüller C, Karlsson EK, Hytönen MK *et al.* (2008) A mutation in hairless dogs implicates FOX13 in ectodermal development. *Science* **321**, 1462–1471

Falk EF, Lam ATH, Barber LG and Ferrer L (2017) Clinical characteristics of doxorubicin-associated alopecia in 28 dogs. *Veterinary Dermatology* **28**, 207–212

Frank LA, Hnilica KA, Rohrbach BW and Oliver JW (2003) Retrospective evaluation of sex hormones and steroid hormone intermediates in dogs with alopecia. *Veterinary Dermatology* **14**, 91–97

Guaguère E, Degorce-Rubiales F, Poujade A *et al.* (2000) Genetic follicular dysplasia in Pont Audemer spaniel dogs: a report of eight cases. *Veterinary Dermatology* **11(S1)**, 14–40

Laffort-Dassot C, Beco L and Carlotti D (2002) Follicular dysplasia in five Weimaraners. *Veterinary Dermatology* **13**, 253–257

Linek M, Boss C, Haemmerling R and Mecklenburg L (2005) Effects of cyclosporine A on clinical and histologic abnormalities in dogs with sebaceous adenitis. *Journal of the American Veterinary Medical Association* **226**, 59–64

May ER, Frank LA and Sula MM (2019) Description and characterization of a hair coat disorder in schipperkes. *Veterinary Dermatology* **30**, 36–43

Mecklenburg L (2009) Canine hyperoestrogenism. In: *Hair Loss Disorders in Domestic Animals*, ed. L Mecklenburg *et al.*, pp. 142–148. Wiley-Blackwell, Iowa

Miller WH, Griffin CE and Campbell K (2013) *Muller and Kirk's Small Animal Dermatology 7th edn.* Elsevier Saunders, St. Louis, Missouri

Miller WH and Scott DW (1995) Follicular dysplasia of the Portuguese Water Dog. *Veterinary Dermatology* **6**, 67–74

Mooney CT (2016) Chapter 299: Hypothyroidism. In: *Textbook of Veterinary Internal Medicine, 7th edn*. ed. SJ Ettinger and EC Feldman, pp. 1731–11742. WB Saunders, Philadelphia

Paradis M (1999) Melatonin therapy in canine alopecia. In: *Kirk's Current Veterinary Therapy XIII*, ed. JD Bonagura, pp. 546–549. WB Saunders, Philadelphia

Paradis M (2019a) Alopecia X. In: *Clinical Veterinary Advisor Dogs and Cats. 4th edn*. ed. Cohn and Coté, pp. 44-45. Elsevier Saunders, St-Louis, Missouri

Paradis M (2019b) Canine pattern alopecia. In: *Clinical Veterinary Advisor Dogs and Cats, 4th edn*. ed. Cohn and Coté, pp. 766–767, Elsevier Saunders, St. Louis, Missouri

Paradis M (2019c) Canine recurrent flank alopecia. In: *Clinical Veterinary Advisor Dogs and Cats, 4th edn*. ed. Cohn and Coté, pp. 869–870. Elsevier, St-Louis

Paradis M and Cerundolo R (2005) Genodermatoses: alopecia and hypotrichoses. In: *Advances in Veterinary Dermatology Vol. 5*, ed. A Hillier *et al*., pp. 360–364. Blackwell, Oxford

Parker HG, Harris A, Dreger DL *et al*. (2017) The bald and the beautiful: hairlessness in domestic dog breeds. *Philosophical Transaction Research Society*, doi.org/10.1098/rstb.2015.0488

Pérez-Alenza D and Melian C (2017) Chapter 306: Hyperadrenocorticism in Dogs. *Textbook of Veterinary Internal Medicine, 8th edn*. ed. SJ Ettinger, EC Feldman and E Coté, pp. 1795–1811, WB Saunders, Philadelphia

Welle M, Philipp U, Fenacht SR *et al*. (2009) MLPH genotype–melanin phenotype correlation in dilute dogs. *Journal of Heredity* **100**, S75–S79

Chapter 19

An approach to otitis

Emmanuel Bensignor

Otitis is a very frequent clinical presentation in veterinary practice, estimated to affect up to 15–20% of the canine population (Bensignor et al., 2008; Harvey and Haar, 2017). It is often underestimated in the acute phase both by the owner and the veterinary surgeon (veterinarian), which may lead to chronicity and, in some cases, irreversible damage and deafness. Recurrent or chronic otitis externa is one of the most frustrating diseases encountered in daily practice and can adversely affect the quality of life of both patients and owners. Otitis should always be considered as a consequence of an underlying disease, and the investigation and management of ear disease should therefore be considered in the context of a dermatological disease. This chapter provides an oriented approach to otitis, relevant to general practitioners. Treatment is covered in Chapter 20.

Definitions

Otitis

Otitis is defined as inflammation of the pinna and ear, which includes the ear canal (otitis externa), middle ear cavity (otitis media) and inner ear (otitis interna). The history and clinical examination are important to determine which part of the ear is affected (Miller et al., 2012).

Otitis externa

Otitis externa is defined as an inflammatory condition affecting the external auditory canal, extending from the pinna to the tympanic membrane. It can be subdivided into different conditions depending on the time of onset of clinical signs, the rate of relapse and/or the clinical presentation (Figure 19.1). Otitis externa is very common in dogs and cats, with its incidence being reported as between 5 and 12% of consultations in dogs and up to 2% of cats referred to a dermatologist (Carlotti and Taillieu-Leroy, 1997; Bensignor et al., 2000; Aymeric and Bensignor, 2018).

Otitis media: spontaneous

Otitis media is defined as inflammation within the middle ear. The reported prevalence of otitis media varies widely, but in dogs and cats is usually a consequence of otitis externa. In one study of 214 dogs presenting with signs of middle ear disease, 40% of those which underwent

Classification	Duration	Clinical signs
Acute	<7 days	Erythema, inflammation of the ear canal, no discharge. Commonly associated with acute flares of atopic dermatitis
Subacute	7–30 days	Inflammation and discharge present with significant pruritus
Chronic: episodes may respond partially to treatment but relapse quickly	>30 days	Usually associated with significant, often suppurative, discharge. Pruritus may be present but these cases are often painful. Hyperplastic changes result in significant stenosis

19.1 Various clinical presentations of otitis externa in dogs and cats.

computed tomography (CT) examination had changes on the images and these were most frequently associated with a history of chronic suppurative otitis (Belmudes et al., 2018). However, some cases can occur directly due to increased production of exudate in the middle ear and/or from decreased draining through the auditory tube (e.g. primary secretory otitis media seen in brachycephalic dogs and spoontaneous primary otitis media in cats) (Harvey and Haar, 2017).

Otitis interna

Otitis interna is defined as inflammation within the inner ear. Otitis interna generally results from an extension of otitis media, but the route of infection may (rarely) be meningogenic or haematogenic. Clinical signs are principally neurological, identical to those seen with peripheral vestibular disease, or deafness may occur (Harvey and Haar, 2017).

Pathogenesis

Otitis is usually not only a local phenomenon, but rather one manifestation of an underlying dermatosis with consequences on the ear canal. It has a complex and multifactorial aetiology and a number of authors have proposed that the causes should be classified as primary, secondary, predisposing and perpetuating factors (Griffin, 1993; Saridomichelakis et al., 2007) (Figure 19.2).

- Primary factors are directly responsible for the inflammation and by themselves are sufficient to cause a problem.

Primary factors
• Ectoparasites
• Allergic dermatitis
• Keratinization disorders
• Autoimmune dermatosis
• Foreign bodies
• Neoplasia
Secondary factors
• *Malassezia*
• Bacteria
• Ulcerations
Predisposing factors
• Conformation of the ear
• Humidity
• Inappropriate cleaning
• Irritant treatments
• Excessive hair growth in auditory canals
• Pyrexia
• Immunocompromising disorders
Perpetuating factors
• Proliferative and hyperplastic changes
• Otitis media
• Over treatment

19.2 Primary, secondary, predisposing and perpetuating factors of otitis in dogs and cats.

(Data from Griffin, 1993)

- Infections are common secondary factors.
- Predisposing factors are conditions that increase the risk of otitis but by themselves are not sufficient to cause otitis (Scott *et al.*, 2001).
- Perpetuating factors are responsible for the chronicity in the sense that they prevent the resolution of the otitis externa (e.g. otitis media).

The successful management of otitis relies on the identification and treatment of all the above factors.

Irrespective of the cause of inflammation, if left untreated hyperplasia of the epidermal lining and ceruminous glands occurs, resulting in excess cerumen production and narrowing of the ear canals. The speed of development of these changes can vary according to the breed of dog. Cocker Spaniels are the best example of a breed prone to develop a rapid onset of glandular hyperplasia as a result of inflammation. Chronic changes also impair the normal otic housekeeping mechanism that results in movement of cerumen up and out of the ear canal, further contributing to the accumulation of discharge within the auditory canal (Harvey and Haar, 2017). This leads to an environment favourable for the growth of, and infection with, commensal microorganisms such as yeasts and bacteria, leading to further inflammation.

In most chronic cases, extensive epidermal hyperplasia develops and the diameter of the ear canal decreases as the apocrine glands become hyperplastic and dilated. A dense dermal inflammatory infiltrate occurs, followed by fibroplasia, which further exacerbates the canal obstruction (Bensignor *et al.*, 2008; Harvey and Haar, 2017). Ossification of the cartilages and associated skin may occur in longstanding cases. When the infection becomes chronic and/or when there is a high quantity of exudate in the ear canal, the tympanic membrane may be ruptured and otitis media develops, which further contributes to the clinical signs and is a factor in recurrence of disease following apparently successful therapy. Finally, it has been demonstrated recently that certain bacteria can produce a biofilm in which they become relatively quiescent.

In these cases, most antibiotics are ineffective as they cannot penetrate the biofilm, allowing the bacteria to multiply, which contributes to the chronicity of the disease. This may also be true in some cases of *Malassezia* infection.

Clinical scoring of otitis in dogs

A study has described the use of a clinical scoring system for otitis (Otitis Index Score, OTIS). This scoring system has been demonostrated to be clinically relevant with good inter- and intra-observer reliability, sensitivity to change, and the ability to distinguish between affected ears, healthy ears and ears in remission (Nuttall and Bensignor, 2014). The scoring system may be used in clinical practice or for studies regarding the diagnosis and management of canine otitis.

Clinical approach

History

In acute cases, a brief history should be taken as this can be of value in establishing possible contributory factors. This is important because early identification of predisposing and primary factors can help to prevent chronicity. Key questions should include:

- Is there evidence of pruritus or pain? Is it unilateral or bilateral?
- Where does the dog exercise? Is there the possibility of a foreign body, such as grass awn?
- Does the dog swim?
- Has there been evidence of generalized skin disease, pruritus and/or skin eruptions?
- Is there any previous history of skin disease, particularly atopic dermatitis?
- Has there been any change in the animal's hearing or balance?

In more chronic cases, a thorough history is imperative (Figure 19.3) and can provide vital clues as to the underlying aetiology. For example, a presentation of gradual onset unilateral otitis externa in an older animal should raise the index of suspicion for neoplasia, whereas a history of recurrent otitis along with clinical signs of facial and pedal pruritus would suggest chronic atopic dermatitis. In chronic cases, assessment of pain and for the presence of otitis media are imperative. The owner should be asked specific questions relating to the animal's hearing, balance and the pain associated with bullae/temperomandibular articulation.

General questions
• Any history suggestive of systemic disease?
• Management: diet, exercise, swimming?
• Evidence of contagion or zoonosis?
• Evidence of more generalized pruritus or skin disease?
Specific to ear disease
• When did the ear disease start?
• How often does it recur?
• Evidence of seasonality?
• Unilateral or bilateral disease?
• Nature of discharge/odour – how has this has changed over time?
• Pain on eating/opening mouth?
• Neurological clinical signs?
• Previous treatment and response?

19.3 Questions that should be asked when obtaining a history in cases of chronic otitis.

Physical and dermatological examination

A general physical and dermatological examination should be performed, including assessment of the ventral abdomen and skin fold areas (e.g. the feet and perianal area) for signs of erythema, which should orientate the clinician towards atopic dermatitis or a food-responsive dermatosis (also known as a food allergy or adverse food reaction). The pinnae and external ear canals should be examined for signs of erythema and excoriation (Figure 19.4).

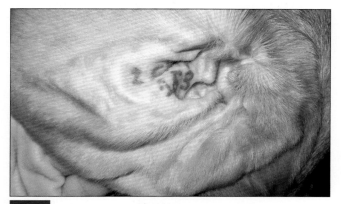

19.4 Acute otitis externa. Note the erythema of the ear canal.

Otoscopic examination

An otoscopic examination is indicated in every case of otits (Figure 19.5) and where discomfort is present, sedation and analgesia are required. Both ears should be examined, even in cases with a unilateral presentation. Where the problem appears to be unilateral, the unaffected ear should be examined first to avoid transferring infectious agents from one ear to another. The clinician should make every effort not to cause the animal further discomfort and the practice of inserting a cold, hard otoscope cone into a painful inflamed ear is to be discouraged.

The following should be assessed during an otoscopic examination:

- The presence of foreign bodies
- The presence of *Otodectes cynotis*
- The presence and nature of any discharge
- The patency of the ear canal and the degree of stenosis
- The appearance of the ear canal lining and the presence of ulceration
- The appearance of the tympanic membrane (which is normally thin and translucent with a visible manubrium of the malleus)
- The presence of neoplasms or polyps.

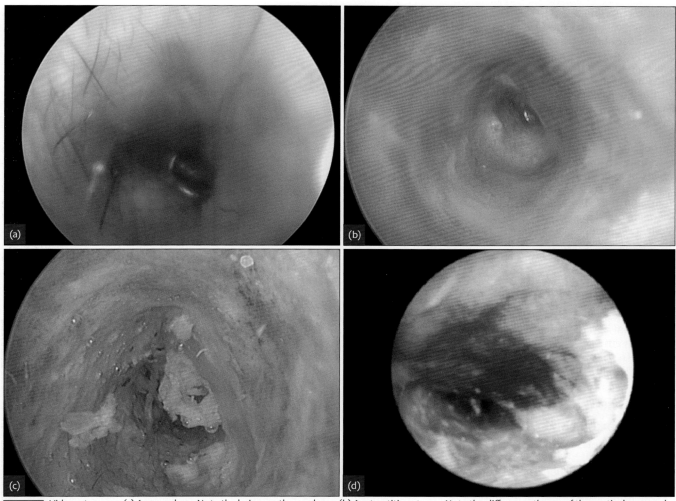

19.5 Video-otoscopy. (a) A normal ear. Note the hair near the eardrum. (b) Acute otitis externa. Note the diffuse erythema of the vertical ear canal. (c) Chronic otitis externa. Note the erythema, erosions and exudate. (d) Chronic otitis externa. Note the large ulcerations.
(b, Courtesy of Dr Prélaud)

The ears may need to be cleaned prior to otoscopic examination, as the accumulation of secretions can prevent assessment of the ear canal and tympanic membrane (Bensignor et al., 2008; Harvey and Haar, 2017). Manual cleaning using a propietary ear cleaner is appropriate in most cases of acute otitis, provided this does not result in pain. Following application of the ear cleaner, the ear canal should be massaged for 30–60 seconds before the discharge is wiped away from the external ear canal using a gauze swab or cotton buds. A wide variety of topical ear cleaners are available for use in practice, including ceruminolytics and surfactants that dissolve and soften cerumen, astringents that have a drying effect within the ear canal and antimicrobial agents (see Chapter 20). Some ear cleaners are contraindicated in the presence of a ruptured tympanic membrane.

However, it should be noted that manual ear cleaning will not remove tightly adherent or material deep within the ear canal and consideration should be given to ear flushing under general anaesthesia if there is a significant accumulation of discharge. Ear flushing can be performed using either a standard handheld otoscope or a video-otoscope. Soaking the ears in a proprietary ceruminolytic ear cleaner prior to flushing facilitates removal of the discharge. A retrograde technique is used to flush the ears: fluid, usually water or sterile saline, is delivered via a giving set, three-way tap, 20 ml syringe and 4 G nasogastric feeding tube (see Chapter 20). The feeding tube is inserted through the otoscope cone into the ear canal to the level of the tympanic membrane. Fluid is then instilled and aspirated using the syringe until all the discharge has been removed from the ear canal. The tip of the catheter may be used to gently dislodge adherent material. Loups and curettes are also available for this purpose. All traces of fluid should be aspirated from the ear canal following cleaning.

Ear flushing is crucial in all cases of otits media as it helps remove the accumulation of bacteria, debris and inflammatory cells from the bulla and disrupts the bacterial biofilm. However, it should be noted that in many cases of chronic erythematoceruminous otitis (see below) there is moderate to marked stenosis of the external ear canal, which precludes thorough cleaning and examination (and prevents the subsequent administration of topical medication), and this should be resolved prior to the procedure. Prednisolone at a dose of 0.5–1 mg/kg orally q24h or methylprednisolone at a dose of 0.4–0.8 mg/kg orally q24h for a period of a few days is usually effective in improving the stenosis.

Neurological examination

A neurological examination should be performed to assess for evidence of Horner's syndrome, nystagmus and facial paralysis, indicating involvement of the middle and inner ear cavity. These cases are serious and referral for diagnostic imaging and specialist evaluation is indicated.

Diagnostic tests

Cerumen examination

Direct examination of the cerumen (collected via a cotton swab or curette) should be performed in cases where a parasitic cause is suspected because otocariosis is still a frequent clinical presentation, especially in cats and young dogs (Bensignor et al., 2000). Mites are usually easily visualized under the low power lens (X4) of the microscope.

Cytology

A cytological examination should be performed in all cases of otitis externa (see Chapters 3 and 4). This allows the clinician to record which microorganisms (if any) are present and for more appropriate targeting of treatment. Furthermore, at follow-up consultations or during subsequent episodes of otitis, cytology facilitates assessment of the efficacy of therapy and progression of the disease over time.

To obtain a sample for cytology, a cotton bud should be inserted into the vertical canal, usually to the level of the junction of the vertical and horizontal canals. The cotton bud should then be rolled gently on to a glass slide. The same glass slide can be used for samples from both ears. The slide should be air-dried and stained with a modified Romanovsky-type stain (e.g. Diff-Quik®, Rapi-Diff® or RAL®). It is possible to heat-fix very ceruminous samples by passing them through a flame prior to staining. Samples should not be placed into an alcohol fixative because this tends to dissolve the material that has been collected. Following staining, a coverslip can be applied using a drop of immersion oil. It is possible to use only the third (blue) stain after air drying; this decreases the time taken to perform the procedure whilst still allowing visualization of inflammatory cells and microbial agents, but is less effective in cases of eosinophilic inflammation (Deschamps and Bensignor, 2009).

There are many different cytological presentations seen with acute otitis externa. Typically, in cases of acute otitis externa associated with underlying atopic dermatitis (a common clinical presentation), there may be an increased number of squames but no evidence of microbial infection. In cases of acute otitis exerna associated with infection, there may be Malassezia overgrowth (peanut-shaped yeasts) (Figure 19.6) or numerous cocci (usually Staphylococcus pseudintermedius) present with or without a purulent infiltrate. Cocci appear as round, often grouped, bacteria, whereas rods are enlongated. It is unusual to see rod-shaped infections with acute otitis externa (Aymeric and Bensignor, 2018).

Bacterial culture and sensitivity testing

It is advisable to obtain samples for bacterial culture and sensitivity testing in cases of chronic otitis under the following circumstances:

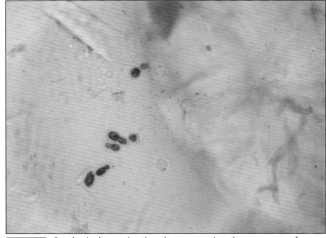

19.6 Cytological examination demonstrating the presence of *Malassezia* pachydermatis. (Original magnification X1000)

- Rods are seen on cytological examination because the spectrum of antibacterial sensitivity for rod infections is unpredicatable
- Cocci are seen on cytological examination and multiple previous treatments have been administered without success
- If there is evidence of otits media (see below).

It should be noted that samples for bacterial culture and sensitivity testing are not as useful in cases of otitis externa because discrepancies exist between *in vivo* and *in vitro* data and because the high drug concentrations achieved by topical therapy can sometimes overcome apparent *in vitro* resistance. This is particularly true for concentration-dependent antibiotics such as fluoroquinolones. It has been recently demonstrated that the use of concentrations above the clinical breakpoints are effective in inhibiting and in some cases killing resistant isolates, which highlights the potential for routine susceptibility tests to mislead the clinician in the choice of topical antimicrobials in cases of otitis externa in dogs and cats (Boyd *et al.*, 2019).

Diagnostic imaging

Diagnostic imaging is useful for chronic cases where canal stenosis is present and/or when calcification and/or otitis media are suspected (Bensignor *et al.*, 2008; Harvey and Haar, 2017). These cases are expected to respond poorly to medical management and may be candidates for surgical intervention. Ventrodorsal, lateral, right and left oblique lateral and rostrocaudal open mouth radiographic views are useful but have been largely replaced by CT and magentic resonance imaging (MRI), which are considered to be more sensitive for the detection of fluid within the tympanic bullae (Dickie *et al.*, 2003; Griffiths *et al.*, 2003; Belmudes *et al.*, 2018). Positive contrast ear canalography has also been described for the detection of otitis media (Trower *et al.*, 1998): 2–5 ml of a positive contrast medium should be infused into the ear canal. The presence of contrast medium within the tympanic bulla indicates a ruptured tympanic membrane and otitis media. Impedance audiometry is available in specialized centres. Brainstem auditory evoked response (BAER) may also be a useful technique to assess hearing (Figure 19.7).

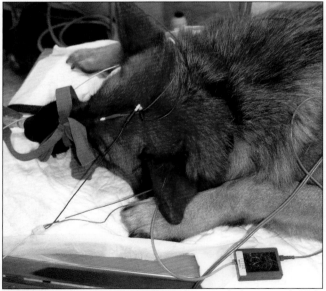

19.7 Measurement of brainstem auditory evoked response (BAER). Note the electrodes on this German Shepherd Dog.

Further investigations

Otits externa is usually a manifestation of generalized dermatosis. The successful management of the associated skin disease is the key to prevention of further episodes of otitis and thus additional investigations may be required. If the animal has a history and clinical signs consistent with atopic dermatitis, diet trials to rule out a food-responsive dermatosis and intradermal testing or immunoglobulin (Ig)E serology to identify causative allergens with the view of using allergen-specific immunotherapy is indicated (Miller *et al.*, 2012). It may be necessary to perform these tests early on in the investigation as glucocorticoid therapy will affect the results. Additional tests that may be indicated in cases of chronic otitis include histopathological examination, haematology, biochemistry, urinalysis and an endocrine work-up.

Chronic erythematoceruminous otitis externa

This clinical presentation is characterized by erythema, ceruminous discharge, pruritus, malodour and variable stenosis of the external ear canal (Figure 19.8). The most common complaint from owners is one of persistent or recurrent aural pruritus with head shaking, but other complaints such as a bad smell or pain can also occur. In these cases, the discharge is generally creamy yellow to dark brown and is obviously ceruminous rather than purulent in nature. The most common primary cause for chronic erythematoceruminous otitis is an underlying atopic dermatitis, but other primary diseases include a food-responsive dermatosis, otodectic and demodectic otitis, primary keratinization defects, endocrinopathies and neoplasia (Griffin, 1993).

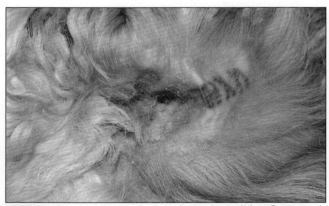

19.8 Chronic otitis externa. Note the erythema, lichenification and slight hyperpigmentation of the ear pinna and the ear canal.

Suppurative otitis externa

Suppurative otitis externa is seen less frequently than chronic erythematoceruminous otitis, respresenting 21% of all cases of otitis externa in a recent study (Aymeric and Bensignor, 2018). These cases are characterized by the presence of a malodourous, often liquid, discharge (Figure 19.9). The colour of the exudate varies depending on the type of bacteria involved (from dark grey to green/yellow – the latter is often seen with *Pseudomonas aeruginosa*);

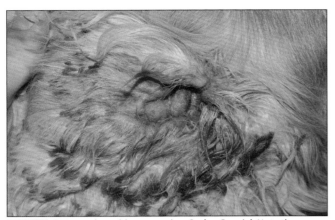

19.9 Suppurative otitis externa in a Cocker Spaniel. Note the purulent discharge on the ear pinna.

however, the colour by itself is not a reliable method for predicting the type of microbial involvement. Pus draining from the ear canal may be seen on the ear pinna and/or on the cheek. Purulent otitis is frequently accompanied by ear canal erosions or ulceration, especially in the case of Gram-negative microbial infection. The chief complaint of owners is variable: some animals are presented for malodour, others for head shaking or pain. The pain is often acute and pruritus minimal, which may help to differentiate this condition from erythematoceruminous otitis externa.

Feline otitis externa

Acute and chronic otitis externa are rare in cats but do occur and can be challenging to manage. The most common cause of otitis externa, particularly in younger animals, is *Otodectes cynotis* infestation, which accounts for up to 50% of cases (as opposed to 5% of cases in dogs) (Figure 19.10), but *Demodex cati* may also be responsible for otoacariasis (Miller *et al.*, 2012). Cats are susceptible to *Malassezia* spp. and bacterial otitis, sometimes secondary to underlying hypersensitivity disorders. Although atopic dermatitis and cutaneous food-responsive dermatosis are less common causes of otitis externa in cats compared with dogs, they do occur, and some dermatologists consider that recurrent pruritic otitis externa is a fifth pruritic feline cutaneous reaction pattern alongside symmetrical alopecia, miliary dermatitis, eosinophilic granuloma complex and head and neck pruritus.

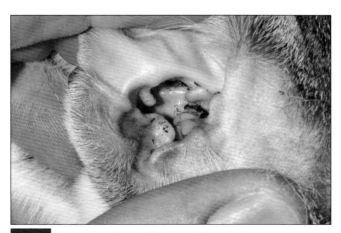

19.10 Otoacariasis in a cat. Note the dark brown cerumen.

Ceruminous gland cysts (ceruminous cystadenomatosis) is not rare in the older cat. The clinician should also be aware that suppurative otitis externa in cats, especially if it is unilateral, is often associated with the presence of a nasopharyngeal polyp or neoplasm (ceruminous gland adenoma (Figure 19.11) or adenocarcinoma) in the external ear canal and/or tympanic bulla. In addition, idiopathic ceruminous otitis externa is becoming an increasingly recognized problem. This condition is characterized by an excess amount of cerumen production, with waxy brown debris filling the ear canal (Kennis, 2013).

The investigation and treatment of feline otitis externa is similar to that of the dog. However, the clinician should be aware of the anatomical differences between the species. The feline tympanic bulla has an incomplete bony septum that divides the ventral tympanic chamber into ventrodorsal and dorsolateral portions. Axons of the sympathetic trunk course rostrally through the tympanic cavity and are exposed as they cross the promontory and thus vulnerable to damage (Harvey and Haar, 2017). Accordingly, there is an increased risk of Horner's syndrome in cats with otitis media and in those undergoing ear flushing procedures. Due to the frequency of occurence of nasopharyngeal polpys in cats, the author routinely recommends a CT and/or MRI examination in cases with chronic relapsing episodes. In addition, the clinician should be aware that cats appear to be more susceptible than dogs to ototoxicity and that the use of topical medications should be undertaken with caution (Kennis, 2013).

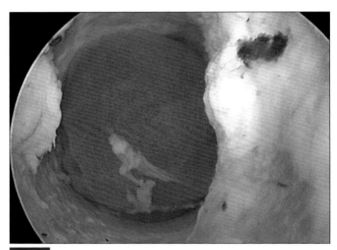

19.11 A polyp in the horizontal part of the ear canal in a cat.

Treatment

The treatment of otitis is covered in Chapter 20.

Key points

- Recurrent otitis externa is usually associated with an underlying disease, commonly atopic dermatitis in the dog
- Successful management involves the identification and treatment of primary, secondary, predisposing and perpetuating factors
- Due to anatomical differences, cats are more prone to neurological damage if otitis media develops

---

References and further reading

August JR (1988) Otitis externa: a disease of multifactorial etiology. *Veterinary Clinics of North America: Small Animal Practice* **18**, 731–742

Aymeric E and Bensignor E (2018) A prospective study of canine otitis in general practice. *Revue Veterinaire Clinique* **53**, 3–9

Belmudes A, Pressanti C, Barthez PY *et al.* (2018) Computed tomographic findings in 205 dogs with clinical signs compatible with middle ear disease: a retrospective study. *Veterinary Dermatology* **29**, 45-e20

Bensignor E, Germain PA and Gautier O (2008) *Les maladies de l'oreille du chien et du chat*. Point Vétérinaire, Rueil Malmaison

Bensignor E, Legeay D and Medaille C (2000) Etude prospective sur les otites externes du chien adulte en France. *Pratique Medicale et Chirurgicale de l'Animal de Compagnie* **35**, 405–414

Boyd M, Santoro D and Gram D (2019) *In vitro* antimicrobial activity of topical otological antimicrobails and Tris-EDTA against resistant *Staphylococcus pseudintermedius* and *Pseudomonas aeruginosa* isolates from dogs. *Veterinary Dermatology* **30**, 139-e40

Carlotti DN and Taillieu-Leroy S (1997) L'otite externe chez le chien: étiologie et clinique, revue bibliographique et étude rétrospective portant sur 752 cas. *Pratique Médicale et Chirurgicale de l' Animal de Compagnie* **32**, 243–257

Cole LK, Kwochka KW, Kpwalski JJ and Hillier A (1998) Microbial flora and antimicrobial susceptibility patterns of isolated pathogens from the horizontal ear canal and middle ear in dogs with otitis media. *Journal of the American Animal Hospital Association* **212**, 534–538

Deschamps V and Bensignor E (2009) Comparaison de trois techniques de fixation et de coloration pour l'évaluation cytologique des otites érythémato-cérumineuses du chien. *Informations Dermatologiques Vétérinaires* **22**, 7–12

Dickie AM, Doust R, Cromarty L *et al.* (2003) Comparison of ultrasonography, radiography and a single computed tomography slice for the identification of fluid within the canine tympanic bulla. *Research in Veterinary Science* **75**, 209–216.

Griffin CE (1993) Otitis externa and otitis media. In: *Current Veterinary Dermatology, the science and art of therapy*, ed. CE Griffin *et al.*, pp 245–264. Mosby Year Book, St Louis

Griffiths LG, Sullivan M, O'Neill T and Reid SW (2003) Ultrasonography versus radiography for detection of fluid in the canine tympanic bulla. *Veterinary Radiology and Ultrasound* **44**, 210–213

Harvey RG and Haar G (2017) Ear, nose and throat diseases of the dog and cat. *CRC Press Boca Raton* **28**, 422

Kennis RA (2013) Feline otitis. *Veterinary Clinics of North America: Small Animal Practice* **43**, 51–56

Miller WH, Griffin CE and Campbell KA (2012). *Muller and Kirk's Small Animal Dermatology, 7th edn*, pp 948. W.B. Saunders, Philadelphia

Nuttal T and Bensignor E (2014) A pilot study to develop an objective clinical score for canine otitis externa. *Veterinary Dermatology* **25**, 530–537

Nuttall T and Cole L (2007) Evidence-based veterinary dermatology: a systematic review of interventions for treatment of *Pseudomonas* otitis in dogs. *Veterinary Dermatology* **18**, 69–77

Nuttall T and Cole L (2007) Ear cleaning: the UK and US perspective. *Veterinary Dermatology* **15**, 127–136

Radlinsky MAG (2016) Advances in otoscopy. *Veterinary Clinics of North America: Small Animal Practice* **46**, 171–179

Roth L (1988) Pathologic changes in otitis externa. *Veterinary Clinics of North America: Small Animal Practice* **18**, 755–764

Saridomichelakis MN, Farmaki R, Leontides LS and Koutinas AF (2007) Aetiology of canine otitis externa: a retrospective study of 100 cases. *Veterinary Dermatology* **18**, 341–347

Scott DW, Miller WH and Griffin CE (2001) Diseases of eyelids, claws, anal sacs, and ears. In: *Muller & Kirk's Small Animal Dermatology, 6th edn.*, ed. DW Scott, WH Miller and CE Griffin, pp. 1185–1235. W.B. Saunders, Philadelphia

Trower ND, Gregory SP and Lamb CR (1998) Evaluation of the canine tympanic membrane by positive contrast ear canalography. *Veterinary Record* **142**, 78–81

Chapter 20

Management of otitis

Peter J. Forsythe

Otitis externa is a complex multifactorial condition involving primary and secondary causes of inflammation and various predisposing and perpetuating factors (see Chapter 19). Treatment, therefore, involves more than just identifying and treating the infection and, in fact, this approach is likely to lead to failure of therapy or recurrence of disease. Instead, the clinician should make every effort to identify and address as many of the causes and factors involved. This chapter covers the general principles of treating otitis externa as well as the distinctions between managing acute *versus* chronic disease. The management of otitis media is also discussed in this chapter.

General principles

Otitis externa can be classified as acute, subacute or chronic, depending on the duration of disease. The general principles for the management of acute and chronic otitis externa are similar and include:

- Relieving inflammation, pain and pruritus
- Cleaning of the ear canals and addressing other perpetuating factors
- Elimination of microbial infection
- Maintaining a clean ear canal and addressing primary causes of inflammation.

However, perpetuating factors will be more marked in chronic disease and necessitate more aggressive and prolonged therapy. One important aim when treating acute disease is to prevent the onset of chronic changes.

Relieving and preventing inflammation, pain and pruritus

In referral dermatology practice, it is common to be presented with ear phobic dogs that will no longer tolerate examination of the ears or topical therapy. This unfortunate situation can arise through careless use of a handhold otoscope or the forced application of topical therapy to painful and inflamed ears. Whilst this situation can be addressed, it creates difficulties in the management of otitis externa. The risk of creating ear phobia should be at the forefront of the clinician's mind when approaching any case of otitis externa. One of the first considerations should be to relieve discomfort and inflammation, which

results in a dog that is more tolerant of topical therapy and makes it easier for the owner to apply treatment. Systemic glucocorticoid therapy is the treatment of choice for resolving inflammation and pruritus. This is discussed in more detail below, but the author favours the use of oral prednisolone or methylprednisolone given for not more than 2–3 days at anti-inflammatory doses. Consideration should also be given to the use of analgesia, which should be mandatory in cases where there is ulceration of the ear canals.

Ear cleaning

It is suspected that epithelial cell migration is impaired in otitis externa, resulting in the accumulation of cerumen, which may predispose to secondary infection and prevent exposure of the ear canal lining to topical therapies. Ear cleaning is indicated if there is discharge within the ear canal preventing visualization of the tympanic membrane or areas of the ear canal lining and may be the single most important aspect of managing otitis externa. As well as exposing the lining of the ear canal to topical medication, cleaning facilitates examination of the ear canal, removes material that can harbour microorganisms and inactivate topical medications, and removes small foreign bodies, toxins, and damaged and degenerated cells. Regular ear cleaning is frequently part of long-term management of otitis externa.

Manual ear cleaning in the conscious dog

Manual cleaning using a proprietary ear cleaner is appropriate in most cases of acute otitis externa and may be sufficient in more chronic disease. There is a wide variety of topical ear cleaners available with different actions, including ceruminolytics and surfactants, astringents and antimicrobial agents (Nuttall and Cole, 2004). The veterinary surgeon (veterinarian) should be aware that some components of ear cleaners are contraindicated in the presence of a ruptured tympanic membrane. It is worth stating that there may be a sufficient ear cleaning effect from excipient oils in topical antimicrobial/glucocorticoid preparations in mildly affected ears to negate the requirement for an additional ear cleaner.

- **Cerumenolytic products** – these products contain organic oils and solvents that soften and dissolve cerumen. They include propylene glycol, lanolin, glycerine, squalene, butylated hydroxytoluene, ocamidopropyl betaine and mineral oils. They are useful in mildly waxy or dirty ears. Some ear cleaners contain surfactants (dioctyl Na/Ca sulphosuccinate), which help the cleaning process by emulsifying and breaking up debris. Foaming agents, such as carbamyl peroxide or urea, have a similar effect. The author does not use foaming agents in conscious dogs as they can cause distress/anxiety.

- **Astringent cleaners** – these products dry the lining of the ear canal to prevent further maceration. Ear cleaning ingredients with astringent/drying effects include isopropyl alcohol, acetic acid, boric acid, benzoic acid, salicylic acid, sulphur, aluminium acetate and silicon dioxide.
- **Antimicrobial effects** – many ear cleaners also have antimicrobial effects, including those containing parachlorometaxylenol (PCMX), chlorhexidine, tris-EDTA, *N*-acetylcysteine and acetic acid.

It is important to choose an appropriate product for the individual case. Cerumenolytic ear cleaners should be used where there are waxy discharges. A cleaner with aqueous properties (such as saline or tris-EDTA) is indicated in cases of suppurative otitis. Acidic cleaners should be avoided if the ear canal is eroded or ulcerated. Most cleaners (with the exception of tris-EDTA, acetic acid, boric acid and squalene) are contraindicated if there is rupture of the tympanic membrane.

As mentioned above, manual ear cleaning in a conscious dog should be avoided when the ears are markedly painful or pruritic. In all cases, the minimum of restraint should be used and ear cleaning avoided if it causes the dog any distress.

Owners need to be instructed carefully on how to use the cleaner effectively. In the author's practice, this is done by means of a practical demonstration on the dog by an experienced veterinary nurse. Following application of an ear cleaner, the vertical ear canal should be massaged for 30–60 seconds with the aim of creating turbulence in the horizontal canal to break up any accumulated material. Any discharge is wiped away from the external ear canal using a gauze swab or cotton wool, but the practice of inserting cotton buds into the vertical canal should be discouraged because this may impact material within the canals.

Cleaning undertaken by the owner at home is unlikely to remove adherent material or secretions impacted deep within the ear canal and is ineffective in chronically diseased stenotic ears. In these circumstances, consideration should be given to retrograde ear flushing under general anaesthesia.

Retrograde ear cleaning under general anaesthesia

Deep ear cleaning under general anaesthesia is indicated if home cleaning is ineffective, if there is significant material impacted within the horizontal canal, or if the patient will not tolerate home ear cleaning. The author always performs this procedure under general anaesthesia using a retrograde flushing technique (see Chapter 19). In the author's practice, sterile saline is delivered via a giving set, three-way tap, 20 ml syringe and 6 G nasogastric feeding tube, which is passed through the working channel of the video-otoscope. A wider catheter allows aspiration of larger clumps of material but cannot be used with a video-otoscope. Ear flushing creates inflammation and can be painful, therefore, systemic prednisolone or methylprednisolone should be administered for up to 5 days after the

procedure, along with appropriate analgesia. Following retrograde ear cleaning, the owner should continue to clean the ears at home using an appropriate product. To start with, twice-weekly cleaning is sufficient but should be reduced over time to perhaps weekly or fortnightly. Over-cleaning should be avoided as the continued maceration of the ear canal can predispose to further inflammation and infection.

Video-otoscopy

The use of a video-otoscope greatly improves the management of otitis externa, as it allows vastly improved visualization of the structures within the ear canal, as well as real-time examination during the ear cleaning process. In addition, video-otoscope attachments such as loups, forceps and curettes facilitate the removal of foreign bodies, cerumenoliths, small tumours and polyps.

Elimination of microbial infections

Antimicrobial therapy is indicated if infection is identified on cytology. Topical antimicrobial therapy is the mainstay of treatment for infection in otitis externa because systemic antimicrobials are unlikely to reach the lining of the ear canal in sufficient concentration to be effective (Morris, 2004). Topical therapy achieves a far higher concentration of antimicrobial within the ear canal compared with systemic administration and can often overcome apparent *in vitro* resistance.

Reflecting the complex aetiology of otitis externa, most proprietary topical antimicrobial therapies contain a combination of an antibacterial, an antifungal and a glucocorticoid. Some also contain an antiparasitic. Clinicians should be familiar with the various active ingredients. The constituents of the proprietary topical aural preparations available in the UK are listed in Figure 20.1. It is important to use a sufficient volume of any proprietary topical antimicrobial product. Pump dispensers and single use tubes deliver a measured amount, but the use of dropper bottles can result in under-dosing. A syringe may be used to draw up a measured dose for each application (0.5–1 ml should be sufficient for most ears).

Selection of a topical antimicrobial product should be based on the results of a cytological examination, as well as taking into consideration the ability of the owner to apply topical therapy, how the patient is likely to react to such therapy and, above all, good antibiotic stewardship. Thus, antimicrobials with efficacy against Gram-negative bacteria should be reserved for those cases where rods are identified on cytology.

Topical antimicrobials

Products containing nystatin, miconazole, clotrimazole, posaconazole and terbinafine are effective for the treatment of *Malassezia* infections. Miconazole and other azoles also have significant activity against some Gram-positive bacteria (Frosini and Bond, 2017).

Fusidic acid: This is effective against Gram-positive bacteria, but Gram-negative bacteria are highly resistant.

Florfenicol: This is a thiamphenicol analogue. It is effective against Gram-positive and some Gram-negative bacteria. It is available in a once-weekly topical therapy combined with terbinafine and betamethasone for otitis externa, although this product is currently only licensed for the treatment of *Malassezia* and staphylococcal otitis.

Product	Antibacterial	Antibacterial spectrum	Antifungal	Glucocorticoid and potency	Contraindicated if TM perforated
Canaural®	Diethanolamine fusidate Framycetin	Gram-positive Gram-negative	Nystatin	Prednisolone Low	Yes
Surolan®-suspension	Polymyxin B Miconazole	Gram-negative Gram-positive	Miconazole	Prednisolone Low	Yes
Otomax®	Gentamicin	Gram-positive Gram-negative	Clotrimazole	Betamethasone valerate Medium	Yes
EasOtic®	Gentamicin	Gram-positive Gram-negative	Miconazole	Hydrocortisone aceponate Medium	Yes
Osurnia®	Florfenicol	Gram-positive	Terbinafine	Betamethasone acetate Medium	Yes
Neptra	Florfenicol	Gram-positive	Terbinafine	Mometasone High	Yes
Aurizon® Marbodex aural®	Marbofloxacin[a]	Gram-positive Gram-negative	Clotrimazole	Dexamethasone acetate Medium	Yes
Posatex®	Orbifloxacin[a]	Gram-positive Gram-negative	Posaconazole	Mometasone furoate High	Yes
Recicort®				Triamcinolone Medium	Yes

20.1 Topical aural products and glucocorticoid potencies. [a] It is prudent to reserve fluoroquinolones for the treatment of clinical conditions that have responded poorly, or are expected to respond poorly, to other classes of antibiotics. TM = tympanic membrane.

Polymyxin B: This is an effective antibiotic against the majority of Gram-negative organisms, but may not be effective against *Proteus* spp. It is inactivated by purulent exudates. It is also ototoxic and should not be used if the tympanic membrane is perforated.

Aminoglycosides: These include neomycin, framycetin, gentamicin, amikacin and tobramycin. They are effective against some Gram-positive and many Gram-negative bacteria. They are ineffective against anaerobes. They will only work effectively in a clean ear. They are more effective in an alkaline environment (use at least an hour after an acidifying ear cleaner). They are variably ototoxic, but gentamicin seems to be safe when instilled into the middle ear cavity as an aqueous solution (Strain *et al.*, 1995). Tobramycin is reported to be ototoxic in dogs (Nuttall and Carr, 2010).

Fluoroquinolones: These are bactericidal and broad spectrum in effect. There is a strong argument for reserving the fluoroquinolones for Gram-negative infections. Several studies have investigated the sensitivity of *Pseudomonas aeruginosa* isolates to different fluoroquinolones and, in general, fewer were resistant to marbofloxacin compared with enrofloxacin or ciprofloxacin (Martin Barrasa *et al.*, 2000; McKay *et al.*, 2007; Rubin *et al.*, 2008). Off-label recipes for mixing fluoroquinolones with ear cleaning products have been described (Metry *et al.*, 2012). Fluoroquinolones are not reported to be ototoxic. Soluble aqueous products (not oily polypharmaceuticals) should be safe to use where the tympanic membrane is ruptured.

Antiseptics

With increasing concerns about antibiotic resistance, it is worth considering the use of antiseptics rather than always resorting to antibiotic use. The key is to use antiseptics frequently (several times daily), so compliance may be a problem.

Silver sulfadiazine: This is active *in vitro* against various Gram-negative and Gram-positive organisms, including *Pseudomonas aeruginosa* (von Silva-Tarouca *et al.*, 2019).

Silver sulfadiazine 1% cream may be diluted in water (1.5 ml of cream in 13.5 ml water gives a 0.1% suspension). It has been used topically to treat Gram-negative otitis externa effectively. There are no reports of ototoxicity and most dermatologists consider it safe to use if the tympanic membrane is ruptured (Barnard and Foster, 2017).

Tris-EDTA: This has a direct effect against bacteria by chelating metal ions important for bacterial cell wall structure. It is reported to potentiate the effect of antibiotics when treating Gram-negative and Gram-positive bacteria involved in otitis, but *in vitro*, as a sole ingredient, it has minimal to no antibacterial effect (Buckley *et al.*, 2013). It is available as a sole ingredient or combined with chlorhexidine in various proprietary ear cleaners. The combination of tris-EDTA and 0.15% chlorhexidine has been shown to have effect against organisms commonly involved in otitis externa (Guardabassi *et al.*, 2010). It is considered safe to use in cases where the tympanic membrane is perforated. As an aqueous product, it is useful as a flush when treating suppurative otitis externa. It does not exacerbate discomfort in ulcerated ear canals.

Other disinfectants: There are a number of other disinfectants that are available in proprietary ear cleaning formulations, including organic acids (acetic, boric, citric, lactic), alcohols, chlorhexidine (<0.25%) and povidone–iodine.

Glucocorticoids

The majority of otitis externa cases benefit from treatment with glucocorticoids. Glucocorticoids may be administered topically, systemically or by intralesional injection. Glucocorticoids may be useful in the following circumstances:

- To relieve pruritus and pain (facilitating examination, cleaning and topical therapy)
- Ear canal stenosis due to soft tissue swelling and epithelial hyperplasia
- Stenosis resulting from cerumenal gland hyperplasia (Figure 20.2) and other proliferative responses

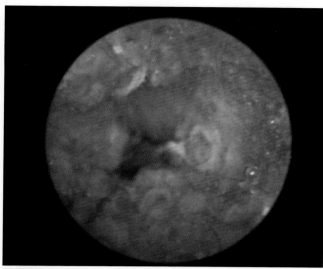

20.2 Severe cerumenal gland hyperplasia in a Welsh Springer Spaniel. These changes are commonly found in spaniel breeds with chronic otitis externa.

- Reduction of exudate production and glandular secretion
- *Pseudomonas* otitis
- Long-term management of atopic otitis.

For more severe clinical signs, systemic prednisolone or methylprednisolone should be administered at 0.5–1 mg/kg until resolution. Higher dosages may be required for resolution of severe stenosis due to fibrosis (see below).

Addressing primary causes of otitis

It is beyond the scope of this chapter to discuss in detail the management of the many primary causes of inflammation in otitis externa. However, every effort should be made to identify and address these causes and the reader, in particular, is referred to the chapters on atopic dermatitis (see Chapters 9 and 10), as this is the most common primary cause. In many cases where there is evidence of more generalized skin disease, a thorough work-up for pruritus is indicated but in those cases where disease is confined to the ears, it may simply be appropriate to manage the ear disease alone (see 'Allergic otitis externa' below).

Management of acute otitis externa

Acute otitis externa is defined as disease that has been present for up to 7 days. The implication is that these cases will not have developed significant perpetuating factors. As already discussed, an important aim when presented with a case of acute otitis externa, is to put in place measures to prevent repeated episodes that can lead to the onset of chronic disease. Thus, it is worth discussing this concern with the owner early on in the course of the disease, clarifying that simply supplying further topical medication without addressing the causes and factors is likely to result in the onset of chronicity, and they may be more likely to accept the clinician's advice regarding further investigation and preventive measures.

Allergic otitis externa

Allergic otitis externa is a common presentation. The dog presents with a pruritic, often erythematous, ear but the ear canal is clean and there is no cytological evidence of infection. There may or may not be additional signs suggestive of atopic dermatitis, such as pedal and ventral pruritus. The use of topical antimicrobials in these cases is unnecessary and inappropriate. Where the disease is confined solely to the ears, these dogs often respond to topical glucocorticoid therapy or any of the standard systemic therapies for atopic dermatitis. A topical ear drop containing triamcinolone is available in the UK. In some cases, there may be an accumulation of cerumen within the ear canals, which predisposes to secondary infection and cleaning with a cerumenolytic ear cleaner is indicated. This may be sufficient to prevent secondary infections but if not, the off-licence addition of a soluble glucocorticoid (such as an aqueous dexamethasone injectable) to the ear cleaner can be very effective. As a guide, the concentration of dexamethasone should be no greater that 0.2%. Weekly to fortnightly ear cleaning may be sufficient. Lifelong management will be required and a more in-depth work-up for atopic dermatitis may be indicated.

Acute otitis externa associated with microbial infection

These cases usually present with head shaking and ear scratching, along with a ceruminous discharge often accompanied by malodour. Cytological evaluation identifies the presence of infection. The majority of acute or subacute otitis externa cases present with *Malassezia* or staphylococcal infections. These cases are generally treated with a proprietary polypharmaceutical topical product containing an antifungal, an antibiotic and a glucocorticoid (see Figure 20.1) according to manufacturer's datasheet directions.

Client compliance is a major factor in the treatment of otitis externa and the ease of application of any product should be considered. Once-daily *versus* twice-daily treatment can have a significant impact on compliance. There is also the option of using a long-acting product that may be applied twice at weekly intervals (Osurnia) or once monthly (Neptra). These products are particularly helpful in dogs that are already starting to show signs of ear phobia or those that might be at risk.

The glucocorticoid content of the product should also be considered (see Figure 20.1). A more potent glucocorticoid would be advantageous if there is marked inflammation and soft tissue swelling or early signs of hyperplastic changes within the ear canal.

Duration of therapy

Treatment duration can vary considerably from a few days to several weeks, depending on the disease presentation. Revisits should be scheduled for every 1–2 weeks. Antimicrobial therapy should be continued until there is complete clinical and cytological resolution of both the infection and inflammation. Otoscopic examination and cytology should be part of the re-examination process. The follow-up otoscopic examination should reveal a clean ear canal and it should be possible to visualize the tympanic membrane (Figure 20.3). If a significant discharge is evident, client compliance and ear cleaning techniques should be appraised. Retrograde ear flushing under general anaesthesia is indicated if manual cleaning is ineffective in achieving a clean ear canal. Repeat cytology should reveal no microorganisms and no evidence of inflammation (i.e. neutrophils or neutrophilic debris; Figure 20.4).

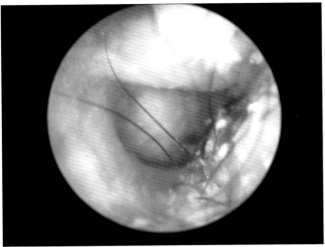

20.3 Clean ear canal and visible tympanic membrane on follow-up examination after treatment for otitis externa.

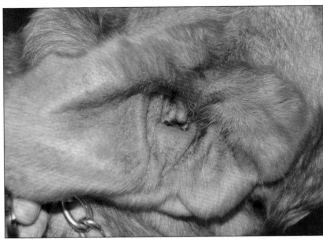

20.5 Erythematoceruminous otitis in a Dogue de Bordeaux associated with *Malassezia* spp. infection and underlying atopic dermatitis.

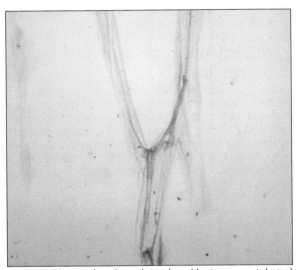

20.4 The purple-coloured streaks evident on ear cytology during treatment of bacterial otitis represent neutrophilic debris indicating ongoing inflammation. Occasional cocci can be seen. Antimicrobial therapy should be continued until there is complete cytological resolution of both the infection and inflammation. (Original magnification X1000)

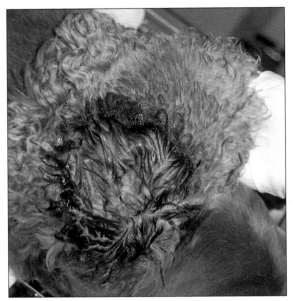

20.6 Suppurative otitis externa associated with severe cerumenal gland hyperplasia and *Pseudomonas aeruginosa* infection in a 12-year-old Cocker Spaniel.

Ongoing ear cleaning may be required as epithelial cell migration can take a prolonged period of time to re-establish or may never recover. However, it is also important to remember that over-cleaning should be avoided. A healthy, clean tympanic membrane is a sign that epithelial cell migration is returning to normal, but some ears require lifelong cleaning, perhaps on a weekly or fortnightly basis. In recurrent cases, every attempt should be made to address primary causes of inflammation.

Management of chronic otitis externa

Chronic otitis externa is defined as disease that has been present for more than 30 days. It generally presents as either erythematoceruminous otitis (Figure 20.5) or suppurative otitis (Figure 20.6). The greater the duration of disease, the more marked the perpetuating factors are likely to be, including soft tissue swelling, discharge, epithelial hyperplasia, cholesteatoma, fibrosis, calcification, cerumenal gland hyperplasia and otitis media. It is these perpetuating factors that present much of the challenge to treatment, and failure to identify and address them is a common reason for treatment failure.

Managing chronic otitis externa is an involved and costly undertaking. A successful outcome is highly dependent on having a committed and compliant client. The dependence on the involvement of the owner, costs and potential long-term outcomes should be discussed prior to starting therapy. For some clients and patients, surgery may be the better option. In many cases of chronic otitis externa, it is worth considering referral to a veterinary dermatologist.

Erythematoceruminous otitis externa

In addition to a profuse ceruminous discharge, erythematoceruminous otitis is often associated with soft tissue swelling, epithelial hyperplasia, cerumenal gland hyperplasia and other proliferative changes that result in stenosis. These changes throw the ear canal lining into folds (Figure 20.7), providing crevices that act as a safe haven for microbes and prevent exposure to topical antimicrobials, and can result in almost complete occlusion of the ear canal lumen. These changes also prevent effective cleaning and administration of topical medications and therefore need to be resolved.

The mainstay of treatment is aggressive systemic and, possibly, topical glucocorticoid therapy. Prednisolone (or methylprednisolone) may be used at a dosage of 1–3 mg/kg q24h for up to 3 weeks. An intralesional injection can be attempted, although this is likely to be a referral procedure. Failure of the changes to resolve following glucocorticoid therapy is an indication that this is a surgical problem. At initial presentation, the ears may be severely infected (e.g. with Gram-negative microorganisms) but antibiotic treatment is not required at this stage. Once the stenosis has been reversed, deep ear cleaning under general anaesthesia followed by appropriate topical antimicrobial therapy and ongoing ear cleaning (see above) is indicated.

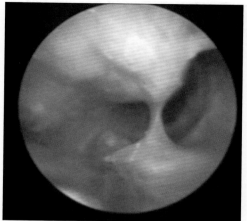

20.8 Biofilm formation in a Cocker Spaniel with *Pseudomonas* otitis externa.

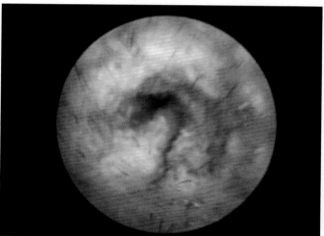

20.7 Soft tissue swelling and epithelial hyperplasia have thrown the ear canal lining into folds, creating a safe haven for microorganisms. Systemic glucocorticoids completely reversed these changes.

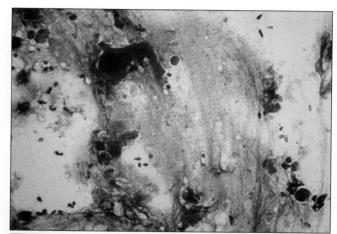

20.9 Photomicrograph showing the biofilm associated with suppurative *Malassezia* otitis externa. Note the halo around the microorganisms consistent with a biofilm. (Original magnification X1000)

Suppurative otitis externa

Suppurative otitis externa is most commonly associated with Gram-negative bacterial infection, particularly *Pseudomonas aeruginosa*, but is also seen less commonly in cases of *Malassezia* infection. *Pseudomonas aeruginosa* is the most common Gram-negative isolate in cases of canine otitis externa and causes a particular problem because many strains are resistant to multiple groups of antimicrobials.

Bacterial biofilms

Suppurative otitis externa is often associated with biofilm formation (Figure 20.8). This is a variably coloured (often brown to black), slimy gelatinous discharge produced by sessile bacteria, which not only impairs the host's response to the bacteria but can result in a minimal inhibitory concentration of antibiotic that is 100–1000 times greater than that required for free-living bacteria. Biofilm production has been reported in 40% of *Pseudomonas* spp. isolates from canine otitis cases (Robinson *et al.*, 2019). On cytology, suppurative otitis may be identified as variably thick lace-like material (Figure 20.9).

Treatment

As with other forms of otitis externa, topical therapy is the mainstay of treatment for suppurative otitis. Purulent discharges and bacterial biofilms within the external ear canal can render topical antimicrobials inactive and thorough ear cleaning under general anaesthesia prior to topical therapy is probably the single most important factor in achieving resolution of infection. This process has been described above, but in the author's practice, prior to the flushing procedure, the ear canal is filled with a tris-EDTA and chlorhexidine product and allowed to soak for 5–10 minutes.

Many Gram-negative bacteria are typically multiple drug resistant and this is often of great concern to veterinary surgeons. However, culture and sensitivity testing is only a guide and the use of topical therapy may overcome apparent *in vitro* resistance. Thus, the results of culture and sensitivity testing can be misleading. Topical antibiotics available as proprietary preparations in the UK that have activity against *Pseudomonas aeruginosa* include marbofloxacin, orbifloxacin, gentamicin and polymyxin B (Figure 20.11). Proprietary preparations containing these antibiotics are contraindicated if the tympanic membrane is perforated and alternatives that may be considered in this circumstance are listed in Figure 20.10. Additional therapies useful in the management of *Pseudomonas* otitis are listed in Figure 20.11.

Antibacterial	Dose	Ototoxicity
Ciprofloxacin	0.2% solution at 0.15–0.3 ml/ear q24h	No
Enrofloxacin	2.5% injectable solution diluted 1:4 with saline applied topically q24h; 22.7 mg/ml solution at 0.15–0.3 ml/ear q24h	No
Marbofloxacin	2% injectable solution diluted 1:4 with saline applied topically q24h; 20 mg/ml injectable solution at 0.15–0.3 ml/ear q24h	No
Silver sulfadiazine	0.1–0.5% solution diluted with saline/water	No
Amikacin	50 mg/ml solution at 0.15–0.3 ml/ear q24h	
Gentamicin	0.27% aqueous solution	No

20.10 Topical antimicrobial drugs useful against *Pseudomonas* infection that may be used when tympanic membrane is ruptured.
(Adapted from Nuttall, 2016)

Drug	Comments
Silver sulfadiazine	An alternative topical antimicrobial therapy that has been used to good effect for the treatment of *Pseudomonas* otitis. Silver has been reported to disrupt bacterial biofilms
Tris-EDTA	Potentiates the effect of antibiotics, particularly fluoroquinolones and gentamicin[a] and should be used as an ear flush 20–30 minutes prior to application of the antimicrobial
N-acetylcysteine	Can inhibit and destroy bacterial biofilms, allowing the penetration of antibiotics[b]. May be useful for the management of canine otitis externa associated with biofilm production[c]. A tris-EDTA/N-acetylcysteine-containing proprietary ear cleaner is now available
Systemic and topical glucocorticoids	Can have a markedly beneficial effect on the pain, inflammation and ulceration associated with *Pseudomonas* otitis and are indicated in the majority of cases

20.11 Treatment options for suppurative otitis externa in cases where the tympanic membrane has ruptured.
[a] (Buckley *et al.*, 2013); [b] (Dinicola *et al.*, 2014); [c] (Chan *et al.*, 2019)

Suppurative *Malassezia* otitis cases present in the same way as suppurative bacterial otitis, often with ulceration of the ear canals and occasionally biofilm formation, but cytology reveals the presence of neutrophils and *Malassezia* spp. yeasts. In some cases, the yeast can be scarce and quite difficult to identify on cytology. These cases tend to be quite refractory to treatment and the owner should be prepared for a prolonged treatment course. Thorough cleaning, the use of tris-EDTA with or without N-acetylcysteine, topical antifungals and systemic glucocorticoids are indicated.

With both bacterial and yeast suppurative otitis, as the infection and inflammation resolve, the nature of the discharge usually changes from purulent to ceruminous and the ear cleaner should be changed accordingly to a cerumenolytic product. Careful follow-up every 2 weeks with repeat cytology is essential in these cases. Many weeks of therapy may be required in cases of suppurative otitis to achieve both clinical and cytological resolution of both the infection and the inflammation.

Tympanic membrane perforation

Perforations of the tympanic membrane (Figure 20.12) are most commonly associated with Gram-negative bacterial

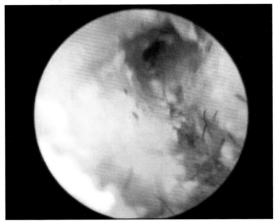

20.12 Perforation of the tympanic membrane in a French Bulldog with otitis media.

suppurative otitis, but may be seen with other chronic disease presentations. In cases where there has been prolonged impaction of material within the horizontal canal, the tympanic membrane may be friable and weakened, resulting in perforation during the cleaning process even with a very gentle technique.

Often the first indication of a tympanic membrane perforation are bubbles that arise from deep within the ear canal, which represent air escaping from the middle ear cavity (Figure 20.13). These perforations tend to take the form of small slits in the tympanic membrane that generally heal within 1–2 weeks. The concern is that infection may enter the middle ear cavity from the horizontal canal. The ear canal should be thoroughly cleaned to minimize this risk. There are no licensed products for use in this situation and aqueous products should be used until the tympanic membrane has healed. Preparations that may be used if the tympanic membrane is ruptured include aqueous injectable marbofloxacin, enrofloxacin, silver sulfadiazine, tris-EDTA and soluble injectable dexamethasone (Barnard and Foster, 2017).

In cases of *Malassezia* otitis with tympanic membrane perforation, clotrimazole, miconazole and nystatin have been shown to be non-ototoxic in guinea pigs when instilled into the middle ear cavity (Tom, 2000) and in a World Small Animal Veterinary Association (WSAVA) Congress workshop, clotrimazole cream diluted 50:50 with water was reported to be safe when used in dogs with visibly ruptured tympanic membranes (Nuttall and Carr, 2010).

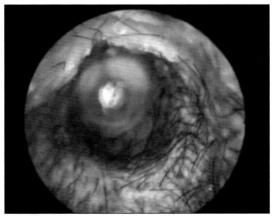

20.13 Air bubble escaping from the middle ear cavity through a perforation in the tympanic membrane (same case as Figure 20.8).

Otitis media

Otitis media implies infection within the middle ear cavity and different treatment strategies are indicated. There are three components to treating otitis media: lavage, treating the otitis externa and the use of systemic therapy.

Lavage

Flushing of the tympanic bulla with copious amounts of fluid to try and thoroughly lavage the middle ear to remove as much material as possible is the single most important therapeutic measure in the treatment of otitis media. This is performed under general anaesthesia, usually as part of the initial cleaning and evaluation of the otitis externa. Water, saline, tris-EDTA and acetic acid/boric acid are the safest fluids for flushing the middle ear. Most cerumenolytics have the potential to cause ototoxicity and should be avoided.

To effectively flush the middle ear, it is necessary to introduce a catheter into the tympanic bulla. If the tympanic membrane is intact, a myringotomy should be performed. A 6 G nasogastric feeding tube is generally used to flush the bulla and an attempt should be made to direct the tip of the catheter ventrally into the tympanic bulla, so as to achieve retrograde flushing of material. This is made difficult by the presence of the septum bulla. Following thorough flushing, the middle ear should be soaked in tris-EDTA for 10 minutes prior to introduction of an antibiotic. These procedures carry significant risk of contact with the underlying promontory and damage to the round or oval windows. Referral to a trained veterinary dermatologist is advisable.

Treatment of otitis externa

It is important to treat the otitis externa to reverse proliferative disease and other perpetuating factors. The procedure is as discussed above: thorough cleaning, glucocorticoid therapy if required and the use of appropriate topical antimicrobial therapy. An antimicrobial should be inserted into the tympanic bulla at the time of the initial flushing procedure. This is then 'trapped' within the bulla and should provide prolonged therapy. Potentially ototoxic products should be avoided, which means the off-license use of drugs as discussed in the section on perforations of the tympanic membrane. The benefit of using aqueous topical antimicrobials is that there is an increased chance that the product will pass down through a perforated tympanum to the middle ear cavity where it will have a direct effect on the infection.

Systemic therapy

Whilst topical therapy is the mainstay of treatment for otitis externa, it is generally accepted that systemic therapy is required for the treatment of otitis media, although opinions differ. This is because the middle ear cavity is comparatively inaccessible to topical therapy, but it is lined by a vascular respiratory epithelium which should allow penetration of drugs from the circulation across the membrane and into the cavity. If otitis media is suspected, samples should be obtained from the tympanic cavity by myringotomy, if necessary, for cytology and bacterial culture and sensitivity testing. The choice of antimicrobial therapy should be based initially on cytological findings and, if necessary, later changed depending on the results of bacterial culture and sensitivity testing. Antimicrobial therapy should be continued until all discharge has resolved, there is no evidence of bacteria or inflammation on cytology and, ideally, once a normal tympanic membrane has re-established. In some cases, the tympanic membrane never reforms. In one study, the mean time to resolution of chronic otitis media in 44 dogs was 117 ± 86.7 days (range 30–360 days) (Morris, 2004). Systemic glucocorticoids are also useful in the management of otitis media to reduce swelling and secretion within the middle ear.

Surgical management

With improved medical management, surgery should be considered as a salvage procedure for otitis that involves irreversible pathological changes (Bradley, 1988). It should be appreciated that surgery does not address the primary causes of otitis and, although improving drainage may help to control infection, inflammation due to underlying diseases (such as atopic dermatitis) will persist. In addition, some forms of surgery that aim to improve drainage can actually make topical therapy more difficult for owners because of the loss of the 'filler funnel' effect of the vertical canal.

Lateral wall resection and vertical canal ablation

Lateral wall resection (LWR) is indicated to improve ear canal drainage or to gain access to the vertical canal for the removal of polyps or neoplastic lesions. The procedure is contraindicated if there is already irreversible disease or otitis media present. Thus, it is contraindicated in the majority of long-standing otitis cases, but may be of benefit if used as a preventative measure in dogs with congenitally stenotic ear canals, such as the Shar Pei. Vertical canal ablation (VCA) may be of benefit if there is intractable disease of the vertical canal, but the horizontal canal and tympanic bullae are unaffected. However, in reality, this is a fairly unlikely scenario. Complications of these procedures involve wound dehiscence, stenosis of the remaining ear canal and failure to alter the course of the otitis.

Total ear canal ablation and lateral bulla osteotomy

This procedure is indicated in chronic end-stage otitis and some neoplastic diseases. This technique excises the entire ear canal, the lateral wall of the tympanic bulla and the mucoperiosteum of the middle ear canal. Surgical complications include Horner's syndrome, facial nerve paralysis and para-aural abscessation. In addition, the animal will be deaf. However, many dogs are already deaf before this procedure and some patients still feel vibrations; therefore, the thought of a deaf dog should not discourage owners from considering this procedure when it is in the best interest of the animal.

Feline otitis externa

The treatment of feline otitis externa is similar to that in the dog. Feline otitis externa is frequently a manifestation of feline hypersensitivity dermatitis (see Chapter 19). These cats often present with acute otitis externa and secondary bacterial or yeast infections. There may be a profuse ceruminous aural discharge and pruritus may be intense. There are topical proprietary antimicrobials licensed for use in cats, but some animals are exquisitely sensitive to topical medications and seem to be more likely than dogs to develop contact reactions (Kennis, 2013). This should be considered if signs seem to deteriorate following topical application in cases of feline otitis externa.

Glucocorticoids can be invaluable in the early stages of treatment of these cases to reduce inflammation and facilitate topical therapy. Many cases benefit from ear cleaning under general anaesthesia. However, the anatomy of the feline ear means that cats with otitis media are at an increased risk of developing Horner's syndrome from ear flushing procedures (see Chapter 19). Warmed saline is probably the safest cleaning agent in cats.

A common clinical presentation in middle-aged to older cats is suppurative, malodourous otitis externa that is frequently unilateral. In these cases, the clinician should suspect a mass within the ear canal, either a cerumenal adenoma, adenocarcinoma or inflammatory polyp. Histopathological examination is advisable to ascertain the type of mass present. Some polyps may be removed by traction; adenomas originating from the wall of the vertical or horizontal canal may be removed with a snare via video-otoscopy, but in other cases ear canal ablation or ventral bulla osteotomy are required.

Key points

- A primary consideration in animals with chronic otitis is to manage the inflammation and pain to prevent ear phobia developing
- Regular ear cleaning is an important component of long-term management of chronic otitis externa
- Topical antimicrobial therapy is optimal for the treatment of otitis externa and systemic therapy is only added when otitis media has developed

---

References and further reading

Barnard N and Foster A (2017) *Pseudomonas* otitis in dogs: a general practitioner's guide to treatment. *In Practice* **39**, 386–398

Bradley RL (1988) Surgical management of otitis externa. *Veterinary Clinics of North America: Small Animal Practice* **18**, 813–819

Buckley LM, McEwan NA and Nuttall T (2013) Tris-EDTA significantly enhances antibiotic efficacy against multidrug-resistant *Pseudomonas aeruginosa in vitro*. *Veterinary Dermatology* **24**, 519–e122

Chan WY, Khazandi M, Hickey EE *et al.* (2019) *In vitro* antimicrobial activity of seven adjuvants against common pathogens associated with canine otitis externa. *Veterinary Dermatology* **30**, 133–e138

Dinicola S, De Grazia S, Carlomagno G and Pintucci JP (2014) N-acetylcysteine as a powerful molecule to destroy bacterial biofilms. A systematic review. *European Review for Medical and Pharmacological Sciences* **18**, 2942–2948

Frosini SM and Bond R (2017) Activity *in vitro* of clotrimazole against canine methicillin-resistant and susceptible *Staphylococcus pseudintermedius*. *Antibiotics* **6**, 29

Guardabassi L, Ghibaudo G and Damborg P (2010) *In vitro* antimicrobial activity of a commercial ear antiseptic containing chlorhexidine and tris-EDTA. *Veterinary Dermatology* **21**, 282–286

Kennis RA (2013) Feline otitis: diagnosis and treatment. *Veterinary Clinics of North America: Small Animal Practice* **43**, 51–56

Martin Barrasa JL, Lupiola Gomez P, Gonzalez Lama Z and Tejedor Junco MT (2000) Antibacterial susceptibility patterns of *Pseudomonas* strains isolated from chronic canine otitis externa. *Journal of Veterinary Medicine B Infectious Disease and Veterinary Public Health* **47**, 191–196

McKay L, Rose CD, Matousek JL *et al.* (2007) Antimicrobial testing of selected fluoroquinolones against *Pseudomonas aeruginosa* isolated from canine otitis. *Journal of the American Animal Hospital Association* **43**, 307–312

Metry CA, Maddox CW, Dirikolu L, Johnson YJ and Campbell KL (2012) Determination of enrofloxacin stability and *in vitro* efficacy against *Staphylococcus pseudintermedius* and *Pseudomonas aeruginosa* in four ear cleaner solutions over a 28 day period. *Veterinary Dermatology* **23**, 23–28, e26

Morris DO (2004) Medical therapy of otitis externa and otitis media. *Veterinary Clinics of North America: Small Animal Practice* **34**, 541–555

Nuttall T (2016) Successful management of otitis externa. *In Practice* **38**, 17–21

Nuttall T and Carr MN (2010) Topical and systemic antimicrobial therapy for ear infections. In: *Advances in Veterinary Dermatology 6th edn.*, ed. DJ Deboer, VK Affolter, PB Hill, pp 402–407. Wiley-Blackwell, Oxford

Nuttall T and Cole LK (2004) Ear cleaning: the UK and US perspective. *Veterinary Dermatology* **15**, 127–136

Paterson S and Matyskiewicz W (2018) A study to evaluate the primary causes associated with *Pseudomonas* otitis in 60 dogs. *Journal of Small Animal Practice* **59**, 238–242

Robinson VH, Paterson S, Bennett C and Steen SI (2019) Biofilm production of *Pseudomonas* spp. isolates from canine otitis in three different enrichment broths. *Veterinary Dermatology* **30**, 218–e267

Rubin J, Walker RD, Blickenstaff K, Bodeis-jones S and Zhao S (2008) Antimicrobial resistance and genetic characterization of fluoroquinolone resistance of *Pseudomonas aeruginosa* isolated from canine infections. *Veterinary Microbiology* **131**, 164–172

Strain GM, Merchant SR, Neer TM and Tedford BL (1995) Ototoxicity assessment of a gentamicin sulfate otic preparation in dogs. *American Journal of Veterinary Research* **56**, 532–538

Tom LW (2000) Ototoxicity of common topical antimycotic preparations. *Laryngoscope* **110**, 509–516

Von Silva-Tarouca MSE, Wolf G and Mueller RS (2019) Determination of minimum inhibitory concentrations for silver sulfadiazine and other topical antimicrobial agents against strains of *Pseudomonas aeruginosa* isolated from canine otitis externa. *Veterinary Dermatology* **30**, 145–e142

Chapter 21

An approach to superficial and deep pyoderma

Daniel O. Morris and Anette Loeffler

Clinical presentations

The word 'pyoderma' literally means 'pus in the skin'. While many disease processes can cause an accumulation of inflammatory cells within the skin, colloquial use of the word often replaces the more descriptive term 'bacterial pyoderma'. Recognizing the presence of pyoderma in a dog is one of the most essential skills necessary for the successful practice of small animal medicine. This is because canine pyoderma is an extremely common clinical problem and typically associated with an underlying disease process. By comparison, feline pyoderma is relatively uncommon (with the exception of abscesses that result from fighting behaviour). Pyoderma is capable of producing a very wide spectrum of clinical lesions in both species. This variability is dependent upon the depth of the infection involving the skin and its appendages, and the hair coat type of the individual animal. Pyoderma is classified according to its depth in the skin as surface, superficial or deep infection.

Surface pyoderma

Surface pyoderma occurs when bacteria proliferate on the surface of the epidermis but do not invade deeper tissues. Surface infections are usually managed successfully with topical therapy alone (see Chapter 22). There are three major types of surface pyoderma recognized in veterinary medicine:

- **Intertrigo (skin fold infection):** Intertrigo refers to an overgrowth of microbes (bacteria, yeasts or both) within the warm/moist environment of a skin fold. It is common in brachycephalic dogs and cats (within facial and tail folds), around the vulva in bitches with deep perivulvar folds (Figure 21.1), and other intertriginous areas on obese animals. Primary inflammation, such as that caused by allergic diseases, exacerbates intertrigo, inflammatory cells and a mixed microbial overgrowth are common cytological findings
- **Acute moist dermatitis, pyotraumatic dermatitis ('hot spots'):** As the name implies, this is an acute lesion caused by self-trauma (licking) associated with pruritus in dogs. A very common cause is flea bite allergy, but any irritant can initiate this reaction pattern. Bacterial overgrowth on the surface of the traumatized, denuded skin occurs rapidly. If the pruritus is not interrupted (and the skin surface cleansed and dried),

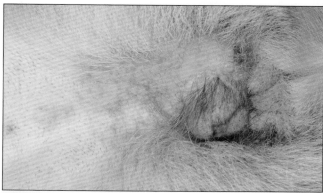

21.1 Intertrigo. Note the deep perivulvar folds. When the skin is stretched to reveal the lesional area, erythema with exudation, and in some cases erosions, may be noted. Pruritus is common.

the bacterial overgrowth may progress to pyotraumatic bacterial folliculitis (see below). In cats, eosinophilic plaques may present a similar clinical picture to canine 'hot spots'
- **Bacterial overgrowth syndrome:** Bacterial overgrowth syndrome in dogs is not considered to be a true form of pyoderma due to its lack of neutrophilic inflammation. However, like true pyoderma, the aetiology is bacterial – usually involving staphylococci. Lesions associated with bacterial overgrowth syndrome, which are typically intensely pruritic and malodourous, include greasy seborrhoea, erythema, excoriations, alopecia, and, in chronic cases, lichenification and hyperpigmentation (Pin *et al.*, 2006). Ventral aspects of the body are most commonly affected, especially intertriginous areas.

Superficial pyoderma

Superficial pyoderma is defined as the presence of infection within the hair follicle (bacterial folliculitis), within the epidermis but between hair follicles (forming subcorneal pustules, i.e. impetigo), or dissecting through layers of the stratum corneum (exfoliative superficial pyoderma). Superficial infections result from disruption of the skin/mucous membrane barrier defense mechanisms, due to physical or immunological compromise (see 'Differential diagnosis' below). Widespread or generalized superficial pyoderma may require systemic antimicrobial therapy, although topical therapy alone can be successful when due diligence is paid to frequency of application (see Chapter 22).

Bacterial folliculitis

Of the various types of pyoderma, bacterial folliculitis is the one that has the most variable clinical picture and its diagnosis can be quite elusive, especially for less experienced clinicians. The most common lesions caused by folliculitis in dogs are papules and/or pustules. Since these primary lesions are fleeting, only secondary crusts, follicular plugs or small epidermal collarettes will be seen in some cases (Figure 21.2). Crusts are caused by dried exudate, whereas epidermal collarettes are either the 'footprint' of a ruptured pustule (in which case they are quite small) or due to the centrifugal advancement of staphylococcal infection, which lifts up the leading edge of stratum corneum.

Bacterial folliculitis can be extremely subtle in some canine cases, where it produces no obvious primary or secondary lesions. In short-haired dog breeds (e.g. Dalmatians and Bulldogs), it may produce only a 'moth-eaten' appearance (referred to as 'short coat pyoderma'; Figure 21.3), whilst in silky-coated breeds (e.g. Irish Setters and Yorkshire Terriers) it may produce only a vague thinning of hair in patches. In heavily-coated (e.g. Akitas and Huskies) and wire-haired breeds, bacterial folliculitis may affect the secondary hairs disproportionally, resulting in a thinning of the undercoat.

Folliculitis is also subtle when the patient is receiving glucocorticoids, as evidence of inflammatory changes is removed. Thus, any multifocal alopecia, even without obvious evidence of papules, pustules and collarettes, should prompt the consideration of superficial pyoderma. When alopecia is the primary complaint, it is often helpful to examine areas of glabrous (sparsely-haired) skin, such as the groin and axillae, as it is in these areas that primary and secondary pyoderma lesions are most obvious. In the absence of such lesions, it may be quite helpful to shave some of the remaining hair around an alopecic area in order to better appreciate the clinical lesions and inflammatory changes centred on the hair follicle pores.

Exfoliative superficial pyoderma

Clinical lesions of exfoliative superficial pyoderma (ESP) are caused by staphylococcal bacteria disseminated throughout the stratum cornea and are characterized by rapidly expanding erythematous rings with peripheral peeling (epidermal collarettes; Figure 21.4). In its more florid form, ESP may present with unusually dramatic and coalescent collarettes, where extensive centrifugal peeling, alopecia and post-inflammatory hyperpigmentation

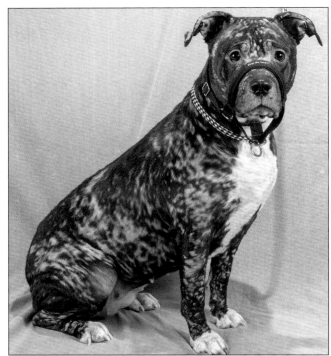

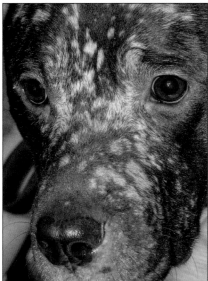

21.3 Bacterial folliculitis in a dog. Patches of alopecia in a 'moth-eaten' pattern with minimal visible inflammation and lacking primary lesions (e.g. papules and pustules) characterize this presentation of 'short coat pyoderma'. Only mild erythema and scale accompany the extensive alopecia.
(Courtesy of Dr David Duclos)

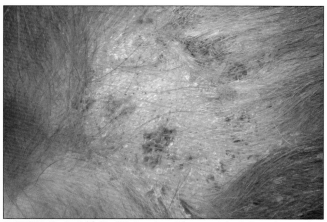

21.2 Bacterial folliculitis in a dog. A large patch of alopecia reveals plugging of the follicular ostia (also known as comedones), crusted exudate and scale at the advancing edge of the lesion.

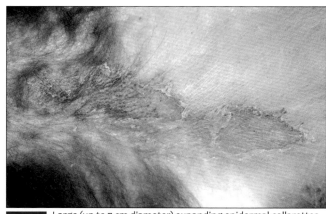

21.4 Large (up to 7 cm diameter) expanding epidermal collarettes are typical lesions associated with exfoliative superficial pyoderma.
(Courtesy of Dr David Duclos)

are hallmarks. Lesions may be highly pruritic. This form has been compared with human staphylococcal scalded skin syndrome, which is mediated by exfoliative toxins, and toxins produced by *Staphylococcus pseudintermedius* have been implicated in ESP of dogs (Banovic *et al.*, 2017). The more severe phenotype is most common in heavily-coated herding breeds (Shetland Sheepdogs, Border Collies, Australian Shepherds and collies) and has a predilection for the trunk and ventrum. ESP is not a direct consequence of bacterial folliculitis, but may occur concurrently in some cases (Banovic *et al.*, 2017).

Impetigo

The term impetigo should be reserved for the description of pustules that are not centred on the hair follicle pores. It is most common in puppies (also known as 'puppy pyoderma') and associated with an immature immune response. In adult dogs, impetigo is most commonly associated with underlying immunosuppression (Cushing's disease or iatrogenic hyperglucocorticoidism). Bullous impetigo is a term that refers to large, flaccid pustules, typically ranging from 5 to 15 mm in diameter. The lesions are much larger than the typical transient pustules seen with superficial bacterial folliculitis and are usually non-pruritic. The pustules may appear white, yellow or light green in colour and are often surrounded by a rim of erythema (Figure 21.5). These large pustules rupture easily to form yellow crusts and footprint collarettes.

Deep pyoderma

Deep pyoderma is defined by the presence of infection outside the confines of the epidermis or its contiguous hair follicle epithelium. Deep infections result from rupture of the hair follicle wall, penetrating wounds or haematogenous spread (sepsis). Deep pyoderma requires systemic antimicrobial therapy based upon culture and antimicrobial susceptibility testing, although topical treatment can be a valuable adjunct (see Chapter 22).

Furunculosis

Furunculosis is preceded by folliculitis and created by the rupture of hair follicles. The inflammatory response to free keratin in the dermis is entirely out of proportion to the number of bacteria present. Folliculitis/furunculosis may occur anywhere on the body, but there are several clinical terms used for common presentations:

- **Nasal folliculitis/furunculosis** – affects the haired skin of the dorsal muzzle (Figure 21.6)
- **Chin folliculitis/furunculosis** – also known as 'canine acne' (Figure 21.7)
- **Interdigital folliculitis/furunculosis** (Figure 21.8)
- **Post-grooming folliculitis/furunculosis**.

Localized patches of folliculitis/furunculosis on the limbs may result from self-trauma, known as 'acral lick dermatitis' (Figure 21.9). German Shepherd Dogs are particularly prone to widespread severe furunculosis and cellulitis, and the term 'German Shepherd pyoderma' is used to describe this poorly understood syndrome (Figure 21.10).

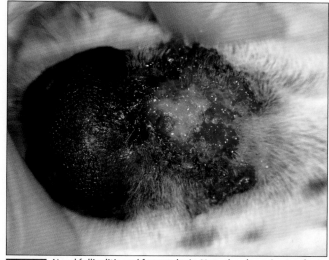

21.6 Nasal folliculitis and furunculosis. Note the alopecia, purulent exudate and haemorrhage, and heavy crusting on the bridge of the nose. Note similarities to eosinophilic furunculosis of the face (see Figure 21.16).

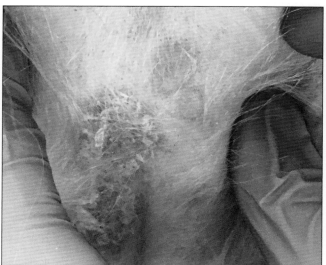

21.5 Large flaccid pustules (impetigo) and 'footprint' collarettes in an adult dog on long-term immunosuppressive therapy.

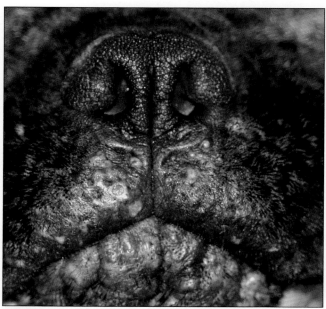

21.7 Folliculitis and furunculosis of the muzzle (also known as 'canine acne').

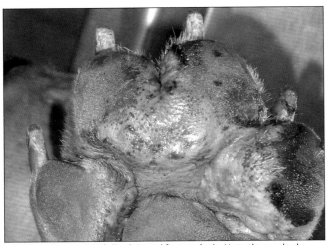

21.8 Interdigital folliculitis and furunculosis. Note the marked tissue swelling, plugging of the follicular ostia (comedones) and loss of the normal footpad architecture. Tissue culture should be performed to confirm a bacterial aetiology and select an optimum antimicrobial therapy.

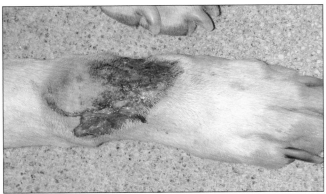

21.9 Localized folliculitis and furunculosis over the carpus (also known as canine 'acral lick granuloma')

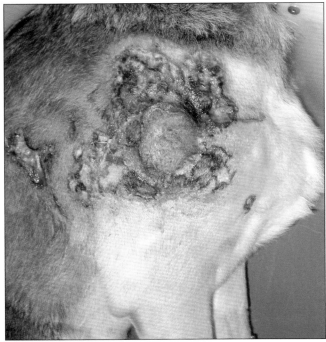

21.10 Regional folliculitis, furunculosis and cellulitis in a German Shepherd Dog (also known as 'German Shepherd pyoderma').

Cellulitis

Cellulitis is inflammation of the deep subcutaneous connective tissues, and common usage of the term in human medicine has come to imply bacterial infection.

Abscesses

Abscesses are created by pooling of suppurative material within pockets of tissue (dermal or subcuticular). Abscesses are the most common form of deep pyoderma that occurs in cats, likely due to their very supple/pliant skin.

Atypical presentations of canine pyoderma

There are two less common presentations of canine pyoderma that deserve special mention, since they have unique or syndromic presentations.

Mucocutaneous pyoderma

Mucocutaneous pyoderma (MCP) is a form of surface pyoderma that most commonly affects the lips and perioral skin, nasal planum and nares. Less commonly, it may involve the mucocutaneous junctions of the eyelids, vulva, prepuce and anus (Bassett *et al.*, 2004). The clinical appearance of the disease, which can mimic cutaneous lupus (see Chapter 28), is variable but may begin with erythema and oedema that progresses to crusts, erosions, ulcers, fissures, and focal depigmentation (Figure 21.11). German Shepherd Dogs and their crossbreeds appear to be at increased risk for MCP.

Post-grooming furunculosis

This uncommon but distinctive form of deep pyoderma is characterized by the acute onset of clinical signs within 7 days (median 2 days) after bathing, hand stripping or traumatic brushing of the hair coat (Cain and Mauldin, 2015). Lesions may include pustules, haemorrhagic bullae and fistulae, and are most commonly located on the dorsal trunk (Figure 21.12). Most affected dogs are in extreme pain and this may be mistaken for back pain, since constitutional signs (pain, fever, malaise) may precede the onset of grossly visible skin lesions. Minor trauma to the hair follicles combined with contaminated bathing products,

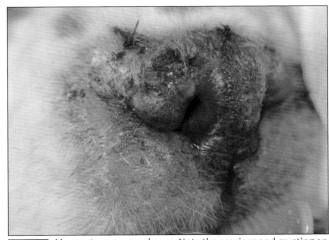

21.11 Mucocutaneous pyoderma. Note the erosions and crusting on the nasal planum extending on to the mucocutaneous junctions and continuing (as bacterial folliculitis) on to the haired skin of the muzzle. The primary differential diagnoses for this complex of lesions include autoimmune skin diseases and atypical dermatophytosis.

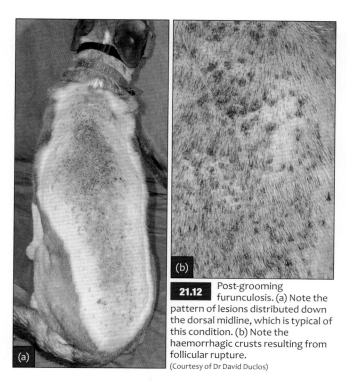

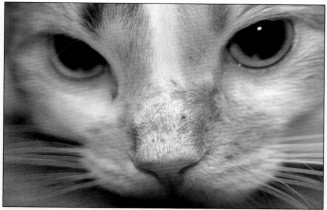

21.14 Feline bacterial folliculitis. Small patches of alopecia with marked erythema are the only signs of bacterial folliculitis in this cat, for which the primary differential diagnoses should be dermatophytosis and demodicosis (caused by *Demodex cati*).

21.12 Post-grooming furunculosis. (a) Note the pattern of lesions distributed down the dorsal midline, which is typical of this condition. (b) Note the haemorrhagic crusts resulting from follicular rupture.
(Courtesy of Dr David Duclos)

such as shampoos and crème rinses, may initiate the infection. In particular, self-service dog bathing facilities and grooming parlours, which use communal bathing products that have been diluted with tap water, have been implicated. Gram-negative bacteria, such as *Pseudomonas aeruginosa*, are often isolated from lesions via culture, and this condition has a distinctive histopathological appearance when a biopsy is performed.

Special considerations for cats

The most common presentations of feline staphylococcal infection are otitis externa, facial acne and surface pyoderma superimposed upon eosinophilic plaques and indolent lip ulcers (Morris *et al.*, 2006). It is widely accepted that feline bacterial folliculitis is uncommon to rare compared with dogs, although some authors believe that it is underdiagnosed. In cats, bacterial folliculitis may manifest as milia (small crusted papules), larger crusts (Figure 21.13) or alopecia with minimal inflammation visible grossly (Figure 21.14). Therefore, cats exhibiting

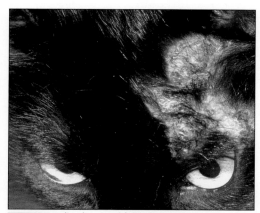

21.13 Feline bacterial folliculitis with crusting. Large patches of alopecia with exudation and serocellular crusts are formed by self-trauma and secondary bacterial folliculitis in this cat with facial pruritus due to a food-responsive dermatosis (also known as food allergy or adverse food reaction).

focal/multifocal alopecia, or any of the feline inflammatory reaction patterns commonly associated with allergic and ectoparasitic diseases (see Chapter 23), should be sampled cytologically for evidence of bacterial involvement before treatment.

Aetiology

The most common aetiological agents of pyoderma are *Staphylococcus* spp., which are also normal inhabitants of the skin and mucous membranes of all mammals and birds.

Coagulase-positive staphylococci

Coagulase-positive staphylococci have traditionally been considered to be the 'true' pathogens:

- **S. pseudintermedius** – This is the most common cause of pyoderma in dogs and cats (and is of low pathogenicity to humans). Domestic animal species are the primary reservoirs
- **S. schleiferi** subspecies **coagulans** – This is the second most common pathogen of dogs (which are likely to be a natural reservoir). It is rare in cats and humans, but may cause skin disease indistinguishable from that caused by *S. pseudintermedius* and *S. aureus*. *S. schleiferi* is coagulase-variable and has a coagulase-negative variant (see 'Clinical approach' below)
- **S. aureus** – Humans are the primary reservoir for most strains, and this is the most common pathogen of people. It is a less common pathogen of dogs and cats, and most *S. aureus* infections in pets are thought to represent 'spill over' from humans
- **S. hyicus** – Pigs are the primary reservoir, but infections of dogs and cats do occur rarely.

Coagulase-negative staphylococci

Coagulase-negative staphylococci (CoNS) have traditionally been considered to be non-pathogenic residents or transient commensals. However, this viewpoint is likely oversimplified and in human medicine the paradigm is shifting (Morris *et al.*, 2017). This is in part due to the increasing prevalence of immunosuppression within the human population, which has allowed greater susceptibility to less pathogenic organisms on a population-wide basis. To compound the problem, CoNS commonly express multiple antimicrobial drug resistance patterns (see Chapter 22).

Coagulase-negative variant of *S. schleiferi*

The coagulase-negative variant of *S. schleiferi* should always be considered pathogenic when isolated by culture from a lesion thought to be infected. Due to this, it is now more important than ever for veterinary microbiology laboratories to fully speciate CoNS, so that clinicians can make informed therapeutic decisions (Morris *et al.*, 2017).

Other CoNS species

Since most CoNS are still thought to be only marginally pathogenic, a common question posed by clinicians is what should be done when a laboratory reports that a CoNS has been isolated from a clinical sample. This should largely depend upon how confident one is that the 'true' aetiological agent has been isolated. Again, coagulase-negative *S. schleiferi* should always be considered pathogenic when isolated from a lesion compatible with a clinical diagnosis of pyoderma. For other CoNS, the solution is much less clear. The following are general guidelines for determining pathogenicity:

- If the culture sample was obtained from an intact primary skin lesion (pustule, bulla, closed abscess), treatment should be recommended based on susceptibility results
- If the sample was obtained from a 'contaminated' secondary lesion (skin surface swab, open wound, crust or collarette), the result should be interpreted with caution and the clinician should consider repeating the culture, especially if multiple drug resistance presents a therapeutic dilemma
- The clinical microbiologist should be consulted, as the laboratory may have isolated only a single colony, in which case the relevance of the isolate may be questioned.

Non-staphylococci

Less commonly, pyoderma may be caused by Gram-negative bacteria and/or non-staphylococcal Gram-positive cocci. This is quite rare for superficial pyoderma, but much more likely in cases of surface bacterial overgrowth and deep infection. Still, although quite rare, pustular pyoderma caused by Gram-negative bacterial species is possible. If bacterial rods are noted on cytology from a primary lesion, culture/susceptibility testing should be recommended. The same is true for cases of deep pyoderma. Since surface infections are typically treated with topical antimicrobial agents only, culture/susceptibility testing of these cases is less useful (see 'Diagnostic tests' below).

Differential diagnosis

Skin lesions

The differential diagnoses for skin lesions caused by bacterial pyoderma may be extensive, since pyoderma can masquerade as many clinical forms. Therefore, specific considerations will vary according to the clinical appearance of lesions presented by any particular case.

Surface pyoderma

A very important differential diagnosis for most forms of surface pyoderma is *Malassezia* dermatitis (see Chapter 26). This is especially true for both intertrigo and bacterial overgrowth syndrome. In fact, bacteria and yeast may be admixed on the surface of skin lesions. When occurring around the mouth, MCP may be easily confused with lip fold intertrigo, as they affect the same area. However, intertrigo does not typically cause ulceration. Lip fold intertrigo of the lips is most common in breeds with deep lip folds (e.g. spaniels and setters). When MCP affects the nasal planum, it can closely resemble discoid lupus erythematosus both clinically and histopathologically (Wiemelt *et al.*, 2004). An antimicrobial therapeutic trial is advised prior to taking biopsy samples from the affected area.

Superficial pyoderma

Superficial bacterial folliculitis is by far the most common clinical presentation in dogs. Although some lesions of bacterial folliculitis (e.g. moth-eaten alopecia) may closely resemble dermatophytosis and demodicosis, 'ringworm' is quite uncommon in dogs compared with pyoderma. Simple in-house diagnostic tests (skin surface cytology, scrapings and dermatophyte screening tests) are needed to rule in/out each differential diagnosis (see Chapter 3).

When papules and/or pustules are the dominant clinical lesion, the approach to investigation should follow the recommendations in Chapter 13. When alopecia is the dominant clinical manifestation, the differential diagnosis may depend on the pattern and extent of the alopecia (see Chapter 17). For highly pustular presentations, sterile pustular diseases, such as sterile granulomatous dermatitis and lymphadenitis (juvenile cellulitis; Figure 21.15) and pemphigus foliaceus, should be ruled out both by cytology and histopathology. It has now been shown that sterile granulomatous dermatitis and lymphadenitis may occur in older adult dogs and it is no longer considered to be a differential diagnosis restricted to puppies (Inga *et al.*, 2019; see Chapter 28).

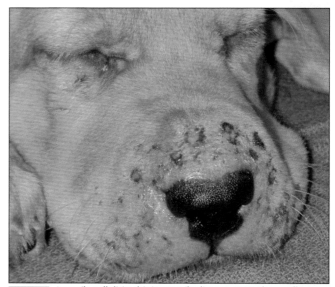

21.15 Juvenile cellulitis: this is a sterile disease. Note the swelling, alopecia, ulceration and exudation of the muzzle, which can easily be confused with folliculitis and furunculosis, especially if it occurs in an adult animal.

Deep pyoderma

The many different forms of folliculitis/furunculosis may invoke specific differential diagnosis lists. For all forms, it is important to rule out demodicosis and dermatophytosis, as both of these follicular diseases can be complicated by secondary bacterial furunculosis and accurate identification and correction of the underlying disease is critical for a successful treatment outcome.

- For furunculosis limited to the face, or for localized lesions on the trunk, canine eosinophilic furunculosis should be ruled out by cytology and biopsy. This is a sterile eosinophilic process invoked by the bites or stings of insects (Figure 21.16) and presents a unique histopathological picture. In some cases, the pet owner will have witnessed the envenomation.
- Furunculosis of the paws in dogs (interdigital spaces often called interdigital 'cysts') starts as a sterile process, which only becomes infected when the lesions rupture and are subject to trauma, often by licking. The aetiology of these lesions is multifactorial and include allergic inflammation, abnormal weight bearing associated with orthopaedic conditions, obesity and endocrine disease. In addition, neoplastic processes and foreign bodies may need to be considered for individual lesions. A thorough evaluation of the contributing causes and appropriate long-term management is indicated (Nuttall, 2019).
- In cases presenting with nodules and draining tracts refractory to routine management (true for both dogs and cats), atypical bacterial organisms such as actinomycetes and mycobacteria, deep/systemic fungal infections (e.g. sporotrichosis, blastomycosis, cryptococcosis, etc.) and protozoal diseases (e.g. leishmaniosis) should be ruled out by histopathology, appropriate culture methods and/or molecular diagnostics.

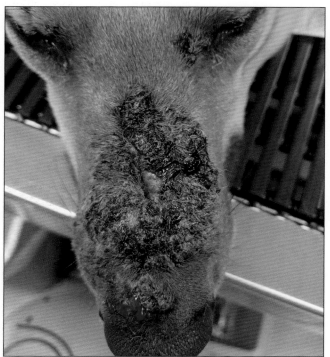

21.16 Eosinophilic furunculosis of the face. Haemorrhage, ulceration and heavy crusting can be seen on the face of this dog, which had been stung/bitten by an unknown type of insect. Note the swelling of the muzzle due to inflammation and oedema. Multiple dogs in the kennel presented with similar lesions.

Primary (predisposing) diseases

The overwhelming majority of pyoderma cases are due to an underlying disease process. This is true for most superficial pyodermas and bacterial folliculitis (with or without furunculosis) and may be present in cases of recurrent surface pyoderma. In both the dog and the cat, pruritic skin diseases (especially allergic dermatoses) should be primary suspects (see Chapter 6). It has been well established that dogs with atopic dermatitis are highly predisposed to bacterial pyoderma (see Chapter 9). However, any pruritic disorder may lead to self-trauma and disruption of stratum corneum barrier function, which predisposes to bacterial overgrowth and infection. Although less common on a day-to-day basis, immunosuppressive conditions, such as hyperadrenocorticism in dogs and retroviral infection in cats, may also predispose to pyoderma. This is also true for patients undergoing immunosuppressive therapies for management of neoplasia and systemic immune-mediated diseases.

Clinical approach

History

The clinical approach should begin with a comprehensive case history, including patient signalment, origin, travel history, prior treatments (including antipruritic, antimicrobial and parasite control interventions) and any evidence of contagion or zoonosis. A description of the initial (gross) appearance of lesions and how they have progressed is also often helpful since skin lesions have 'life spans' and change over time. As it has been estimated that >90% of pyoderma cases are secondary to other factors, it is imperative to identify and mitigate the effects of underlying disease processes in order to prevent recurrence of the pyoderma and reduce obstacles to effective antimicrobial therapy.

Diagnostic tests

Cytology

The diagnosis of pyoderma is often a clinical judgement. Confirmation by cytology is always worth pursuing to:

- Rule out the presence of acantholytic cells (the calling card of pemphigus; see Chapter 28)
- Confirm the presence of inflammatory cells and bacteria (see Chapter 4 for descriptions of cytological techniques).

In general, a cytological examination should be performed on papular, pustular and erosive lesions, and from beneath secondary skin lesions such as crusts and epidermal collarettes. However, it is important to understand that with folliculitis, the bacteria may not be within reach. In cases of bacterial folliculitis that are minimally inflammatory (especially where alopecia is the only grossly visible lesion), there may be no exudate on the surface of the epidermis and the bacteria may be confined within the follicular unit. Therefore, failure to identify bacteria and inflammatory cells from the surface of the skin does not exclude the diagnosis of bacterial pyoderma.

Bacterial culture and susceptibility testing

Bacterial culture and susceptibility testing should be performed by a laboratory with experience handling veterinary samples. Minimum reporting by microbiology laboratories should include complete speciation of all staphylococci (regardless of coagulase status) and an antibiogram for all cultured isolates (Morris *et al.*, 2017). Bacterial culture and susceptibility testing is critical under any of the following conditions:

- Superficial pyoderma that fails to respond to appropriate empirical therapy
- History of repeated administration of antimicrobials
- History of prior isolation of meticillin-resistant *Staphylococcus* spp.
- Rod-shaped or filamentous bacteria on cytology
- Nodular/granulomatous lesions
- All cases of deep pyoderma and draining tracts
- When uncommon bacterial species are suspected (e.g. actinomycetes, mycobacteria).

Sampling techniques for bacterial culture: There are several techniques for sampling, based upon the lesions present:

- **Primary lesions:** Direct swab inoculation from a primary lesion (papule/pustule or non-draining furuncle or abscess) is always preferable. In a dog with dorsally distributed folliculitis, where crusts and collarettes are the only lesions present, the glabrous skin of the groin and axillae should be checked for intact pustules/papules; these are the best places to find them
- **Secondary lesions:** When there are no primary lesions present, a moistened swab can be rolled under the leading edge of an epidermal collarette to obtain a sample. Removing a crust can also be effective if the skin is moist underneath. The authors prefer to streak the swab on to a sterile glass slide to look for cocci (using Diff-Quik® or Gram stain) before submitting the sample for culture. This provides some assurance that the bacteria have been harvested from the lesion. But of course, it is possible to have a cytology-negative/culture-positive sample, since the microbiology laboratory will amplify organisms that are present on the swab
- **No primary or secondary lesions present:** For cases of folliculitis with neither primary nor secondary lesions, a small skin punch biopsy for macerated tissue culture is usually effective. The surface of the lesion should not be aggressively scrubbed because residual antimicrobials may be incorporated into the tissue slurry and inhibit growth *in vitro*. Blotting the surface with an alcohol swab (allowing it to air dry) helps to reduce contamination. The tissue sample should be submitted to the laboratory in a culturette, a sterile glass tube, or in transport media supplied by the laboratory. Balanced salt solution or sterile water should not be used as a transport medium unless instructed to do so by the laboratory.

Biopsy and histopathology

Skin biopsy has a place in the diagnostic process for pyoderma because some lesion types have important differential diagnoses that must be ruled out histologically. These include:

- Pemphigus foliaceus and juvenile cellulitis (for pustular lesions)
- Cutaneous lupus (for mucocutaneous and nasal lesions)
- Sterile eosinophilic furunculosis (for facial or localized truncal furunculosis)
- Sterile panniculitis and fungal, protozoal or atypical bacterial infections (for deep lesions with draining tracts)
- Deep interdigital lesions (which may also represent a sterile inflammatory process or even deep-seated *Demodex* mites).

The reader is referred to Chapter 3 for discussion of appropriate skin biopsy techniques and procedures.

Key points
- Bacterial pyoderma can present with varied clinical signs. The majority of infections occur secondary to an underlying problem
- Confirmation of bacterial involvement should be made by collecting samples for cytology
- Bacterial culture and sensitivity testing should always be performed if a deep pyoderma is present and in most cases of chronic recurrent superficial infections

---

References and further reading

Banovic F, Linder K and Olivry T (2017) Clinical, microscopic and microbial characterization of exfoliative superficial pyoderma-associated epidermal collarettes in dogs. *Veterinary Dermatology* **28**, 107–e23

Bassett RJ, Burton GG and Robson DC (2004) Antibiotic responsive ulcerative dermatoses in German Shepherd Dogs with mucocutaneous pyoderma. *Australian Veterinary Journal* **82**, 485–489

Cain CL and Mauldin EA (2015) Clinical and histopathologic features of dorsally located furunculosis in dogs following water immersion or exposure to grooming products: 22 cases (2005–2013). *Journal of the American Veterinary Medical Association* **246**, 522–529

Inga A, Griffeth GC, Drobatz KJ *et al.* (2019) Sterile granulomatous dermatitis and lymphadenitis (juvenile cellulitis) in adult dogs: a retrospective analysis of 90 cases (2004–2018). *Veterinary Dermatology* **30**, 302–303

Morris DO, Loeffler A, Davis MF *et al.* (2017) Recommendations for approaches to methicillin-resistant staphylococcal infections in small animals: diagnosis, therapeutic considerations and preventative measures. Clinical Consensus Guidelines of the World Association for Veterinary Dermatology. *Veterinary Dermatology* **28**, 304–e69

Morris DO, Rook KA, Shofer FS *et al.* (2006) Screening of *Staphylococcus aureus*, *S. intermedius*, and *S. schleiferi* isolates obtained from small companion animals for antimicrobial resistance: a retrospective review of 749 isolates (2003–2004). *Veterinary Dermatology* **17**, 332–337

Nuttall T (2019) Chronic pododermatitis and interdigital furunculosis in dogs. *Companion Animal* **24**, doi.org/10.12968/coan.2019.24.4.194

Pin D, Carlotti DN, Jasmin P *et al.* (2006) Prospective study of bacterial overgrowth syndrome in eight dogs. *Veterinary Record* **158**, 437–441

Wiemelt SP, Goldschmidt MH, Greek JS *et al.* (2004) A retrospective study comparing the histopathological features and response to treatment in two canine nasal dermatoses, DLE and MCP. *Veterinary Dermatology* **15**, 341–348

Chapter 22

Management of superficial and deep pyoderma

Anette Loeffler and Daniel O. Morris

With the emergence of meticillin-resistant, multiple drug resistant staphylococci (MDRS) as small animal pathogens, reliance on empirical drug choices is no longer appropriate. The globally continuing spread of antimicrobial resistance amongst bacterial pathogens is one of the biggest threats to human and animal health. There is an urgent need to reduce antimicrobial use in order to preserve currently available drugs for the most critically ill patients.

In many countries, restrictions for small animal veterinary surgeons (veterinarians) are already in place to minimize inappropriate prescribing of certain antimicrobial classes of drugs. In other countries (e.g. currently the UK), veterinary surgeons are free to use antimicrobial drugs within a prescribing cascade, and adherence to good antimicrobial stewardship principles and published guidelines is expected on a voluntary basis.

Pyoderma remains amongst the top three indications for which antimicrobials are prescribed in small animal practice, but the recognition of multiple drug resistance in pyoderma pathogens (see 'Meticillin-resistant staphylococcal pyoderma' below) has prompted a re-think of treatment recommendations. The skin provides unique opportunities for the responsible use of antimicrobials through its accessibility to easy sampling and topical therapy. Figure 22.1 highlights the key recommendations for the successful management of pyoderma. Client education is also of key importance to effect resolution of the infection and prevent future recurrence.

Antibacterial therapy

Guidelines

There are currently two sets of guidelines specific for pyoderma (Beco *et al.*, 2013; Hillier *et al.*, 2014) and another on meticillin-resistant staphylococcal infections largely concerned with pyoderma (Morris *et al.*, 2017), which are all free to access online. In addition, there are many national and international antimicrobial use guidance documents that include advice on the management of skin infections. In the UK, for example, the BSAVA PROTECT ME poster (updated in 2019) and the European FECAVA Advice on Responsible Use of Antimicrobials poster both include a list of common indications for which systemic antimicrobial use is considered unnecessary. There are no consensus guidelines dealing with deep pyoderma or with feline infections at present. In addition to pyoderma-specific guidance, general prescribing rules for antimicrobials (e.g. accurate dosing, selection of narrow-spectrum over broad-spectrum agents) also apply to the management of skin infections.

General principles

Drug delivery to the skin is tricky by both the systemic and the topical route. For topically applied medications, the epidermis (and the lumen of the hair follicle by extension) are protected by the effective barrier action of the stratum

Opportunities	Action	Advantages
Confirm the diagnosis (see Chapter 3)	Cytology to identify bacteria and phagocytosis	In-house, rapid, inexpensive
Prevent recurrence of pyoderma (see 'Recurrent pyoderma' in the text)	Identify and correct underlying primary causes	Reduces antimicrobial use
Make use of accessibility of the skin	Topical therapy (see 'Topical antibacterial therapy' in the text and Chapter 27)	Uses biocides and antimicrobials not needed for systemic therapy
Culture-based prescribing for systemic therapy (see 'Systemic antibacterial therapy' in the text)	Avoid empirical drug choice	Reduces overall morbidity and cost, identifies MDRS early
Awareness of risk factors for MDRS and regional prevalence (see 'Meticillin-resistant staphylococcal pyoderma' below)	Early submission for bacterial culture and susceptibility testing (see Chapter 3)	Early identification to reduce risk of transmission and practice contagion
Good follow-up	Re-examination before stopping therapy (clinician needs to determine whether lesions have resolved, not owner). Cytology should be employed	Facilitates identification of primary disease

22.1 Opportunities for responsible antimicrobial prescribing in canine and feline pyoderma. MDRS = multiple drug resistant staphylococci.

corneum and do not receive a direct blood supply. The drug carrier, or vehicle, can therefore be critically important in the delivery of an active ingredient molecule to the infection site. While topical therapy is intuitive and effective for surface infections, a degree of intercellular distribution between layers is required and highlights the importance of clinical studies in drug development. On the other hand, drugs administered orally or by injection will eventually distribute to the skin via blood vessels in the dermis. However, since only 4% of cardiac output reaches the dermis, drug doses need to be chosen towards the higher end of recommended ranges for skin infections. Furthermore, staphylococci associated with pyoderma can be located both extra- and intracellularly and the selection of drugs that accumulate in cells can be valuable.

Since pyoderma is frequently secondary to pruritic or chronic diseases (or both), a combination of antimicrobial therapy and antipruritic treatment may often seem desirable. Antimicrobial drugs will either slow bacterial growth (traditionally referred to as 'bacteriostatic') or kill most bacteria, for example. by disrupting the cell walls ('bacteriocidal'). However, cure of clinical infection relies on collaboration with the host's immune system and any medication that interferes with the normal immune response may therefore cause delays in the clearance of infection. While glucocorticoids have always been contraindicated in the face of infection, effects are less clear for the newer anti-inflammatory molecules authorized for the management of allergic skin disease.

As a general rule and in the interest of successful long-term management, pyoderma should always be resolved before the underlying disease process is assessed. Likewise, any identified or suspected parasites should be treated. It is only at this stage that proper determination of an underlying pruritic or non-pruritic disorder can be made and further investigations and specific treatments instigated. Exceptions to this rule are surface pyoderma where a primarily inflammatory problem leads to microbial overgrowth (e.g. acute moist dermatitis/pyotraumatic dermatitis), and a diagnosis of sarcoptic mange where welfare concerns due to intense pruritus may warrant glucocorticoid therapy whilst acaricides and antimicrobials are used.

Topical or systemic application?

The most important decision before prescribing antibacterial medication is whether systemic drugs are needed, either alone or in combination with topical therapy. Accurate identification of the depth of infection (see Chapter 21) is essential and will inform the best mode of application (Figure 22.2). Other factors that should be considered include the severity of disease (lesion number and distribution), patient factors (such as hair coat, temperament and environment), concurrent disease and the owner's ability to undertake topical or systemic therapy.

Duration of treatment and follow-up

It is currently recommended to treat superficial pyoderma for 3 weeks or 1 week beyond clinical cure, and deep pyoderma for 4–8 weeks or 2 weeks beyond clinical cure. These recommendations are currently based on clinical expertise rather than scientific evidence, but where shorter courses may be prescribed, plans for close monitoring of progress by the veterinary surgeon rather than the owner should be in place. It should be emphasized that the use of cytology before and during treatment is an invaluable adjunctive guide to the success of therapy.

Depth/type of pyoderma	Mode of application
Surface: • Acute moist dermatitis/hot spot • Intertrigo/fold pyoderma • Bacterial overgrowth syndrome/pyotraumatic dermatitis	Always topical therapy alone
Superficial: • Bacterial folliculitis • Impetigo • Mucocutaneous pyoderma	Topical therapy alone In combination with systemic first-tier antimicrobial drugs if extensive or severe
Deep: • Chin acne • Acral lick dermatitis • Furunculosis • Interdigital infected nodules	Always systemic therapy Always based on bacterial culture and antimicrobial susceptibility test results Combine with supportive topical therapy where practical and tolerated

22.2 Recommended treatment modalities for different types of pyoderma.

Owner education

It is important to involve owners in discussions relating to good antimicrobial stewardship in order to improve compliance and monitoring of treatment progress. With antimicrobial resistance nowadays discussed in mainstream media, many owners will be familiar with the context. However, this may be an abstract concept compared with decisions and emotions related to the treatment of their pet, and owners should be reminded of the importance of completing courses and keeping follow-up appointments.

Topical antibacterial therapy

The role of topical antimicrobial therapy has shifted from supportive towards mainstay therapy and is indicated in almost every case of pyoderma as:

- Sole antibacterial therapy for:
  - Surface pyoderma
  - Most cases of superficial pyoderma (including meticillin-resistant *Staphylococcus pseudintermedius* (MRSP) pyoderma)
- Adjunctive to systemic therapy for:
  - Severe or extensive superficial pyoderma
  - Deep pyoderma
- Preventative or supportive use for:
  - Recurrent (relapsing) superficial pyoderma
  - Reducing contagion and zoonotic transmission from MRSP carried on hair, skin and mucosae – during and after infection has resolved.

The use of topical antibacterial agents inevitably relies more extensively on anecdotal information and a degree of 'trial and error' than systemic therapy. It is, therefore, important to keep in mind that authorized products will have undergone efficacy and safety trials in order to be licensed for a specific indication, such as bacterial skin infection. The authorization process would also have included documentation of a controlled manufacturing process to provide stability in potency of the active ingredient. Products authorized for bacterial skin disease should be the first choice, at least when starting treatment, to facilitate assessment of suitability and compliance. If a licensed product with proven efficacy fails despite appropriate prescription and good compliance, then other factors may be involved and alternatives need to be considered. In addition, skin irritation may occur in any dog or cat with any product.

Active ingredients

A range of antibacterial compounds are available, either as prescription-only medicines or as 'over-the-counter' preparations marketed as antibacterial and accessible to owners without prescription. Molecules used as active ingredients come from a wide background of original uses (e.g. antiseptics, antibiotics, disinfectants, household detergents, herbal extracts) and the associated terminology is not always clearly distinctive. Some of the most widely used ingredients are listed in Figure 22.3.

When looking for evidence supporting the choice of topical antibacterials, it is important to distinguish between clinical studies providing data on resolution of pyoderma and *in vitro* studies that typically report on minimum inhibitory concentrations or other parameters

Active ingredient	Chemical or formulation particulars	Best known use	Supporting evidence	Comments
Benzoyl peroxide	2.5%	Human acne medication and industrial bleaching agent	RCT in dogs with pyoderma (Mueller *et al.*, 2011)	Oxidizing agent that damages bacterial membranes May irritate skin and has a drying effect
Bleach (sodium hypochlorite, NaOCl)	Current recommendation for clinical use in dogs is 0.1% dilution	Disinfectant Broad spectrum	Fadok and Irwin, 2019	Bleach baths used in the management of human eczema but no evidence for efficacy demonstrated in a 2019 Cochrane review Household bleach typically contains 3–8% sodium hypochlorite
Chlorhexidine	Gluconate or digluconate (typically used interchangeably) 2–4% shampoo, scrub solution, spray, wipes Also available in combination with tromethamine (Tris)	Antiseptic (synthetic biguanide) Broad spectrum	RCT (Mueller *et al.*, 2011) No controlled studies for Tris combination	Damages cytoplasmic membrane and coagulates cytoplasm Rarely irritating, not inactivated by organic material
Chloroxylenol	PCMX	Household disinfectant and antiseptic	Ineffective *in vitro* against *Staphylococcus pseudintermedius* (Young *et al.*, 2012) No clinical studies	Likely mechanism of antibacterial action through phenol effect on cell membrane
Ethyl lactate	10% shampoo		Conflicting (Mueller *et al.*, 2011)	*In vitro*, 30–60 minutes incubation required for bacterial killing (Young *et al.*, 2012)
Fusidic acid [a]	2% cream or ointment Combination product 0.5% fusidic acid with 0.1% betamethasone	Antibiotic Narrow spectrum anti-staphylococcal	As combination: comparable efficacy to parenteral dexamethasone and oral clavulanate-potentiated amoxicillin in dogs with acute moist dermatitis (hot spots) (Cobb *et al.*, 2005)	In dogs, topical only (systemic route not appropriate)
Hypochlorous acid (HOCl)	HOCl Water-based spray	Endogenous antibacterial molecule	No controlled studies	
Medical honey	Hygroscopic properties, which dehydrate bacteria	Antimicrobial	*In vivo* efficacy comparable to chlorhexidine in 36 dogs with intertrigo (Mueller *et al.*, 2011)	Non-toxic but may sting in wounds Only products that have been sterilized should be used to avoid contamination with, for example, spores of *Clostridium botulinum*
Mupirocin [a]	2% ointment (USA)	Antibiotic Narrow spectrum anti-staphylococcal	Good (Mueller *et al.*, 2011)	Topical only
Polymixin B	Sulphate Cutaneous suspension combination with miconazole and prednisolone	Broad spectrum but mainly against Gram-negative bacteria		Inactivated by organic material Rarely irritating
Povidone–iodine	Shampoo, scrub	Antiseptic		Prevents hydrogen bonding Contact sensitization
Sulphur and salicylic acid	Synergistic effect			
Silver sulfadiazine	1% cream	Broad spectrum	Limited (based on Mueller *et al.*, 2011)	Pyoderma caused by *P. aeruginosa*. Poor efficacy against Gram-positive bacteria
Triclosan	Shampoo	Antiseptic		

22.3 Selection of active antibacterial ingredients commonly recommended for the management of canine pyoderma (alphabetical order). RCT = Randomized controlled trial. [a] Fusidic acid and mupirocin are both anti-staphylococcal compounds with unfortunate national differences in authorization and recommendations for use. Fusidic acid is licensed in European countries and in Canada for use in dogs. Mupirocin ointment is authorized in the USA for dogs (and is commonly used off-label in cats) but reserved for use in human medicine in most of Europe to treat multiple drug resistant staphylococcal infections and eliminate meticillin-resistant *Staphylococcus aureus* carriage.
(From Morris *et al.*, 2017)

that give an indication of bacterial killing under laboratory conditions. Unfortunately, data from randomized controlled clinical studies specifically in canine pyoderma is still extremely sparse as summarized in a systematic review on topically-used antimicrobials (Mueller *et al.*, 2011).

For canine pyoderma, the review found good evidence (several open clinical trials) for efficacy of products containing 2–3% chlorhexidine and benzoyl peroxide and fair evidence (one open clinical trial) for fusidic acid, silver sulfadiazine and medical honey. In addition, *in vivo* studies have shown efficacy for two 4% chlorhexidine products (Borio *et al.*, 2015) and for a combination shampoo containing sodium hypochlorite (bleach) (Fadok and Irwin, 2019) and tolerance of 0.05 and 0.005% diluted bleach on healthy canine skin (Banovic *et al.*, 2018). Other active ingredients such as acetic and boric acid (available as a shampoo, solution, wipes) have been tested and marketed for skin infections, but *in vitro* and clinical studies have produced conflicting results.

In contrast, there is a wealth of *in vitro* study data for well-known compounds, some combination products and for some novel molecules (plant extracts, antimicrobial peptides, anti-biofilm agents); hopefully these have the potential for clinical use in the future, as the need for alternative topical antibacterial treatment options is likely to increase.

Formulations

Active ingredients are available in different formulations (see Chapter 27). This provides further opportunity to improve outcome by choosing a formulation to suit the particular type of infection, location, coat type and owners' ability to apply the product.

- **Shampoos** – best for widespread infections affecting hairy areas; mechanical cleansing helps to reduce pruritus and malodour and removes debris and crust. Contact time typically 10–15 minutes.
- **Creams, gels and suspensions** – for localized lesions and targeted treatment of affected skin.
- **Sprays** – helpful for painful areas where direct touch is not tolerated.
- **Wipes** – practical and effective for management of microbial overgrowth (surface pyoderma) in facial or other folds; easy for daily use.
- **Mousse or foam preparations** – facilitate drug application to interdigital areas due to their 'leave on' instructions.
- **Soaks or applications of undiluted antiseptic solutions** – wipe-on or spray-on without rinsing.

Resistance and compliance

Resistance is frequently discussed in the context of topical antibacterials. However, treatment failure (clinical resistance) in cases of pyoderma (non-biofilm), of appropriately applied products, has not been convincingly reported to date. Laboratory test reports are of limited value when selecting topical antibacterial agents for pyoderma. Results of 'resistant/intermediate/susceptible' as reported by the microbiology laboratory rely on the availability of clinical breakpoints, which are defined by taking into account pharmacokinetics and pharmacodynamics of a drug at a specific infection site and in a defined host species. No such breakpoints have yet been defined for topical antimicrobial therapy. With topical applications, the active ingredient bypasses the metabolic effects of the liver and the diluting effect of blood perfusion. Instead,

high drug concentrations can be achieved directly at the site of infection. If a poor response is seen, other factors such as compliance, co-morbidities or product formulation need to be considered.

Good owner and pet compliance are crucial for the success of topical therapy, and the effort and time required to engage owners in the process should not be underestimated. Owners need to understand and welcome the benefits of topical therapy. Beyond outlining the safety aspect (topical therapy allows targeted treatment of only the affected organ or even lesion) and the reduced risk for selecting multiple drug resistant pathogens, it can be helpful to mention possibly more familiar examples of topical treatments used in human medicine, such as widely used eczema creams. Furthermore, topical therapy can provide owners with a degree of control over their animal's treatment (to be used as prescribed, but for long-term management it is easier to tailor to the dog's needs) and additional value, such as removal of dirt, improvement of coat quality and smell or mechanical disruption of biofilm (e.g. in lip fold). Monitoring compliance (and efficacy) and supporting owners in making topical treatment work (e.g. by involving veterinary nurses or referring owners to online visual guidance for shampooing dogs) can further improve the outcome.

Systemic antibacterial therapy

A wide range of antimicrobial drugs is available for use in dogs and cats, many with an authorization for skin infections. For canine pyoderma, only a few efficacy studies documenting outcome have been published (Summers *et al.*, 2012).

Tier system and priority lists

When prescribing antimicrobial drugs for dogs, it is important to remember that most are also used in human medicine, either as identical or related molecules. Although small animal medicine receives less attention with regard to the risk of antimicrobial resistance transmission than livestock, the close contact between humans and pets inevitably heightens such transmission concerns. Antimicrobials have been classified and prioritized by several Public Health organizations in order to mitigate the risk from antimicrobial use in animals to humans, and the key antimicrobials recommended for canine pyoderma are all listed by the World Health Organization (WHO) as 'highly important' or 'critically important antimicrobials for human medicine' (WHO, 2019). Tier systems or classification of antimicrobials into first- and second-line drugs are available in veterinary published guidelines and are proposed for the skin infections described in this chapter (Figure 22.4) to help responsible decision-making in practice. Such tier systems are specific for the type of infection or infected organ and try to take into account the impact on public health and microbiome, as far as published evidence allows.

Empirical or culture-based drug choice

First-tier drugs are those that may be chosen empirically, i.e. without prior culture and susceptibility testing. With the majority of skin infections involving *Staphylococcus pseudintermedius*, empirical drug selection may seem a reasonable approach where the cost of laboratory testing is of concern. However, empirical choices for *S. pseudintermedius* infections are not appropriate in regions with

Tier	Appropriate use	Antimicrobial class/group/drug		Dose	Classification and prioritization according to WHO[a]
First	May be chosen empirically for superficial pyoderma First choice for deep (and superficial) pyoderma if *in vitro* tests indicate susceptibility	Lincosamides	Clindamycin Lincomycin	5.5–10 mg/kg orally q12–24h 15–25 mg/kg orally q12h	HI
		Beta-lactams	First-generation cephalosporins: Cefalexin (cefadroxil)	15–30 mg/kg orally q12h	HI
			Amoxicillin/clavulanate	12.5–25.0 mg/kg orally q12h	CIA
		Potentiated sulphonamides	Trimethoprim-sulfamethoxazole (Ormetoprim-potentiated sulphonamides)	15–30 mg/kg orally q12h 55 mg/kg on first day, then 27.5 mg/kg orally q24h	HI
Second	Use only after *in vitro* tests indicate susceptibility	Tetracyclines	Doxycycline (Minocycline) (Oxytetracycline)	5 mg/kg orally q12h or 10 mg/kg orally q24h 5 mg/kg orally q24h with food 10 mg/kg orally q12h	HI HI HI
		Third-generation cephalosporins	Cefovecin (Cefpodoxime proxetil)	8 mg/kg s.c. once, repeat after 14 days if infection improved but not fully resolved 5–10 mg/kg orally q24h	CIA with highest priority
		Fluoroquinolones	Enrofloxacin Marbofloxacin Pradofloxacin	5–20 mg/kg orally q24h 2.75–5.5 mg/kg orally q24h 3 mg/kg orally q24h	CIAs with highest priority

22.4 Antimicrobial drugs for systemic use in deep pyoderma or extensive, severe superficial pyoderma in the dog and suggested tier system to guide choice. Drugs not licensed for use in dogs in the UK are shown in brackets. [a]World Health Organization Advisory Group on Integrated Surveillance of Antimicrobial Resistance (AGISAR). CIA = critically important antimicrobial; HI = highly important antimicrobial.
(Adapted from Hillier *et al.*, 2014 using the UK prescribing cascade)

high levels of MRSP (>5%) and where patients have received multiple courses of antibiotics in the past. In addition, for deep pyoderma, laboratory testing is always indicated. In approximately 40% of deep infection cases, other bacteria are isolated on culture, including occasionally Gram-negative pathogens, and inappropriate antibacterial choices will delay effective treatment for the patient and will not be cost-effective for the owner. If topical therapy alone is to be prescribed, susceptibility testing is not relevant (see 'Topical antibacterial therapy' above) but may still be helpful to identify multiple drug resistant pathogens early for infection control purposes.

Interim treatment

Bacterial culture and antimicrobial susceptibility test results will take at least 2 days after the sample is received by the laboratory, even if matrix-assisted laser desorption ionization–time of flight (MALDI-ToF) machines and automated minimum inhibitory concentration (MIC) testing are used. If selective steps or extensive sub-culturing are required, then results may not be available for up to 7 days. If clinical signs are severe, or if there is a risk of rapid progression without intervention, 5–7 days of systemic therapy should be prescribed while culture results are pending. Cytology needs to inform choices for interim treatment. If cocci predominate, a first-tier drug (see Figure 22.4) can be administered on the expectation of a staphylococcal infection. With a predominance of rods, more drug-resistant Gram-negative bacteria are likely and a fluoroquinolone may be prescribed. Interim medication should be dispensed for the period during which results are pending, and owner contact scheduled within days so that treatment can be extended or changed (escalated or de-escalated) as required.

Third-tier antimicrobials

In most countries, none of the agents in this group are licensed for use in dogs and all are associated

with potentially significant adverse effects. Referral for specialist treatment and comprehensive infection control measures is recommended. Third-tier antimicrobials that may occasionally be considered for dogs with MRSP deep pyoderma include (all off-label, require careful review and discussion of risks prior to prescribing) (Plumb, 2015):

- Rifampicin: 5 mg/kg orally q12h or 10 mg/kg orally q24h (hepatotoxic; causes orange/red urine, tears and saliva during treatment)
- Amikacin: 15–30 mg/kg i.v., i.m. or s.c. q24h for dogs (nephrotoxic; avoid in animals with renal insufficiency; follow guidelines from the International Renal Interest Society for the prevention of aminoglycoside-induced acute kidney injury)
- Chloramphenicol: 40–50 mg/kg orally, i.v., s.c., i.m. q8h (bone marrow suppression; hepatotoxic; nephrotoxic; risk of aplastic (fatal) anaemia in humans – avoid direct contact with the medication).

As all three drugs are considered of either high importance (chloramphenicol) or critical importance (rifampicin, amikacin) for human health by the WHO, certain conditions of use should apply:

- *In vitro* tests indicate susceptibility
- First- and second-tier drugs are not appropriate
- Infection would not be treatable with topical antibacterial therapy alone
- Infection is severe
- Owner is committed and compliant and able to fund repeat follow-up examination and sampling, including for carriage status after infection has resolved.

With the number of untreatable human infections increasing worldwide, the use of glycopeptides, linezolid and potentially new anti-meticillin-resistant *Staphylococcus aureus* (MRSA) drugs in pets with pyoderma cannot be justified.

Meticillin-resistant staphylococcal pyoderma

MRSA and MRSP have emerged as the two most problematic multiple drug resistant pyoderma pathogens in small animal practice. Treatment options may be substantially limited for MDRS infections but, importantly, additional management considerations will be required to minimize contagion and deal with their zoonotic potential. Nevertheless, MDRS are no more virulent than their meticillin-susceptible counterparts and the prognosis for MDRS infections can be good, depending on the underlying cause and diligence in care.

Resistance, epidemiology and zoonotic potential

Meticillin is a semi-synthetic beta-lactam antibiotic no longer in clinical use, but meticillin resistance is used as a marker for multiple drug resistance in coagulase-positive staphylococci. Amongst coagulase-negative species, meticillin resistance may be widespread but is infrequently associated with multiple drug resistance and rarely clinically relevant.

On a molecular level, resistance to meticillin is encoded by a small genetic element (*mecA*), which results in an altered cell wall protein that confers low affinity (and clinical resistance) to all beta-lactam antibiotics, including the cephalosporins, the potentiated beta-lactams and the carbapenems. Since this broad beta-lactam resistance typically occurs in clinical isolates from infected patients, treatment selects for resistance to other antimicrobial classes with subsequent spread through clonally expanding lineages.

Previous antimicrobial therapy, repeated visits to veterinary establishments and invasive procedures have been described as the main risk factors for MDRS infections in pets. Knowledge of risk factors helps to raise suspicion of MDRS involvement, but diagnosis is by laboratory testing. There are no clinical markers for MDRS pyoderma from currently circulating lineages.

The spread of MDRS is largely determined by host adaptation and environmental resilience. Staphylococci, irrespective of their meticillin resistance, have host preferences but are not host-specific and can, therefore, be transmitted between pets and humans in both directions and cause opportunistic infections. Furthermore, staphylococci can survive on dry surfaces for many months and thus contaminate the practice and home environment.

MRSA is primarily a human pathogen and, if found in pets, isolates are indistinguishable from human hospital-associated trails ('spill-over' from human hospitals). Rapid spread between pets or rates above 10% even in areas with high MRSA rates in human hospitals have not been observed. Although pets can be considered as 'innocent bystanders' in the transmission of MRSA, it is prudent to recommend that owners inform their medical practitioner of MRSA isolation from their pet, so that the medical practitioner can determine any risk to humans in light of their patient's medical history.

In contrast, MRSP is well adapted to dogs (like its *mecA*-negative counterpart), but rare human infections occur when opportunity arises. MRSP is expected to be easily transmitted amongst dogs through direct and indirect contact and, combined with its treatment-related risk factors, needs to be considered as a veterinary nosocomial pathogen. MRSP prevalence varies substantially between countries (reported from <5% to >50% of *S. pseudintermedius* laboratory submissions). It is important for veterinary practitioners to be familiar with their local and regional resistance patterns to inform an appropriate level of suspicion.

A third coagulase-positive staphylococcal pathogen, *S. schleiferi* (MRSS, seen as a coagulase-positive and a coagulase-negative variant, both involved in clinical disease), has also received attention for its not infrequent meticillin resistance in some countries.

Treatment of MDRS infection

All cases of surface and superficial pyoderma should be treated with topical antibacterial therapy alone, and all efforts should be made to avoid systemic therapy even if *in vitro* testing indicates that some antimicrobials may still work. With superficial pyoderma frequently recurrent due to chronic underlying conditions, and due to the often persistent nature of MRSP at carriage sites and in the environment, future isolates are likely to be even more drug-resistant. Owners need to understand that good compliance is paramount and that, at least for surface and superficial infections, multiple drug resistance can still be overcome by topical therapy.

For deep MDRS infections, treatment decisions must still follow the prioritization recommended in the tier system (see Figure 22.4) and general prescribing rules (narrow spectrum, accurate dosing, monitoring and good follow-up). Since numerous MDRS isolates may be involved concurrently, and as susceptibility patterns can change over time, only recent test results should be used to inform treatment choices. Repeated testing may be indicated if progress during therapy becomes slow. Laboratory reports will require careful interpretation, largely as animal-specific laboratory standards and breakpoints are still being developed. At present, the following recommendations apply:

- No representatives of beta-lactam antibiotics should be used for MRSP infections, even if *in vitro* testing indicates susceptibility for individual agents of this class
- Testing for inducible resistance to clindamycin is recommended for MDRS to avoid treatment failure during therapy
- Extrapolation of results from one type of tetracycline to another may be unreliable as resistance is mediated by a number of different genes
- Resistance to one fluoroquinolone is likely to indicate resistance to others in MRSP; MIC determination may then help to inform treatment decisions.

Most canine and feline MRSA infections involve the globally successful human hospital-associated lineage EMRSA-15, which often shows susceptibility to several first-tier drugs. Tetracyclines, trimethoprim-potentiated sulphonamides and clindamycin (50% of MRSA susceptible) should be effective clinically if *in vitro* susceptibility is predicted. Treatment of MRSA infections in pets is therefore rarely problematic and the outcome depends on primary and concurrent diseases.

With MRSP and MRSS isolates, an alarmingly broader resistance profile is often identified. If individual susceptibilities for authorized drugs are reported (occasionally to a tetracycline or a fluoroquinolone), their use is preferable due to their tested safety profile. If no authorized antimicrobial is reported with predicted susceptibility, the laboratory can be asked to undertake extended susceptibility testing, provided the isolate is still available. The use of amikacin, rifampicin or chloramphenicol (see 'Systemic antibacterial therapy' above) is most frequently described for deep MRSP infections (Frank and Loeffler, 2012; Papich, 2012). Due to additional toxicity concerns, prescriptions need to be preceded by appropriate dose calculations, monitoring of adverse health events, and detailed owner education about associated risks and the need for compliance, including advice on infection control measures to limit spread (Morris *et al*., 2017). More detailed information specifically on the treatment of MDRS infections and appropriate hygiene recommendations is freely accessible in the Clinical Consensus Guidelines on MDRS infections (Morris *et al*., 2017).

Practice hygiene and follow-up

After resolution of MDRS infection, most animals continue to carry MDRS on the skin and mucosae (swabs from mucosal and skin sites should be submitted for MDRS enrichment culture). MDRS carriage can resolve naturally if animals are kept in a clean environment and provided further selection pressure from antimicrobial therapy can be avoided. However, in some animals, carriage can persist for over 1 year. While carrying MDRS (and during active infection), animals have the potential to spread the bacteria to other animals and humans and will continue to contaminate their environment. Although no specific evidence-based recommendations are available at present, implementation of infection control measures until at least one carriage site sample is MRSP-negative seems sensible.

Identification and correction of primary triggers

Although the diagnosis of underlying triggers may not seem a priority for owners compared with the urgency of resolving pyoderma lesions, identification of primary disease is an integral part of successful pyoderma management (see Chapter 21). As a minimum, every time antibacterial therapy is prescribed, diagnostic and preventative efforts should include the following to investigate or prevent the most commonly suspected and easily manageable underlying triggers and avoid inappropriate antibiosis:

- A thorough history and physical examination, at first presentation and at re-examination when pyoderma lesions have resolved, can reveal skin lesions and other clinical signs that provide further diagnostic clues as to the primary causative disease and guide subsequent tests
- In-house tests to rule out ectoparasitic diseases (curable) that might resemble or occur at the same time as pyoderma; in particular, hair plucks and skin scrapes for demodicosis (see Chapter 3) should be undertaken each time a deep pyoderma is diagnosed. It should be noted that follicular damage in demodicosis is a well recognized cause of deep pyoderma and requires acaricidal treatment
- Comprehensive ectoparasite prophylaxis should be in place whenever pyoderma is diagnosed
- The most problematic cases at re-examination, in the authors' opinion, are those dogs that in the absence of pyoderma (i.e. when the infection has been resolved)

present either with no clinical signs suggestive of underlying triggers or with signs compatible with very mild allergic skin disease. In these cases, provided the history and signalment are in line with allergic skin disease (and ectoparasite control is in place), trial anti-inflammatory medication (low dose prednisolone on alternate days or ciclosporin) may help to prevent pyoderma flares. If successful, this approach can subsequently be optimized (Olivry *et al*., 2015)
- Endocrine, neoplastic and immune-mediated underlying causes (see Chapter 21) should be investigated, depending on the presence of other clinical signs recorded during the initial physical examination.

A small number of skin infections may present as 'one off' episodes and therefore do not require further diagnostic efforts. However, true idiopathic aetiologies are questionable. Most skin infections involve opportunistic normal skin commensals (staphylococci) and for infection to occur, an imbalance between microbes and the host's skin defences (physical, chemical, immunological) is to be expected, even if it cannot always be diagnosed.

Recurrent pyoderma

Pyoderma, especially canine superficial pyoderma, often recurs after successful treatment unless underlying primary causes have self-resolved or are identified and corrected. Recurrences can be seen within a few weeks or months after initial resolution, often lead to repeated antimicrobial prescribing and can be extremely frustrating for all involved (pet, veterinary staff and owner).

It is important to differentiate recurrence, where clinical signs truly resolve with treatment and then reappear, from resistance (and from non-infectious skin diseases resembling pyoderma, see Chapter 13). Recurrent pyoderma can be confirmed based on historical information and cytology, whilst bacterial culture and susceptibility testing (or skin biopsy for other differential diagnoses) are required if resistance is suspected. Unfortunately, primary causes cannot always be diagnosed using available diagnostic tests. Management of dogs with recurrent pyoderma should include efforts to:

- **Resolve presenting pyoderma flare** – especially in cases presenting within a few weeks, it is critical to shift from systemic therapy to topical therapy wherever possible. There is good evidence for repeated systemic antibacterial therapy being the main risk factor for the acquisition of multiple drug resistant staphylococci. At a time of increasing MRSP levels in most countries, such a treatment plan needs to be considered as high risk. If systemic therapy is deemed necessary due to severity or practicalities, drugs should be prescribed only after cytological confirmation of infection, based on culture and susceptibility testing and taking into consideration the general rules for good antimicrobial stewardship (narrow spectrum, accurate dosing)
- **Prevent relapse** – staphylococcal bacterins aid the management of recurrent pyoderma. They are thought to stimulate innate immunity, although their mechanism of action is not fully understood. Bacterins are available either as *S. aureus* lysate (Delmont Laboratories) or as autogenous *S. pseudintermedius* preparations (prepared by some laboratories on demand from the dog's own infecting bacterial isolate). Bacterins need to

be injected subcutaneously, twice weekly initially, then weekly or fortnightly long term. Efficacy has been reported in up to 40% of dogs with superficial pyoderma in controlled studies, albeit involving small numbers of animals. However, due to their consistently excellent safety record and in the absence of other alternatives, bacterins warrant consideration and further assessment (Glos and Mueller, 2011; Wilson *et al.*, 2019)

- **Continue search for primary triggers** – investigations into causative diseases, e.g. repeated endocrine testing every 3–6 months, is preferable to repeat prescribing and the associated risk of MRSP acquisition. Comprehensive flea prophylaxis should remain in place. It should be noted that some cases of atopic dermatitis manifest with recurrent superficial pyoderma (particularly in large-breed, short-coated dogs) and consideration should be given to diet trials and specific allergen testing for environmental hypersensitivities with a view to long-term allergen-specific immunotherapy
- **Manage owner expectations** – it should be explained to the owner that relapses occur secondary to elusive primary triggers and a plan outlined for proposed management. Although extended or repeated testing may occasionally reveal a primary aetiology and lead to a cure, lifelong management may be required in some cases. The risks and often hidden costs of repeated antibiotic prescribing need to be weighed against repeat diagnostic testing and the continuous efforts of topical therapy.

Pyoderma in cats

Although superficial bacterial pyoderma (folliculitis) is likely underdiagnosed in cats (estimated prevalence of 4–20% in cats with skin lesions), it remains uncertain (and controversial) whether antibacterial treatment is required to achieve clinical improvement in all cases. A small number of feline pyoderma cases have been described where antibacterial treatment alone (systemic, topical, or in combination) led to a reduction in lesion size or number and associated pruritus. In contrast, most older efficacy studies on anti-inflammatory treatment did not exclude secondary bacterial complications specifically, suggesting that anti-inflammatory treatment alone can also lead to normalization of bacterial numbers and resolution of infection in some treated allergic cats.

There is little published information on the treatment of feline pyoderma and prescribing decisions are probably too often governed primarily by safety and practical concerns, such as true or perceived difficulties of drug administration. For surface and superficial lesions where bacterial infection is suspected (e.g. crusted papules (milia) or eosinophilic plaques), infection should be confirmed by cytological examination before treatment is started.

Opportunities for topical therapy in cats may be limited by temperament, grooming behaviour and the lack of products authorized for use in this species. Shampoo treatment is rarely tolerated, but for localized lesions (e.g. chin acne, infected eosinophilic plaques) antibiotic creams or suspensions with or without prednisolone may be suitable if an Elizabethan collar can be fitted for a few minutes after application to prevent immediate removal by the cat.

If systemic therapy is indicated, antimicrobials categorized as first-tier choices, such amoxicillin/clavulanic acid (15–25 mg/kg orally q12h), cefalexin (20–30 mg/kg orally q12h) or clindamycin (11 mg/kg orally q24h), may be chosen empirically. As for dogs, second-tier drugs need to be reserved for those infections where susceptibility testing has indicated resistance to first-tier drugs.

Of note in cats with pyoderma:

- MDRS infections, particularly MRSA, are recognized in cats and a lack of improvement in clinical signs after 3–4 days should always prompt sampling for bacterial culture and antimicrobial susceptibility testing
- The availability of a long-acting injectable formulation of cefovecin, which is licensed for cats, must not lead to inappropriate use for skin infections due to convenience. Cefovecin may be confused with the first-line drugs cefalexin or cefadroxil (both first-generation cephalosporins) but, as a third-generation cephalosporin, cefovecin has a substantially broader spectrum that includes Gram-negative pathogens. Thus, it resembles the fluoroquinolones in indications and should be reserved for infections where laboratory testing has shown involvement of such pathogens.

Key points

- In cases of recurrent pyoderma, the focus should be on managing the underlying primary disease to prevent future infections
- Topical antimicrobial therapy is indicated in every case of pyoderma. In the majority of cases with superficial disease, resolution can be achieved with good topical therapy alone
- When systemic agents are prescribed, they should be done so in the context of recommended tier system and, in many cases, based on culture and sensitivity testing

---

References and further reading

Banovic F, Olivry T, Baumer W *et al.* (2018) Diluted sodium hypochlorite (bleach) in dogs: antiseptic efficacy, local tolerability and *in vitro* effect on skin barrier function and inflammation. *Veterinary Dermatology* **29**, 6–e6

Beco L, Guaguère E, Lorente Méndez C *et al.* (2013b) Suggested guidelines for using systemic antimicrobials in bacterial skin infections: part 2 – antimicrobial choice, treatment regimens and compliance. *Veterinary Record* **172**, 156–160

Borio S, Colombo S, La Rosa G *et al.* (2015) Effectiveness of a combined (4% chlorhexidine digluconate shampoo and solution) protocol in MRS and non-MRS canine superficial pyoderma: a randomized, blinded, antibiotic-controlled study. *Veterinary Dermatology* **26**, 339–344

Cobb MA, Edwards HJ, Jagger TD *et al.* (2005) Topical fusidic acid/betamethasone-containing gel compared to systemic therapy in the treatment of canine acute moist dermatitis. *The Veterinary Journal* **169**, 276–280

Fadok VA and Irwin K (2019) Sodium hypochlorite/salicylic acid shampoo for treatment of canine staphylococcal pyoderma. *Journal of the American Animal Hospital Association* **55**, 117–123

Frank LA and Loeffler A (2012) Meticillin-resistant *Staphylococcus pseudintermedius*: clinical challenge and treatment options. *Veterinary Dermatology* **23**, 283–291

Glos K and Mueller RS (2011) Treatment of chronic recurrent idiopathic pyoderma in the dog with vaccines containing bacterial antigens. *Tierärztliche Praxis Ausgabe Kleintiere und Heimtiere* **39**, 425–428.

Hillier A, Lloyd DH, Weese JS *et al.* (2014) Guidelines for the diagnosis and antimicrobial therapy of canine superficial bacterial folliculitis (Antimicrobial Guidelines Working Group of the International Society for Companion Animal Infectious Diseases). *Veterinary Dermatology* **25**, 163–e43

Morris DO, Loeffler A, Davis MF *et al.* (2017) Recommendations for approaches to meticillin-resistant staphylococcal infections of small animals: diagnosis, therapeutic considerations and preventative measures. Clinical Consensus Guidelines of the World Association for Veterinary Dermatology. *Veterinary Dermatology* **28**, 304–e69

Mueller RS, Bensignor E, Ferrer L *et al.* (2011) Treatment of demodicosis in dogs: 2011 clinical practice guidelines. *Veterinary Dermatology* **23**, 86–96

Olivry T, DeBoer DJ, Favrot C *et al.* (2015) Treatment of canine atopic dermatitis: 2015 updated guidelines from the International Committee on Allergic Diseases of Animals (ICADA). *BMC Veterinary Research* **11**, 210

Papich MG (2012) Selection of antibiotics for meticillin-resistant *Staphylococcus pseudintermedius*: time to revisit some old drugs? *Veterinary Dermatology* **23**, 352–360

Plumb DC (2015) *Plumb's Veterinary Drug Handbook, 8th edn*, eds. Davidson G, Powell L. Wiley-Blackwell, New Jersey

Summers JF, Brodbelt DC, Forsythe PJ *et al.* (2012) The effectiveness of systemic antimicrobial treatment in canine superficial and deep pyoderma: a systematic review. *Veterinary Dermatology* **23**, 305–329

Wilson A, Allers N, Lloyd DH *et al.* (2019) Reduced antimicrobial prescribing during autogenous staphylococcal bacterin therapy: a retrospective study in dogs with pyoderma. *Veterinary Record* **184**, 739

Young R, Buckley L, McEwan N and Nuttall T (2012) Comparative *in vitro* efficacy of antimicrobial shampoos: a pilot study. *Veterinary Dermatology* **23**, 36–40

Useful websites

BSAVA (British Small Animal Veterinary Association) PROTECT ME poster, 2018:
www.bsavalibrary.com/content/chapter/10.22233/9781910443644.chap6_1

IRIS Preventing Aminoglycoside-induced AKI:
www.iris-kidney.com/education/prevention.html

FECAVA (Federation of European Companion Animal Veterinary Associations) Advice on responsible use of antimicrobials:
www.fecava.org/wp-content/uploads/2020/01/FECAVA-Advice-on-Responsible-use-of-Antimicrobials-ENGLISH.pdf

WHO Critically Important Antimicrobials for Human Medicine, 6th revision, 2018:
www.who.int/publications/i/item/9789241515528

Worms and Germs blog, University of Guelph, including information on contagious disease and infection control tips, with useful advice for owners on MRSA and MRSP:
www.wormsandgermsblog.com/articles/diseases/mrsamrsp/

Chapter 23

An approach to feline-specific conditions

Mandy Burrows

Alopecia

Alopecia is common in cats and may be self-induced or result from spontaneous hair loss. Self-induced alopecia is caused by excessive licking and, less commonly, by chewing, pulling or plucking hair, or scratching due to pruritus, pain or behavioural disorders (Figure 23.1). Spontaneous alopecia occurs either as a result of inflammation or infection, targeting the hair follicle and/or the hair shaft, or because the hair follicle is dysplastic or atrophic, thus not able to produce a normal hair shaft (Figure 23.2). Unlike dogs, this is an unusual occurrence in cats.

The diagnostic approach to alopecia in a cat must initially differentiate spontaneous from self-induced alopecia. This can be achieved by collecting a detailed history, careful clinical examination and by performing a microscopic examination of the hair. Some owners find it difficult to distinguish excessive licking from normal grooming behaviour and do not always interpret over-grooming as a sign of pruritus, pain or stress. The diagnostic investigation of self-induced traumatic alopecia differs from that for spontaneous alopecia, and thus it is important that the clinician makes this distinction early in the diagnostic process.

Cause	Aetiological agent/disease
Ectoparasites	• *Notoedres cati* • Cheyletiellosis • Demodicosis (*Demodex gatoi*) • *Otodectes cynotis* • *Sarcoptes scabiei* • *Lynxacarus radovskii*
Allergic	• Flea bite hypersensitivity • Food-responsive dermatosis (also known as food allergy or adverse food reaction) • Feline atopic skin syndrome
Infectious	• Superficial bacterial pyoderma • Dermatophytes • *Malassezia* dermatitis
Neoplasia	• Epitheliotrophic lymphoma • Feline lymphocytosis
Immune-mediated	• Pemphigus foliaceus • Cutaneous drug eruptions (carbimazole)
Behavioural	• Psychogenic alopecia
Neurological/pain	• Feline hyperaesthesia syndrome • Feline idiopathic cystitis

23.1 Causes of self-induced alopecia in the cat.

Cause	Aetiological agent/disease
Infectious	• Superficial bacterial pyoderma • Dermatophytes • Demodicosis (*Demodex gatoi*)
Immune-mediated (rare)	• Pseudopelade • Lymphocytic mural folliculitis • Alopecia areata
Dysplasia/atrophy	• Topical glucocorticoid administration • Topical/systemic adverse drug reaction • Telogen effluvium
Endocrine	• Spontaneous/iatrogenic hyperadrenocorticism
Neoplasia	• Paraneoplastic alopecia
Genetic	• Congenital hypotrichosis • Pili torti

23.2 Causes of spontaneous alopecia in the cat.

Self-induced alopecia

Self-induced alopecia is commonly caused by excessive licking. Licking in cats is a major component of grooming. Grooming is a normal feline behaviour, but can be exhibited by cats as a manifestation of displacement associated with stress and emotional conflict. Under these circumstances, grooming can increase in frequency and intensity and become a compulsive behaviour.

After microscopic examination of hair shafts has confirmed self-induced alopecia (the presence of fractured hair shafts), the clinician should evaluate the history to consider a medical problem. If the alopecia affects the ventral inguinal region only, urinalysis and bacterial culture, sensitivity testing and abdominal ultrasonography should be performed to investigate feline idiopathic cystitis, urolithiasis and/or lower urinary tract disease. If the alopecia is focal and located on a single limb, then radiographic evaluation may be indicated, particularly if there is a history of previous trauma. Self-induced alopecia in an old cat may be caused by hyperthyroidism, and haematology, biochemistry and endocrine testing should be performed.

Clinical approach

History and signalment: In very young cats, ectoparasites and dermatophytosis are common, especially with stray or adopted kittens. In adult cats, allergic and immune-mediated skin diseases are common, whilst in older cats, hyperthyroidism may be a cause of overgrooming. Older

BSAVA Manual of Canine and Feline Dermatology, fourth edition. Edited by Hilary Jackson and Rosanna Marsella. ©BSAVA 2021

cats can also present with pruritus due to *Malassezia* overgrowth as a cutaneous marker of an underlying systemic disease or paraneoplastic syndrome. The severity of the pruritus should be noted, as some skin diseases are characterized by severe pruritus (e.g. notoedric mange) compared with others where pruritus is very mild (e.g. cheyletiellosis, dermatophytosis). Allergic skin disease in cats is a diagnosis of elimination. It should be noted that cats with feline atopic skin syndrome (FASS) or a cutaneous food-responsive dermatosis can present with one or more reaction patterns (see below). Importantly, clinical presentations of allergic skin disease are not specific for a particular trigger, thus no diagnosis of an underlying trigger can be made based on the clinical signs. Clinicians need to rely on the history and rule out other pruritic causes before making a diagnosis of allergic skin disease. Extracutaneous clinical signs may be present, such as sneezing, conjunctivitis or asthma and, in the case of food-responsive dermatoses, vomiting and/or diarrhoea.

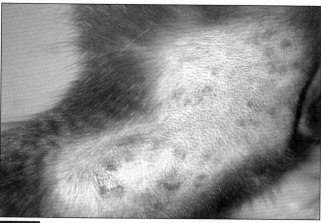

23.4 Miliary dermatitis (note that the region has been clipped).

Feline reaction patterns

Reaction patterns seen in pruritic cats include:

- Self-induced alopecia
- Eosinophilic diseases
- Head and neck pruritus
- Miliary dermatitis

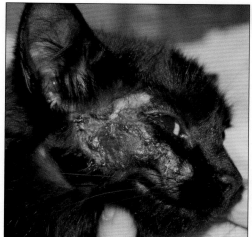

23.5 Head and neck pruritus.

Physical examination: Self-induced, non-inflammatory alopecia caused by overgrooming may be associated with very short, broken hair shafts and an absence of skin lesions. The alopecic regions are usually well demarcated (Figure 23.3). With broken hairs, the residual hair can be palpated or seen with a magnifying lens as it leaves the follicular ostia. Hair cannot be easily epilated. Alopecia can also accompany inflammatory pruritic reaction patterns. The clinical examination may reveal small, erythematous, crusted, non-follicular papules with variable alopecia in cats with miliary dermatitis (Figure 23.4). Erosive and crusting facial dermatitis presents with alopecia, crusting, excoriations, erosions and ulceration affecting the head and neck region, resulting from marked pruritus and self-trauma (Figure 23.5).

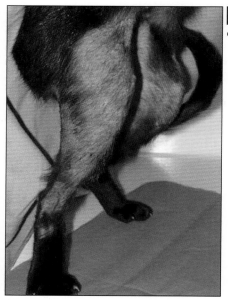

23.3 Alopecia in an overgrooming cat.

Microscopic hair examination: A microscopic examination of plucked hair shafts is the initial investigation indicated for any case of alopecia in the cat. The hair tips should be examined to determine whether the hair loss is a result of traumatic or spontaneous epilation. With traumatic hair loss, the hairs are fractured and the usual slender tapering tips are absent. After the microscopic examination of the hair shafts has confirmed self-induced alopecia, the clinician should construct a list of differential diagnoses and their order of priority, and then diagnostic tests should be performed to rule out or confirm these diagnoses.

Diagnostic tests: From a clinical point of view, pruritus in cats is usually caused by ectoparasites, allergies, infections or immune-mediated diseases, which can be exacerbated by concurrent factors, such as stress, boredom, dry skin or high environmental temperature (see Figure 23.1). The approach to the diagnosis of pruritus is best achieved using a logical step-by-step approach.

Step 1 – Coat combing, superficial and deep skin scraping, acetate tape testing and microscopic examination of ear cerumen: The clinician should begin with simple tests to diagnose or rule out ectoparasites. Coat combing, multiple superficial and deep skin scrapings and acetate tape testing should be performed to evaluate for ectoparasites (fleas, *Demodex*, *Cheyletiella*, *Otodectes*, *Notoedres*, *Sarcoptes* and *Lynxacarus* species). If pruritus is mainly affecting the ears and head, a microscopic examination of ear cerumen should be performed to evaluate for *Otodectes cynotis* and *Demodex cati* mites. *Notoedres* mites are usually easy to detect on skin scrapings but *Demodex*, *Cheyletiella*, *Otodectes* and *Sarcoptes* mites can be more challenging to locate in cats. If no mites are detected but there is a high index of clinical suspicion for an ectoparasite, then an acaricidal trial should be implemented using a broad-spectrum isoxazoline acaricide (e.g. fluralaner) to rule out the diagnosis.

Step 2 – Wood's lamp examination and fungal culture: The second step is to rule out or diagnose dermatophytosis. A microscopic examination may reveal fungal arthrospores surrounding and invading fragments of the hair shafts. A Wood's lamp examination should be performed. When present, fluorescent hairs should be plucked for fungal culture. If the Wood's lamp examination is negative, then a hair sample should be obtained using a soft bristle toothbrush and submitted for fungal culture and polymerase chain reaction (PCR) analysis.

Step 3 – Cytology: This is a cheap, simple and rapid method for evaluating bacterial and yeast overgrowth on the skin or in the ears, which complicates the primary disease and increases the severity of pruritus. These infections are often overlooked by clinicians in the diagnostic evaluation of pruritic cats, and their importance is underestimated. Samples may be collected by impression smear, using a cotton swab or a piece of acetate tape, to evaluate for *Malassezia* yeast, bacteria and inflammatory cells.

Step 4 – Therapeutic trial to rule out fleas: The first step in determining the primary cause of the pruritus is a therapeutic trial for flea control, which may have not been identified during the initial investigations for ectoparasites. It is important to identify the type of ectoparasite control the owner uses, which exact product is administered, how often and to which of the animals in the household. A diagnosis of flea infestation or flea bite hypersensitivity can be confirmed by observing a resolution of clinical signs with complete flea eradication. The time taken for clinical improvement depends on the severity and chronicity of the disease; the degree of hypersensitivity and the magnitude of the flea challenge are usually evaluated within 6–8 weeks of initiation of treatment. The veterinary surgeon (veterinarian) should select a single or combination of oral insecticides, which rapidly reduce flea feeding times (e.g. spinosad, nitenpyram) to reduce allergen exposure. Topical endectocides (e.g. indoxacarb or an isoxazoline) can be used when the administration of oral medication is prohibited. With large numbers of immature stages in a warm and humid environment, spraying the house or apartment with an insect growth regulator, such as *S*-methoprene or pyriproxyfen, will hasten clinical improvement in affected cats.

Step 5 – Elimination diet: If the therapeutic trial for fleas is unrewarding, the second step is to perform an elimination diet with a home-cooked or extensively hydrolysed diet for the diagnosis of a food-responsive dermatosis. Cats are obligate carnivores, so when choosing a home-cooked diet, they can be fed pure protein. A carbohydrate source is not essential for cats and may decrease palatability and compliance. The diet should be fed exclusively for approximately 8 weeks and more than 90% of cats with food-responsive dermatosis will improve over this time.

After documenting a marked improvement or resolution of clinical signs, confirming a diagnosis of food-responsive dermatosis requires demonstrating a clinical flare after feeding the original diet (provocative challenge) for up to 7 days, followed by subsequent resolution of clinical signs with further feeding of the elimination diet. It is optimal, in cases where provocation does cause a relapse of clinical signs, that a sequential re-challenge with individual proteins is implemented to identify the offending protein(s). Each protein should be fed for approximately 7 days. If the offending allergen(s) can be identified, then the cat can be fed a commercial hydrolysed or selected protein diet.

Some owners are reluctant to perform a sequential re-challenge and the causative protein cannot be identified. If the elimination diet is used as a long-term maintenance diet, it is recommended that a veterinary nutritionist is consulted in order to balance the diet and avoid nutritional deficiencies.

Step 6 – Investigation for feline atopic skin syndrome: The diagnosis of FASS is based on the exclusion of other pruritic diseases, such as ectoparasites, dermatophytosis and bacterial infections, as well as evaluation of the role of flea and food allergens as flare factors, compatible clinical signs and a positive response to appropriate therapy.

Allergy testing can be performed to select the allergens for an immunotherapy regime and to implement allergen avoidance measures. Two methods of allergy testing are available for the investigation of FASS:

- Intradermal allergy test (IDT)
- *In vitro* allergen-specific immunoglobulin (Ig)E serology testing (ASIS).

IDT demonstrates the presence of hypersensitivity based on skin reactivity to various environmental allergens (mites (house dust mites and storage mites); insects (cockroaches, moths, ants and houseflies); pollens (trees, weeds and grasses) and moulds). Intradermal testing is usually performed by veterinary dermatologists or clinicians with a specific interest in dermatology. Clinically relevant reactions can then be used to select allergens for specific immunotherapy (see Chapter 11 for more information).

A number of ASIS tests are now commercially available and easy to use in practice. However, the value of these diagnostic tests is controversial and all the studies to date have failed to demonstrate their reliability in discriminating cats affected with FASS from either healthy cats or cats affected with other pruritic skin disorders.

If an owner elects not to pursue an investigation of allergic skin disease, then the most appropriate course of action is to commence with medical therapy to control the clinical signs.

Step 7 – Psychogenic factors: Self-induced alopecia resulting from an underlying behavioural cause is referred to as psychogenic alopecia in cats. The regions typically affected include the thorax, groin, ventrum, medial or caudal thighs, flanks and front limbs. The repetitive behaviour can cause focal or diffuse depilation, excoriations, crusts and non-healing ulcers with symmetrical or asymmetrical lesions and peripheral lymphadenopathy due to inflammation and/or secondary infection. The diagnosis is one of exclusion and primary pruritic skin diseases and conditions causing pain (orthopaedic disease, low urinary tract disease, abdominal pain) and neurological disease (hyperaesthesia) should be ruled out. Consulting a veterinary behaviourist may be helpful in such cases.

Spontaneous alopecia

Spontaneous alopecia is typically due to infection or inflammation affecting the hair follicle or hair shaft, or due to the inability to produce a normal hair shaft (see Figure 23.2). However, spontaneous alopecia can also be caused by factors that interfere with the hair follicle cycle, such as hormonal imbalances (e.g. hypercortisolism), stress or systemic disease (e.g. telogen effluvium). All these factors can induce arrest of hair growth and loss of hair.

Clinical approach

Spontaneous alopecia may be partial or complete, and hair can be easily epilated from the periphery of the alopecic region with traction. The skin appears glabrous and smooth. A few short fragments of hair can be seen emerging from the follicular ostia in cases of spontaneous alopecia due to inflammatory causes such as dermatophytosis.

History and signalment: Infectious and ectoparasitic diseases, such as dermatophytosis, are commonly observed in kittens or in animals housed in crowded environmental conditions, such as breeding colonies or pet shops. Paraneoplastic syndromes and neoplasia are typically seen in older cats. In an old cat presenting with alopecia and systemic signs, such as polyuria/polydipsia, polyphagia, vomiting or weight loss, the clinician should consider the possibility of alopecia being caused by a systemic disease. If the alopecic skin appears thin, with bruising and/or tears developing after minimal traction, the cat should be investigated for hyperadrenocorticism. The history may suggest iatrogenic hyperadrenocorticism, if glucocorticoids have been administered for a long time, or spontaneous hyperadrenocorticism, if there is no history of glucocorticoid administration or the cat is diabetic. Ventrally distributed alopecia with shiny skin in a cat presenting with concurrent weight loss, depression, vomiting, and/or diarrhoea may point towards a diagnosis of paraneoplastic alopecia and should prompt to perform an abdominal ultrasound examination.

Diagnostic tests: As with self-induced alopecia, the diagnosis of spontaneous alopecia is best achieved using a logical step-by step approach.

Step 1 – Skin scrapings: Skin scrapings are indicated for the investigation of demodicosis.

Step 2 – Microscopic examination of hair, Wood's lamp examination and fungal culture: The microscopic examination of hair may reveal arthrospores and fungal hyphae and be strongly suggestive of dermatophytosis. A Wood's lamp examination, fungal culture and PCR of affected hair are used to confirm or rule out a diagnosis of dermatophytosis (see Chapter 25 for more information). Since dermatophytosis is the most common cause of alopecia in cats, a fungal culture is appropriate in all cases presenting in this manner.

Step 3 – Skin biopsy: Some rare diseases presenting with spontaneous alopecia can only be diagnosed with histopathology (e.g. pseudopelade, sebaceous adenitis, congenital hypotrichosis and adverse drug reactions), thus skin biopsy samples should be collected and submitted for examination.

Step 4 – Complete blood count and serum biochemistry: These may be of value as screening tests for cats with an underlying systemic disease. Specific hormonal evaluation for hyperadrenocorticism may be indicated.

Feline eosinophilic dermatitis

Feline eosinophilic dermatitis presents as a number of distinct clinical lesions: eosinophilic (indolent) ulcers, eosinophilic plaques and eosinophilic (collagenolytic/linear) granulomas. These represent a cutaneous reaction pattern incited by underlying allergic causes, most commonly hypersensitivity reactions to fleas, environmental and food allergens (Figure 23.6). In some cases, no external inciting stimuli can be identified and the feline eosinophilic lesions are described as idiopathic. A combined genetic and allergic aetiopathogenesis has also been suggested. Eosinophilic dermatitis is confirmed by cytology and/or biopsy.

Mechanism	Aetiological agent/disease
Allergic	• Flea bite hypersensitivity • Food-responsive dermatosis • Feline atopic skin syndrome

Infectious	• Bacterial
	• Viral
	  • Feline herpesvirus
	• Fungal
	  • Dermatophytes

Miscellaneous	• Foreign body
	  • Exogenous (insect)
	  • Endogenous (hair)
	• Genetic
	• Idiopathic

23.6 Underlying causes of feline eosinophilic dermatoses.

Clinical presentation and differential diagnoses

Eosinophilic ulcer/indolent ulcer

This is a well circumscribed, red–brown ulcer often covered with a yellow exudate, which usually occurs unilaterally or bilaterally on the upper lip at the mucosal margin at the philtrum or adjacent to the upper canine tooth (Figure 23.7). There can be marked swelling, but pain and pruritus are not usually observed. The differential diagnoses for eosinophilic ulcers include neoplasia (squamous cell carcinoma), deep fungal infection, especially cryptococcosis, and trauma.

Eosinophilic plaque

This is a well demarcated, flat-topped, erythematous plaque with a moist surface, which is usually alopecic, eroded to ulcerated and highly pruritic (Figure 23.8). Lesions are most common on the ventral abdomen, thorax and medial aspect of the hind limbs, but can occur anywhere on the body. Secondary bacterial infection and regional lymphadenopathy are common. The differential diagnoses include neoplasia (squamous cell carcinoma, lymphoma, mast cell tumour, metastatic mammary adenocarcinoma), dermatophytosis, cutaneous viral disease (herpesvirus, calicivirus or feline cowpox), mycobacterial infection and cryptococcosis.

Eosinophilic granuloma

These are well defined, firm, alopecic, yellow to pink, crusting papular to nodular lesions located anywhere on the body, including the chin (Figure 23.9), mid-lower

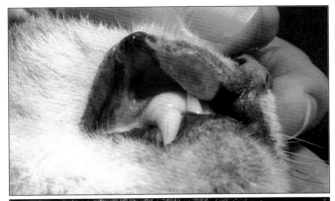

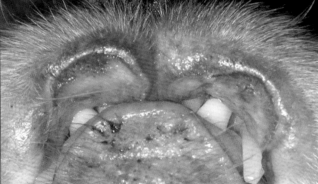

23.7 Eosinophilic/indolent ulcers.

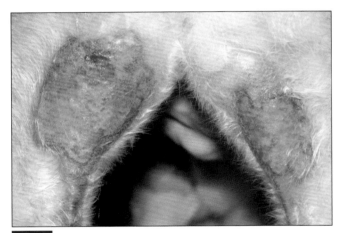

23.8 Eosinophilic plaques on the lips of a cat.

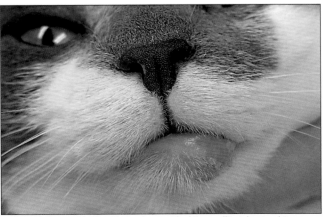

23.9 Domestic Shorthaired cat with chin swelling due to chin eosinophilic granuloma.

lip, tongue, hard palate, caudal hind limbs (linear) (Figure 23.10), and footpads. Alopecia and ulceration are common, with white to yellow stippling of the lesion corresponding to foci of eosinophilic degranulation seen in the centre of ulcerated lesions. Pedal lesions are frequently ulcerated and crusted, whereas mucosal lesions appear as irregular yellowish nodules, frequently located on the tongue and the palate (Figure 23.11). Oral lesions may cause drooling and dysphagia and are usually non-pruritic. There may be a local lymphadenopathy. The differential diagnoses include neoplasia (squamous cell carcinoma, lymphoma, mast cell tumour, metastatic mammary adenocarcinoma), dermatophytosis, cutaneous viral disease (herpesvirus, calicivirus or feline cowpox), mycobacterial infection, deep fungal infection and sterile granulomatous disease.

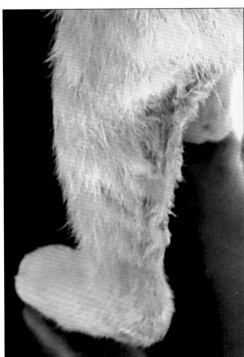

23.10 Domestic Shorthaired cat with a linear granuloma.

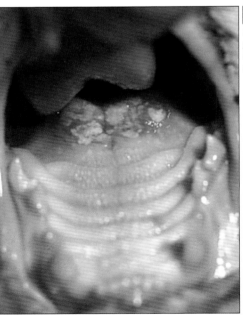

23.11 Eosinophilic granuloma in the oral cavity of a cat.

Clinical approach
History

A thorough general and dermatological history is essential to identify possible underlying allergic factors for feline eosinophilic dermatitis. Flea bite hypersensitivity is a common underlying trigger, and this differential diagnosis should always be evaluated before a more extensive diagnostic investigation is undertaken in cats with eosinophilic skin disease. Cats with flea bite hypersensitivity may present with eosinophilic lesions in the absence of other clinical evidence of pruritic skin disease.

Diagnostic tests

The initial diagnostic approach should clarify whether bacterial infection is playing a role. The next stage of the investigation should focus on confirming whether the lesion is an eosinophilic ulcer, eosinophilic plaque or eosinophilic granuloma. The presence of bacterial colonization can confuse the clinical picture, hence the initial approach.

Cytology: Cytological evaluation of direct or acetate tape impression smears from the lesional surface should be performed on all skin lesions to investigate the role of secondary bacterial infection. The back of a scalpel blade can be a used to obtain a sample from eosinophilic ulcers: the surface of the lesion should be gently scraped with the back of a blade to make an impression smear with the retrieved debris. The sample should be evaluated for the presence of inflammatory cells and intracellular and/ or extracellular bacteria (Figure 23.12). If intracellular or extracellular bacteria and degenerate neutrophils are observed, then bacterial colonization and/or infection is confirmed. Topical antimicrobials and occasionally systemic antibiotics are indicated. Bacterial culture and sensitivity testing are not recommended as a routine diagnostic investigation, unless antimicrobial resistance is suspected (history of multiple antimicrobial treatment interventions; failure of empirical antimicrobial therapy) or rod-shaped bacteria are detected.

Histology: Clinical signs and cytological evaluation of an impression smear from the lesional surface demonstrating large numbers of eosinophils are highly suggestive of eosinophilic dermatitis. A tissue biopsy sample collected using a 4–6 mm biopsy punch should be submitted for histological examination and bacterial and fungal culture from ulcers, plaques, nodules or tumours to rule out the non-allergic

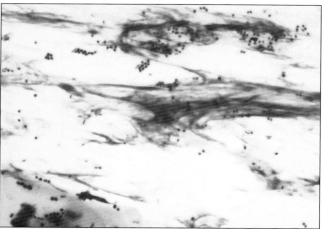

23.12 Cytological examination revealing coccoid bacteria. (Original magnification X1000)

differential diagnoses, particularly deep fungal infections, viral disease and neoplasia. The main histopathological features are varying degrees of epidermal hyperplasia and erosion or ulceration, and a prominent eosinophilic dermal infiltrate. Small foci, known as flame figures, in which collagen fibres are surrounded by degranulated eosinophils, are a common feature.

Elimination diet trial: Feline eosinophilic skin disease can be associated with a cutaneous food-responsive dermatosis. The diagnosis should be based on the exclusion of the other triggers, a positive response to an elimination diet trial and subsequent flare with a provocative food challenge. Elimination diet trials can be very challenging for owners to implement. The typical problems encountered include: cats refusing to eat the diet consistently due to lack of palatability; outdoor cats gaining access to alternative food sources; and gastrointestinal adverse effects (vomiting and/or diarrhoea) associated with a dietary transition. If there is no response to appropriate flea control measures and an elimination diet, then the cat should be evaluated for feline atopic skin syndrome. A clinical diagnosis should be made on the basis of a compatible history and by ruling out a food-responsive dermatosis and flea bite hypersensitivity dermatitis.

Feline mosquito bite hypersensitivity

Feline mosquito bite hypersensitivity is an uncommon, seasonal, pruritic dermatitis associated with a Type I hypersensitivity reaction to mosquito antigens. There is no age, sex or breed predilection. Short-haired, free-roaming, dark-coloured cats in geographical regions where mosquitoes are endemic are more commonly affected. The disease is seasonal, occurring in spring and summer and abating in winter.

Clinical presentation and other differential diagnoses

The typical clinical manifestations of mosquito bite hypersensitivity may include:

* Papules to small nodules with focal crusting on the haired convex surface of the pinnae
* Multifocal punctate ulcers to severely crusted lesions on the nasal bridge (Figure 23.13). The pinnae and interdigital skin may also be affected
* Erythema, ulceration and depigmentation of the nasal planum.

The peripheral margins of the footpads can also be affected with erythema, scaling and crusting. Regional submandibular lymph nodes may be enlarged. The degree of pruritus can be variable, ranging from mild to very intense.

The clinical features are sufficiently characteristic to make a diagnosis in typical cases. However, other important differential diagnoses that need to be taken into consideration include:

* Feline herpesvirus dermatitis
* Pemphigus foliaceus
* Photo-induced dermatitis (e.g. actinic dermatitis and squamous cell carcinoma).

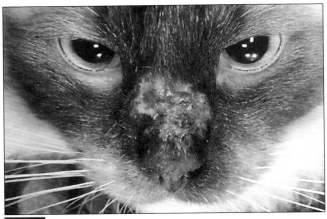

23.13 Mosquito bite hypersensitivity on the nasal bridge of a cat.

Herpesvirus dermatitis

Herpesvirus dermatitis can present with large crusts on the nasal bridge with erosions and ulceration affecting the face and nasal planum (Figure 23.14). Lesions can be painful and/or pruritic. Cats with feline herpesvirus dermatitis are sometimes misdiagnosed as having mosquito bite hypersensitivity or other eosinophilic feline skin diseases based on the clinical appearance and histopathology (see below). Exacerbation of lesions following corticosteroid or ciclosporin therapy due to this erroneous diagnosis may be an important diagnostic clue.

Squamous cell carcinoma

In cases of squamous cell carcinoma, erosive, crusted lesions on the tips of the pinnae and nasal planum may develop, particularly in white-haired cats (see Chapter 33).

Clinical approach
Diagnostic tests

Cytology: Cytological evaluation of impression smears from erosive lesions may demonstrate marked eosinophil infiltration with mild to moderate numbers of lymphocytes, macrophages, basophils and/or mast cells.

Histology: Histopathological findings include a marked eosinophilic infiltration into the dermis and hair follicle walls with flame figures (small to moderate sized foci of degenerated eosinophils) often with overlying crusting, erosion and ulceration. However, it can be difficult to

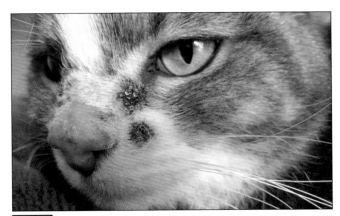

23.14 Facial dermatitis associated with herpesvirus infection.

differentiate these histological changes from those seen with herpesvirus dermatitis. Amphophilic, intranuclear viral inclusion bodies in the epithelium may be present with herpesvirus infection, but not in all cases.

Other tests: Tissue PCR identification of the herpesvirus genome has a high sensitivity and specificity. Immunohistochemistry (IHC) for feline herpesvirus antigen is also commercially available and may be preferable for formalin-fixed tissue samples. It should be appreciated, however, that many cats carry herpesvirus, and a positive reaction should be interpreted in conjunction with the history, clinical signs and histopathological findings. Both of these investigations are recommended to eliminate the potential diagnosis of herpesvirus dermatitis for cats with presumptive mosquito bite hypersensitivity that do not respond to routine anti-inflammatory treatment. Intradermal and serological testing may be supportive if mosquito antigen is available.

Feline nodular skin diseases
Feline sarcoid

Sarcoids are uncommon and most often seen in male cats with access to the outdoors. Affected animals present with one or more discrete nodules often on the face or limbs. The lesions are caused by non-replicating bovine papilloma virus in the dermis and are histologically similar to equine sarcoids.

Plasma cell pododermatitis

Whilst the exact pathogenesis of feline plasma cell pododermatitis is uncertain, an immune-mediated process is suspected. Affected individuals present with a violaceus swelling of one or more footpads. Ulceration can occur and pain is variable. Diagnosis relies on biopsy and histopathology demonstrating an accumulation of non-neoplastic plasma cells.

Key points
- Pruritus in the cat can have a variable clinical presentation, but the clinician should perform a logical work-up, which should rule out fleas as a causative agent
- Secondary bacterial and *Malassezia* skin infections are less common in the cat than the dog; however, cats should be evaluated for their contribution to the presenting skin disease
- Endocrine disease as a cause of alopecia in the cat is rare

References and further reading

Hobi S, Linek M, Marignac G et al. (2011) Clinical characteristics and causes of pruritus in cats: a multicentre study on feline hypersensitivity-associated dermatoses. Veterinary Dermatology 22, 406–413

Mason KV and Evans AG (1991) Mosquito bite-caused eosinophilic dermatitis in cats. Journal of the American Veterinary Medical Association 198, 2086–2088

Olivry T, Mueller RS and Prelaud P (2015) Critically appraised topic on adverse food reactions of companion animals (1): duration of elimination diets. BMC Veterinary Research 11, 225

Ravens PA, Xu BJ and Vogelnest LJ (2014) Feline atopic dermatitis: a retrospective study of 45 cases (2001–2012). Veterinary Dermatology 25, 95–102

Chapter 24

Management of feline-specific conditions

Alison Diesel

Cats develop unique dermatological conditions such as feline eosinophilic dermatitis and miliary dermatitis. These clinical syndromes can be caused by a variety of underlying diseases (see Chapter 23). The management of these conditions relies on the correct identification of the underlying disease. For example, the management of miliary dermatitis caused by flea allergy is different from that due to dermatophytosis. In cases of feline eosinophilic dermatitis (indolent ulcers, eosinophilic granulomas and eosinophilic plaques), it is accepted that the dermatological syndromes are often triggered by allergic stimuli. However, as no correlation exists between the type of allergy and the resulting clinical syndrome, it is important for clinicians to identify and correct the trigger. This is based on the patient's history (e.g. seasonality, use of flea products, environment) and a process of elimination. If parasites are suspected, they need to be treated and, if no seasonality is detected in the history, a food trial should be considered to rule out dietary triggers. This is necessary because the diagnosis of environmental allergies is one of exclusion and cannot be determined using a test.

Feline atopic skin syndrome

The diagnosis of feline atopic skin syndrome (FASS) is based on the exclusion of other causes of pruritic diseases, such as ectoparasites, dermatophytes and bacterial infections, as well as evaluation of the role of flea and food allergens as flare factors, compatible clinical signs and a positive response to appropriate therapy. As with atopic dermatitis in other species, there is no cure for FASS. Thus, the goal for management should be to decrease the severity and frequency of the pruritic flares, whilst minimizing the side effects of therapy. The initial approach should be to identify and manage any secondary diseases (e.g. parasites and skin infections), as these will compound the degree of pruritus present. In addition, other flare factors (such as food) should be recognized and addressed. It is common for patients to have multiple triggers and it is important to systematically identify and correct each one.

Various therapeutic options are available for managing FASS. The majority of cases require a multimodal approach, which should be tailored to the specific needs of the patient and the ability of the owner to administer treatment.

Medical management

Medical intervention to manage the clinical signs of FASS includes both conservative (essential fatty acid supplementation, antihistamines) and more aggressive (glucocorticoids, ciclosporin, oclacitinib) options. The decision regarding treatment should be weighed in light of the severity of the clinical disease, side effects and client/patient factors.

Essential fatty acids

Essential fatty acid (EFA) supplementation may lead to improvement in epidermal barrier function, decreased production of inflammatory molecules and/or improvements in hair coat quality. In addition, synergistic benefit may be noted with concurrent antihistamine administration. Side effects of EFA supplementation are minimal and limited to occasional gastrointestinal disturbance. Common EFAs include supplements derived from fish, evening primrose, sunflower and safflower oils. Formulations may be added to food (capsule, oil, spray) or applied topically. It should be noted that many diets for skin disease are fortified with these EFAs. Administration for 6–8 weeks is recommended to assess efficacy (see Chapter 31 for more information).

Antihistamines

Antihistamines show variable efficacy for managing FASS. Currently, there is not sufficient evidence to support the use of cetirizine for pruritus in cats. Anecdotally, these medications may be more effective in cats that also show non-cutaneous manifestations of disease, such as sneezing, conjunctivitis or asthma (Wildermuth et al., 2013). Several options may be considered for cats with FASS (Figure 24.1); it is recommended to trial an antihistamine for approximately 2–3 weeks to determine possible efficacy. Sequential administration of different antihistamines may be necessary to determine the best option for an individual cat; as with dogs and humans, there is no one 'best antihistamine' for allergic cats. As with EFAs, synergy may be observed when antihistamines are administered with other therapeutics (e.g. EFAs, glucocorticoids); improved efficacy and/or the ability to reduce of the dose of other medications may be observed.

Glucocorticoids

Glucocorticoids are still considered to be key for managing FASS, especially during an allergic flare. For cats with seasonal or intermittent clinical signs, steroids are often

Drug	Dosage	Notes on therapy
Amitriptyline	5–10 mg/cat orally q12–24h	
Clemastine	0.25–0.68 mg/cat orally q12h	Possible side effects: diarrhoea, lethargy and drug eruption
Chlorpheniramine	2–4 mg/cat orally q8–24h	May cause drowsiness. Noted to be unpalatable (bitter)
Cyproheptadine	2 mg/cat orally q12h	May cause gastrointestinal disturbances (increased appetite, vomiting), vocalization, sedation or behavioural changes (increased affection)
Diphenhydramine	2–4 mg/cat orally q12h 1–2 mg/kg orally q8–12h	Noted to be unpalatable; liquid form exists in alcohol base
Fexofenadine	30–60 mg/cat orally q24h 2 mg/kg orally q12–24h	
Hydroxyzine	5–10 mg/cat orally q8–12h	May cause behavioural changes (hyperexcitability, depression). Noted to be teratogenic

24.1 Antihistamines that can be used for the treatment of feline atopic skin syndrome (FASS).

the mainstay of maintenance therapy due to their rapid onset of action and effective control of allergic skin disease. Although cats typically show better tolerance of glucocorticoids compared with dogs, with fewer adverse reactions reported even with long-term administration, they are certainly not without side effects and may become less effective with regards to disease management over time (tachyphylaxis).

> ## Side effects of glucocorticoids in cats
> - Polyuria/polydipsia
> - Weight gain
> - Diabetes mellitus (particularly in obese cats)
> - Cutaneous atrophy, resulting in severe skin fragility
> - Congestive cardiac disease in cats with pre-existing heart problems

Steroids are available in topical, oral and injectable preparations.

- **Topical glucocorticoids** – while frequently used for managing focal flares of atopic dermatitis in dogs, this option is often not efficacious in cats due to their fastidious grooming behaviour and often general intolerance of topical products. However, the consideration of rapidly absorbed products may be beneficial for FASS. A 0.0584% hydrocortisone aceponate spray has demonstrated efficacy for managing feline allergic skin disease. While minimal to no systemic absorption is appreciated with this preparation (metabolized almost exclusively in the epidermis), cutaneous atrophy can develop with frequent and repeated application to the same location. Although the product is not currently licensed for use in cats, it appears to be efficacious and well-tolerated.

- **Oral glucocorticoids** – when systemic therapy is required, oral glucocorticoids should be chosen where possible to allow for tapering to the lowest effective dose to manage the clinical signs. Dosing recommendations for feline allergic skin disease are most frequently based on clinical experience and extrapolation from canine pharmacokinetic studies (Figure 24.2). One important difference, however, is the preference for use of prednisolone in cats compared with prednisone. The latter has decreased bioavailability in cats due to their reduced capacity to glucuronidize and thereby metabolize the pro-drug to its active form. It should also be noted that triamcinolone appears to be less potent in cats than dogs. Ideally, whichever steroid is chosen, the dose should be tapered over time to the minimum effective dose that maintains comfort whilst decreasing the risk of adverse effects, especially in cases that require long-term administration. While there is no single tapering regimen, dose reduction is typically started 7–10 days following initiation of therapy. The goal should be to administer the steroid at the lowest possible dose on alternate days (or even less frequently in the case of potent steroids such as dexamethasone; see Chapter 28 for further information).

- **Injectable glucocorticoids** – in cases where oral medication is not an option, injectable steroids can be used. However, care should be exercised in these cases as repeated injections (particularly of repository formulations) can heighten the risk of diabetes mellitus, heart failure and skin fragility syndrome. In cats where frequent and repeated steroid injections are warranted to manage FASS, alternative treatments with fewer side effects (e.g. ciclosporin, allergy-specific immunotherapy) should be considered.

Drug	Dosage
Prednisolone	1–2 mg/kg/day initially, tapered to 0.5–1 mg/kg q48h
Methylprednisolone	1–2 mg/kg/day initially, tapered to 0.5–1 mg/kg q48h
Triamcinolone	0.1–0.2 mg/kg/day initially, tapered to 0.1–0.2 mg/kg q48–72h
Dexamethasone	0.1–0.2 mg/kg q72h

24.2 Oral steroids that can be used for the treatment of feline allergic skin disease.

Ciclosporin

Ciclosporin in a good alternative to steroids for the medical management of FASS and has an overall enhanced safety profile. The microemulsion formulation of this calcineurin inhibitor (ciclosporin (modified)) is available as a liquid and is approved for the treatment of feline cutaneous allergy. This formulation has more predicable pharmacokinetics with good bioavailability in both dogs and cats than generic preparations. Ciclosporin has anti-inflammatory activity and a targeted effect on T lymphocytes. In addition, it stabilizes eosinophils and mast cells, thereby decreasing inflammatory cytokine production in the skin. It has relatively good tolerability in cats for long-term management of allergic skin disease. Common side effects include gastrointestinal upset (vomiting, diarrhoea, decreased appetite); these are often transient and typically noted during the initiation of therapy. Rarely, fatal toxoplasmosis has been reported in cats receiving ciclosporin therapy. Although clinical trials are lacking, there is also concern for an increased risk of contracting certain viral diseases (e.g. feline leukaemia virus (FeLV), feline immunodeficiency virus (FIV)) with the use of ciclosporin.

The recommended dose is 7 mg/kg/day; although efficacy has been shown with doses between 5 and 10 mg/kg/day in allergic cats. Ciclosporin has a delayed onset of action compared with steroids; patient improvement is typically noted from 2–3 weeks following the initiation of treatment and reaches a steady state from 4–6 weeks. At this time, dose reduction is frequently feasible; most cats with FASS can be managed at the same dose administered on alternate days (or less frequently) without a recurrence of clinical signs. It should be noted that the liquid formation is known to be somewhat unpalatable; the medication can be mixed with food without a decrease in efficacy. An injectable formulation for cats that do not tolerate oral ciclosporin has been explored. A small pilot study showed efficacy with administration of subcutaneous ciclosporin at initial doses of 2.5–5 mg/kg q24–48h (Koch et al., 2018). Larger clinical trials are needed to further evaluate this therapeutic option and track side effects long term.

Oclacitinib

Oclacitinib, a Janus kinase inhibitor, is licensed for the treatment of allergic skin disease in dogs. Whilst not licensed for cats, it has been shown to be somewhat effective and well tolerated for short-term use. Oclacitinib has not been well studied in cats and the ideal dose range and recommendations have yet to be established in this species. Cats metabolize the drug more rapidly than dogs, often necessitating a higher dose (1 mg/kg administered twice daily) initially with the intent to taper to the lowest effective dose. Anecdotally, it may be beneficial for some feline patients when alternative medical options have been deemed ineffective and/or are not well tolerated. Any feline patient prescribed this treatment should be monitored carefully (clinical signs, bloodwork and urinalysis), as the long-term side effects in cats are unknown.

Allergen-specific immunotherapy

Allergen-specific immunotherapy may be effective, either alone or combined with other medical treatment, for the management of cats with FASS or feline asthma. Much of what is understood with regards to allergen-specific immunotherapy for the allergic cat is extrapolated from canine studies and based on clinical preferences and anecdotal evidence with reference to efficacy. Although the exact mechanism of action is unknown, allergy immunotherapy works to retrain the immune response and decrease hyperreactivity to inciting environmental allergens. This retraining takes time to become clinically apparent; it can take approximately 3–6 months to start seeing improvements, whilst maximum efficacy may take about 12 months. This therapy is imperfect and does not work for all patients; various studies have shown efficacy of 50–70% of companion animal patients improving on immunotherapy. Anecdotally, cats may have a higher response rate compared with other species. Currently, allergen-specific immunotherapy is the safest option available for managing FASS. Side effects are minimal and often limited to injection site pruritus (see Chapter 11 for

further information on immunotherapy). For clients interested in this treatment option, referral to a veterinary dermatologist is recommended due to the intricacies of immunotherapy manipulation to achieve maximal benefit.

Feline eosinophilic dermatitis

It is important to remember that eosinophilic lesions (granulomas, plaques, indolent ulcers) are not pathognomonic for a specific dermatopathology. Rather, they are cutaneous reaction patterns with a myriad of aetiological agents that may lead to their manifestation (see Chapter 23). Some lesions (particularly plaques and indolent ulcers) may be associated with bacterial infection, which should be confirmed by cytology. Other lesions may be associated with an underlying allergic skin disease.

In cases associated with bacterial infection, antimicrobial therapy should be considered as the first line of treatment. The location of the lesion (e.g. in the case of indolent ulcers) and behaviour of the cat can prohibit topical treatment and thus systemic antibiotic therapy may be indicated (Figure 23.3). Superficial lesions (such as eosinophilic plaques) necessitate 3–4 weeks of appropriate antibiotic therapy, whereas deeper lesions (such as indolent ulcers and eosinophilic granulomas) require a minimum of 6–8 weeks of treatment. Cats should be reassessed after 3–4 weeks to check for improvement in the clinical signs and determine whether a longer course of therapy is required for full resolution of the lesions. If a lack of improvement is appreciated, bacterial culture and sensitivity testing is warranted.

If lesions persist following resolution of the bacterial infection (as seen on cytology), then investigation for an underlying allergy is prudent (see Chapter 33). As flea allergy is the most common allergic skin disease in cats, year-round use of adulticidal flea prevention is recommended. However, some eosinophilic lesions (particularly granulomas) may be refractory to the standard recommended therapy. Alternative options that may be considered when standard antipruritic therapy is deemed ineffective include:

- Chlorambucil (at a dose of 0.05–0.1 mg/kg orally q24h; tapering may not be possible until after 4–8 weeks of therapy. Any side effects noted during treatment should be thoroughly evaluated)
- Interferon-alpha (at a dose of 30 IU orally q24h)
- Surgical excision
- Cryotherapy
- Laser ablation
- Radiation therapy.

Drug	Dosage
Co-amoxiclav	20 mg/kg orally q12h
Cefalexin	22–30 mg/kg orally q12h
Cefpodoxime	10 mg/kg orally q24h
Cefovecin	8 mg/kg s.c. q14d
Clindamycin	5.5 mg/kg orally q12h or 11 mg/kg orally q24h
Lincomycin	10 mg/kg orally q12h
Ormethoprim-sulfadimethoxine	55 mg/kg orally on day 1, then 27.5 mg/kg orally q24h
Trimethoprim-sulfadiazine or sulfamethoxazole	15–30 mg/kg orally q12h

24.3 Systemic antibiotic therapy that can be used for the treatment of the bacterial component of feline eosinophilic dermatitis (see Chapter 22).

Infectious diseases

Viral infections

There is no specific therapeutic protocol for treating cutaneous viral infections in cats and supportive therapy is generally recommended. Steroid administration is not advised. In cases of feline herpesvirus infection, systemic antiviral medication may be beneficial to decrease the severity of the clinical signs. Famciclovir at a dose of 90 mg/kg orally q12h has been reported as optimal for cats. This dose may need to be adjusted in patients with concurrent renal impairment. There is no evidence that oral lysine is effective. Good nursing care and management of secondary bacterial upper respiratory tract infections are imperative in cats with herpesvirus and calicivirus infections. Broad-spectrum antibiotics may be required in cases with concurrent bacterial respiratory disease. In cats with upper respiratory tract signs, appetite needs to be carefully monitored. In addition, topical antiviral ophthalmic medications (e.g. trifluridine, cidofovir, idoxuridine) may be indicated in cats that present with ocular manifestations of disease, and topical antibacterial ophthalmic drugs may be warranted in cases of secondary bacterial conjunctivitis. Although not commonly seen outside of Western Europe and Asia, cats with feline cowpox infection also require supportive treatment. This infectious agent is potentially zoonotic to immunocompromised individuals and appropriate care should be taken.

Bacterial pyoderma

The reader is referred to Chapter 22 for more information on the management of superficial pyoderma in the cat.

Fungal infections

Cats are prone to fungal infections (most commonly dermatophytosis), particularly in catteries. Fungal disease can be categorized as superficial/intermediate infections (e.g. *Malassezia*, dermatophytosis) and deeper infections ± systemic mycoses (e.g. *Cryptococcus neoformans*, *Sporothrix schenckii*, dermatophytic pseudomycetoma/granuloma, phaeohyphomycosis) (see Chapters 25, 26 and 30 for further information).

Mycobacterial infections

Cats are more susceptible to atypical mycobacterial infections than dogs. This condition is seen particularly in cats allowed to roam outside (i.e. due to the potential of getting into a fight and the accidental inoculation of these saprophytic organisms, which thrive in the panniculus of cats) (see Chapter 30 for further information).

Protozoal infections

Depending on geographical region, various *Leishmania* species can cause cutaneous infection in the cat; however, it is considered rare compared with the incidence of canine infection. In the USA, *Leishmania mexicana* is most commonly isolated. In other regions, infections caused by the *L. donovani* complex (particularly *L. infantum*) are more common. Whilst cutaneous manifestations are most commonly seen in cats, visceral spread has also been observed. The use of flumethrin/imidacloprid collars has been shown to effectively decrease transmission of the infectious agent from sandfly vectors. These should be recommended for cats living in endemic areas.

If focal lesions are present, surgical excision has the potential to debulk the disease; however, lesions can recur. Combination therapy may be the best approach, which might need to be continued indefinitely. Most of the treatment recommendations for cats have been extrapolated from canine protocols for manging the disease. It is important to note that not all therapeutic options are available in all geographical regions (e.g. meglumine antimoniate and miltefosine are not available in the USA). Novel therapeutics may need to be considered in some cases where the side effects of more standard therapy impact the treatment course. Monitoring for the adverse effects of medication administration is recommended periodically. Treatment options for cats are shown in Figure 24.4.

Drug	Dosage
Allopurinol	10–20 mg/kg orally q12–24h
Meglumine antimoniate	5–50 mg/kg or 375 mg/cat s.c., i.m. q24h
Marbofloxacin	2.75–5.5 mg/kg orally q24h
Miltefosine	2 mg/kg orally q24h[a]
Imiquimod 5% cream	Topically three times a week[a]
Artemisinin	50 mg/cat orally q24h for 11 days, followed by discontinuation for 3 days (repeat in cycles)[a]

24.4 Therapeutic options for cats with leishmaniosis. [a] Novel therapeutics.

Feline nodular skin diseases

Feline sarcoid

Associated with bovine papilloma virus infection, feline sarcoids are considered to be rare dermal neoplasms in the cat. Surgical excision with wide margins is recommended for these tumours; incomplete excision is often associated with recurrence of the disease. However, in some cases surgery may not be feasible based on lesion location. When disease is noted to have recurred and/or when incomplete excision is reported on histopathological evaluation, adjunct or alternative therapies should be considered. Although information is limited in the veterinary literature, options to consider include:

- Radiation therapy
- Cryotherapy
- Strontium plesiotherapy
- Chemotherapy
  - Toceranib (with prednisolone after cycle completion)
  - Doxorubicin/carboplatin combination therapy
- Immunotherapy
  - Interferon
  - Imiquimod 5% cream.

Plasma cell pododermatitis

Whilst the exact pathogenesis of feline plasma cell pododermatitis is uncertain, an immune-mediated process is suspected. In some cases where the disease is mild and the cat is asymptomatic or minimally affected, lesions may spontaneously regress without the need for medical intervention. However, in most cases, therapy is typically indicated. It is not uncommon for lesions to be painful and/or ulcerated, leading to marked discomfort. With ulcerated pads, bacterial infection may occur, and this should be identified by cytology and/or culture. In addition, any allergic triggers should be identified and managed (including flea allergy dermatitis) as this can potentially exacerbate clinical disease.

Medical management

Steroids are typically indicated for initial management. Prednisolone at a dose of 4 mg/kg orally q24h until resolution and then gradually tapered is effective in most cases. Alternatively, triamcinolone at a dose of 0.8 mg/kg orally q24h or dexamethasone at a dose of 2 mg/cat orally q1–3d followed by tapering may be used. In most cases, improvement should be seen within 3 weeks, with complete resolution in approximately 10–14 weeks.

However, some cats have a more smouldering presentation or recurrent disease, necessitating long-term therapy. Whilst steroids are effective in these cases as well, alternative therapeutic options may be warranted to minimize the long-term adverse effects of steroids. The addition of ciclosporin at a dose of 5–10 mg/kg orally q24h initially, then decreased to every 48–72h afterwards for approximately 4–6 weeks can be effective for managing disease and can act as a steroid-sparing agent. Doxycycline has also been used in cats with this condition for its immunomodulatory properties: 5–10 mg/kg q12h is effective for most cats and may be a good option for persistent mild disease. The risk of oesophageal stricture should be minimized by using either an oral suspension or following administration of a tablet or capsule with water or food. The long-term use of antimicrobials is not recommended.

Surgical management

Cats with large nodular lesions may require surgery to remove the masses, as they can interfere with the ability of the animal to ambulate. Surgery should always be combined with management of any underlying triggers to maximize success and reduce the likelihood of relapse.

Key points

- Successful management of FASS relies on identifying the underlying triggers and causes of treatment flares
- Treatment options for the allergic cat are more limited than in the dog, and the clinician should also be aware of species differences in drug doses and side effects
- Unlike dogs, cutaneous viral diseases are occasionally seen in cats and the clinician should be aware of this possibility prior to initiating anti-inflammatory treatment

References and further reading

Diesel A and Moriello KA (2008) A busy clinician's review of cyclosporine. *Veterinary Medicine* **103**, 266–274

Koch SN, Torres SMF, Diaz S *et al.* (2018) Subcutaneous administration of ciclosporin in 11 allergic cats – a pilot open-label uncontrolled clinical trial. *Veterinary Dermatology* **29**, 107–e43

Lowe AD, Campbell KL and Graves T (2008) Glucocorticoids in the cat. *Veterinary Dermatology* **19**, 340–347

Morris DO, Loeffler A, Davis MF *et al.* (2017) Recommendations for approaches to methicillin-resistant staphylococcal infections in small animals: diagnosis, therapeutic considerations and preventative measures. *Veterinary Dermatology* **28**, 304–e69

Pennisi MG, Hartmann K, Lloret A *et al.* (2013) Leishmaniosis in cats – ABCD guidelines on prevention and management. *Journal of Feline Medicine and Surgery* **15**, 638–642

Wildermuth K, Zabel S and Rosychuk RA (2013) The efficacy of cetirizine hydrochloride on the pruritus of cats with atopic dermatitis: a randomized, double-blind, placebo-controlled, crossover study. *Veterinary Dermatology* **24**, 576–581

Wood CJ, Selmic LE, Schlag AN *et al.* (2020) Biological behavior and clinical outcome in 42 cats with sarcoids (cutaneous fibropapillomas). *Veterinary and Comparative Oncology*, doi: 10.1111/vco.12598

Chapter 25

Dermatophytosis

Karen A. Moriello

Dermatophytosis is a contagious superficial fungal skin disease of keratinized structures (hair, skin, claws). It is a non-life-threatening, treatable and curable disease, as well as a low-level zoonotic disease (i.e. it does not cause death and is easily treated). In otherwise healthy animals, the disease will self-resolve, but this can take weeks to months. Treatment is recommended to shorten the course of the disease and to limit contagion to other animals and people.

Pathogens of importance

Dermatophytes are aerobic fungi that invade keratin and are classified by host preference:

- Anthropophilic (humans)
- Zoophilic (animals)
- Geophilic (soil).

Dermatophytes are also classified and named by whether or not they are in an asexual state (anamorph) or sexual state (teleomorph). However, dermatophyte species are in the process of being reclassified into a one fungus = one name system, via molecular testing. For example, the genera Trichophyton and Microsporum are being reclassified into the genus Arthroderma. For the purposes of this chapter traditional names will be used.

The most commonly isolated pathogens from cats and dogs are *Microsporum canis*, *Trichophyton* spp., and *M. gypseum*. In cats, *Trichophyton* spp. and *M. gypseum* infections are very uncommon. *Trichophyton* spp. infections are more common in winter months (Moriello *et al.*, 2020). In dogs, these pathogens are more common in working or hunting animals (Cornegliani *et al.*, 2009).

Prevalence

Dermatophytosis is not a reportable disease, so the true prevalence is unknown. Although there are hundreds of studies reporting on the prevalence of isolation of dermatophytes from the hair coat, these are unreliable indicators of true prevalence because culture findings were not correlated with clinical findings (i.e. true disease). A recent critical review of published studies, which did correlate culture findings and true disease and/or data from electronic medical records, found the prevalence to be less than 4% in dogs and cats (Moriello *et al.*, 2017).

Risk factors

Although dermatophytosis is uncommon, there are factors that increase disease risk in dogs and cats. The disease is more common in warm, humid environments, as moisture is important in the pathogenesis. It is most common in puppies and kittens and is a major differential diagnosis for skin lesions in this age group. With regard to older pets, in the absence of direct exposure to an infected animal, there is no evidence that older pets are at increased risk of infection. It is more common in dogs and cats that are under physiological stress, in high density situations and/or where overall animal husbandry is poor (e.g. hoarding situations; Polak *et al.*, 2014). Nodular dermatophytosis is more common in Persian cats, Yorkshire Terriers are at increased risk of dermatophyte infection, and inflammatory nodular dermatophytosis (i.e. kerion reactions) is more common in hunting and working dogs (Cornegliani *et al.*, 2009).

Pathogenesis

Dermatophytes are not part of the normal fungal flora of cats and dogs. Isolation of these organisms indicates either true disease or fomite carriage. Lesions develop as follows:

- The infective form is called an arthrospore, which is formed from fragmentation of infective hyphae
- Infection requires being exposed to a critical mass of naturally infective material. The infective spores must first evade the host's innate protective mechanisms, such as the hair coat, grooming, fungistatic properties of sebum and the immune system
- Successful inoculation and subsequent infection require skin microtrauma and moisture to facilitate sporulation of the arthrospores
- Arthrospores adhere to corneocytes and start germinating. This can happen within 6–8 hours under optimum conditions
- Germ tubes penetrate the stratum corneum and start to grow. Fungal hyphae start to grow in all directions and shed infective material
- Foci of lesions can develop within 5–7 days.

Transmission

The primary mode of transmission is via direct contact with another infected animal. Transmission from a contaminated environment or fomites can occur but only if there is concurrent microtrauma. This could be from scratching due to an ectoparasite infestation (*Otodectes*, fleas, ticks) or trauma from clipper blades/grooming tools. Handling of animals while wearing contaminated gloves (e.g. 'scruffing' of cats), can cause sufficient microtrauma to create lesions. The development of true disease by mere exposure to a contaminated environment is rare (Moriello *et al*., 2017).

Clinical presentation

The development of clinical signs reflects an interaction of the overall health of the animal and the disease pathogenesis.

- Simple infections in otherwise healthy animals can be easily treated. These infections are also most likely to self-resolve if left undetected or untreated. These animals have the least complications associated with treatment and cure most readily.
- Complicated infections are widespread and inflammatory and occur because the overall health of the dog or cat is poor. In addition, infections can be considered 'complicated' if other underlying health conditions are present or if there are obstacles to treatment (e.g. animal cannot be bathed, long hair or the animal is non-compliant with treatment).
- Culture-positive/lesion-free. Cases occur when the positive culture status of the animal is due to either fomite carriage or an early infection that was missed at the time of initial sampling.

Common lesions

Any combination of the following dermatological lesions may be observed:

- Focal to widespread distribution of lesions (Figures 25.1 to 25.4)
- Focal to widespread alopecia
  - Note bacterial pyoderma in adult dogs is commonly misdiagnosed as dermatophytosis
- Scaling and crusting (mild to severe)
- Erythema
- Hyperpigmentation
- Follicular plugging
- Variable pruritus (none to severe).

Lesions may be asymmetrical and can mimic pyotraumatic dermatitis (dogs) or eosinophilic lesions (cats).

Uncommon presentations

Uncommon presentations include:

- Nodular dermatophytosis in long-haired cats
- Inflammatory nodules in dogs (kerion reactions)
- Pustular lesions or lesions that resemble pemphigus foliaceus
- Pustular dermatophytosis
- Exudative paronychia in cats.

Lesions may be present on multiple animals in the household and, since this is a zoonotic disease, human involvement is also possible.

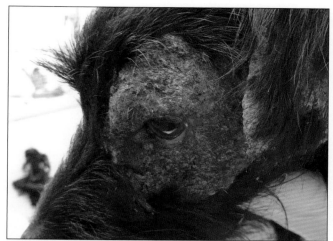

25.1 Localized dermatophytosis around the eye of a dog. Note the crusting that results from dry pustules and the demarcated alopecia.

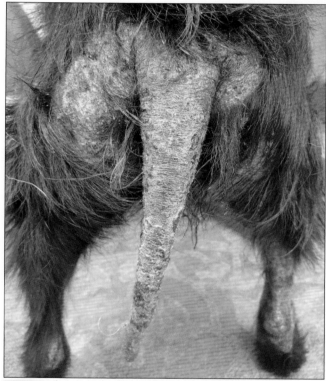

25.2 Chronic *Trichophyton* infection in a terrier. Note the focal draining tracts associated with folliculitis/furunculosis.

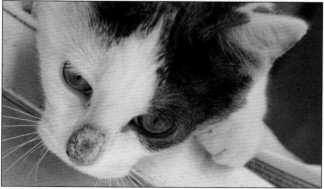

25.3 Localized dermatophytosis on the nose of a cat. The crusting and alopecia are sharply demarcated in this patient.

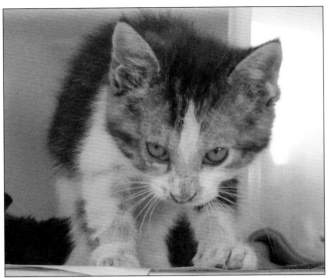

25.4 Kitten with dermatophytosis. In this patient, the erythema is present on most of the muzzle and on the legs.

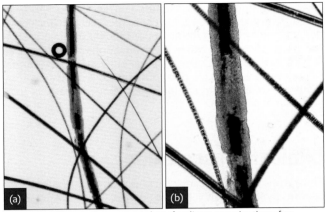

25.5 Mineral oil mount cytology for direct examination of an infected hair. (a) There is one infected hair in the field; note how much thicker and wider it is than the other hairs present (4X). (b) Close-up of the sample (10X).

Clinical approach

An evidence-based review of the diagnostic tests associated with dermatophytosis concluded that there is no 'gold standard test' (Moriello *et al.*, 2017). From a clinical perspective, all tests are subject to false-positive and false-negative results. In addition, only two diagnostic tests truly confirm the presence of active infection within the hair follicle or skin: direct examination of hair and scales and skin biopsy. Fungal culture, so often called 'the gold standard test', merely answers the question of whether or not there are fungal spores on the hair coat. Another major finding in the critical review is that much of the information about Wood's lamp examinations is incorrect.

For dermatophytosis, diagnostic tests are divided into two major groups: point of care (POC) and reference laboratory (RL) diagnostics. Unless the animal is otherwise ill, complete blood counts, serum chemistry panels and urinalysis are not cost-effective or needed.

Point of care diagnostic tests

Cytology of hair and scales

The one POC test that can confirm a dermatophyte infection is direct examination of the hair and scales. If infection can be confirmed, treatment can be initiated immediately. Skin scraping and plucking hairs from the margin of suspected lesions are the best way to collect specimens for direct examination. In one study, when the two techniques were combined, infection was confirmed in 84% of dogs and 90% of cats (Colombo *et al.*, 2010). Hairs should be plucked in the direction of growth. A dermoscope or Wood's lamp can help find suspect hairs in *Microsporum canis* infections (see below).

Lesions should be gently scraped using a skin spatula and the sample mounted in mineral oil on a glass microscope slide. A coverslip should be applied to the slide to improve visualization of the sample. Using mineral oil allows the specimen to be examined for abnormal hair shafts (Figure 25.5) and mites at the same time. This makes cytology a very time- and cost-effective diagnostic test. In addition, if it is difficult to find suspect hairs on the

specimen, the Wood's lamp can be held over the sample and since mineral oil does not damage fluorescence, the glowing hairs can be easily found. In animals, there is no evidence that 'clearing agents' which are caustic help improve visualization of infected hairs. Finally, mineral oil will not damage skin or the microscope lens.

Dermoscope: A dermoscope is a hand-held tool that both magnifies and illuminates the skin surface and hairs. It is used to examine suspect lesions and look for abnormal hairs which appear wider, frayed, broken or opaque. These suspect hairs would be plucked or scraped off the surface for direct examination in mineral oil or for fungal culture.

Wood's lamp: A Wood's lamp is *not* a diagnostic test but rather a diagnostic tool that helps find abnormal hairs for direct examination or fungal culture. Many clinicians have been mistakenly taught that this is a 'diagnostic test' and that 'less than 50% of *M. canis* strains fluoresce'. These comments stem from retrospective studies from diagnostic laboratories and not studies on spontaneous disease. When data from animals with spontaneous disease or experimentally induced infections were evaluated, it was found that fluorescence was very common in untreated animals (>90%) and not unexpectedly less common in animals under treatment. Experimental infection studies revealed that this is a good tool to monitor response to treatment in animals with *M. canis* infection. Key points about the use of this tool include the following:

- The only veterinary pathogen of importance that fluoresces is *M. canis*. Since this is the most common pathogen for which a Wood's lamp is used to find suspect hairs, it is cost- and time-effective
- Only a plug-in medical grade lamp with an ultraviolet (UV) spectrum of 320–400 nm wavelength should be used; do not use battery operated lamps or 'black lights', as these are not the same as a true Wood's lamp
- A lamp with built-in magnification should be used as this will improve visualization of suspect hairs (Figure 25.6)
- The lamp does not need to warm up but allow your eyes to adapt to the light
- The lamp should be held close to the skin (2–4 cm) to minimize distracting fluorescence of scale and dust on the hair coat, which appears blue/white; sebum appears yellow/green

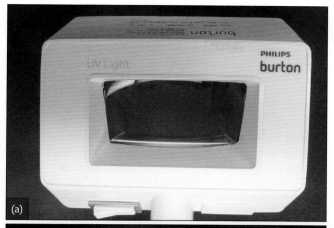

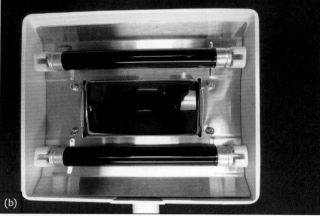

25.6 (a) Plug in Wood's lamp with built-in magnification. (b) This lamp has two replaceable bulbs.

- The examination should start at the head, moving the lamp slowly, as this is the most common site of lesions
- Only hair shafts fluoresce the characteristic apple green (Figure 25.7); crusts should be lifted to look beneath for glowing hairs
- A positive control slide should be used for training and for determining whether your eyes have adapted to the light. This is easily made by pressing clear sticky tape to an area of fluorescing hairs and then mounting it directly to a clean glass microscope slide. Hairs will retain their fluorescence for years.

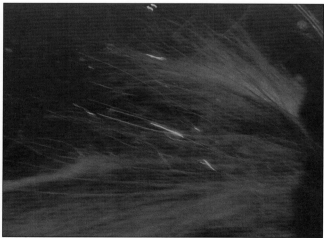

25.7 Example of hairs with positive fluorescence as seen under a Wood's lamp with magnification. These hairs would be ideal for sampling for direct examination and/or culture.

Impression smear cytology

Macroconidia are never observed on skin cytology specimens. Organisms that resemble macroconidia are invariably pollen granules or mould spores. Although uncommon, it is sometimes possible to see fungal arthrospores extra- and intracellularly in neutrophils or macrophages in animals with exudative lesions. If observed, additional samples should be obtained and sent to a clinical veterinary pathologist for confirmation as it requires a high level of confidence to confirm that these are arthrospores. However, if these organisms are observed, the clinician should be much more aggressive in obtaining skin scraping and hair plucking samples for direct examination.

Fungal culture

Fungal culture is used to confirm the dermatophyte species. This can be a POC test or an RL test. A recent study found good correlation between POC and RL fungal culture findings, if fungal culture medium was stored properly before use, and individuals performing the POC fungal cultures were trained. The key to optimal performance was daily examination of the plates, use of gross characteristics to identify suspect colonies, and confirmation of the pathogen on microscopic examination of suspect colonies (Kaufmann *et al.*, 2016). Another helpful finding from a recent study is that fungal cultures can be finalized as negative if there is no growth at day 14 of culture, regardless of whether it is a pre- or post-treatment sample (Stuntebeck *et al.*, 2018). Finally, another reason POC fungal cultures are helpful is that they allow for daily examination of plates and determination of colony forming units (CFU) per plate. It is no longer adequate to report fungal cultures as 'positive' or 'negative'; the number of CFU/plate contains valuable information before and during treatment monitoring. It is not within the scope of this chapter to review in detail how to perform, monitor and interpret in-house cultures, however, the following are key points to remember:

- A new toothbrush in the wrapping is sterile and is the recommended sampling tool. Use only a soft bristled toothbrush
- Dermatophyte test medium flat plates should be used as these are easy to open, inoculate and sample
- Suspect colonies are pale and have a red colour change in the medium around them. Pigmented colonies are not pathogens
- Only suspect lesions should be sampled, ensuring that the bristles reach the skin surface. Hairs should be visible in the bristles. In some young kittens, hairs are very short and in these cases at least 20 brushings should be performed to obtain a sample
- Room temperature plates should be inoculated by gently stabbing the bristles on to the surface. There should be a small amount of medium on the bristles. Do not over inoculate the plates, as this may lead to only the growth of hyphae. The author makes 5–8 stabs on a 90 mm fungal culture plate. Do not pluck hairs from the bristles as this has been shown to result in increased contamination and false-negative cultures (Di Mattia, *et al.*, 2019)
- Inoculated plates should be incubated at 25–30° C and stored medium side up to prevent condensation forming on the surface. The author stores individual plates in plastic bags to prevent cross-contamination and dehydration

- When examining plates, do not open the plates but rather hold the plate up to the light to examine for the presence or absence of growth plates should be opened only when there is sufficient growth to obtain a clear acetate tape preparation using lactophenol cotton blue stain
- Counting CFU/plate should be considered to help monitor response to treatment and solve treatment-related problems (Figure 25.8).

Monitor growth on POC DTM plates and record growth

• No growth
• Contaminant growth
   • If there is heavy contamination, resample the lesion/patient
• Pathogen
   • Identify microscopically

Count the number of CFU/plate for pathogens
• Pathogen score 1 (P1): 1–4 CFU/plate • Pathogen score 2 (P2): 5–9 CFU/plate • Pathogen score 3 (P3): ≥10 CFU/plate
Clinical usefulness

• **Untreated pets and pets under treatment**
   • Untreated pets with active infections tend to have P3 scores. Often the growth will be confluent and may be recorded as too many to count CFU/plate
   • As treatment progresses and the infection is eradicated the number of CFU/plate and density will decrease, i.e. P score will decrease
   • Cured animals will a have no growth, contaminant growth or P1 scores. If the latter, it is likely from environmental contamination
   • Cultures with fluctuating growth (no growth and P1 growth) are a common pattern in animals exposed to a contaminated environment
• **Factors causing sudden increase in P score**
   • Development of new lesions, especially around the eyes and ears
   • Fomite exposure
   • Inadequate disinfection of hair coat, especially around the face
• **Factors causing persistent P2/P3 scores in clinically cured animals**
   • Lack of disinfection of the hair coat
   • Subclinical infection, mostly on the face and ears
   • Fomite carriage
• **Factors causing persistent P2/P3 scores in the presence of persistent lesions**
   • Too short of a treatment period (continue treatment)
   • Concurrent systemic illness
   • Treatment compliance problems

25.8 Using colony forming units from point of care (POC) fungal cultures. CFU = colony forming units; DTM = dermatophyte test medium; POC = point of care.
(Adapted from Moriello and DeBoer, 2012)

Reference laboratory diagnostic tests
Skin biopsy

Dermatophytosis may be identified by histological examination of the skin in the following situations:

- During the work-up of an animal with a nodular, non-healing or markedly exudative lesion
- During the work-up of an animal with suspect pemphigus. There is a form of dermatophytosis that can present as pustular dermatophytosis
- During the work-up of an animal with chronic skin lesions that are unusual and dermatophytosis was not a considered differential diagnosis or, possibly, missed during POC testing.

With regard to skin biopsy specimens, a sample at least 6–8 mm in diameter should be obtained or an excisional biopsy performed. It is important to tell the pathologist that dermatophytosis is a considered differential diagnosis, so that extra sections can be ordered for special fungal stains as the fungal elements can be hard to find on routine haematoxylin and eosin (H&E) sections. If dermatophytosis is a truly suspect differential, a 6 mm punch or wedge biopsy specimen should be submitted in sterile transport medium for fungal culture.

Fungal polymerase chain reaction

Polymerase chain reaction (PCR) testing detects the presence of fungal deoxyribonucleic acid (DNA) on the hair coat. The major advantage of PCR testing compared with fungal culture is that the turn-around time is shorter. Key points to remember include:

- It is necessary to use a RL that has established laboratory protocols for testing animal specimens
- This can be a useful test in clinical practice (Moriello and Leutenegger, 2018)
- It is very sensitive and PCR will detect both viable and non-viable fungal DNA. It has the same weaknesses as toothbrush fungal cultures, in that sample acquisition is critical. It cannot distinguish between fomite carriage and true disease
- Negative results can occur in truly infected animals due to sample acquisition and/or if the laboratory is not familiar with handling toothbrush cultures and/or harvesting hairs (Jacobson et al., 2018)
- If submitting specimens, only the lesion should be sampled and the clinician should ensure that crusts, scale and at least 20 hairs with bulbs are submitted, if possible, to ensure the laboratory has adequate samples
- When using this test to monitor animals for mycological cure, it may be helpful to bathe the animal to remove non-viable spores and fomite carriage to minimize a false-positive result.

Treatment

This disease will spontaneously resolve, but treatment is recommended to shorten the course of the infection and minimize transmission to humans and other animals.

Confinement

With regard to confinement, this needs to be carefully considered, as it is an animal welfare concern. This disease occurs at a critical time in the life of young or newly adopted animals, when socialization is required. If animals are over confined, this can lead to life-long behavioural problems. The following are key things to remember:

- The primary mode of transmission is not via contact with the environment, but rather from direct contact with infective spores on the hair coat of the animal
- The purpose of confinement is to minimize the area that requires cleaning during the treatment period
- Cleaning is necessary to remove shed hairs and spores in the environment that can lead to false-positive test results on fungal culture or PCR monitoring for determining mycological cure
- The confinement room(s) should allow the animal to freely play and move
- It is not acceptable to cage or crate an animal for the duration of therapy.

Clipping of the hair coat

Clipping of the hair coat is not necessary in every case of dermatophytosis. Whole body clipping requires sedation and can lead to microtrauma that worsens the severity of the disease. It can also lead to thermal burns from contact with electric clipper blades. The following are recommended:

- Only children's metal blunt-tipped scissors should be used
- Hair matts should be removed from the hair coat to facilitate bathing and topical therapy
- It is acceptable to scissor clip the margins of lesions, if this can be done safely
- It is often easier and safer to 'debulk' hairs by combing the hair coat.

Environmental cleaning

The primary reason for cleaning is to minimize problems with false-positive fungal culture or PCR test results that make determination of mycological cure difficult. Contrary to the older literature, evidence-based studies have shown that spores can be easily removed from the environment. In a study of 70 homes exposed to *M. canis* infected cats, 69 of 70 were decontaminated following the instructions below (Moriello, 2019a). The only home not decontaminated was due to admitted owner non-compliance. The key to disinfection is the mechanical removal of hair and debris and washing surfaces until they are visibly clean.

Key points to stress to clients to counter myths are:

- Spores do not multiply in the environment and they do not 'invade' home structures like mould and mildew. They are like 'dust'
- Spores are easily removed via routine cleaning
- Spores are not 'alive'; spores are a normal dormant life stage
- Infection from the environment is rare
- Environmental sampling is not cost-effective or needed, unless there is concern about fomite contamination.

Specific cleaning recommendations include:

- **Laundry:** Pet laundry should be kept separate from home laundry. It should be washed twice in a washing machine on the longest cycle. Do not overfill the washing machine. Hot water and bleach are not needed (Moriello, 2016)
- **Rugs:** Pets should be kept off rugs or they should be vacuumed daily. Carpet can be decontaminated via commercial steam cleaning or using a beater brush cleaner (Moriello, 2017)
- **Pet room:** The focus should be on mechanical removal of debris. Floors should be mopped two to three times a week; disposable cloths and/or disinfectant wipes should be used for dusting
- **Mechanical cleaning of hard surfaces:** Debris should be removed and the hard surfaces washed with a detergent until visibly clean, then rinsed with water and any excess water removed. This alone can disinfect most hard, non-porous surfaces and is recommended for pet food bowls (Moriello, 2019b)
- **Disinfectants:** The use of disinfectants does not take the place of mechanical cleaning. Disinfectants are intended for spores not removed by cleaning. For safety **only** use ready-to-use commercial disinfectants labelled as efficacious against *Trichophyton* spp. The most readily available products are bathroom disinfectants
- **Carriers:** Animal carriers should be cleaned
- **Bleach:** Household bleach should not be used as this has no detergency and is an animal and human health hazard.

> The author's cleaning mantras:
> *'If you can wash it, you can decontaminate it'*
> *'Clean as if company is coming'.*

Topical antifungal treatment

Topical therapy is as important as systemic therapy in the treatment of dermatophytosis. It is the only way to kill infective spores on the hair coat, which transmit the disease. The following may be helpful in facilitating topical therapy:

- The hair coat should be combed before applying topical therapy. This will remove loose hairs, help prevent matting of the hair coat and facilitate topical application of a whole body product
- A whole body antifungal rinse or shampoo should be applied twice a week, making sure to soak hairs and the skin
- Clients should be instructed to use warm water and to pat dry the animal in towels. Care should be taken that small animals do not suffer from hypothermia. Transferring small kittens to a clean carrier with warm towels immediately removed from a clothes dryer is practical in a home situation
- The following topical antifungals are recommended because they have been shown to be sporicidal, consistently efficacious in field studies and to decrease spore load in the environment with continued use:
  - **Lime sulphur leave-on solution:** A 1:16 dilution in warm water prepared freshly for each application should be used. Ensure that the hair coat and skin are soaked. This product is odorous when wet and will discolour the hair coat temporarily. This product has residual activity
  - **Enilconazole topical leave-on solution diluted as per label instructions:** This product is an emulsion and needs to be frequently agitated during application. It can leave the hair coat with an oily residue. This product has residual activity
  - **2% Miconazole/2% chlorhexidine shampoo (not available worldwide):** This should be diluted 1:1 with water; shampoo for at least 3 minutes or longer if possible.
- Leave-on mousse products that contain chlorhexidine and miconazole, ketoconazole or climbazole can be used in patients that cannot be wetted (e.g. cats with upper respiratory infection)
- Adjuvant focal topical therapy may be indicated in animals with lesions on the face and in or around the ears. Owners are reluctant to apply whole body topical products to these areas:
  - For ears: otic medications containing miconazole or ketoconazole applied daily can be used. It is important not to use products that contain glucocorticoids or antibiotics
  - For the face: 2% miconazole vaginal cream can be applied to the face and is safe to use around the eyes (Gyanfosu *et al.*, 2018).

Systemic antifungal treatment

Systemic antifungal treatment is used to eradicate the infection within the hair follicle and is used in conjunction with topical antifungal therapy and environmental cleaning. Unless there are contra-indications, it is indicated in all confirmed cases. The current drugs of choice are terbinafine or itraconazole.

Terbinafine

Terbinafine has the lowest minimum inhibitory concentration (MIC) against dermatophytes. It is the drug of choice for medium to large dogs and, although unlicensed, is an alternative treatment option for cats. Unless a veterinary formulation is used, the human tablets are large and can be difficult to administer to small cats.

Key treatment points include:

- Terbinafine dose is 30–40 mg/kg orally once daily or week on/week off until mycological cure
- The most common side effects are vomiting or diarrhoea
- Routine laboratory monitoring is not needed, unless the animal has a concurrent comorbid disease that requires it.

Itraconazole

Itraconazole is the treatment of choice for cats and small dogs. This drug accumulates within the adipose tissue, sebaceous glands and hair for weeks after administration, which makes pulse therapy possible (Vlaminck and Engelen, 2005). Compounded formulations should not be used, as studies in both dogs and cats have shown that these formulations have poor bioavailability (Mawby et al., 2014, 2018).

Key treatment points include:

- Itraconazole suspension treatment protocol for cats is 5 mg/kg orally once daily week on/week off (i.e. 7 days of treatment, 7 days without treatment; Puls et al., 2018). Many animals will achieve mycological cure with three cycles of treatment as part of a comprehensive treatment plan. Animals should be treated until mycological cure
- There is no weight restriction on the product. Experimental studies have used it safely in kittens as young as 10 days of age (Vlaminck and Engelen, 2005)
- The formulation is well tolerated in the majority animals with the most common adverse effect being temporary gastrointestinal upset
- Severe adverse effects have not been associated with the use of the drug at doses for dermatophytosis, but rather with long-term high dose use for the treatment of systemic or intermediate fungal diseases (Moriello et al., 2017)
- Routine laboratory monitoring is not needed in simple infection cases
- This drug should be administered with food.

Ketoconazole

Ketoconazole at a dose of 5 mg/kg orally once daily is the licensed drug option for dogs in the UK but has higher MIC than terbinafine or itraconazole. Its use should be avoided in cats, as it is not well tolerated. It should be administered with food.

Not recommended

The following drugs are not recommended for the treatment of dermatophytosis:

- **Griseofulvin:** This was the first systemic antifungal developed. It is less effective than itraconazole and terbinafine. It is associated with a higher number of side effects and is not recommended for use
- **Fluconazole:** This has poor antifungal efficacy against dermatophytes and has the highest MIC compared with terbinafine, itraconazole, ketoconazole and griseofulvin. It should not be used
- **Lufenuron:** This is not effective for the treatment or prevention of disease and should not be used
- **Fungal vaccines:** These are not recommended for the treatment of dermatophytosis.

Monitoring and mycological cure

Clinical cure precedes mycological cure. A lack of response to treatment and/or the development of new lesions indicates treatment-related problems or an incorrect diagnosis. If the diagnosis is correct and there is good adherence to treatment, it could be an indication of the development of a concurrent medical problem.

A recent retrospective study reported that in shelter cats with simple infections the mean time to cure was 4.3 weeks (range 3–12 weeks) and in cats with complicated infections the mean time was 11.9 weeks (range 8–28 weeks) (Stuntebeck and Moriello, 2019). In the latter group, cure did not occur until the underlying medical problem was resolved. Data for dogs is not available.

It is accepted to treat until animals have achieved 'mycological cure'. This term was introduced into the veterinary literature in a 1959 study describing the use of griseofulvin in the treatment of Persian cats (n = 22) with chronic dermatophytosis (Kaplan and Ajello, 1959) and was defined as 'two successive negative cultures taken at 2 weeks apart'. This requirement of two negative cultures has become entrenched in the veterinary literature, but never investigated or challenged. In a recent study, it was found that, when there has been high compliance with cleaning, topical therapy and systemic therapy, the first negative culture was predictive of mycological cure in 90.3% of cats (Stuntebeck and Moriello, 2019).

Current recommendations are as follows:

- Monitor for clinical cure and resolution of lesions
- In *M. canis* infected animals, perform a Wood's lamp evaluation to look for residual sites of infection
- If there are no new lesions and no glowing hair shafts, obtain a post-treatment fungal culture. Continue topical therapy until the results are available. If the fungal culture is positive, review cleaning protocols with the client and do one of the following:
  - Continue treatment for another 4–6 weeks, then repeat the culture
  - Continue topical therapy and have the client aggressively clean the environment and then obtain another sample for culture from the pet
- If animals are ill or unthrifty at the time of diagnosis, the first post-treatment fungal culture is best delayed until there is both a clinical cure and resolution of the underlying medical problem.

Lesion-free/culture-positive animals

The question here is whether the animal is a fomite carrier or truly infected:

- As soon as the culture results are available, the animal should be examined in room light and with a Wood's lamp. If lesions are found, samples should be obtained for direct examination to confirm infection
- If no lesions are found, the most likely explanation is that the animal is a fomite carrier. This can be confirmed by bathing the animal in an antifungal shampoo and repeating the culture after 24 hours. Pending culture results, topical therapy should be continued.

Public health concerns

Dermatophytosis is an animal-associated zoonotic skin disease. At one point, this disease was of major public health significance because effective systemic and/or topical treatments were not available. Key client education points include:

- Dermatophytosis causes skin lesions and is treatable and curable in humans. It is not life threatening. It is important to educate clients that this is a different disease entirely to respiratory mould-associated illnesses they may have heard about in buildings
- This disease is common in humans but the terms 'toenail fungus' or 'athlete's foot fungus' are used. The human diseases are caused by a different pathogen, not an animal-sourced pathogen
- Transmission from animals to humans is via direct contact and simple measures can minimize transmission
- In animals, it is treatable and curable, and euthanasia is not necessary
- The most common complication of animal-associated infections in immunosuppressed humans is prolonged treatment time (Moriello et al., 2017).

Key points

- Dermatophytosis is more common in puppies and kittens and in warm, humid environments
- There is no 'gold standard' diagnostic test and a definitive diagnosis is achieved by performing a combination of various tests, which should be interpreted in the context of the clinical picture
- Effective management requires a combination of topical, systemic and environmental treatments

---

References and further reading

Colombo S, Cornegliani L, Beccati M et al. (2010) Comparison of two sampling methods for microscopic examination of hair shafts in feline and canine dermatophytosis. Veterinaria (Cremona) 24, 27–33

Cornegliani L, Persico P and Colombo S (2009) Canine nodular dermatophytosis (Kerion): 23 cases. Veterinay Dermatology 20, 185–190

Di Mattia D, Fondati A, Monaco M et al. (2019) Comparison of two inoculation methods for Microsporum canis culture using the toothbrush sampling technique. Veterinary Dermatology 30, 60–e17

Gyanfosu L, Koffuor GA, Kyei S et al. (2018) Efficacy and safety of extemporaneously prepared miconazole eye drops in Candida albicans-induced keratomycosis. International Ophthalmology 38, 2089–2100

Jacobson LS, Mcintyre L and Mykusz J (2018) Comparison of real-time PCR with fungal culture for the diagnosis of Microsporum canis dermatophytosis in shelter cats: a field study. Journal of Feline Medicine and Surgery 20, 103–107

Kaplan W and Ajello L (1959) Oral treatment of spontaneous ringworm in cats with griseofulvin. Journal of the American Veterinary Medical Association 135, 253–261

Kaufmann R, Blum SE, Elad D et al. (2016) Comparison between point-of-care dermatophyte test medium and mycology laboratory culture for diagnosis of dermatophytosis in dogs and cats. Veterinary Dermatology 27, 284–e68

Mawby D, Whittemore JC, Fowler LE et al. (2018) Comparison of absorption characteristics of oral reference and compounded itraconazole formulations in healthy cats. Journal of the American Veterinary Medical Association 252, 195–200

Mawby D, Whittemore JC, Genger S et al. (2014) Bioequivalence of orally administered generic, compounded, and linnovator-formulated itraconazole in healthy dogs. Journal of Veterinary Internal Medicine 28, 72–77

Moriello KA (2016) Decontamination of laundry exposed to Microsporum canis hairs and spores. Journal of Feline Medicine and Surgery 18, 457–461

Moriello KA (2017) Decontamination of carpet exposed to Microsporum Canis hairs and spores. Journal of Feline Medicine and Surgery 19, 435–439

Moriello KA (2019a) Dermatophytosis in cats and dogs: A practical guide to diagnosis and treatment. In Practice 41, 138–147

Moriello KA (2019b) Mechanical washing of pet food bowls is effective for Microsporum canis decontamination. Veterinary Dermatology 30, 428–e130

Moriello KA , Coyner K, Paterson S et al. (2017) Diagnosis and treatment of dermatophytosis in dogs and cats. Clinical Consensus Guidelines of the World Association for Veterinary Dermatology. Veterinary Dermatology 28, 266–e268

Moriello KA and deBoer DJ (2012) Cutaneous fungal infections: dermatophytosis. In: Infectious diseases of the dog and cat, 4th edn., pp 588–602. Ed. C Green, Elsevier Saunders, St. Louis

Moriello KA and Leutenegger CM (2018) Use of a commercial qPCR assay in 52 high risk shelter cats for disease identification of dermatophytosis and mycological cure. Veterinary Dermatology 29, 66–e26

Moriello KA, StuntebecK R and Mullen L (2020) Trichophyton species and Microsporum gypseum infection and fomite carriage in cats from three animal shelters: a retrospective case series. Journal of Feline Medicine and Surgery, 22, 391–394

Polak K, Levy J, Crawford P et al. (2014) Infectious diseases in large-scale cat hoarding investigations. Veterinary Journal 201, 189–195

Puls C, Johnson A, Young K et al. (2018) Efficacy of itraconazole oral solution using an alternating-week pulse therapy regimen for treatment of cats with experimental Microsporum canis infection. Journal of Feline Medicine and Surgery 20, 869–874

Stuntebeck R and Moriello KA (2020) One versus two negative fungal cultures to confirm mycological cure in shelter cats treated for Microsporum canis dermatophytosis: a retrospective study. Journal of Feline Medicine and Surgery, 22, 598–601

Stuntebeck R, Moriello KA and Verbrugge M (2018) Evaluation of incubation time for Microsporum canis dermatophyte cultures. Journal of Feline Medicine and Surgery 20, 997–1000

Vlaminck K and Engelen M (2005) An overview of pharmacokinetic and pharmacodynamic studies in the development of itraconazole for feline Microsporum canis dermatophytosis. Advances in Veterinary Dermatology 5, 130–136

Chapter 26

Malassezia dermatitis

Tim Nuttall

Malassezia are commensals but are capable of opportunistic skin and ear infections. Atopic dogs may also become sensitized to *Malassezia* allergens. Understanding their biology, prompt identification and effective treatment are therefore important.

Malassezia spp. and ecology

Species and nomenclature

Malassezia spp. yeasts are commensals on mammalian skin. They are single-cell yeasts with a thick cell wall. Individual cells are ovoid, globular or cylindrical and bud to form characteristic 'peanut'/'Russian doll' shapes (Figure 26.1). *Malassezia* can also form hyphae-like structures. At least 14 *Malassezia* spp. are recognized, although molecular techniques are revising their relationships and nomenclature. Most are highly lipid-dependent but *M. pachydermatis* is less dependent on lipid supplements for *in vitro* culture. However, it is considered lipophilic and there are some lipid-dependent strains (Puig *et al.*, 2017).

Ecology

Malassezia are acquired at birth and in early life through skin contact and licking. They colonize the superficial epidermal and infundibular stratum corneum. Culture-based studies found that *Malassezia* preferred lipid-rich areas (e.g. ear canals, anal sacs, interdigital skin and mucocutaneous junctions) in healthy animals, but that atopic dogs were colonized on lesional and non-lesional skin at a variety of body sites. However, culture-independent quantitative

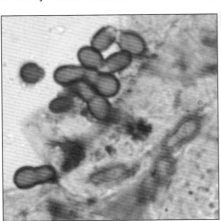

26.1 The characteristic 'peanut', 'Russian doll' or 'snowman' shapes of budding *Malassezia pachydermatis* from a dog (Diff-Quik® stain; original magnification X1000).

polymerase chain reactions (qPCR) and next generation sequencing (NGS) are now revolutionizing the study of the cutaneous mycobiota.

In humans, *Malassezia* dominate most body sites apart from contact areas (e.g. feet) where environmental fungi are more prevalent. An early study in healthy dogs also showed that the mycobiota was dominated by environmental fungi, particularly *Alternaria* and *Cladosporium*, although this varied between dogs (Meason-Smith *et al.*, 2015). Samples from atopic dogs were similar, although significantly less rich in species. More recently, however, it has been shown that *Malassezia* are also prevalent in the mycobiota of healthy, atopic and experimentally sensitized dogs. *M. globosa* and *M. restricta* are more abundant on healthy skin, whereas *M. pachydermatis* is more abundant on naturally affected and allergen-induced atopic skin lesions (Meason-Smith *et al.*, 2019). The otic mycobiota is similar, again with a loss of richness and a *Malassezia* dysbiosis in atopic dermatitis (Korbelik *et al.*, 2018). The shift from highly to less lipid-dependent species suggests that the skin lipid profile may play a role in *Malassezia* dysbiosis.

In cats, the most abundant fungi were also *Alternaria* and *Cladosporium* (Meason-Smith *et al.*, 2016), although more *Malassezia* are seen in Devon Rex cats (Older *et al.*, 2019). The mycobiota varied between cats, but there were few differences between body sites. Cats with allergic skin disease had a similarly diverse mycobiota, but with more *Agaricomycetes* and *Sordariomycetes* and less *Epicoccum*. However, *Malassezia* was only isolated from 30% of the healthy and 21% of allergic cats with low abundance in both groups. *M. pachydermatis* strains differ from those in dogs (Puig *et al.*, 2016), which may explain the differences in colonization and virulence.

Virulence factors and host susceptibility

Malassezia can be significant pathogens when a combination of host and microbial virulence factors allow the yeasts to overwhelm the host's physical, chemical and immunological defences. *Malassezia* dermatitis and/or otitis are therefore usually secondary to an underlying condition (Figure 26.2). However, distinct disease-associated *M. pachydermatis* genotypes and phenotypes have been identified (Czyzewska *et al.*, 2018, 2019). This suggests that host factors enable both a *Malassezia* dysbiosis and a shift towards more pathogenic strains.

Differential diagnoses
• Demodicosis
• Other ectoparasites
• Dermatophytosis
• Staphylococcal pyoderma
• Atopic dermatitis
• Atopic-like dermatitis
• Food-responsive dermatosis (also known as food allergy or adverse food reaction)
• Contact dermatitis
• Seborrhoeic dermatitis
• Primary keratinization disorders
• Feline acne/facial dermatitis
• Drug reactions
• Epitheliotrophic lymphoma

Possible underlying conditions
• Demodicosis
• Other ectoparasites
• Atopic dermatitis
• Atopic-like dermatitis
• Food-responsive dermatosis
• Endocrinopathies
• Superficial necrolytic dermatitis
• Zinc-responsive dermatosis
• Feline paraneoplastic alopecia
• Feline thymoma
• Mural folliculitis
• Primary keratinization disorders
• Feline acne/facial dermatitis
• Skin fold dermatitis (intertrigo)
• Feline leukaemia virus or feline immunodeficiency virus
• Other immunosuppressive conditions or treatment

26.2 Comparison of the differential diagnoses and underlying conditions in *Malassezia* dermatitis and otitis.

Virulence factors

Malassezia express protein and glycoprotein adhesion molecules that bind to carbohydrate ligands on canine corneocytes. They also secrete proteases, lipases, phospholipases, lipoxygenases and other enzymes that cause proteolysis and lipolysis, alter cutaneous pH, activate complement and trigger the release of inflammatory mediators. The dysbiosis and shift to *M. pachydermatis* may be significant. Multiple *M. pachydermatis* genotypes can be cultured from healthy dogs and dogs with skin lesions, with some associated with particular locations and lesions. In one study, isolates from skin lesions had higher phospholipase activity than those from non-lesional skin, and a low phospholipase genotype was recovered only from healthy skin (Cafarchia *et al.*, 2008). In contrast, a disease-associated genotype exhibited greater biofilm formation, phospholipase production and pro-inflammatory cytokine release from human keratinocytes *in vitro* (Buommino *et al.*, 2016). *M. restricta* and *M. globosa* can also form biofilms (Zareei *et al.*, 2018).

Host factors and underlying diseases

Anatomical features (skin folds, pendulous lips, hairy feet), inflammation, exudates and licking can create a warm, lipid-rich microenvironment that favour *Malassezia*. Keratinization defects and endocrine disorders may increase humidity and alter sebum lipids. Furthermore, disruption to the stratum corneum by self-trauma, keratinization or metabolic defects could alter expression of adhesion molecules and facilitate *Malassezia* colonization.

Malassezia has been associated with a number of primary conditions in dogs and cats (see Figure 26.2). In dogs, it is most commonly associated with underlying hypersensitivity disorders (particularly atopic dermatitis and food-responsive dermatosis; Figure 26.3). Treatment with glucocorticoids or ciclosporin does not alter *Malassezia* populations (Widmer *et al.*, 2018).

Breed susceptibility

Certain breeds are predisposed to *Malassezia* dermatitis. This could be due to anatomical features or other host factors and/or predisposition to diseases with secondary *Malassezia* involvement. However, mucosal and cutaneous *Malassezia* populations are elevated in healthy Basset Hounds and Devon Rex cats, which suggests that specific factors facilitate *Malassezia* colonization in these breeds.

Immune response

Immune responses to *Malassezia* can be detected in both healthy and affected dogs. At least 14 different protein antigens have been identified. Dogs with *Malassezia* dermatitis tend to recognize more antigens than healthy dogs, but no association between the pattern of antigen recognition and any particular *Malassezia* strain or virulence has been demonstrated (Chen and Hill, 2005). Protective immunity appears to be associated with cell-mediated rather than humoral responses and elevated immunoglobulin levels (Bond *et al.*, 1998).

The results of specific intradermal test (IDT) reactivity, immunoglobulin (Ig)G and IgE serology, lymphocyte proliferation and passive transfer suggest that *M. pachydermatis* can act as an allergen in some dogs with atopic dermatitis (Nuttall and Halliwell, 2001; Morris and DeBoer, 2003; Chen and Hill, 2005). Extracts for IDTs and *Malassezia*-specific IgE serology tests are now commercially available, although the results must be interpreted with care and in the light of the clinical signs and cytology findings (Farver *et al.*, 2005).

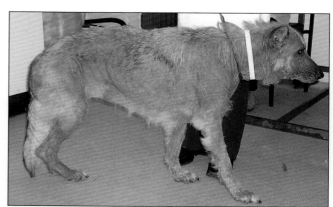

26.3 German Shepherd Dog suffering from severe atopic dermatitis and secondary *Malassezia* dermatitis. The dog responded well to twice weekly bathing with a 2% chlorhexidine/2% miconazole shampoo and ciclosporin at a dose of 5 mg/kg orally q24h.

Zoonotic potential

Canine *M. pachydermatis* can colonize transiently in-contact humans (Morris *et al.*, 2005). This is of little consequence to healthy humans, but zoonotic infections have been reported in immunocompromised neonates and adults. This underlines the need to observe hygiene precautions when handling healthy animals, as well as those affected by *Malassezia* dermatitis.

Clinical presentation

Dogs

Malassezia dermatitis can occur in any breed (although some are predisposed), age or sex. Pruritus is common and can be severe enough to be misinterpreted as a neurological problem. In the early stages, there is erythema and greasy exudation, scaling and crusting (Figure 26.4a). Chronic *Malassezia* dermatitis is characterized by greasy alopecia, lichenification and hyperpigmentation (Figure 26.4b). Clinical signs can be focal, multifocal or generalized and diffuse or well demarcated. Commonly affected sites include the ears, lips, muzzle, interdigital skin, flexor surfaces, ventral neck and body, axillae, medial limbs and perineum. Affected dogs often have a rancid, musty or yeasty odour. However, the clinical picture can be complicated by the underlying condition (see Figure 26.2) and/or concurrent staphylococcal infection.

Malassezia are commonly associated with erythroceruminous otitis externa (i.e. characterized by erythema, swelling and a waxy discharge). The discharge is often dark brown but may be lighter or tan-yellow (Figure 26.5). *Malassezia* are uncommon in suppurative otitis with a purulent discharge (see Chapters 19 and 20). *Malassezia* can also cause paronychia with a waxy exudate and brownish discoloration of the nails. *Malassezia* can also be a rare cause of stomatitis, pharyngitis and tonsillitis.

Cats

Malassezia dermatitis is less common in cats than in dogs and pruritus is a less constant feature. *Malassezia* infections can be found in otitis externa, feline (chin) acne, seborrhoeic and scaling facial dermatitis (Figure 26.6a), and paronychia with discoloration of the nails (particularly in Devon Rex cats; Figure 26.6b). Generalized erythema and scaling (Figure 26.6c) has been associated with *Malassezia* dermatitis in cats with thymoma, lymphocytic mural folliculitis and paraneoplastic alopecia.

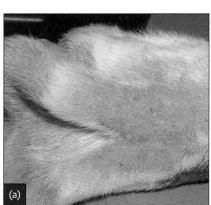
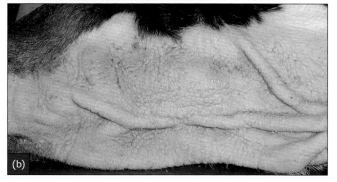

26.4

(a) Erythema, alopecia and scaling of the foot of a Boxer with *Malassezia* dermatitis secondary to hyperadrenocorticism. The skin was also greasy and malodorous.
(b) Chronic *Malassezia* dermatitis of the ventral neck in an atopic Staffordshire Bull Terrier. The affected skin is erythematous, alopecic, lichenified and seborrhoeic.

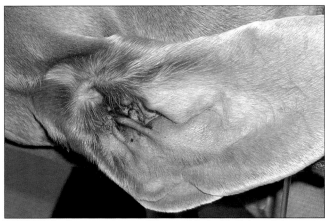

26.5 Erythroceruminous otitis associated with *Malassezia* in a Weimeraner with a cutaneous food-responsive dermatosis. There is diffuse erythema of the ventral pinna with a dark brown waxy discharge around the opening of the vertical ear canal.

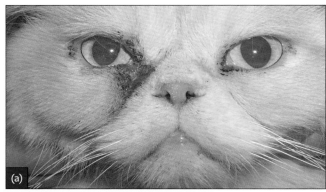
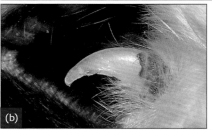
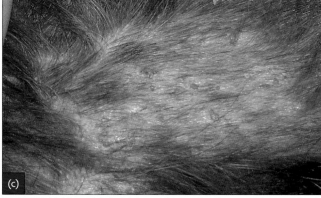

26.6 (a) Idiopathic facial dermatitis in a Persian cat. This condition is often associated with *Malassezia* dermatitis, although even aggressive topical or systemic anti-*Malassezia* treatment can have little impact. (b) Build-up of brown waxy material on the proximal claw of a cat with *Malassezia paronychia*. Generalized exfoliative *Malassezia* dermatitis in cats is often associated with severe systemic disease. However, the mural folliculitis and *Malassezia* dermatitis spontaneously resolved in this cat. (c) Generalized alopecia and scaling associated with *Malassezia* overgrowth in a Domestic Shorthaired cat with lymphocytic mural folliculitis.

Diagnostic tests

The differential diagnosis list is extensive (see Figure 26.2) and is complicated by the fact that many conditions considered to be differentials are also risk factors for secondary *Malassezia* dermatitis. Essentially, *Malassezia* should be considered in any case of pruritic dermatitis, particularly if it is associated with erythema, scaling, seborrhoea, hyperpigmentation and lichenification. It should be remembered that identifying *Malassezia* organisms should prompt further diagnostic steps to determine the underlying condition.

Cytology

Cytology is quick, easy, cheap and non-invasive (see Chapter 4). Adhesive tape strips are effective unless the skin is very moist. Direct impression on to a glass slide is possible on accessible skin; it is helpful if the skin is very moist or waxy. Blunt scalpel blades, spatulas, cotton swabs or toothpicks can be used to collect waxy exudate from the ears, nail folds, skin folds and feet (see Chapters 3 and 4).

Air-drying and conventional alcohol fixing is suitable in most cases. Heat-fixing can be used for very waxy or oily samples, but can damage cells and organisms, and has not been shown to be a superior technique. Samples can be stained using a modified Wright-Giemsa stain (such as Diff-Quik®) using the two-stain or one-stain method. The one-stain method is quicker, avoids losing material during fixing and rinsing, and results in more intense staining. However, the staining is more monochrome (Figure 26.7). Tape strips should not be fixed before staining because fixatives usually destroy the adhesive layer with the sample. The stains may also damage the tape and it is necessary to find one that resists the stain being used. The pots should be cleaned and the staining solutions changed regularly (at least every 7–14 days) because yeasts can collect in them, leading to false-positive diagnoses.

Slides are scanned initially under low power (X40–X100) to check staining efficiency and to select areas with plenty of squames for closer inspection. *Malassezia* appear as small oval to 'peanut'/'snowman'/'Russian doll' shapes, often forming rafts on the surface of squames (see Figures 26.1 and 26.8). They stain most frequently blue–purple but can appear red–pink or pale blue. Some *Malassezia* fail to

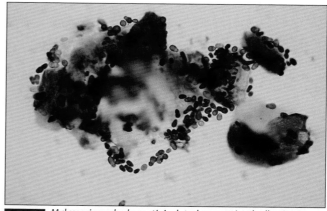

26.8 *Malassezia pachydermatis* isolated on a stained adhesive tape strip preparation from a dog. This sample was stained with the eosinophilic (pot 2) and basophilic (pot 3) Diff-Quik® stains. Compare the staining with that in Figure 26.7, where the preparation was stained with only the basophilic stain. (Original magnification X400)

stain, but their refractile cell wall can be seen with a closed condenser diaphragm. Using the oil immersion lens (X1000) is the most accurate way to find *Malassezia*, but with practice they can be identified easily using the dry lens (X400).

There is no standard accepted number of organisms needed to diagnose *Malassezia* dermatitis. Estimates of commensal *Malassezia* populations range from <8 yeasts/cm² to <1 yeast per high power field (X400) and clinically significant numbers from >2 yeasts per high power field to >10 yeasts per oil immersion field (X1000). It is likely that these figures reflect differences in technique, breed and body site. In addition, *Malassezia* are often found in rafts associated with squames and may not be distributed uniformly across a slide. Finally, low numbers of *Malassezia* may still be clinically significant in sensitized dogs. Hence, clinical experience and acumen is as important as relying upon numbers.

Culture

M. pachydermatis will grow on Sabouraud's medium, although the lipid-dependent species require supplemented media, such as modified Dixon's agar. Colonies are small, cream to yellow, dome-shaped, smooth to slightly wrinkled, with a regular to slightly lobed edge. However, because *Malassezia* are commensal organisms, isolation is not necessarily significant. Typically, <1 colony forming unit can be isolated from healthy canine skin, but much higher populations can be isolated from the lips and interdigital skin.

Skin biopsy and histopathology

Malassezia can be present in the overlying keratin crust and hair follicles, but organisms are often removed by processing. *Malassezia* can also be an incidental finding in biopsy samples from other dermatoses. *Malassezia* dermatitis histopathology is characterized by acanthosis, hyperkeratosis (often including parakeratosis with nucleated keratinocytes) and a superficial inflammatory infiltrate.

Response to treatment

Given the uncertainties surrounding the significance of the presence of *Malassezia*, the final diagnosis relies on the response to treatment. However, the systematic prescription of antifungal drugs to every dog with atopic dermatitis

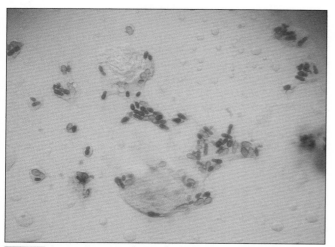

26.7 Impression smear from a dog's skin stained with the Diff-Quik® basophilic stain (pot 3) only. The *Malassezia* organisms have clearly stained well but note the monochrome image. Compare with Figures 26.1 and 26.8, which have been stained with both the eosinophilic (pot 2) and basophilic stains. (Original magnification X400)

or other skin conditions is not recommended because this is likely to increase the prevalence of drug-resistant microorganisms. The International Committee on Atopic Disease in Animals (ICADA; www.icada.org) recommends that a series of steps should be followed to determine whether *Malassezia* are contributing to the clinical signs of atopic dermatitis:

- Identification of appropriate skin lesions
- Documentation of *Malassezia* at these lesional sites by cytology
- Specific antifungal treatment
- Reduction in the number of *Malassezia* on cytology following treatment
- Amelioration of skin lesions at the affected sites following treatment.

The response to treatment should be interpreted with caution. For example, topical treatment may also eliminate staphylococcal pyoderma (e.g. miconazole/chlorhexidine) or parasites (e.g. selenium sulphide), and systemic treatment may modulate immune responses (e.g. ketoconazole). In some animals, clinical signs are not associated with elevated *Malassezia* numbers, but they do respond to antifungal agents. It is not clear whether this response indicates other actions of antifungal agents or an alternative pathogenesis, such as hypersensitivity to *Malassezia*.

Treatment and prognosis

Evidence-based medicine

Several topical and systemic treatment options are available to treat *Malassezia* dermatitis. However, the evidence to support many of these is anecdotal or of low quality. There are two evidence-based reviews of treatment: one for *Malassezia* dermatitis (Negre *et al.*, 2008) and one for topical antimicrobial treatment (Mueller *et al.*, 2012). These reviews concluded that there was good evidence to support the use of:

- 2% miconazole/2% chlorhexidine shampoo for 5–10 minutes, twice weekly for 3 weeks
- Ketoconazole at 5–10 mg/kg orally q24h for 3 weeks
- Itraconazole at 5 mg/kg orally q24h on 2 consecutive days each week for 3 weeks.

There was insufficient evidence to recommend the use of systemic terbinafine or topical miconazole, enilconazole, chlorhexidine, piroctone olamine, benzalkonium chloride or other products. Nevertheless, clinicians should also consider more recent publications, the owner's resources and expectations, tolerance, adverse effects and medicines legislation. This chapter describes many of these treatment options, but readers are directed to the evidence-based reviews and other publications for further details of published efficacy and safety. Concurrent bacterial infections can complicate *Malassezia* dermatitis and otitis, and treatment regimens that also reduce bacterial numbers may be superior to those with antifungal action only in these cases.

Topical treatment

Topical therapy is generally the most cost-effective and safest treatment. However, it is also the most labour-intensive and, therefore, not necessarily appropriate in all cases. This is especially true for shampoos, which may limit compliance. Foams, sprays and wipes are easier to use and do not need rinsing. Chlorhexidine/imidazole shampoos are effective against *Malassezia in vitro* (Young *et al.*, 2012), and shampoos, foams and sprays with these ingredients show persistent antibacterial activity on the skin and hairs (Kloos *et al.*, 2013; Mesman *et al.*, 2016; Ramos *et al.*, 2019); 3% chlorhexidine/0.5% climbazole wipes show *in vitro* (Rafferty *et al.*, 2019) and *in vivo* (Cavana *et al.*, 2015) efficacy against *Malassezia*, although there was no residual activity.

Localized *Malassezia* dermatitis can be treated with focal application of an antifungal product, but the whole body should be treated in cases of multifocal or generalized *Malassezia*. It is particularly important to treat the ears, mucocutaneous junctions and feet because these areas are likely to be reservoirs for *Malassezia*. Treatment should be continued daily to twice weekly until resolution, then as necessary to maintain the improvement. Treatment with degreasing shampoos or antibacterial products may also be necessary initially. Adverse reactions are uncommon, although most antifungal products can be drying and may need to be combined with emollient products. This is especially true in dogs with atopic dermatitis because the skin barrier is often compromised.

Ear cleaners with proven anti-*Malassezia* activity (Swinney *et al.*, 2008) can be used regularly to help prevent *Malassezia*-associated otitis externa. In the author's experience, a non-licensed 50% mixture of 0.0584% hydrocortisone aceponate and 1% clotrimazole solutions is effective in managing and preventing *Malassezia* otitis in atopic dogs.

Other treatment options include imidazole-containing shampoos, lotions, ointments and creams authorized for medical use (e.g. ketoconazole, clotrimazole and terbinafine). These are not licensed for use in animals, but the creams can be useful for treating focal lesions. Recent studies have shown *in vitro* anti-*Malassezia* efficacy of plant-derived essential oils (Sim *et al.*, 2019) and a honey-based otic gel (Oliveira *et al.*, 2018). Tris-EDTA and disodium EDTA also show *in vitro* activity against *Malassezia* (Chan *et al.*, 2019) and may potentiate the efficacy of antifungals.

Systemic treatment

Systemic antifungals are appropriate if topical therapy is impractical or ineffective. Ketoconazole (5–10 mg/kg orally q24h; licensed for dermatophytosis in dogs) or itraconazole (5 mg/kg orally q24h; licensed for dermatophytosis in cats) are effective in most cases. Their bioavailability is increased when administered with food. Treatment should be administered daily until clinical and cytological resolution.

Ketoconazole and itraconazole inhibit the fungal cytochrome P450 enzyme system, but either drug (particularly ketoconazole) can also affect the canine P450 system. This may necessitate dose alterations for other drugs metabolized through the P450 system (e.g. ciclosporin). Azole side effects can include anorexia, vomiting, diarrhoea, liver damage, vasculitis, thrombocytopenia and teratogenicity. Itraconazole is better tolerated than ketoconazole, and adverse effects in reported trials were limited to infrequent vomiting and decreased appetite (Negre *et al.*, 2008). However, vasculitis has been seen at doses ≥10 mg/kg.

The allylamine terbinafine is not authorized for use in dogs, but systemic treatment with 30 mg/kg orally q24h is reported to be effective and well tolerated. However, another trial reported poor efficacy with this dose. A further study showed a good response to 25 mg/kg/day, although this was in combination with topical 1% terbinafine and selenium sulphide (Negre *et al.*, 2008). Terbinafine does not achieve high concentrations in the stratum corneum or sebum in dogs, and to exceed the *Malassezia* minimum inhibitory concentration (MIC)90, doses higher than 30 mg/kg orally q24h are required (Gimmler *et al.*, 2015).

Antifungal resistance

The long persistence of azole drugs and terbinafine in the stratum corneum following administration allows long-term pulse dosing (e.g. every other week or 2 days each week). However, it is likely that long-term pulse dosing increases the risk of resistance. Miconazole-resistant *Malassezia* isolates have been selected for in a laboratory study (Kano *et al.*, 2019), and chronic topical and systemic azole treatment resulting in resistance and treatment failure has been reported (Angileri *et al.*, 2019). In addition, biofilm formation should be considered when planning treatment, as this increases the MIC at the site of infection (Nogueira Brilhante *et al.*, 2018). Therefore, effective management of the underlying disease and topical therapy to manage the fungal dysbiosis associated with *Malassezia* dermatitis and otitis is preferred.

Allergen-specific immunotherapy

Allergen-specific immunotherapy (ASIT) can be considered in atopic dogs with *Malassezia* hypersensitivity demonstrated on intradermal tests or serology (Figure 26.9) (see Chapter 11). In one study, 16 atopic dogs mono-sensitized to *Malassezia* were treated with subcutaneous ASIT (SCIT) for at least 10 months (Aberg *et al.*, 2017). Nine dogs (56%) had a >50% reduction in pruritus, as well as decreased antifungal and/or anti-inflammatory medication. No adverse

effects were reported. *Malassezia*-specific SCIT could therefore be considered in appropriate cases. However, it is unknown whether similar efficacy will be seen in atopic dogs also sensitized to environmental allergens or with other ASIT protocols (e.g. rush SCIT, sublingual (SLIT) or intralymphatic (ILIT)).

Prognosis

The prognosis with either systemic or topical treatment is very good in most cases. However, unless an underlying cause is diagnosed and treated, it is likely that lifelong maintenance therapy will be necessary. A greater understanding of *Malassezia* dermatitis and otitis may allow us to explore targeted treatment of the epidermal lipid barrier, immunotherapy or colonization with non-pathogenic strains in the future.

Key points

- *Malassezia* dermatitis is a common skin infection in the dog, less common in the cat and, generally, develops secondary to an underlying disease in both species
- Topical therapy is the initial treatment of choice
- Atopic dogs can develop a hypersensitivity to *Malassezia*. Affected individuals are often intensely pruritic when even small numbers of *Malassezia* are present on the skin

---

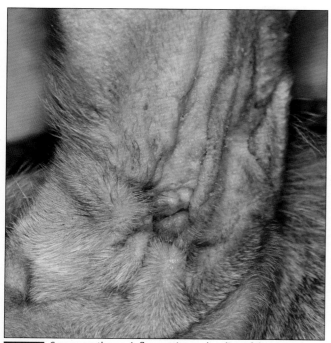

26.9 Severe erythema, inflammation and scaling of the ventral pinna in a crossbreed dog with atopic dermatitis. Similar lesions were present in the interdigital skin, muzzle, axillae and groin. An intradermal allergen test was positive for *Malassezia* only. The dog had a good response to *Malassezia*-specific subcutaneous immunotherapy and topical anti-*Malassezia* treatment.
(Courtesy of Hilary Jackson)

References and further reading

Aberg L, Varjonen K and Ahman S (2017) Results of allergen-specific immunotherapy in atopic dogs with *Malassezia* hypersensitivity: a retrosective study of 16 cases. *Veterinary Dermatology* **28**, 633–e157

Angileri M, Pasquetti M, De Lucia M *et al.* (2019) Azole resistance of *Malassezia pachydermatis* causing treatment failure in a dog. *Medical Mycology Case Reports* **23**, 58–61

Bond R, Elwood CM, Littler RM *et al.* (1998) Humoral and cell mediated responses to *Malassezia pachydermatis* in healthy dogs and dogs with *Malassezia* dermatitis. *Veterinary Record* **143**, 381–384

Buommino E, Nocera FP, Paris, A *et al.* (2016) Correlation between genetic variability and virulence factors in clinical strains of *Malassezia pachydermatis* of animal origin. *New Microbiologica* **39**, 216–223

Cafarchia C, Gasser RB, Latrofa MS *et al.* (2008) Genetic variants of *Malassezia pachydermatis* from canine skin: body distribution and phospholipase activity. *FEMS Yeast Research* **8**, 451–459

Cavana P, Peano A, Petit J-Y *et al.* (2015) A pilot study of the efficacy of wipes containing chlorhexidine 0.3%, climbazole 0.5% and Tris-EDTA to reduce *Malassezia pachydermatis* populations on canine skin. *Veterinary Dermatology* **26**, 278–e261

Chan WY, Khazandi M, Hickey EE *et al.* (2019) *In vitro* antimicrobial activity of seven adjuvants against common pathogens associated with canine otitis externa. *Veterinary Dermatology* **30**, 133–e38

Chen TA and Hill PB (2005) The biology of *Malassezia* organisms and their ability to induce responses and skin disease. *Veterinary Dermatology* **16**, 4–26

Czyzewska U, Bartoszewicz M, Siemieniuk M *et al.* (2018) Genetic relationships and population structure of *Malassezia pachydermatis* strains isolated from dogs with otitis externa and healthy dogs. *Mycologia* **110**, 666–676

Czyzewska U, Karkowska-Kuleta J, Bartoszewicz M *et al.* (2019) Differences in protein profiles between *Malassezia pachydermatis* strains obtained from healthy and infected dogs. *Mycologia* **111**, 624–631

Farver K, Morris DO, Shofer F *et al.* (2005) Humoral measurement of type-1 hypersensitivity reactions to a commercial *Malassezia* allergen. *Veterinary Dermatology* **16**, 261–268

Gimmler JR, White AG, Kennis RA *et al.* (2015) Determining canine skin concentrations of terbinafine to guide the treatment of *Malassezia* dermatitis. *Veterinary Dermatology* **26**, 411–e496

Kano R, Aramaki C, Murayama N *et al.* (2020) High multi-azole-resistant *Malassezia pachydermatis* clinical isolates from canine *Malassezia* dermatitis. *Medical Mycology* **58**, 197–200

Kloos I, Straubinger RK, Werckenthin C *et al.* (2013) Residual antibacterial activity of dog hairs after therapy with antimicrobial shampoos. *Veterinary Dermatology* **24**, 250–e254

Korbelik J, Singh A, Rousseau J *et al.* (2018) Analysis of the otic mycobiota in dogs with otitis externa compared to healthy individuals. *Veterinary Dermatology* **29**, 417–e138

Meason-Smith C, Diesel A, Paterson A *et al.* (2015) What is living on your dog's skin? Characterization of the canine cutaneous mycobiota and fungal dysbiosis in canine allergic dermatitis. *FEMS Microbiology Ecology* **91**, 1–12

Meason-Smith C, Diesel A, Patterson AP *et al.* (2016) Characterization of the cutaneous mycobiota in healthy and allergic cats using next generation sequencing. *Veterinary Dermatology* **28**, 71–e17

Meason-Smith C, Olivry T, Lawhon SD *et al.* (2019) *Malassezia* species dysbiosis in natural and allergen-induced atopic dermatitis in dogs. *Medical Mycology* **58**, 756–765

Mesman ML, Kirby AL, Rosenkrantz WS *et al.* (2016) Residual antibacterial activity of canine hair treated with topical antimicrobial sprays against *Staphylococcus pseudintermedius in vitro*. *Veterinary Dermatology* **27**, 261–e261

Morris DO and DeBoer DJ (2003) Evaluation of serum obtained from atopic dogs with dermatitis attributable to *Malassezia pachydermatis* for passive transfer of immediate hypersensitivity to that organism. *American Journal of Veterinary Research* **64**, 262–266

Morris DO, O'Shea K, Shofer FS *et al.* (2005) *Malassezia pachydermatis* carriage in dog owners. *Emerging Infectious Diseases* **11**, 83–88

Mueller RS, Bergvall K, Bensignor E *et al.* (2012) A review of topical therapy for skin infections with bacteria and yeast. *Veterinary Dermatology* **23**, 330–e362

Negre A, Bensignor E and Guillot J (2008) Evidence-based veterinary dermatology: a systematic review of interventions for *Malassezia* dermatitis in dogs. *Veterinary Dermatology* **20**, 1–12

Nogueira Brilhante RS, da Rocha MG, de Melo Guedes GM *et al.* (2018) *Malassezia pachydermatis* from animals: Planktonic and biofilm antifungal susceptibility and its virulence arsenal. *Veterinary Microbiology* **220**, 47–52

Nuttall TJ and Halliwell REW (2001) Serum antibodies to *Malassezia* yeasts in canine atopic dermatitis. *Veterinary Dermatology* **12**, 327–332

Older CE, Diesel AB, Lawhon SD *et al.* (2019) The feline cutaneous and oral microbiota are influenced by breed and environment. *Plos One* **14**, e0220463

Oliveira AMP, Devesa J and Hill PB (2018) *In vitro* efficacy of a honey-based gel against canine clinical isolates of *Staphylococcus pseudintermedius* and *Malassezia pachydermatis*. *Veterinary Dermatology* **29**, 180–e65

Puig L, Castella G and Cabaes FJ (2016) Cryptic Diversity of *Malassezia pachydermatis* from healthy and diseased domestic animals. *Mycopathologia* **181**, 681–688

Puig L, Rosa Bragulat M, Castella G *et al.* (2017) Characterization of the species *Malassezia pachydermatis* and re-evaluation of its lipid dependence using a synthetic agar medium. *Plos One* **12**, e0179148

Rafferty R, Robinson VH, Harris J *et al.* (2019) A pilot study of the *in vitro* antimicrobial activity and *in vivo* residual activity of chlorhexidine and acetic acid/boric acid impregnated cleansing wipes. *BMC Veterinary Research* **15**, 382

Ramos SJ, Woodward M, Hoppers SM *et al.* (2019) Residual antibacterial activity of canine hair treated with five mousse products against *Staphylococcus pseudintermedius in vitro*. *Veterinary Dermatology* **30**, 183–e157

Sim JXF, Khazandi M, Chan WY *et al.* (2019) Antimicrobial activity of thyme oil, oregano oil, thymol and carvacrol against sensitive and resistant microbial isolates from dogs with otitis externa. *Veterinary Dermatology* **30**, 524–e159

Swinney A, Fazakerley J, McEwan NA *et al.* (2008) Comparative *in vitro* antimicrobial efficacy of commercial ear cleaners. *Veterinary Dermatology* **19**, 373–379

Widmer G, Ferrer L, Favrot C *et al.* (2018) Glucocorticosteroids and ciclosporin do not significantly impact canine cutaneous microbiota. *BMC Veterinary Research* **14**

Young R, Buckley L, McEwan NA *et al.* (2012) Comparative *in vitro* efficacy of antimicrobial shampoos: a pilot study. *Veterinary Dermatology* **23**, 36–40

Zareei M, Mohammadi SR, Shahbazi S *et al.* (2018) Evaluation of the ability of *Malassezia* species in biofilm formation. *Archives of Clinical Infectious Diseases* **13**

Chapter 27

Topical treatments

Carly Mason and Darren Berger

Topical therapies have an increasingly important role in managing small animal dermatology patients. They offer good access to the target tissue and, depending on the skin condition, may be used as a sole therapeutic agent or as part of a multimodal treatment regime. There are regional variations in availability and prescribing authorization worldwide. The clinician should take this into consideration and use locally approved products. It should also be noted that some topical products are not licensed for medicinal use. Subsequently, there are many *in vitro* studies describing benefits of a variety of agents, but good evidence from double-blinded placebo controlled *in vivo* clinical trials is lacking. It is therefore recommended that products with published *in vivo* efficacy are sought for use.

Aim of topical treatments

Many dermatoses will benefit from topical therapy. For example, canine atopic dermatitis cases commonly suffer from secondary infections, such as recurrent pyoderma (*Staphylococcus pseudintermedius*) or *Malassezia* dermatitis. Therefore, routine topical antimicrobial therapy is an important long-term management consideration for patients with canine atopic dermatitis, alongside control of the inflammatory aspects of the disease. Examples of diseases, where topical supportive treatments are useful, are summarized in Figure 27.1.

The active ingredients and formulation prescribed should be appropriate to the dermatosis present, hair coat

Disease	Comment
Parasitic: Routine prophylactic treatment for ectoparasites and endoparasites Demodicosis	• Spot-on, spray, rinse (see Chapter 8) • Removal of follicular debris • Treatment of secondary infection
Fungal: *Malassezia* dermatitis Dermatophytosis	• Fungicidal • Removal of organisms and debris • Prevention of relapse • Primary or concurrent therapy option • Sporicidal • Removal of scale/debris • Reduction of environmental contamination • Concurrent therapy with systemic treatment
Allergic skin disease: Canine and feline allergic skin diseases (e.g. canine atopic dermatitis; feline atopic syndrome[a])	• Treatment of secondary infections • Prevention of recurrent infections • Soothing/reduction of pruritus • Removal of allergens • Improve epidermal barrier function
Pyoderma: Secondary to any dermatitis disturbing the skin barrier ± immune system (primary pyoderma is very rare)	• Primary treatment option for superficial infections • More rapid lesion resolution when used as an adjunctive therapy with systemic antimicrobials • Minimal adverse events • Decrease bacterial burden on skin surface • Prevention of recurrent infections • Reduced potential for development of resistant bacterial strains
Keratinization: Primary or secondary disorders	• Treatment of secondary infections • Removal of scale • Improve epidermal barrier function
Autoimmune and immune-mediated	• Some disorders can be treated topically • Treatment of secondary infection until underlying disease process is controlled

27.1 Examples of diseases where topical therapy can be useful. [a] Cats are less commonly topically treated due to their general dislike of water. They are, however, often relatively easily treated with spot bathing of lesions.

type (length and density), location and type or extent of lesions. The active components may be antibacterial, antifungal, antipruritic, antiparasitic, antiseborrhoeic, astringent or moisturizing. Topical formulations commonly used include: shampoos, spot-on products, mousses/foams, sprays, rinses, wipes, creams, gels and ointments.

Time should be taken with the owner during a consultation to consider the suitability of topical therapy. It is important to discuss the method of application, ability of the owner to perform the advised regime, patient temperament, treatment cost and affordability. The advantages and disadvantages of topical therapy are summarized in Figure 27.2.

Once topical therapy is applied, it must have adequate contact time (product and formulation dependent) to penetrate and diffuse through the epidermis to take effect. Products that can penetrate the epidermal barrier may gain access to the dermal vascular system, which may potentially result in systemic side effects. This is particularly important to consider when more potent topical glucocorticoids are prescribed.

Advantages
• Treatment applied directly to the target organ
• Minimal adverse events (typically well tolerated)
• May reduce the requirement or shorten the duration of systemic medication (e.g. antibiotics)
• May reduce the exposure of bystander organisms or microbiota in other organ systems to antibiotics
• Reduces odour
• Removes allergens, microbial organisms, scale and debris
• Aids drainage of deep lesions
• May improve patient comfort
• Normally effective and potentially safer therapeutic option in cases with meticillin-resistant staphylococcal infections
• Often more economical than systemic treatment

Disadvantages
• Labour intensive, which may result in decreased owner compliance
• Local side effects possible for pet and owner (e.g. uncommon chlorhexidine sensitivity of owner or pet)
• Unsuitable if pet temperament is poor
• Owner health and ability must be considered
• Can be difficult to perform in cats
• Clinician must spend time educating the owner on proper use

27.2 Advantages and disadvantages of topical therapy.

Shampoos

Shampoos are the mainstay of topical therapy for dogs. They typically contain cleansing and therapeutic agents. Shampoos mechanically remove superficial scale, crust, inflammatory cells, exudate, glandular products, microbial organisms, debris, pollen and allergens from the skin. They are particularly useful when generalized disease is present and when the patient's hair coat is long or dense. Shampoos may also be used in cases of localized disease, but other formulations, such as wipes or mousses, may offer additional advantages. Cats tend to be resentful of whole body bathing, but localized spot bathing can be useful and well tolerated for focal lesions.

When using a shampoo, it is important to understand that efficacy likely correlates with contact time, as the active agents are typically removed when the patient is rinsed. The exact contact time varies by active ingredient, commercial product and the condition being treated. This will typically vary from 5–15 minutes, but a good general

guideline for antimicrobial treatment or infection preventatives is 10–15 minutes. It is recommended that owners use a clock or timer as most will overestimate the time when not monitored. To work around the issue of contact time, some companies have utilized microvesicle technology to potentially improve stability, binding and sustained release of active agents over time.

There is currently a plethora of products available to the veterinary surgeon (veterinarian) the therapeutic qualities of which are influenced by the ingredients they contain. A shampoo formulation may be drying, rehydrating, keratolytic, keratoplastic, antibacterial, antifungal, antipruritic or antiparasitic (antiparasitic shampoos tend to have poor residual action and are therefore not routinely recommended). It is important that the various components of these products be understood, so that the correct shampoo can be selected for the disorder being treated. Although in most cases a single product may be sufficient, there are instances where multiple products, or a transition to a different product, may be required. One such circumstance commonly occurs in canine patients with atopic dermatitis. Initially, an antiseptic shampoo may be required to resolve or prevent secondary infections, but once the patient is adequately controlled, they may benefit from adjustment to a hydrating, moisturizing, antipruritic or barrier replacement shampoo.

Antiseptic shampoos

Examples of lesions that may benefit from antiseptic shampoo treatment are shown in Figures 27.3 and 27.4.

Chlorhexidine (2–4%)

This active agent tends to be the most common antiseptic selected for therapy as it has the best evidence to support its use. It has good broad-spectrum antibacterial and antifungal activity above 3% concentration against *Malassezia* yeast (Maynard *et al.*, 2011). There is good evidence for using 2–4% chlorhexidine shampoos for superficial pyoderma, including those involving meticillin-resistant *Staphylococcus pseudintermedius* (MRSP) strains (Mueller *et al.*, 2012; Borio *et al.*, 2015; Morris *et al.*, 2017). When used as sole therapeutic agent, twice weekly shampooing may improve rather than resolve pyoderma (Murayama *et al.*, 2010; Loeffler *et al.*, 2011), although it does have

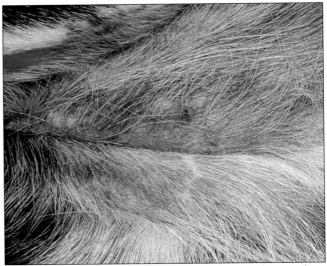

27.3 Epidermal collarettes, papules and pustules on the ventral abdomen of a dog.

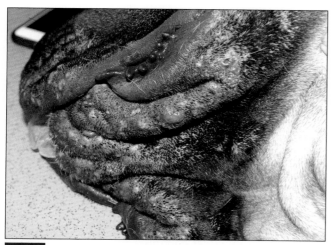

27.4 Deep pyoderma chin acne lesions in a Boerboel Dog.

some residual activity (Kloos *et al.*, 2013). However, more frequent use (up to daily) or use alongside supportive chlorhexidine-containing spray or mousse has been demonstrated to effectively resolve clinical signs, similar to the use of systemic antibiotics (Bryan *et al.*, 2012). Regardless of whether it is used in sole or combination therapeutic protocols, topical therapy is indicated until seven days post clinical resolution and cytological cure.

Chlorhexidine shampoo efficacy and stability may be formulation-dependent due to the cationic nature of the agent. A recent *in vitro* study demonstrated this concept, where a shampoo containing 2% chlorhexidine and 2% miconazole had superior *in vitro* performance over some higher chlorhexidine-containing products (Kloos *et al.*, 2013). Adverse effects as a result of chlorhexidine shampoos are uncommon and primarily consist of irritant or contact dermatitis, reported in dogs and humans. Prolonged use for wounds at >0.5% should be avoided as it can slow granulation tissue formation. Miconazole has some anti-staphylococcal activity and has demonstrated *in vitro* synergistic action with chlorhexidine. There is good evidence for use of 2% chlorhexidine and 2% miconazole shampoo, and some evidence for 3% chlorhexidine and 0.5% climbazole shampoo, for *Malassezia* dermatitis (Bourdeau *et al.*, 2011; Mueller *et al.*, 2012).

Benzoyl peroxide (2–3%, USA only)

This is a second line antiseptic agent with some evidence for use in superficial pyoderma (Mueller *et al.*, 2012). It is reported to have broad-spectrum antibacterial activity. Efficacy for bacterial pyoderma and residual action are described when used 2–3 times weekly (Kwochka *et al.*, 1991; Viaud *et al.*, 2012). Other studies did not support efficacy for superficial pyoderma (Loeffler *et al.*, 2011), nor residual action (Kloos *et al.*, 2013), when used twice weekly.

Ethyl lactate (10%)

This agent has reported antibacterial and keratoplastic activity, but there are some reports of unsatisfactory action *in vivo* and *in vitro*. Therefore, further evidence of clinical efficacy is required before its use can be routinely recommended for treatment of bacterial pyoderma as a sole therapeutic agent (Mueller *et al.*, 2012). However, ethyl lactate containing products may offer benefit when used in combination with systemic cephalexin to reduce duration of treatment (De Jaham, 2003).

Acetic acid (2%) and boric acid (2%)

There are anecdotal claims for treatment of bacterial and yeast dermatitis with these agents, and *in vitro* studies have shown mixed results with regards to efficacy against *Staphylococcus pseudintermedius*, *Malassezia pachydermatis* and *Pseudomonas aeruginosa*. As a result, more controlled *in vivo* studies are required to document clinical efficacy before use over other proven active agents can be recommended (Mueller *et al.*, 2012).

Other agents

Triclosan is present in some antiseptic shampoos but no supportive studies of efficacy have been performed in animals to recommend use. Povidone–iodine has evidence for antibacterial efficacy but adverse effects, including irritation, make it less suitable for routine use. Piroctone olamine inhibits adherence of bacteria and *Malassezia* to canine keratinocytes *in vitro*. Clinical effect *in vivo* is unproven. Sodium hypochlorite (active ingredient of bleach) is also found in a shampoo combined with salicylic acid (USA only). Sodium hypochlorite has excellent *in vitro* activity against a wide array of microbes. However, at this time there is only a single pilot investigation showing potential *in vivo* benefit that needs to be validated in larger controlled trials before routine use can be recommended (Fadok and Irwin, 2019).

Antiseborrhoeic (descaling) shampoos

These are selected for management of primary or secondary keratinization disorders. Descaling agents may be keratolytic or keratoplastic. Keratolytic agents decrease corneocyte adhesion and aid scale removal. Keratoplastic agents normalize aberrant keratinization by reducing basal cell turnover, and many have unproven mechanisms of action. Different products should be selected for use in cases of dry seborrhoea (seborrhoea sicca) and greasy seborrhoea (seborrhoea oleosa). Examples of dry and greasy seborrhoea that may benefit from descaling shampoo are given in Figures 27.5 and 27.6.

Benzoyl peroxide (2–3%, USA only)

This agent is keratolytic, keratoplastic, degreasing and has follicular flushing actions. Indications include seborrhoea oleosa, demodicosis and chin acne. Disadvantages include its strong drying nature, bleaching of dark hair and fabrics, and irritant contact dermatitis (avoid using high concentrations in cats). Applying moisturizing agents after use can be useful to reduce excessive drying.

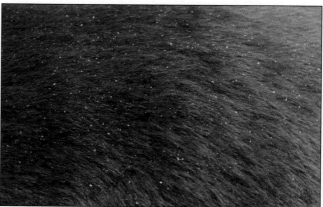

27.5 Seborrhoea sicca on the dorsum of a dog with atopic dermatitis.

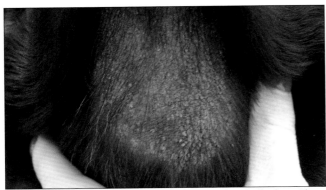

27.6 Seborrhoea oleosa involving the ventral neck of a dog with atopic dermatitis and secondary *Malassezia* overgrowth and pyoderma.

Salicylic acid (2%)

Salicylic acid is keratolytic (above 3% concentration), keratoplastic, bacteriostatic and mildly antipruritic. It is synergistic with sulphur. Indications include primary and secondary keratinization disorders.

Sulphur (0.25–2%)

Sulphur is keratolytic, keratoplastic, antifungal, antibacterial and antiparasitic. It is a poor degreaser. Indications include dry seborrhoea in primary keratinization disorders and seborrhoeic dermatitis. It is synergistic with 2% salicylic acid. It can be drying and irritating.

Other agents

Some agents previously marketed for animals are now only available in human medicinal formulations. These include coal tar and selenium sulphide that have keratolytic and keratoplastic actions, but are very drying and irritating. Selenium sulphide (1%) has good antifungal action. They are only appropriate for intermittent use in patients with excessively greasy, scaly skin. Coal tar is potentially carcinogenic and is toxic to cats.

Moisturizing shampoos

Products containing colloidal oatmeal are useful moisturizing agents for slightly dry scaly skin, or for gentle routine bathing of sensitive skin. They are soothing and have a mild antipruritic action.

Spot-on products

These products are popular with pet owners due to convenience and ease of use (see Chapter 8 for more information regarding products containing ecto-/endoparasiticides). Lipid complex spot-on products marketed for canine atopic dermatitis and seborrhoeic disease are lipophilic and diffuse through the intercellular stratum corneum matrix for slow release of the active ingredients. There is evidence of abnormalities in epidermal barrier function in canine atopic dermatitis that may increase transepidermal water loss, increase allergen permeability and reduce epidermal defence against microbes. Therefore, safe topical products which improve stratum corneum function are ideal. These spot-on products contain skin barrier constituents and those with evidence for use include:

- Phytosphingosine used weekly. Currently only anecdotal evidence of clinical benefit
- Free fatty acids, cholesterol and ceramides (Allerderm™) used twice weekly (UK only). There is evidence for improvement of microscopic skin barrier abnormalities (Piekutowska *et al.*, 2008; Popa *et al.*, 2012). This product reduced the clinical signs of atopic dermatitis in dogs in one uncontrolled and one controlled trial (Fujimura *et al.* 2011; Marsella *et al.*, 2013), but was ineffective in another controlled trial (Hobi *et al.*, 2017)
- Unsaturated fatty acids and essential oils (Dermoscent® essential 6) used weekly. This product showed some efficacy in canine atopic dermatitis by improving clinical signs and pruritus (Tretter and Mueller, 2011; Blaskovic *et al.*, 2014).

In conclusion, larger controlled studies are needed to determine whether skin barrier repair produces significant clinical benefit in canine atopic dermatitis (Marsella *et al.*, 2013). Potential problems with spot-on use include: product run off the skin and coat, objection to product odour, topical sensitivity and removal by bathing.

Sprays and foams

Many products are now available in a mist spray or foam formulation and are generally well tolerated by cats and dogs. They can be used to apply products to large or localized areas, regions with less hair coat, and intertriginous areas. If applied to haired skin, they may require rubbing in by hand after application to ensure adequate penetration of the product to the epidermal layer. They contain similar ingredients to many shampoo formulations and may be antiseptic, moisturizing or antipruritic in action. They are not rinsed from the skin and provide a convenient rapid alternative to shampoo therapy, especially for owners that find bathing difficult. Care must be taken when applying to sensitive areas such as the periocular and perioral skin (e.g. apply with a cotton pad) to prevent product contact with the eyes or mouth.

Antiseptic spray/foam

These products may contain 2–3% chlorhexidine or antifungal agents (1% ketoconazole, 2% miconazole, 0.5% climbazole). As with shampoos, 2–4% chlorhexidine spray/mousse may have good residual activity and efficacy may be dependent on formulation rather than concentration (Mesman *et al.*, 2016; Ramos *et al.*, 2019). Foams and sprays are often combined with shampoo therapy to reduce the frequency of bathing. They may be used daily to treat superficial and surface pyoderma. They can also be used 2–3 times weekly to prevent bacterial or *Malassezia* infections. As with shampoos, they should be used until 7 days after clinical and cytological cure. Products containing antimicrobial peptides are safe, but currently support for their use in the prevention or treatment of bacterial pyoderma is purely anecdotal. A sodium hypochlorous spray is available and has *in vitro* antimicrobial claims against many pathogens, including meticillin-resistant *Staphylococcus aureus* (MRSA). Controlled studies are lacking but benefit has been seen in the treatment of acute moist dermatitis (pyotraumatic dermatitis), bacterial overgrowth syndrome and pyoderma, including multiple drug resistant (MDR) strains.

Moisturizing spray/foam

Colloidal oatmeal is available in spray/foam products and is useful for treatment when moisturizing is required (e.g. mild dry scale in the hair coat).

Antipruritic and anti-inflammatory spray/foam

Topical steroids are commonly available in a spray formulation for the treatment of pruritus. Commercially available products include the following active ingredients: 0.0584% hydrocortisone aceponate (UK only), 0.015% triamcinolone acetonide (USA only), 1.77 mg/ml triamcinolone acetonide with 17.7 mg/ml salicyclic acid (UK only) and 1% hydrocortisone (see Chapter 10). Other sprays available include 2% diphenhydramine or 1% pramoxine (USA only). A *Hamamelis* (witch hazel) extract with menthol spray can be used for cooling pruritic areas. Phytosphingosine is also available in spray and foam formulations for application. It has some anti-inflammatory effects, alongside skin barrier support. Daily spraying may improve the clinical signs of canine atopic dermatitis (Bourdeau *et al.*, 2007; Tretter and Mueller, 2011) or be beneficial in primary or secondary keratinization disorders.

Wipes

Medicated wipes are very easy to use and owner compliance is often good. They are very useful for focal lesions and to clean intertriginous areas, such as the facial folds, interdigital spaces, inguinal and perineal area (Figure 27.7). They contain similar active antiseptic agents to shampoos, sprays and foams. Enhancing agents (e.g. Tris-EDTA, zinc) or moisturizing agents (glycerine) may be included. These products may be used daily, or as required to resolve secondary infections, or as a preventative therapy for problematic regions (lip folds and interdigital regions). Despite their common use, there are very few supportive studies demonstrating the efficacy of these products. Small investigative studies have revealed the ability of wipes to reduce *Malassezia* spp. populations on canine skin and demonstrated residual action (Cavana *et al.*, 2015).

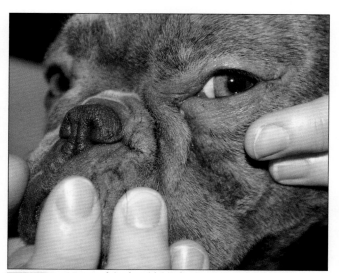

27.7 Intertrigo of the facial fold of a French Bulldog with atopic dermatitis and secondary pyoderma.

Rinses and soaks

Concentrated solutions are diluted and poured or sponged on to the patient. In veterinary dermatology, lime sulphur and enilconazole are the primary agents used in rinse products (see Chapter 25 for information on their use in the treatment of dermatophytosis). Enilconazole rinses are not authorized for use for *Malassezia* dermatitis but have good antifungal activity. They may be toxic to cats. Magnesium sulphate (Epsom salt) soaks are a useful adjunctive treatment for deep pyoderma lesions (e.g. pododermatitis); they aid in the removal of inflammatory discharge and are soothing. Diluted household bleach (sodium hypochlorite) rinses are anecdotally advocated for the treatment and prevention of MDR pyoderma. Further studies are indicated to determine the most effective concentration and frequency of application.

Creams, ointments, gels and balms

These useful topical agents for skin disease are covered in more detail in Chapters 10, 20, 22 and 32. Their use is limited in haired animals to localized relatively small lesions. They are mostly used for the nasal planum, lip folds, paws, elbows, ears and localized pyoderma. They generally contain antimicrobial, anti-inflammatory, moisturizing and ultraviolet (UV) radiation protective agents. Antibacterial agents include fusidic acid, silver sulfadiazine, mupirocin, benzoyl peroxide (USA only) and medicinal honey. Topical steroids and anti-inflammatory agents are commonly present in ointments (e.g. betamethasone combined with fusidic acid, 0.1% tacrolimus) (see Chapters 10 and 29 for more information). Human antifungal creams and ointments (e.g. clotrimazole, miconazole, terbinafine) are not authorized for use for *Malassezia* dermatitis or dermatophytosis, but may be useful to treat focal areas if licensed shampoo use is not possible.

Emollient agents soften the skin and include oils or lanolin. Moisturizing agents increase the water content of the skin and can be applied between baths. Products containing propylene glycol, glycerine, urea (USA only), sodium lactate and lactic acid have moisturizing properties. A moisturizing balm containing essential fatty acids and essential oil has shown benefit in managing canine idiopathic nasal hyperkeratosis (Catarino *et al.*, 2017). Petroleum jelly and salicylic acid gels (USA only) are commonly used for nasal and digital hyperkeratosis. High concentrations of propylene glycol (>60%) are keratolytic and can be used topically to treat focal areas of severe hyperkeratosis, or at 50–75% (diluted with water) can be used as a spray treatment for sebaceous adenitis. This can be messy to handle. This agent also has antibacterial and antifungal actions. Urea is humectant and keratolytic at concentrations over 20%. It may be used for moisturizing calluses, nasodigital hyperkeratosis and ear margin seborrhoea.

How to use topical agents

The properties, indications for use and active ingredients of topical products available are summarized in Figure 27.8. The mechanism of action, formulations and indications for commonly used active agents are summarized in Figure 27.9.

Property	Indications	Active ingredients
Emollient (soften, lubricant, soothe) or moisturizer (hydrate)	Cases requiring frequent bathing Mild dry/scaly hair coats Routine gentle shampoo	Fatty acids Lipids Phytosphingosine[b] Ceramides[b] Urea Glycerine Colloidal oatmeal Chitosanide Propylene glycol
Antiseborrhoeic	Mild to moderate dry or greasy scaling Severe greasy scaling	Salicylic acid Sulphur Benzoyl peroxide (USA only) Zinc gluconate Pyridoxine Phytosphingosine Coal tar Selenium sulphide
Antibacterial	Surface or superficial pyoderma as a sole or adjunctive agent Deep pyoderma as an adjunctive agent	Chlorhexidine[ab] Benzoyl peroxide[ab] (USA only) Ethyl lactate[b] Triclosan Iodine Sulphur Carbohydrates (mannose, D-galactose, L-rhamnose)[b] Hypochlorous acid[b] Sodium hypochlorite[b] Nisin (USA only) Silver sulfadiazine[b]
Antimycotic	Mild Malassezia dermatitis as a sole agent to prevent or treat Adjunctive for moderate to severe Malassezia dermatitis or dermatophytosis	2% miconazole/2% chlorhexidine[a] 3% chlorhexidine Miconazole[a] Climbazole[b] Ketoconazole Enilconazole[a] Selenium sulphide
Antipruritic (moisturizing agents can also provide some antipruritic effect via stratum corneum hydration, e.g. colloidal oatmeal)	Adjunctive support for pruritic skin disease	1% hydrocortisone shampoo (USA only) 0.0584% hydrocortisone aceponate (UK only)[a] 0.015% triamcinolone (USA only)[a] 0.1% tacrolimus Colloidal oatmeal Phytosphingosine Hamamelis/menthol (cooling) 0.01% fluocinolone (USA only) 2% diphenhydramine (USA only) 1% pramoxine (USA only)

27.8 Properties of topical agents, their indications for use and active ingredients. [a] Ingredients with best *in vivo* evidence; [b] Ingredients with *in vitro* evidence.

Active ingredient	Mechanism of action	Formulations	Indications
Chlorhexidine (2–4%)	Cell wall damage and intracellular coagulation at higher concentrations	Shampoo Spray Foam Wipes	Treatment and prevention of bacterial pyoderma
Chlorhexidine (2%) + miconazole (2%) Chlorhexidine (2%) + ketoconazole (1%) Chlorhexidine (3%) + climbazole (0.5%) Chlorhexidine (0.3%), climbazole (0.5%), zinc gluconate (1%), tris-EDTA	Chlorhexidine as above Azoles damage fungal cell wall Cell wall damage	Shampoo Spray Mousse (USA only) Wipes	Treatment and prevention of Malassezia dermatitis Treatment and prevention of bacterial pyoderma and Malassezia dermatitis
Benzoyl peroxide (2–3%)	Potent oxidizing activity produces free radicals and disrupts bacterial cell membranes	Shampoo (USA only) Gel (USA only)	Greasy seborrhoea Demodicosis Pyoderma Chin acne
Ethyl lactate (10%)[a] (combined with 2% salicyclic acid, USA only)	Penetrates epidermis, hair follicle and sebaceous gland and is hydrolysed to lactic acid and ethanol, which have antibacterial properties	Shampoo Mousse (USA only)	Mild scaling Mild superficial pyoderma
Acetic acid (2%) + boric acid (2%)[a]	Acid toxicity to cells	Shampoo Spray Wipes	Treatment and prevention of bacterial pyoderma and Malassezia dermatitis

27.9 The mechanism of action, formulations and indications for commonly used active agents. [a] Products with low *in vivo* evidence.

As some ingredients can be percutaneously absorbed or cause contact hypersensitivity, owners should wear gloves for application. With extensive lesions and long, dense or matted coats, clipping the hair coat or grooming prior to treatment may be required to facilitate penetration and contact of the product with the skin. A gentle cleansing shampoo can be used prior to antiseptic shampoo if the coat contains debris.

With bathing, the animal should be soaked in water until wet. Shampoos are applied to the skin neat or diluted according to the bottle instructions and lathered in (concentrating on the worst affected areas). It is important to note that many antiseptic shampoos will not lather well, which may lead to excessive use of the product by the owner if they are not properly instructed. After lathering, a contact time of 10–15 minutes is needed for active ingredient action and hydration of the stratum corneum. The shampoo is then thoroughly rinsed from the coat and the pet should be towel dried. Insufficient shampoo volume or inadequate duration of contact can lead to treatment failure.

Other topical products (sprays, foams, wipes, ointments) should be applied to the target area. Some require gentle massage to allow contact with the lesions or to disperse through the coat. The area should be allowed to dry and licking prevented using an Elizabethan collar or distraction for 10–15 minutes (e.g. walking, food, play).

Topical therapy for bacterial pyoderma

Canine bacterial pyoderma is one of the most common conditions presented to veterinary surgeons. There is an increasing worldwide incidence of MDR infections, including MRSP. Therefore, many clinicians have shifted towards the use of topical antiseptics as primary alternatives to systemic antimicrobials. Topical therapy can also be a useful adjunctive to systemic antibiotic treatment, by reducing time to clinical resolution and improving drainage of deeper lesions.

There is good evidence that topical antiseptic therapy alone can be effective in preventing and treating pyoderma, and routine use of systemic antibiotics should be challenged. Topical antiseptics are now recommended for surface or superficial pyoderma involving sensitive and MDR staphylococcal strains, when patient and client compliance is expected (Beco *et al.*, 2013; Hillier *et al.*, 2014; Morris *et al.*, 2017). This reduces gut flora exposure and development of resistance to systemic antimicrobials. Systemic antibiotics should be reserved for cases of deep pyoderma, failure of more superficial pyodermas to resolve with topical therapy, cases where owner or pet compliance is problematic, and severe wide-spread lesions that are difficult to treat topically. Concerns exist regarding development of resistance to topical antiseptics. However, there is no conclusive evidence of treatment failures and the currently consistently low staphylococcal minimum inhibitory concentration will be overcome by the high topical concentrations used.

Key points

- Topical therapy is an important component in the management of many dermatoses. The feasibility of applying topical therapies at home should be discussed with the owner to maximize clinical outcome
- Owners should be advised to wear gloves, and clipping long/dense hair coats is recommended to facilitate contact with the skin

References and further reading

Beco L, Guagere E, Lorente Mendex C et al. (2013) Suggested guidelines for using systemic antimicrobials in bacterial skin infections: part 2 – antimicrobial choice, treatment regimens and compliance. *Veterinary Record* 172, 156–160

Blaskovic M, Rosenktrantz W, Neuber A et al. (2014) The effect of a spot-on formulation containing polyunsaturated fatty acids and essential oils on dogs with atopic dermatitis. *Veterinary journal* 199, 39–43

Borio S, Colombo S, La Rosa G et al. (2015) Effectiveness of a combined (4% chlorhexidine digluconate shampoo and solution) protocol in MRS and non-MRS canine superficial pyoderma: a randomized, blinded, antibiotic-controlled study. *Veterinary Dermatology* 26, 339–344

Bourdeau P, Bruet V and Gremillet C (2007) Evaluation of phytosphingosine-containing shampoo and microemulsion spray in the clinical control of allergic dermatoses in dogs: preliminary results of a multicentre study. *Veterinary Dermatology* 18, 177–178

Bourdeau P, Bruet V, Roussel A et al. (2011) Comparative efficacy of two shampoos containing an azole derivative to decrease clinical signs and *Malassezia pachydermatis* counts in basset hounds: a comparative blinded, randomized trial. *Veterinary Dermatology* 22, 467

Bryan J, Frank L, Rohrbach B et al. (2012) Treatment outcome of dogs with meticillin-resistant and meticillin-susceptible *Staphylococcus pseudintermedius* pyoderma. *Veterinary Dermatology* 23, 361–368

Catarino M, Combarros-Garcia D, Mimouni P et al. (2018) Control of canine idiopathic nasal hyperkeratosis with a natural skin restorative balm: a randomised double-blind placebo-controlled study. *Veterinary Dermatology* 29, 134–138

Cavana P, Peano A, Petit JY et al., (2015) A pilot study of the efficacy of wipes containing chlorhexidine 0.3%, climbazole 0.5% and Tris-EDTA to reduce *Malassezia pachydermatis* populations on canine skin. *Veterinary Dermatology* 26, 278–283

De Jaham C (2003) Effects of an ethyl lactate shampoo in conjunction with a systemic antibiotic in the treatment of canine superficial bacterial pyoderma in an open-label, non placebo-controlled study. *Veterinary Therapeutics* 4, 94–100

Fadok VA and Irwin K (2019) Sodium hypochlorite/salicylic acid shampoo for treatment of canine staphylococcal pyoderma. *Journal of the American Animal Hospital Association* 55, 117–123

Fujimura M, Nakatsuji Y, Fujiwara S et al., (2011) Spot-on skin lipid complex as an adjunct therapy in dogs with atopic dermatitis: an open, pilot study. *Veterinary Medicine International* 281846

Hillier A, Lloyd DH, Weese JS et al. (2014) Guidelines for the diagnosis and antimicrobial therapy of canine superficial bacterial folliculitis (Antimicrobial Guidelines working Group of the International Society for Companion Animal Infectious Diseases. *Veterinary Dermatology* 25, 163–e43

Hobi S, Klinger C, Classen J et al. (2017) The effects of a topical lipid complex therapy on dogs with atopic dermatitis: a double blind, randomized, placebo-controlled study. *Veterinary Research* 28, 369–372

Kloos I, Straubinger RK, Werckenthin C et al. (2013) Residual antibacterial activity of dog hairs after therapy with antimicrobial shampoos. *Veterinary Dermatology* 24, 250–255

Kwochka KW and Kowalski JJ (1991) Prophylactic efficacy of four antibacterial shampoos against *Staphylococcus intermedius* in dogs. *American Journal of Veterinary Research* 52, 115–118

Loeffler A, Bond R and Cobb MA (2011) Comparison of a chlorhexidine and a benzoyl peroxide shampoo as a sole treatment in canine superficial pyoderma. *Veterinary Record* 169, 249–253

Marsella R (2013) Fixing the skin barrier: past, present and future – man and dog compared. *Veterinary Dermatology* 24, 73–76

Marsella R, Genovese D, Gilmer L et al. (2013) Investigations on the effects of a topical ceramides-containing emulsion (Allerderm spot on) on clinical signs and skin barrier function in dogs with topic dermatitis: a double-blinded, randomized, controlled study. *International Journal of Applied Research in Veterinary Medicine* 11, 110–116

Maynard L, Reme CA and Viaud S (2011) Comparison of two shampoos for the treatment of canine *Malassezia* dermatitis: a randomised controlled trial. *Journal of Small Animal Practice* 52, 566–572

Mesman M, Kirby A, Rosenkrantz W et al. (2016) Residual antibacterial activity of canine hair treated with topical antimicrobial sprays against *Staphylococcus pseudintermedius* in vitro. *Veterinary Dermatology* 27, 261–267

Morris DO, Loeffler A, Davis MF et al. (2017) Recommendations for approaches to meticillin-resistant staphylococcal infections of small animals: diagnosis, therapeutic considerations and preventative measures. *Clinical Consensus Guidelines of the World Association for Veterinary Dermatology. Veterinary Dermatology* 28, 304–330

Mueller RS, Bergvall K, Bensignor E et al. (2012) A review of topical therapy for skin infections with bacteria and yeast. *Veterinary Dermatology* 23, 330–341

Murayama N and Nagata M (2010) Efficacy of a surgical scrub including 2% chlorexidine acetate for canine superficial pyoderma. *Veterinary Research* 21, 586–592

Piekutowska A, Pin D, Reme CA et al. (2008) Effects of topically applied preparation of epidermal lipids on the stratum corneum barrier of atopic dogs. *Journal of Comparative Pathology* 138, 197–203

Popa I, Remous N, Osta B et al. (2012) The lipid alternations in the stratum corneum of dogs with atopic dermatitis are alleviated by topical application of a sphingolipid containing emulsion. *Clinical and Experimental Dermatology* 37, 665–671

Ramos SJ, Woodward M, Hoppers SM et al. (2019) Residual antibacterial activity of canine hair treated with five mousse products against *Staphylococcus pseudintermedius* in vitro. *Veterinary Dermatology* 30, 183–187

Tretter S and Mueller RS (2011) The influence of topical unsaturated fatty acids and essential oils on normal and atopic dogs. *Journal of the American Animal Hospital Association* 47, 236–240

Viaud S, Maynard L and Sanquer A (2012) Comparison of two shampoos as a sole treatment for canine bacteria overgrowth syndrome. *Veterinary Record* 170, 675–679

Chapter 28

Autoimmune and immune-mediated skin disease

Hilary A. Jackson

Autoimmune and immune-mediated diseases of the skin are uncommon or rare disorders. The severity can vary from mild localized disease to life-threatening conditions. Many diseases are seen more commonly in certain breeds, suggesting an hereditary predisposition. Diagnosis of such disorders is not always easy and usually relies on biopsy for histopathology. Management should never be instituted until a specific diagnosis has been reached and treatment is often difficult.

Features that may be suggestive of autoimmune and immune-mediated skin disease include:

- Unusual, symmetrical distribution of lesions
- Failure to respond completely to appropriate antimicrobial therapy
- Discrete erosions or ulcerations
- Waxing/waning course
- Development of skin disease in a middle-aged animal.

Golden rules for obtaining diagnostic biopsy samples

- Perform cytology on samples from the surface of suspicious skin lesions – if bacteria or *Malassezia* organisms are present, treat for these first
- If skin lesions do not respond completely to appropriate antimicrobial treatment:
  - If bacteria are still present, consider bacterial culture and sensitivity testing
  - If bacteria and *Malassezia* are absent, perform a biopsy
- Biopsy the newest lesions and select primary lesions:
  - Pustules/vesicles or bullae in their entirety
  - If ulcerations/erosions are present then biopsy across the margins using a wedge technique (in many cases the diagnostic material is in the epidermis, therefore, ensure that the sample submitted includes the surface layer)
  - Biopsy the footpads/nasal planum and other sensitive areas under anaesthesia
  - Take multiple biopsy samples from representative areas
- Biopsy samples should be sent with a complete history and clinical description to a pathologist with an interest in dermatohistopathology

---

Autoimmune diseases

Autoimmune skin diseases are characterized by the development of autoantibodies directed at structural proteins in the skin, which result in disruption of the normal architecture. The severity of the disease usually depends on the role and site of the target structure. Thus, antibodies directed at keratinocyte adhesion proteins in canine pemphigus foliaceus result in a superficial pustular disease, crusts and erosions, whereas antibodies directed at structural proteins in the basement membrane, such as collagen VII in epidermolysis bullosa acquisita, result in subepidermal clefting, ulceration and pain (for information on uveodermatological syndrome and vitiligo, see Chapter 16; and for details on alopecia areata, see Chapter 17).

Pemphigus foliaceus

Pemphigus foliaceus (PF) is the most common autoimmune skin disease seen in dogs and cats. In both species it can vary in extent and severity. PF can arise spontaneously, but in some cases drugs, vaccines or neoplasia appear to trigger the disease. Various topical and systemic antibiotics have been implicated along with topical spot-on flea and tick prophylactics. Sunlight may also exacerbate the lesions. Canine PF generally occurs in middle age, although occasionally dogs <12 months old are affected. Akitas and Chow Chows are predisposed to the disease. In most dogs with PF, the antibodies target desmocollin-1 (DSC1), one of several proteins involved in cell–cell adhesion of keratinocytes. The antibody target in cats is not known. A full history should be taken, paying particular attention to any recent or current drug treatment.

Differential diagnosis

The main differential diagnoses of PF include superficial pyoderma and pustular dermatophytosis, and contact dermatitis. Certain species of dermatophyte (usually *Trichophyton*) are corneophilic and produce keratinases that can disrupt keratinocyte adhesion. This results in a disorder that looks identical clinically and histologically to PF. In contrast to bacterial folliculitis, a disease in which lesions at different stages of development are present concurrently (e.g. papules, pustules, epidermal collarettes), in patients with PF, when a wave of lesions occurs, they are all at the same stage of development. The typical truncal distribution of lesions in bacterial folliculitis may also help to rank the differential diagnoses because pemphigus is a disease that usually, although not always, starts on the head.

Clinical approach

The primary lesion is a pustule, which readily ruptures resulting in multifocal crusts. The lesions have a predilection for the face, nasal planum, pinnae (concave and convex aspects) and footpads (Figure 28.1). In some dogs the disease becomes generalized, but the mucous membranes are spared. Pruritus can occur in the crusting phase and when infections develop. The disease typically has a waxing/waning course. Although specific systemic involvement is not present, the dog may be inappetent and lethargic when the disease is active.

Cats also present with facial involvement, but lesions in this species may develop in the claw beds, footpads and around the nipples. As with dogs, some animals will develop generalized disease. Cats are often lethargic, inappetent and may also be febrile.

Diagnostic tests: The key diagnostic tests for PF include:

- Cytology of an intact pustule
- Culture of intact pustular material
- Dermatophyte culture
- Biopsy for histopathology of an intact pustule.

The diagnosis of PF depends on compatible cytology and histopathology and, most importantly, ruling out an infectious cause of the pustule formation. On cytological examination, the pustules contain multiple non-degenerative neutrophils and free-floating acantholytic keratinocytes (Figure 28.2). A culture of the material from an intact pustule should be negative for bacteria, and culture of the scale/crust should be negative for dermatophytes. Multiple biopsy samples should be collected from intact pustules. These will demonstrate subcorneal pustule formation, which contains non-degenerate neutrophils and acantholytic keratinocytes (Figure 28.3). Special stains for dermatophytes should be negative.

Treatment

The management of PF can be difficult and many cases require lifelong therapy. Most published case series suggest that monotherapy with immunosuppressive doses of glucocorticoids should be used initially, but many dogs do not respond completely to this approach and additional therapies such as azathioprine, chlorambucil or ciclosporin have been required to effect control of the disease.

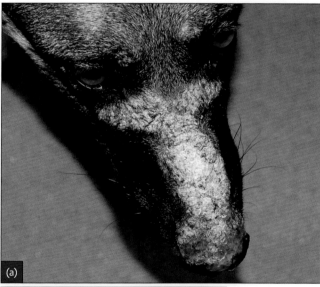

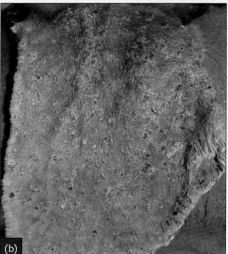

28.1 (a) Symmetrical crusting on the haired skin and nasal planum of a dog with pemphigus foliaceus. (b) Multifocal crusts on the convex pinna of a dog with drug-induced pemphigus foliaceus. (Courtesy of P Forsythe)

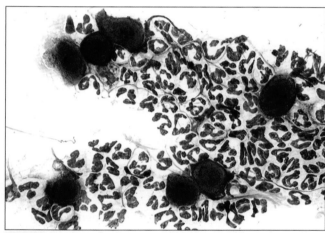

28.2 Cytology of an intact pustule from a case of pemphigus foliaceus. Note the non-degenerate neutrophils and free-floating acantholytic keratinocytes. (Diff-Quik® stain; original magnification X1000)

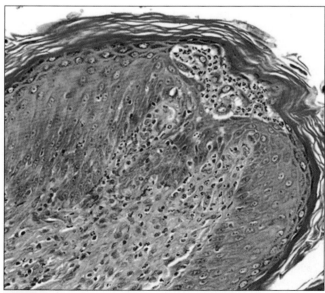

28.3 Histology of pemphigus foliaceus. Note the intact subcorneal pustule. (H&E stain; original magnification X400)

Ciclosporin as a single agent does not appear to be effective. Long-term follow-up has suggested that only about 20% of dogs will go into complete remission, and that some animals have been ultimately euthanized as a result of the adverse side effects of therapy or relapsing disease. In cats, prednisolone or another steroid alone or in combination with chlorambucil is the treatment of choice.

Pemphigus erythematosus

Historically, the term pemphigus erythematosus has been used to describe an autoimmune pustular disease localized to the face. The supporting histology is similar to that seen in PF (subcorneal pustules with acantholytic cells), with the addition of a lichenoid interface dermatitis resembling discoid lupus erythematosus (DLE). In fact, this disease probably represents a subset of PF and the treatment outcomes are similar.

Paraneoplastic pemphigus

Paraneoplastic pemphigus is a rare canine and feline disease in which vesicles develop, progressing to ulceration of the mucocutaneous junctions, haired skin and oral cavity. Animals are generally unwell and internal neoplasia has been identified. The condition is histologically distinct from PF.

Pemphigus vulgaris

Pemphigus vulgaris is a very rare disease of dogs and cats in which autoantibodies are directed at desmoglein-3 (Dsg-3). The resultant clefting lesions occur in the suprabasilar epidermis. Thus, deep erosions and ulcerations develop and typically involve the oral cavity, mucous membranes and sometimes the haired skin. The prognosis for animals with this disease is guarded.

Mucous membrane pemphigoid

In mucous membrane pemphigoid (MMP), autoantibodies are directed at laminin 5 in the basement membrane. Thus, the clinical lesions are deep erosions and ulcers. This uncommon disorder typically affects the mucocutaneous membranes of the face (Figure 28.4), the nasal planum, eyelids, lips and occasionally the pinnae, plus the perianal and perigenital skin. It has been reported in both the dog and the cat. The diagnosis relies on demonstration of clefting at the level of the basement membrane. German Shepherd Dogs are predisposed. Treatment with immunosuppressive doses of prednisolone and/or tetracycline and nicotinamide may be effective. Chronic lesions can result in significant scarring.

Bullous pemphigoid

Bullous pemphigoid is a rare disorder in the dog and cat, which is characterized by the development of autoantibodies to collagen XVII in the basement membrane. This disease involves the oral cavity, mucous membranes and haired skin, where ulcerations are typically seen. On histology, clefting at the level of the basement membrane is present. The disease carries a poor prognosis.

Epidermolysis bullosa acquisita

Epidermolysis bullosa acquisita (EBA) is a rare autoimmune skin disease seen primarily in young Great Danes. Autoantibodies are directed at collagen VII in the basement membrane. This results in subepidermal blistering

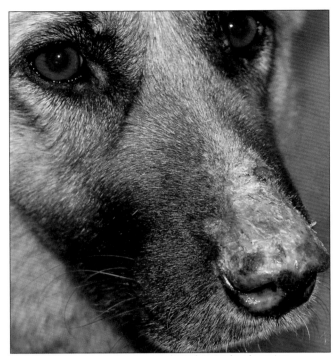

28.4 Mucous membrane pemphigoid. Note the ulceration, crusting, cicatricial alopecia and loss of pigment.

and presents clinically as ulceration, particularly around pressure points. Thus, lesions develop in the oral cavity, axillae, groin and footpads (Figure 28.5). This disease is debilitating and painful and carries a guarded prognosis.

Cutaneous lupus erythematosus

Lupus can be defined as a chronic inflammatory autoimmune disorder that affects many organ systems, including the skin, joints and internal organs. Cutaneous lupus diseases can have a diverse clinical presentation, but are unified by a specific histopathological pattern, namely lymphocytic interface dermatitis with prominent basilar keratinocyte death by apoptosis. All these disorders affect the skin, but some have significant systemic and immunological components.

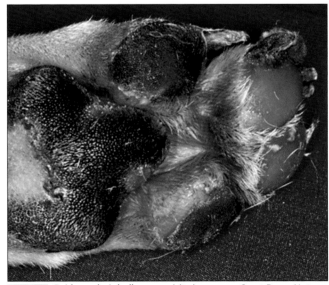

28.5 Epidermolysis bullosa acquisita in a young Great Dane. Note the sloughing of the footpads.

Vesicular cutaneous lupus erythematosus

Vesicular cutaneous lupus erythematosus is a rare disease of the Rough Collie, Shetland Sheepdog and their crosses. A clinically and histologically indistinguishable disease is occasionally noted in unrelated breeds. This disease typically affects middle-aged dogs, and a female predisposition has been noted. The primary lesion is a transient vesicle or bulla that may only be appreciated in histological sections of early lesions because they rupture readily to manifest as annular, polycyclic or serpiginous ulceration (Figure 28.6). The lesions are typically distributed over the groin, axillae and ventral abdomen and often involve the mucocutaneous junctions and medial pinnae. The lesions usually develop during the summer months and can recur annually. There is no systemic involvement in affected dogs unless extensive ulceration has led to secondary complications, such as bacteraemia and septicaemia. Diagnosis relies on the history and clinical presentation and supportive biopsy samples taken across the margin of fresh ulcerations.

Histopathology shows a lymphocyte-rich interface dermatitis and folliculitis. Vesiculation may be present at the dermoepidermal junction. Circulating Ro/SSA and La/SSB antibodies have been demonstrated in a research setting.

The prognosis for successful management of this disease is guarded. Immunosuppressive doses of prednisolone alone or in combination with azathioprine have been effective, but complete remission may not be achieved. Ciclosporin is an effective adjunctive therapy alongside glucocorticoids. Topical and systemic antibacterial therapy is an important adjunct when active lesions are present. Strong sunlight should also be avoided.

Mucocutaneous lupus erythematosus

Mucocutaneous lupus erythematosus (MCLE) affects the mucocutaneous membranes of the nose, lips, eyes, anus and genitalia. It manifests in adult dogs, and of the published cases, 50% were German Shepherd Dogs. Erosions and ulcerations at the mucocutaneous junctions readily become colonized with bacteria. A major differential diagnosis is mucocutaneous pyoderma, which can have a very similar clinical presentation. In the case of mucocutaneous pyoderma, the lesions should completely resolve with topical/systemic antibiosis, whereas in MCLE only partial resolution will occur. The role of bacterial antigens in the development of MCLE has not been determined. Affected dogs appear to respond best to immunosuppressive doses of glucocorticoids.

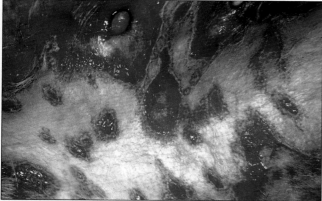

28.6 Vesicular cutaneous lupus erythematosus in a Rough Collie. Note the polycyclic, serpigenous ulcerations on the ventral abdomen.
(Reproduced from Jackson and Olivry (2001) with permission from the publishers)

Discoid lupus erythematosus

In the past, many dogs with nasal dermatitis have been classified as having DLE. Major differential diagnoses for DLE include mucocutaneous pyoderma, MMP, PF and epitheliotrophic lymphoma, and an appropriate therapeutic course of antibiotics is recommended before any further investigation is undertaken. Adult dogs present with depigmentation, erythema and skin atrophy of the nasal planum and dorsal muzzle. Other mucocutaneous junctions of the face may also be affected. Generalized DLE has been reported in the dog and cat. The disease may be exacerbated by sunlight.

The diagnosis depends on biopsy results, which should demonstrate interface dermatitis with basal cell damage, pigmentary incontinence and basement membrane thickening. No systemic abnormalities are present and antinuclear antibodies are not present in the serum.

It is difficult to make specific recommendations for the treatment of DLE because many cases given this diagnosis may not truly have had this disease. Focal lesions may be treated with topical glucocorticoids, such as dexamethasone or betamethasone. In addition, daily topical application of tacrolimus 0.1% was effective in the majority of dogs with DLE in a small case series. Other treatment options include tetracycline or oxytetracycline (250–500 mg/dog orally q8h) with nicotinamide (250–500 mg/dog orally q8h); however, long-term use of antibiotics is discouraged. If topical therapy is ineffective, then systemic glucocorticoids such as prednisolone (2 mg/kg orally q24h) tapered to effect can be used.

Exfoliative cutaneous lupus erythematosus

Exfoliative cutaneous lupus erythematosus is a disease that affects related young adult German Shorthaired Pointers and Vizlas. It is inherited as an autosomal recessive trait. Affected dogs present with scaling, alopecia and follicular casts that typically affect the muzzle, pinnae and dorsum, but lesions are often generalized. In addition, dogs may have lameness, back pain, fever, thrombocytopaenia and lymphadenopathy. Biopsy samples demonstrate an interface dermatitis and sebaceous adenitis. The disease typically waxes and wanes. The prognosis for this disease is guarded as a poor response to various therapies is noted and most dogs are euthanized as a result of disease progression.

Systemic lupus erythematosus

Canine systemic lupus erythematosus (SLE) is a chronic relapsing multi-organ disease. The skin may be involved in approximately 60% of cases. This disease affects adult dogs with no specific gender bias. A breed predisposition for medium to large-breed dogs has been suggested. Clinical signs are diverse and affect many organs, although not necessarily at the same time. The major signs include fever and polyarthritis with renal, haematological and cutaneous involvement. Cutaneous lesions can present as alopecia, scaling, ulceration or erosions. Where cutaneous lesions are present, interface dermatitis may be demonstrated on biopsy samples taken from the affected areas. However, it is also possible that cutaneous lesions may arise from a lupus-induced vasculitis or cryoglobulinaemia.

More than one organ system should be involved and a positive antinuclear antibody (ANA) test demonstrated to make the diagnosis. However, a positive ANA test is not specific for SLE and has been found commonly in other canine inflammatory diseases. Antibodies to extractable nuclear antigens (ENAs) and antihistone antibodies have also been demonstrated in canine SLE. The ANA titres generally fall with improvement in the animal's condition. This disease can typically wax and wane, thus response to therapy may be difficult to determine. Systemic immuno-suppression with prednisolone alone or in combination with azathioprine is the mainstay of treatment.

Immune-mediated diseases

With this group of diseases, the immune system is activated (sometimes presumptively) by endogenous or exogenous neoantigens. The foreign antigen incites an inflammatory process that results in organ-specific damage.

Dermatomyositis

Dermatomyositis is an immune-mediated disease affecting the skin and muscle and most frequently occurs in Shetland Sheepdogs and Collies. It typically has an early age of onset. Skin lesions include ulceration, scarring (cica-tricial) alopecia and scaling, most often affecting the face, ear tips, limbs, paws and tail tip. Muscle involvement may affect mastication and locomotion. It is a complex multi-factorial disease involving both genetic and environmental factors. A combination of genetic mutations, if present, increases the risk of an animal developing the disease.

Vasculitis

The term vasculitis refers to inflammation of the blood vessel walls. The resulting compromise in blood supply, and thus provision of nutrients and oxygen, to the over-lying tissues causes damage.

Aetiology

Vasculitis can arise from a variety of different underlying disorders, including:

- Infectious agents (common):
  - Bacteria – often seeded from an endocarditis
  - Viruses – feline calicivirus and feline infectious peritonitis
  - Vector-borne diseases – Rocky Mountain spotted fever, ehrlichiosis, borelliosis, bartonellosis and leishmaniosis
- Exogenous antigens:
  - Vaccine-associated – rabies
  - Drugs
  - Food (rare)
- Autoimmune diseases:
  - SLE
  - Cryoglobulins
- Neoplasia
- Unknown:
  - Cutaneous and renal glomerular vasculopathy.

A number of specific vasculitides are recognized: these are detailed in Figure 28.7.

Clinical approach

The clinical signs can vary depending on the size and depth of the vessel affected, the acuteness of the insult and the body region involved. Early lesions may be urticarial in

Syndromes	Considerations
Cutaneous and renal glomerular vasculopathy	Unknown aetiology. Incidence in the UK in autumn. Initial presentation with cutaneous ulceration; may develop microangiopathic thromboembolic disease and acute kidney injury. Can be fatal
Dermal arteritis of the nasal philtrum	Intermittent ulceration of the nasal philtrum often associated with significant haemorrhage
Dermatomyositis	Seen in young Rough Collies and Shetland Sheepdogs. Present with ulceration around the head and forelimbs, which heals with cicatricial alopecia. Some dogs also have myositis
Ischaemic dermatopathy	Seen in Bichon Frises. Focal alopecia develops at the site of rabies vaccination 2–3 months after the event due to slow ischaemic damage of the hair follicle
Virulent feline calicivirus	Rare contagious virulent form of feline calicivirus. Often fatal

28.7 Specific syndromes involving vasculitis.

nature, as fluid leaks from the compromised vessels. As the vessel wall becomes damaged further, red blood cells are lost and focal haemorrhage occurs, which results in ecchy-moses and petechiae. Focal necrosis of the overlying tissues results in well circumscribed ulceration or damage to body extremities. More gradual vessel damage may only be sufficient to disrupt certain structures, such as the hair follicle, resulting in a focal area of alopecia.

The clinical signs consistent with vasculitis include:

- Transient focal oedematous plaques and urticaria
- Damage to the extremities (Figures 28.8 and 28.9)
- Petechiae and/or ecchymoses (Figure 28.10)
- Focal well circumscribed ulceration
- Focal cicatricial alopecia
- Intermittent haemorrhage.

Diagnostic tests: The key diagnostic tests for suspected vasculitis include:

- Biochemistry, haematology and urinalysis
- Diascopy
- Skin biopsy
- Screens for infectious agents:
  - Vector-borne disease antibody/antigen
  - Blood culture if a heart murmur is present
  - Viral antibody/antigen.

Focal lesions caused by extravasation of intravascular elements will appear erythematous or purpuric. To confirm vascular compromise, diascopy can be performed. This involves pressing a glass slide over the affected area: inflammatory lesions will typically blanche, whereas those in which extravasation has occurred will not (Figure 28.11). It can be difficult to confirm vasculitis with a skin biopsy as this relies on capturing the damaged vessel(s) in the sample. It is recommended that multiple samples are taken from new lesions.

Treatment

The specific management of vasculitis usually depends on the inciting cause. Judicial use of anti-inflammatory doses of prednisolone is often employed to limit vessel damage. Pentoxifylline (10–15 mg/kg orally q8–12h), a methylxanthine

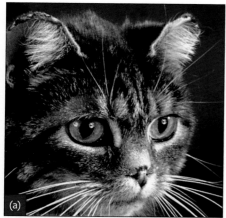

28.8 (a, b) Ischaemic damage to the extremities (ear tips, nose and loss of tail) of a cat with idiopathic vasculitis.

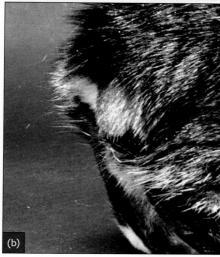

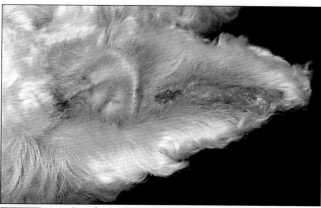

28.9 Vascular infarct of the convex pinna caused by post-vaccination ischaemia.

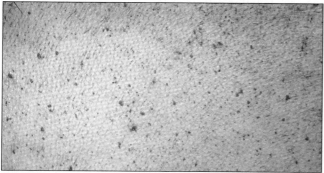

28.10 Petechiae on the lateral flank associated with Rocky Mountain spotted fever (*Rickettsia rickettsii*).

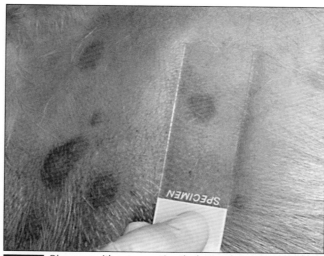

28.11 Diascopy: with extravasation the lesions fail to blanche with pressure.

derivative, has anti-inflammatory and rheological properties and is often used in the management of vasculitis in the dog. It can be used as a steroid-sparing agent. Full efficacy may not be seen for the first few weeks of therapy. This drug should always be given with food to minimize gastro-intestinal upset.

Specific vasculopathies

Cutaneous and renal glomerular vasculopathy: Cutaneous and renal glomerular vasculopathy (CRGV) is an emerging potentially fatal vasculitis of unknown origin. There is a higher incidence of the disease in the autumn months amongst dogs that have been walked in woodland. Although initially reported in southern England, cases have been recognized throughout the UK. Dogs may initially present with multifocal ulcerations on the distal limbs. In some cases these will resolve. Others will progress to develop potentially fatal acute kidney injury.

For dogs presenting with ulcerative skin disease suggestive of a vasculitis, skin biopsy samples may be taken to confirm the diagnosis. It is also recommended that clinical signs, routine haematology, biochemistry and urinalysis be monitored for 4–9 days, as this is the usual time frame in which renal involvement may be observed.

Ischaemic dermatopathy: Affected dogs present with either localized or generalized scaling, crusts and ulcers, which develop into a cicatricial alopecia. Lesions may be seen at the site of vaccination or affecting the distal extremities. The course of the disease may be indolent and smaller breeds are over-represented, including Chihuahuas, Maltese, Yorkshire and Jack Russell Terriers. In some cases, there may be a chronological association with vaccination (within the last 6 months) and these cases usually present with a focal area of alopecia at the site of administration. Many cases are idiopathic.

Dermal arteritis of the nasal philtrum: This is an uncommon disorder in which immune-mediated inflammation of the arterioles supplying the nasal planum is presumed. It affects middle-aged large-breed dogs (St. Bernards are over-represented; Figure 28.12). The clinical appearance is characteristic with ulceration localized to the nasal philtrum. This is often associated with significant haemorrhage. Topical 0.1% tacrolimus as a sole therapy or in conjunction with systemic prednisolone is effective in many cases.

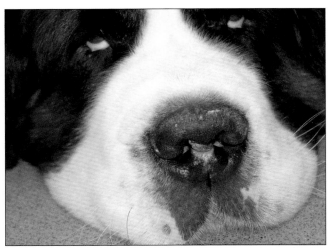

28.12 Nasal arteritis in a St. Bernard. Note the ulceration confined to the nasal philtrum.

Erythema multiforme

Erythema multiforme (EM) is an uncommon skin disease in the dog and cat, which can present in a variety of different ways. Clinical signs include focal or multifocal, flat or raised, target or polycyclic erosions or ulcerations (Figure 28.13). There is some debate as to the pathogenesis of these lesions in small animals. In humans, the eruptions are most commonly associated with herpesvirus antigen. EM has only been associated with viral antigen (parvovirus) in one dog. The lesions are most commonly suggested to be associated with drugs, although this is difficult to prove because the underlying disease, for which the drug has been prescribed, may also play a part. Food antigens are rarely implicated. Neoantigens are thought to incite changes in the keratinocytes, which then undergo T lymphocyte-induced apoptosis.

The severity of EM can also vary from localized lesions to more widespread involvement, including the mucous membranes and oral cavity. It is often classified as EM minor (only one mucosal surface involved) or EM major (more than one mucosal surface involved). The latter is sometimes called Stevens–Johnson syndrome. The diagnosis relies on supportive histopathology from biopsy samples of lesional skin. Interface dermatitis with keratinocyte apoptosis in all layers of the epidermis is present.

Identification and removal of possible triggers is key to the management of EM, but, in the author's experience, the lesions rarely abate. Immunosuppressive doses of prednisolone alone, or in combination with other drugs, may be required.

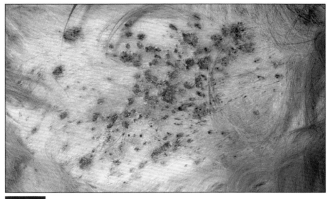

28.13 Multifocal erosions associated with erythema multiforme.

There is debate as to whether toxic epidermal necrosis is a unique entity or a very severe form of EM, in which complete epidermal detachment occurs over significant areas of the body. It carries a very poor prognosis.

Canine acute eosinophilic dermatitis with oedema

Canine acute eosinophilic dermatitis with oedema (Wells-like syndrome) is an uncommon disorder of unknown aetiology. A hypersensitivity reaction is postulated. Cutaneous signs are often preceded by an episode of gastrointestinal upset. Affected dogs develop characteristic erythematous macules most obviously on the ventral abdominal skin. This can progress to oedema affecting the limbs and face. Confirmation of the diagnosis is on histopathology, which shows a diffuse eosinophilic dermatitis with oedema. Most dogs will respond to early intervention with glucocorticoids and generally do not relapse after treatment is withdrawn.

Sterile granulomatous dermatitis and lymphadenitis

Sterile granulomatous dermatitis and lymphadenitis (also known as juvenile cellulitis or puppy strangles) is sporadically seen in puppies from weeks to months of age (Figure 28.14). The typical appearance is of facial swelling, pustular dermatitis and cellulitis. Lesions are often first seen around the mucous membranes and concave pinnae. Affected

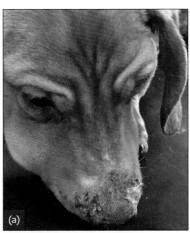

28.14 Juvenile cellulitis in a 4-month-old Dachshund. (a) Crusting and draining tracts around the nose. (b) Swelling and serosanguineous exudate around the muzzle. Note the swelling around the neck due to lymphadenitis.

(a)

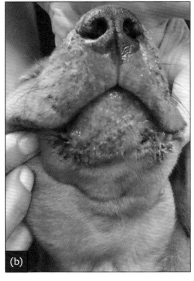

(b)

dogs can be febrile and may present with more generalized disease and joint pain. The condition is also recognized in adult dogs with a similar clinical presentation and histopathology (Inga et al., 2020). The aetiology is unknown. It is important to rule out demodicosis and infectious agents, which may cause dermatitis and cellulitis. Affected dogs respond to glucocorticoids alone or in combination with other immunomodulatory agents such as ciclosporin.

Drug eruptions

Cutaneous drug eruptions can mimic any skin disease in clinical appearance. The histological appearance may be of PF, EM or vasculitis, amongst other patterns. The duration of exposure to the administered drug may be as short as 7 days, or the reaction may occur after months of treatment. There are few published confirmed drug eruptions in companion animals because a definitive diagnosis would require re-administration of the suspected drug to demonstrate recurrence of the eruption. However, there is no doubt that drugs may act as exogenous antigens and have the potential to incite disease. Thus, for any animal presenting with the diseases discussed herein a complete drug history should be obtained and any 'suspicious' treatment discontinued.

Treatment

Successful management of this group of diseases is not easy, even in the hands of an experienced individual, and the practitioner is strongly advised to seek advice from a specialist regarding current management recommendations or to refer the case. The mainstay of treatment is usually immunosuppressive doses of glucocorticoids; however, for many diseases adequate control is not achieved with this alone and other immunosuppressive agents are often combined with glucocorticoid therapy. Selection of the appropriate therapeutic agent or combination of agents for each case is usually based on clinical experience and familiarity with recent literature.

Treatment should be monitored closely with frequent clinical examination of the animal and, where indicated, bloodwork to detect adverse organ-related side effects. Secondary infections commonly develop whilst the animal is on immunosuppressive treatment, and these may occur on the skin, or in the urinary tract or respiratory system. In addition, demodicosis can be a side effect of chronic glucocorticoid therapy. Some diseases may be exacerbated by environmental factors such as ultraviolet light, and this should be taken into consideration when a management programme is designed.

Key points

- Autoimmune and immune-mediated diseases of the skin are rare, and the diagnosis is usually confirmed on histology
- Any secondary bacterial skin infections should be treated prior to taking skin biopsies, and glucocorticoid therapy should be delayed until a definitive diagnosis has been made
- Once therapy is initiated the animal should be carefully monitored for side effects of treatment

---

References and further reading

Backel KA, Bradley CW, Cain CL et al. (2019) Canine ischaemic dermatopathy: a retrospective study of 177 cases (2005–2016). Veterinary Dermatology 30 403–410

Bizikova P and Burrows A (2019) Feline pemphigus foliaceus: original case series and a comprehensive literature review. BMC Veterinary Research 15, 1–15

Bryden SL, White SD, Dunston SM et al. (2005) Clinical, histopathological and immunological characteristics of exfoliative cutaneous lupus erythematosus in 25 German Short-haired Pointers. Veterinary Dermatology 16, 239–252

Evans JM, Noorai RE, Tsai KL et al. (2017) Beyond the MHC: a canine model of dermatomyositis shows a complex pattern of genetic risk involving novel loci. Plos Genetics 13, e1006604

Griffin CE, Stannard AA, Ihrke PJ et al. (1979) Canine discoid lupus erythematosus. Veterinary Immunology and Immunopathology 1, 79–87

Halliwell REW (2004) Systemic lupus erythematosus in domestic animals. In: Systemic Lupus Erythematosus, 4th edn, ed. RG Lahita, pp. 265–278. Elsevier Academic Press, Philadelphia

Holm L and Walker D (2018) Dealing with cutaneous and renal glomerular vasculopathy in dogs. In Practice 40, 426–438

Inga A, Griffeth GC, Drobatz KJ et al. (2020) Sterile granulomatous dermatitis and lymphadenitis (juvenile cellutis) in adult dogs: a retrospective analysis of 90 cases (2004–2018). Veterinary Dermatology 31, 219–e47

Jackson HA (2006) Vesicular cutaneous lupus. Veterinary Clinics of North America: Small Animal Practice 36, 251–255

Jackson HA and Olivry T (2001) Ulcerative dermatosis of the Shetland Sheepdog and Rough Collie dog may represent a vesicular variant of cutaneous lupus erythematosus. Veterinary Dermatology 12, 19–27

Nichols PR, Morris DO and Beale KM (2001) A retrospective study of canine and feline vasculitis. Veterinary Dermatology 12, 255–264

Olivry T (2006) A review of autoimmune skin disease in domestic animals: 1 – superficial pemphigus. Veterinary Dermatology 17, 291–305

Sousa SA (2008) Glucocorticoids in veterinary dermatology. In: Kirk's Current Veterinary Therapy XIV, ed. JD Bonagura and DC Twedt, pp. 400–405. WB Saunders, Philadelphia

Souza CP, Torres SMF, Koch SN and Bernardi de Souza L (2019) Dermal arteritis of the nasal philtrum: a retrospective study of 23 dogs. Veterinary Dermatology 30, 511–e155

Wiemelt SP, Goldschmidt MH, Greek JS et al. (2004) A retrospective study comparing the histopathological features and response to treatment in two canine nasal dermatoses, DLE and MCP. Veterinary Dermatology 15, 341–348

Chapter 29

Management of autoimmune and immune-mediated skin diseases

Hilary A. Jackson and Katharine F. Lunn

Autoimmune diseases of the skin are rare. The diagnosis is based on the signalment, history, appearance of the disease and, in most cases, specific histological features. In many cases, there may be more common, often infectious, diseases, which have a similar appearance. It is also worth remembering that with the loss of skin integrity, secondary bacterial and/or *Malassezia* infection is common. Cytology, in this regard, is a useful diagnostic tool. Infections should be treated prior to obtaining biopsy samples, as they may complicate histological interpretation. Most autoimmune diseases that are confined to the skin are usually not life-threatening, and awaiting a definitive diagnosis prior to instituting treatment is always advised. However, multi-system immune-mediated diseases, in which the skin is one of several organ systems involved, such as systemic lupus erythematosus, do have the potential to be life-threatening.

Treatment goals and strategies

The goals of treatment should be:

- Stop disease progression
- Regression of clinical signs to the point where a good quality of life is restored
- Minimize side effects of treatment.

Note that within this framework the disease may not be completely controlled, but a balance between treatment side effects and disease progression has been achieved. For localized disease, topical therapy may be considered, either as an initial treatment or for maintenance therapy after initial systemic treatment. Whilst glucocorticoids are usually the initial treatment of choice, for more severe and extensive autoimmune disease, combination therapy is usually advised, through the addition of further immunosuppressive agents. An important goal of combination therapy is the reduction of glucocorticoid-related side effects; however, these additional agents do have their own adverse effects, and attention should be directed at monitoring these specifically. When instituting combination therapy with glucocorticoids and additional immunosuppressive agents, it is important to base dosage adjustments on the patient's response, rather than attempting to follow a 'recipe' or pre-conceived plan.

A poor response to therapy after 4 weeks should prompt a review of the management protocol and, possibly, the initial diagnosis. As these diseases are rare, and evidence-based recommendations regarding specific treatment protocols can be difficult to find, it is always worth consulting with, or referring to, a specialist who will have more familiarity with the condition. Any pet being treated for an autoimmune or immune-mediated condition should be inspected regularly. Once the disease is responding to treatment, downward dose adjustments should be conservative, as large dose reductions can be associated with disease flare. In general, when using combination therapy, the dose or frequency of the medication that is causing the more significant adverse effects should be reduced first. It is also important to note that combination therapy with multiple immunosuppressive medications will increase the risk of secondary infections.

In the future, measurement of blood concentrations of immunosuppressive drugs, or their metabolites, as well as pharmacodynamic assessment of specific medications, may lead to more effective targeted therapy of these diseases (Archer *et al.*, 2020).

Autoimmune diseases often wax and wane, and specific trigger factors, such as skin infections, ultraviolet light and oestrus, can exacerbate disease. Any apparent relapse should be assessed for secondary skin infections and/or demodicosis, as these are common occurrences in the immunocompromised patient. Clients feeding raw diets to their pets should also be counselled on the increased risk of disease both to the affected immunocompromised pet and people in contact with the affected animal.

The retrovirus status of cats should also be assessed prior to starting any immunotherapy.

Specific therapeutics

Glucocorticoids

Glucocorticoids are the cornerstone of immunosuppressive therapy for immune-mediated diseases in small animals. Despite their familiarity, low cost, availability and ease of use, they are not benign medications and their adverse effects can significantly affect the patient's quality of life.

Mechanism of action

Immunosuppressive effects are likely to include altered cytokine production, suppression of lymphocyte function, decreased macrophage function and inhibition of leucocyte migration.

Formulations, indications and dosing

Many glucocorticoid products are available for veterinary use as oral, parenteral or topical formulations. These differ in the duration of action, anti-inflammatory potency and mineralocorticoid effects, dependent on the glucocorticoid itself, the specific formulation and how it is administered. Individual glucocorticoid properties can be altered by the addition of esters to the free base of the drug, to change the solubility and duration of action (Figure 29.1).

Drug	Formulation/route	Duration of action
Methylprednisolone	Oral tablets	12–36 hours
Methylprednisolone sodium succinate	Injectable, given i.v.	Minutes
Methylprednisolone acetate	Injectable, given i.m. or s.c.	Days to weeks

29.1 Methylprednisolone can be given as the free base, or its properties can be altered by the addition of esters.

Glucocorticoid selection

In general, the increased anti-inflammatory potency parallels the increased duration of action and biological effects, e.g. suppression of the hypothalamic–pituitary–adrenal (HPA) axis. Short-acting glucocorticoids, such as prednisolone and methylprednisolone (Figure 29.2), suppress the HPA axis for up to 36 hours after a single dose, whereas more potent glucocorticoids such as dexamethasone and betamethasone have a longer duration of action. Using short-acting glucocorticoids on alternate days theoretically leads to less HPA suppression. The anti-inflammatory and immunosuppressive effects of any glucocorticoids, however, last beyond drug withdrawal as a significant mode of action is the up or downregulation of gene expression.

Most glucocorticoids used to treat immune-mediated diseases have minimal mineralocorticoid activity; however, when present, these effects may contribute to some of the adverse effects of glucocorticoids, e.g. sodium retention and polyuria/polydipsia (PU/PD). It is also important to note that prednisolone and prednisone are not necessarily the most effective glucocorticoids in every patient. Clinicians should consider individual response and side effects when selecting a glucocorticoid for a specific animal.

If oral therapy is not possible, injectable glucocorticoids can be used. Injectable dexamethasone can be substituted for prednisolone by using 0.1–0.15 times the desired total daily dose of prednisolone.

Topical glucocorticoids are potentially useful for localized disease. Modification of the steroid molecule to enhance lipophilicity by esterification has led to the development of hydrocortisone aceponate, available as a 0.0584% spray (Cortavance, Virbac).

- Hydrocortisone aceponate is largely metabolized in the skin and has less potential for localized skin atrophy than other potent steroids.

- Patients on regular topical steroid treatment should be closely monitored. Local side effects include skin thinning, bruising and calcinosis cutis. Systemic absorption can result in other side effects (Figure 29.3; see below).

Potential side effects and recommended monitoring

Primary adverse effects of glucocorticoids are signs of iatrogenic hyperadrenocorticism and HPA axis suppression.

Iatrogenic hyperadrenocorticism: The physical examination findings and results of a complete blood count (CBC), serum biochemistry profile and urinalysis will be similar to those in dogs with naturally occurring hyperadrenocorticism.

- Clinical signs in dogs include PU/PD, polyphagia, lethargy, panting, hepatomegaly, pot-bellied appearance, alopecia, thin skin, poor wound healing, calcinosis cutis (Figure 29.4) and muscle weakness.
- Cats are regarded as more resistant to the adverse effects of glucocorticoids, but they are at risk of heart failure and the development of diabetes mellitus (which can be transient).
- Long-term high dose glucocorticoids in cats can cause alopecia, thinning of the skin, risk of tearing secondary to minimal trauma (Figure 29.5) and curling of the ear tips (Figure 29.6).
- More serious complications in both dogs and cats include increased susceptibility to infection, hypertension, proteinuria and hypercoagulability. The latter can lead to life-threatening complications, such as pulmonary thromboembolism (Figure 29.7).

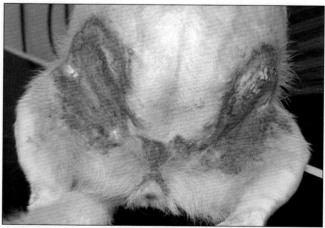

29.3 Localized epidermal atrophy, calcinosis cutis and secondary infection caused by repeated application of a topical glucocorticoid.

Glucocorticoid	Comments	Dogs	Cats
Prednisolone/ prednisone	Prednisolone is the active drug. In cats, the conversion from prednisone to prednisolone is less efficient	1–2 mg/kg q12h Dose at the lower end of the range in large dogs Do not exceed 60 mg total daily dose	Up to 3 mg/kg q12h
Methylprednisolone	May have less mineralocorticoid activity	0.8–1.6 mg/kg q12h	Up to 2.4 mg/kg q12h
Dexamethasone	More potent/longer duration of action Not licensed for oral use in cats/dogs	0.1–0.2 mg/kg q24h	0.2–0.4 mg/kg q24h

29.2 Properties and doses of glucocorticoids in cats and dogs.

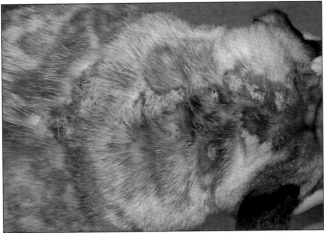

29.4 Calcinosis cutis on the dorsal neck that developed after glucocorticoid therapy for pemphigus foliaceus.

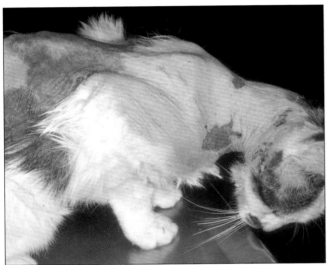

29.5 Epidermal atrophy and skin tearing in a cat after systemic glucocorticoid therapy.

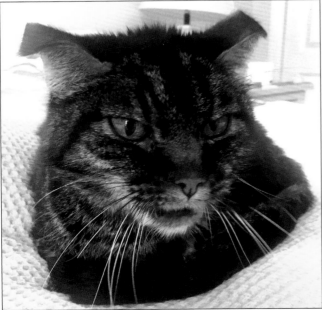

29.6 Ear tip curling as a result of systemic glucocorticoid therapy in a cat.

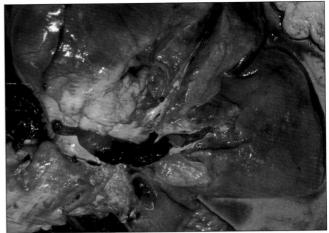

29.7 Fatal thromboembolism resulting from glucocorticoid therapy.

Recommended monitoring includes the following:

- Regular physical examination, blood pressure measurement, CBC, serum biochemistry profile, urinalysis and urine culture should be performed
- Anti-thrombotic agents, such as clopidogrel, should be considered in dogs receiving glucocorticoids, particularly if they develop proteinuria and/or thrombocytosis, or when hypercoagulability is detected with thromboelastography
- Cats that develop diabetes mellitus should be managed with long-acting insulin (such as glargine or protamine zinc insulin) and a low carbohydrate diet. The insulin dose will likely change as the glucocorticoid dose changes and glucose and other parameters should be closely monitored. Remission is possible when glucocorticoids are withdrawn.

When assessing the adverse effects of glucocorticoids, it can be helpful to think in terms of things that affect the patient, concern the owner, or require monitoring (Figure 29.8). To minimize adverse effects of glucocorticoids and HPA axis suppression, wherever possible:

Affects the patient's quality of life
• Lethargy • Panting • Behavioural changes (well documented in humans, less so in dogs and cats) • Muscle weakness • Poor wound healing
Affects the owner's quality of life
• Polyuria/polydipsia • Polyphagia/begging for food • Unable to go for walks or play • Panting • Behavioural changes
Clinician should monitor for
• Hypertension • Proteinuria • Hypercoagulability • Recurrent infections • Calcinosis cutis (dogs) • Insulin resistance (newly-diagnosed diabetes mellitus, or requirement for increased dose of insulin) • Heart failure (cats)

29.8 Adverse effects of glucocorticoids on the patient and the owner, and those the clinician should monitor for.

- Use the lowest dose and lowest potency glucocorticoid that controls the disease
- Combine with other immunosuppressive medications (see below)
- Aim for alternate day therapy
- Use topical therapy
- Withdraw therapy slowly to allow the HPA axis to recover.

Fortunately, the majority of adverse effects will resolve if glucocorticoid medication can be withdrawn. If necessary, the degree of suppression of the HPA axis can be assessed by performing an adrenocorticotropic hormone stimulation test, first ensuring that in the preceding 24 hours the patient has not received medications (prednisone, prednisolone, methylprednisolone, cortisone) that can cross-react with the cortisol assay.

Azathioprine

Although widely used in veterinary medicine, particularly in combination with glucocorticoids, azathioprine (a thiopurine) has only been evaluated in retrospective studies and much information regarding its use is anecdotal.

Mechanism of action

- Acts as a purine antagonist by producing 'false' nucleotides. Interferes with deoxyribonucleic acid (DNA) and ribonucleic acid (RNA) synthesis, causing inhibition of T-cell function. Less effect on humoral immunity.
- Thiopurine methyltransferase (TMTP) is involved in the metabolism of azathioprine; activity of TMTP can be measured. Humans with low TMPT activity are more likely to experience bone marrow suppression; high activity correlates with a poor clinical response to standard doses. TMPT activity is low in cats, variable in dogs, and may be breed-related. However, the measurement of TMPT activity has not been shown to predict clinical outcomes in dogs.

Formulations, indications and dosing

- Oral: 50 mg, 75 mg and 100 mg tablets. 50 mg tablets are most commonly used in dogs.
- Tablets can be compounded into a liquid for more accurate dosing of small dogs.
- Azathioprine **should not** be used in cats due to significant risk of fatal toxicity.
- An injectable product may be available, but there is no veterinary experience with this formulation.
- Azathioprine is often combined with glucocorticoids for the management of immune-mediated disease in dogs.
- If the patient has no adverse effects, azathioprine can be used long term to maintain remission of disease while glucocorticoid doses are reduced.
- The initial dose of azathioprine for control of immune-mediated disease is 1–2 mg/kg q24h; alternatively it can be dosed on a body surface area basis at 50 mg/m² q24h.
- Many clinicians decrease to a q48h schedule after 2–4 weeks, although there is little evidence on which to base this recommendation.
- It is common to aim for alternate day therapy with a glucocorticoid given on one day, and azathioprine on the alternate day.

Potential side effects and recommended monitoring

- Adverse effects include gastrointestinal upset, myelosuppression and hepatotoxicity.
- Gastrointestinal signs are generally mild and often self-limiting.
- Myelosuppression and hepatotoxicity may be idiosyncratic and therefore unpredictable.
- Hepatotoxicity is most likely to occur within the first 2–4 weeks of therapy, whereas the onset of myelosuppression can be delayed (Wallisch and Trepanier, 2015).
- Hepatoxicity and myelosuppression are potentially reversible if detected early.
- CBCs and serum biochemistry panels should be evaluated every 2 weeks during the first 2 months of therapy, and every 1–2 months thereafter.
- If the dog is on combination therapy it can be challenging to differentiate between glucocorticoid-induced increases in liver enzymes (generally benign), and increases in liver enzymes associated with azathioprine hepatotoxicity (not benign).
  - Glucocorticoids typically cause more profound increases in serum alkaline phosphatase (ALP) compared with alanine aminotransferase (ALT).
  - If the magnitude of ALT increase is similar to, or in excess of, the magnitude of ALP increase, azathioprine hepatotoxicity should be suspected and the medication stopped.

Mycophenolate mofetil

This drug was developed as a potentially less toxic alternative to azathioprine for human use. It has been used in a small number of canine and feline immune-mediated diseases.

Mechanism of action

Metabolites inhibit purine biosynthesis, interfering with DNA synthesis. Inhibits T- and B-cell proliferation.

Formulations, indications and dosing

- Oral: 250 mg capsules and 500 mg tablets. Injectable: 500 mg/20 ml vial.
- Has been shown to be a useful adjunctive treatment in immune-mediated skin disease (Ackermann et al., 2017).
- Typical canine/feline dose is 10 mg/kg q12h.

Potential side effects and recommended monitoring

- Gastrointestinal side effects, particularly diarrhoea, are most common, typically occurring early in the course of therapy.
- Mild diarrhoea may be self-limiting or respond to non-specific therapy.
- Myelosuppression is theoretically possible, but not widely reported. CBC should be monitored regularly.

Leflunomide

Previous use of this drug was confined to canine renal transplantation, but it is increasingly used for immune-mediated diseases, although controlled prospective studies are lacking.

Mechanism of action

Metabolites inhibit pyrimidine synthesis. Targets T- and B-cells.

Formulations, indications and dosing

- Oral: 10 mg and 20 mg tablets.
- Has been used for immune-mediated polyarthritis and sporadically reported in other canine diseases, including immune-mediated haemolytic anaemia (IMHA), immune-mediated thrombocytopenia (IMT) and pemphigus foliaceus (Gregory et al., 1998).
- Suggested canine dose: 3–4 mg/kg q24h, or divided q12h.
- Suggested feline dose: 10 mg per cat q24h (but little data on use in cats).

Potential side effects and recommended monitoring

- Gastrointestinal effects, myelotoxicity and hepatotoxicity are possible, but there is little published data on incidence in dogs.
- Clinical signs, CBC and serum biochemistry should be monitored regularly.
- Trough serum levels can be monitored, although the target concentration is unknown.

Chlorambucil

Predominantly used in chemotherapy protocols, but it has some use in immune-mediated or inflammatory diseases in dogs and cats.

Mechanism of action

Alkylating agent. Cytotoxic due to cross-linking of DNA.

Formulations, indications and dosing

- Oral: 2 mg tablets.
- May be used in combination with glucocorticoids to treat immune-mediated diseases such as pemphigus foliaceus.
- Often a preferred immunosuppressive medication in cats.
- Suggested canine dose: 2–4 mg/m^2 q24h; round to the nearest 2 mg.
- Suggested feline dose: 0.1–0.2 mg/kg (1.5–4 mg/m^2) q24h.
- Alternate feline dosing: 2 mg q48h (>4 kg); 2 mg q72h (<4kg).
- Compounding may be necessary for dosing cats and small dogs; this should only be performed at specialized facilities.

Potential side effects and recommended monitoring

- Bone marrow suppression is a potential side effect; CBC should be monitored after 1 month and then every 2–3 months.
- Gastrointestinal side effects may respond to an increased dose interval.

Human intravenous immunoglobulin

Created from pooled plasma from multiple human donors, consisting mainly of purified immunoglobulin (Ig)G. Initially developed to treat human immunodeficiency disorders, but now also used in many immune-mediated and inflammatory conditions. Some reports of use in dogs (Spurlock and Prittie, 2011), but rarely used in cats.

Mechanism of action

Complex and multifactorial, and likely to include:

- B-cell inhibition
- Autoantibody neutralization
- Complement inhibition
- Cytokine modulation
- Fc receptor blockade.

Formulations, indications and dosing

- Intravenous: variety of lyophilized and freeze-dried products requiring reconstitution before administration over 4–6 hours.
- Reported uses include IMHA, IMT, myasthenia gravis and cutaneous diseases.
- Suggested canine dose: 0.5–1.5 g/kg once.

Potential side effects and recommended monitoring

- May promote coagulation and inflammation. Long-term sequelae poorly understood.
- Hypersensitivity, anaphylaxis, fluid overload, hyperviscosity and hypotension may occur during infusion; patients should be monitored as closely as for blood product transfusion.

Nicotinamide

Nicotinamide (niacinamide) is the water-soluble form of vitamin B3. Its use in animals has not been rigorously evaluated.

Mechanism of action

It is essential for the coenzymes required for adenosine triphosphate production in the body. It has anti-inflammatory and antioxidant effects.

Formulations, indications and dosing

Available as 250 mg tablets, nicotinamide has historically been used in combination with tetracycline antibiotics for long-term management of symmetrical lupoid onychodystrophy, discoid lupus, cutaneous reactive histiocytosis and localized pemphigus foliaceus. However, chronic antibiotic therapy is not currently recommended and more recent regimes have combined nicotinamide with omega-3 essential fatty acids and pentoxifylline. Long-term evaluation of the treatment efficacy of these regimes has not been published. Nicotinamide is well tolerated and used at a dose of 250 mg q8h daily for dogs less than 25 kg and 500 mg q8h daily for heavier dogs.

Pentoxifylline
Mechanism of action

Pentoxifylline reduces blood viscosity and has anti-inflammatory effects. It is not licensed for animals in the UK.

Formulations, indications and dosing

It is typically used in the treatment of vasculopathies. In the acute stages, concurrent glucocorticoid therapy may be required and tapered to effect. Pentoxifylline is well tolerated as a maintenance therapy and is dosed in the dog at 15 mg/kg q8h daily. Mild gastrointestinal side effects may occur.

Oclacitinib

Mechanism of action

Oclacitinib is a Janus kinase (JAK) inhibitor with preferential activity for JAK-1 dependent pathways. In this regard, it inhibits the activity of interleukin (IL)-31, a pruritogenic cytokine, but also the activity of various inflammatory cytokines, such as IL-2, IL-4, IL-6 and IL-13. It is licensed in the UK for controlling pruritus in dogs at a dose of 0.4–0.6 mg/kg. A loading dose of twice daily treatment for 2 weeks followed by once daily therapy is recommended.

Formulations, indications and dosing

There is current interest in the use of this drug as an anti-inflammatory treatment for various immune-mediated and autoimmune diseases. However, clinical and *in vitro* studies suggest that a higher dose than that recommended for the control of pruritus would be needed (Aymeric and Bensignor, 2017; Banovic *et al.*, 2019; Levy *et al.*, 2019), and whether this would be effective as a monotherapy or in combination with other treatments is not clear at present. Any off-label use at a higher dose would increase the risk of side effects, such as secondary skin infections, demodicosis, weight gain, histiocytomas, proteinuria and cytopenias. Regular clinical examination and routine haematology, biochemistry and urinalysis are indicated.

Calcineurin inhibitors: ciclosporin and tacrolimus

Mechanism of action

Ciclosporin and tacrolimus are calcineurin inhibitors and the principal mode of action is to inhibit T-cell activation.

Formulations, indications and dosing

Ciclosporin is licensed in the UK and other countries to treat canine and feline atopic dermatitis at a dose of 5 mg/kg q24h for dogs and 7 mg/kg q24h for cats. Tacrolimus is not licensed in the UK for use in animals and the topical 0.1% cream is most commonly prescribed. These drugs have been used alone or in combination with other drugs to treat a variety of other immune-mediated conditions.

Absorption is limited by P-glycoprotein efflux pumps in the intestine, and the drug is metabolized in the liver and intestine by cytochrome P450 (CYP3A). Drugs that competitively inhibit or induce these enzymes will increase ciclosporin serum levels. These include diltiazem, doxycycline, imidazole antifungal drugs, metoclopramide, cimetidine, erythromycin, clindamycin and phenobarbital. Due to the relatively high cost of ciclosporin, this drug interaction is exploited and a combination of 5 mg/kg q24h of ketoconazole alongside 2.5 mg/kg q24h of ciclosporin is sometimes used. Additionally, as ciclosporin is a substrate of the multiple drug resistant mutation (*MDR*)1 P-glycoprotein transporter, co-administration with macrocyclic lactones (and some other drugs) could increase the central nervous system toxicity of this class of drugs.

The most common side effect seen in both dogs and cats is gastrointestinal upset manifesting as diarrhoea and/or vomiting. This is often self-limiting and will settle down after a few days of treatment. If signs persist, then starting with a lower daily dose and titrating the dose slowly upwards or splitting the dose and administering twice daily is often effective.

Long-term side effects include gingival hyperplasia (Figure 29.9), hirsutism (Figure 29.10) and papillomatous growths (Nuttal *et al.*, 2014). Ciclosporin has been shown to increase peripheral insulin resistance and reduce release of this hormone (Kovilak *et al.*, 2011), and whilst the

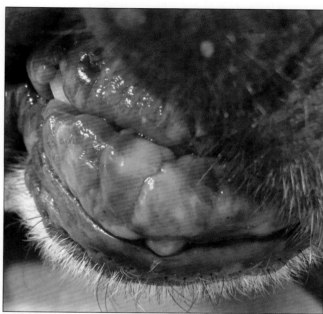

29.9 Gingival hyperplasia resulting from long-term ciclosporin treatment.

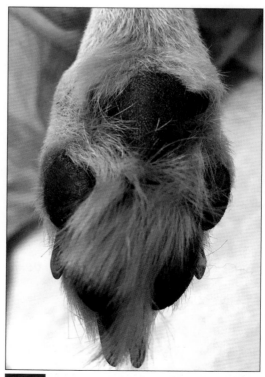

29.10 Hirsutism resulting from long-term ciclosporin treatment.

risk of developing diabetes mellitus on treatment is low, the drug should be used with care, but not necessarily avoided, in diabetic animals. West Highland White Terriers in the UK may be at increased risk (Steffan *et al.*, 2003). Whilst uncommon, the potential for unusual opportunist bacterial and fungal infections in animals on chronic therapy should be considered (Siak and Burrows, 2013; Banovic *et al.*, 2015; McAtee *et al.*, 2017). There are uncommon reports of cats contracting clinical toxoplasmosis whilst on chronic ciclosporin therapy (Lappin *et al.*, 2015). The individuals at risk are those with no previous exposure and an outdoor hunting lifestyle. It is therefore recommended that serology for *Toxoplasma* antibodies be performed prior to starting treatment. A positive titre, representing previous exposure, is protective.

Use of ciclosporin in immune-mediated disease

Sebaceous adenitis: Ciclosporin has been evaluated in the treatment of this immune-mediated disease in dogs. The combination of ciclosporin and topical therapy was shown to be superior to either treatment alone (Lortz *et al.*, 2010).

Symmetrical lupoid onychodystrophy (lupoid onychitis): A Scandinavian study compared the efficacy of a fish oil supplement high in omega-3 fatty acids with ciclosporin. All dogs in the study were on the same diet. After 6 months of treatment, the ciclosporin and fish oil supplement had an equipotent effect (Ziener and Nodtvedt, 2014).

Perianal fistulas and anal furunculosis: Oral ciclosporin at a dose of 5–10 mg/kg q24h is the initial treatment of choice for dogs affected with anal furunculosis. Co-morbidities such as colitis and secondary bacterial colonization of the perianal area should also be addressed. For many affected dogs, the dose can be tapered. Some dogs will go into remission after 8–12 weeks of therapy; others may require a long-term maintenance dose. Once large fistulas are controlled, the addition of topical tacrolimus 0.1%, a related calcineurin inhibitor, may be an effective adjunctive or maintenance treatment (Cain, 2019).

Other uses: Ciclosporin has also been reportedly effective as a sole treatment in cutaneous histiocytosis and metatarsal fistulation. In other immune-mediated diseases, ciclosporin is often effective alongside glucocorticoid therapy, particularly pemphigus foliaceus, sterile nodular panniculitis and cutaneous lupus, and acts as a steroid-sparing agent.

Quinolones

Quinolones are antimalarial drugs used in human medicine, which are also used to treat various forms of human cutaneous lupus erythematosus.

Mechanism of action

Quinolones reduce autoantigen presentation, downregulate proinflammatory cytokines and protect against ultraviolet light-induced cellular damage.

Formulations, indications and dosing

Hydroxychloroquine at a dose of 5–10 mg/kg q24h has been used in a few canine patients with cutaneous lupus with variable efficacy. Dogs should be monitored for retinal damage and cardiotoxicity and haematological abnormalities.

Essential fatty acids

Essential fatty acids (EFAs) are required from dietary sources as they are not synthesized in the body. Omega-6 fatty acids, such as linoleic acid, gamma linoleic acid, arachidonic acid and dihomogammalinoleic acid, are important components of the stratum corneum. Omega-3 fatty acids compete with omega-6 fatty acids for the same enzymes. This results in replacement of omega-6 metabolites in cell membrane phospholipids. Mediators derived from omega-3 fatty acids are less inflammatory, neutral or anti-inflammatory. In this regard, they have often been used as an adjunctive treatment for immune-mediated diseases. Aside from the aforementioned study on the treatment of symmetrical lupoid onychodystrophy, there is a lack of robust evidence for efficacy in autoimmune diseases. However, consideration should be given to using omega-3 EFAs as an adjunctive therapy, given the minimal side effects associated with supplementation or feeding a diet fortified with EFAs.

Pain relief

Consideration should be given to providing adequate pain relief in the acute stages of autoimmune and immune-mediated skin diseases. Severe skin ulceration and diseases affecting the paws, nails and mucosae can cause particular discomfort. Non-steroidal anti-inflammatory medications (NSAIDs) should not be given at the same time as glucocorticoids.

Vaccination whilst on immunosuppressive treatment

- Cats on 7 mg/kg ciclosporin had an adequate humoral response to booster vaccinations, but a poor initial response (Roberts *et al.*, 2015)
- Tetracycline/nicotinamide does not affect titres (Mueller *et al.*, 2002)
- Live vaccinations should not be given to patients on immunosuppressive therapy
- For previously vaccinated patients, booster vaccination may be given with the expectation that the humoral immune response may be blunted. Where possible, vaccination should be delayed until low dose maintenance immunosuppression is achieved

---

Key points

- Glucocorticoids are the cornerstone of immunosuppression in animals with autoimmune disease, but the cumulative effect of treatment can cause many side effects, some of which are life-threatening
- Any animal on long-term therapy for autoimmune disease should have regular clinical examinations and, in many cases, bloodwork and urinalysis should also be monitored
- If an animal on immunosuppressive therapy develops new skin lesions, it should firstly be assessed for bacterial pyoderma, *Malassezia* dermatitis and demodicosis, before assuming that the autoimmune disease has recurred

---

References and further reading

Ackermann AL, May ER, and Frank LA (2017) Use of mycophenolate mofetil to treat immune-mediated skin disease in 14 dogs – a retrospective evaluation. *Veterinary Dermatology* **28**, 195-e44.

Archer TM, Mulligan C, Narayanan L *et al.* (2020) Effects of oral administration of 5 immunosuppressive agents on activated T-cell cytokine expression in healthy dogs. *Journal of Veterinary Internal Medicine* **34**, 1206–1213

Aymeric E and Bensignor E (2017) A case of presumed autoimmune subepidermal blistering dermatosis treated with oclacitinib. *Veterinary Dermatology* **28**, 512–e123

Banovic F, Koch S, Robsin D *et al.* (2015) Deep pyoderma caused by Burkholderia cepacia complex associated with ciclosporin administration in dogs: a case series. *Veterinary Dermatology* **26**, 287–e64

Banovic F, Tarigo J, Gordon H *et al.* (2019) Immunomodulatory *in vitro* effects of oclacitinib on canine T-cell proliferation and cytokine production. *Veterinary Dermatology* **30**, 17–e6.

Cain CL (2019) Canine perianal fistulas. Clinical presentation, pathogenesis and management. *Veterinary Clinics of North America: Small Animal Practice* **49**, 53–65

Dowling SR, Webb J, Foster JD *et al.* (2016) Opportunistic fungal infections in dogs treated with ciclosporin and glucocorticoids: eight cases. *Journal of Small Animal Practice* **57**, 105–109

Gregory CR, Stewart A, Sturges B *et al.* (1988) Leflunomide effectively treats naturally occurring immune-mediated and inflammatory diseases of dogs that are unresponsive to conventional therapy. *Transplantation Proceedings* **30**, 41443–4148

Kovilak M, Thoday KL, Handel IG *et al.* (2011) Ciclosporin A therapy is associated with disturbances in glucose metabolism in dogs with atopic dermatitis. *Veterinary Dermatology* **22**, 173–180

Lappin MR, VanLare KA, Seewald W *et al.* (2015) Effect of oral administration of cyclosporine on *Toxoplasma gondii* infection status of cats. *American Journal of Veterinary Research* **76**, 351–357

Levy BJ, Linder KE and Olivry T (2019) The role of oclacitinib in the management of ischaemic dermatopathy in four dogs. *Veterinary Dermatology* **20**, 201–e63

Lortz J, Favrot C, Mecklenburg L *et al.* (2010) A multicentre placebo-controlled clinical trial on the efficacy of oral ciclosporin A in the treatment of canine idiopathic sebaceous adenitis in comparison with conventional topical treatment. *Veterinary Dermatology* **21**, 593–601

McAtee BB, Cummings KJ, Cook AK *et al.* (2017) Opportunistic invasive cutaneous fungal infections associated with administration of cyclosporine to dogs with immune-mediated disease. *Journal of Veterinary Internal Medicine* **31**, 1724–1729

Mueller RS, Fieseler KV, Bettenay SV and Rosychuk RAW (2002) Influence of long-term treatment with tetracycline and niacinamide on antibody production in dogs with discoid lupus erythematosus. *American Journal of Veterinary Research* **63**, 491–494

Nuttal T, Reece D and Roberts E (2014) Life-long diseases need life-long treatment: long-term safety of ciclosporin in canine atopic dermatitis. *Veterinary Record* **174**, 3–12

Roberts ES, VanLare KA, Roycroft LM and King S (2015) Effect of high-dose ciclosporin on the immune response to primary and booster vaccination in immunocompetent cats. *Journal of Feline Medicine and Surgery* **17**, 101–109

Siak M and Burrows A (2013) Cutaneous Nocardiosis in two dogs receiving ciclosporin therapy for the management of atopic dermatitis. *Veterinary Dermatology* **24**, 453–456

Spurlock NK and Prittie JE (2011) A review of current indications, adverse effects and administration recommendations for intravenous immunoglobulin. *Journal of Veterinary Emergency and Critical Care* **21**, 471–483

Steffan J, Alexander D, Bro Vedani F and FISCH RD (2003) Comparison of cyclosporine A with methylprednisolone for treatment of canine atopic dermatitis: a parallel, blinded randomized controlled trial. *Veterinary Dermatology* **14**, 11–22

Wallisch K and Trepanier L (2015) Incidence, timing and risk factors of azathioprine toxicosis in dogs. *Journal of Veterinary Internal Medicine* **29**, 513–518

Ziener M and Nodtvedt A (2014) A treatment study of canine symmetrical onychomadesis (symmetrical lupoid onychodystrophy) comparing fish oil and cyclosporine supplementation in addition to a diet rich in omega-3 fatty acids. *Acta Veterinaria Scandinavia* **56**, 66

Chapter 30

Subcutaneous, deep and systemic infections

Cecilia Friberg

Cutaneous lesions are prominent in many systemic and deep infectious diseases. When patients present with clinical signs that are compatible with such disorders, a thorough history, especially a travel history, is crucial because many diseases are endemic to certain geographical locations. It should be noted that many of the diseases discussed in this chapter are exotic to the UK. Some of these diseases are also contagious, so the existence of any affected in-contact animals needs to be noted. When gathering samples from these patients, it is recommended that precautions be taken, such as wearing gloves to avoid the transfer of any potentially infectious agents. A complete physical examination, including all organ systems, will help to identify those infections that commonly affect multiple organ systems. Patients on immunosuppressive treatment are particularly susceptible to these types of infections.

Bacterial infections

Atypical mycobacterial infections

Mycobacterium fortuitum, *M. phlei*, *M. smegmatis*, *M. thermoresistibile* and *M. chelonei* are rapidly growing mycobacteria (i.e. non-chromogenic, Gram-positive, acid-fast, aerobic, non-spore forming bacilli, classified as Runyon group IV mycobacteria). These mycobacteria are ubiquitous in nature and can be isolated from soil, dirt and various water sources. Rapidly growing mycobacteria infect cats more often than other species. Infected individuals usually have a history of trauma, and the organisms are introduced through damaged skin. These infections are more common in warm humid climates, but have been reported in many other regions, including parts of Australia, the southern United States, Canada, Finland and Germany.

Mycobacterium avium, *M. ulcerans*, *M. nebraskense*, *M. genavense*, *M. xenopi* and *M. intracellulare* are slow growing mycobacteria (i.e. acid-fast, non-chromogenic, slender rods that may require weeks to months for growth in culture, classified as Runyon group III mycobacteria). These organisms are referred to as the *M. avium* complex because they have similar growth *in vitro*, pigmentation and biochemical characteristics. These mycobacteria are ubiquitous in the environment and infection usually begins with ingestion or percutaneous penetration of the organisms.

Clinical approach

In cats, infection with rapidly growing mycobacteria most commonly presents as chronic or recurrent fistulous tracts and ulcers. Lesions are often found over the ventral abdomen and inguinal fat pads; best described as a mycobacterial panniculitis. The underlying adipose tissue may be palpably thickened, firm and nodular. The infection may migrate along fascial planes. Cats are not affected systemically by this cutaneous disease; although, dissemination may rarely occur. Canine disease is rare and lesions are often associated with trauma, bite wounds or injection sites. Recurrent firm to fluctuant subcutaneous swellings or nodules, or abscesses that ulcerate and drain can be seen in infected dogs. These lesions may spread centrifugally. Disseminated disease and pulmonary disease without cutaneous involvement have been described in the dog. The prognosis for remission with medical and surgical management appears to be better for dogs than for cats.

In cats, infection with slow growing mycobacteria (*M. avium* complex) may present as nodules or diffuse subcutaneous swellings and, in this species, disseminated systemic disease is more common. In dogs, disease usually remains in the visceral organs and cutaneous involvement is rare. Anorexia, weight loss, lymphadenopathy, splenomegaly and anaemia may occur in dogs and cats with disseminated disease.

Diagnostic tests: Culture is preferred for the definitive diagnosis of this disease and antimicrobial sensitivity testing is important for the selection of adequate treatment. The laboratory should be alerted ahead of time that mycobacteria are suspected. Large samples of lesional tissue, including adipose tissue collected under anaesthesia, must be submitted for culture. Deep pockets of purulent material aspirated through intact skin may also be cultured successfully. Exudate from lesions will typically result in negative cultures or the growth of contaminant bacteria. *M. fortuitum* is isolated most commonly, then *M. smegmatis*, *M. phlei* and *M. chelonei*.

Cytological samples from exudates or tissue aspirates are typically pyogranulomatous. Occasionally, special stains will reveal the causative agent in exudate samples. Histopathology shows varying degrees of granuloma formation, pyogranulomatous dermatitis, cellulitis and panniculitis. Organisms are most often visible in the central clear spaces of pyogranulomas, although these acid-fast bacteria are only seen about 50% of the time in affected cases. Organisms of the *M. avium* complex are usually seen in higher numbers and are more likely to be identified on cytology and histopathology compared with rapidly growing mycobacteria.

Treatment

Antimicrobial therapy should be based on culture and sensitivity results. Long courses of antibiotics are required and some patients will relapse after discontinuation of the drugs, necessitating indefinite therapy in these cases. Fluoroquinolone antibiotics (e.g. marbofloxacin, pradofloxacin) and doxycycline (5–10 mg/kg orally q12h) or clarithromycin (10–15 mg/kg orally q12h) are recommended in combination and are preferred for empirical treatment while sensitivity results are pending. High doses of fluoro-quinolone antibiotics are recommended owing to poor perfusion of affected fatty subcutaneous tissue. Pradofloxacin/marbofloxacin is preferred to enrofloxacin use in cats because doses >5 mg/kg orally q24h of enrofloxacin have been associated with blindness. Following preliminary antimicrobial therapy, wide surgical resection of the lesions can be helpful in managing these infections. Antimicrobial therapy should be continued for at least 2 months after clinical resolution. Overall, the prognosis remains guarded.

Feline leprosy syndrome

Feline leprosy has been associated with a variety of mycobacteria, including *Mycobacterium lepraemurium*, *M. lepraefelis*, *M. visibile* and *M. tarwinense* (Figure 30.1). These infections are associated with different clinical presentations and a varied geographical distribution. *M. lepraemurium* is most common in young cats <4 years old and has a wide geographical distribution with an increased prevalence in rural areas, temperate coastal areas and port cities in Canada, the United States, the UK, the Netherlands, France, New Caledonia, Italy, the Greek Islands, Japan, New Zealand and parts of Australia. *M. lepraemurium* is an environmental saprophyte adapted to living in a rodent host, which then infects cats as an incidental 'dead end' host. *M. lepraefelis* has a smaller geographical distribution with infected cats reported in Australia, New Zealand and Canada. Cats infected with *M. lepraefelis* are generally older (mostly over 7 years of age). *M. tarwinense* appears geographically restricted to southeastern Australia and is an environmental sapro-phyte with middle-aged to older cats being incidental 'dead end' hosts.

Clinical approach

Single or multiple, firm to soft, intact or ulcerated, non-painful, freely movable nodules varying in size from a few millimetres to 4 cm in diameter in the skin or subcutis present most frequently on the limbs and head. Regional lymphadenopathy is common, but disseminated disease is rare. Lesions associated with *M. lepraemurium* involve the head and forelimbs and affected cats are usually known hunters and/or fighters. Infected cats tend towards a more protracted disease course over months to years. Infection with *M. lepraefelis* appears to be variable but tends to progress to widespread disseminated cutaneous involvement, sometimes after initially localized disease, with the potential for systemic involvement. Lesions associated with *M. tarwinense* have a predilection to involve the head, especially the ocular, nasal and periocular skin and subcutis.

Diagnostic tests: Biopsy for histopathology is indicated. The histological appearance varies from tuberculoid (with relatively small numbers of acid-fast bacilli) to lepromatous (associated with numerous acid-fast bacilli). However, the absence of growth on routine mycobacterial cultures, along with compatible clinical signs, is the most common diagnostic feature. *M. lepraemurium* is very difficult to grow *in vitro*, even when special microbiological techniques are used. The laboratory should hold the cultures for 3 months before they are considered negative. Inoculation of infected tissue into rats and mice, with resulting localized or disseminated disease, may be helpful in establishing a diagnosis of *M. lepraemurium*. Polymerase chain reaction (PCR)/sequencing assays are needed for species identification.

Treatment

Wide surgical excision of the affected tissue is key to the management of feline leprosy syndrome and may be curative in some cases. If this is not possible, long-term management with a combination of two or more of the following antibiotics should be considered:

- Clofazimine
- Clarithromycin
- Rifampicin
- Moxifloxacin/pradofloxacin.

This is an active area of research and clinicians are encouraged to consult an expert in the field for specific therapeutic advice. Prognosis varies with the type of

Disease feature	Mycobacterium tarwinense	Mycobacterium lepraemurium	Mycobacterium lepraefelis
Age trend	Middle-aged to older adults	Young adults, generally <3 years of age	Middle-aged to older adults, invariably >3 years of age
Gender predilection	No predilection	Male predilection	Male predilection
Clinical disease trend	A few non-ulcerated nodules particularly on the head (often involving ocular and periocular structures). No clinical evidence of haematogenous spread	Can range from localized to widespread disease, likely haematogenous distribution, skin lesions	Typically causes widespread disease, with no anatomical predilection. Systemic signs of illness can develop. Haematogenous spread documented at necropsy
Prognosis with therapy	Variable	Good	Guarded but poor if oedema is present
Disease virulence (risk of death if untreated)	Low	Low	Moderate to high
Geographical distribution of cases	Highly restricted (VIC, Australia, with two outliers in NSW). Never seen outside Australia	Worldwide coastal trend	East coast of mainland Australia, both islands of New Zealand, one suspected case in British Columbia, Canada

30.1 Summary of the comparative qualitative aspects of infection with the three different agents of feline leproid disease. NSW = New South Wales; VIC = Victoria.

(Data from O'Brien et al., 2017a)

infection and immunological status of the patient. Cats infected with *M. tarwinense* respond best to a combination of rifampin plus clarithromycin. In one study, the overall outcome of infection with *M. tarwinense* was typically favourable with complete resolution in 68% of cases (O'Brien *et al.*, 2017b). Cats infected with *M. lepraemurium* tend to respond favourably to surgical excision and use of long-term antibiotics. There are currently no reports of *M. lepraemurium* spread from cat to cat or infection in dogs, ferrets or native wildlife. Infection with *M. lepraefelis* responded less favourably to treatment, with a poor response noted in cats presenting with subcutaneous oedema and/or systemic signs either before or during therapy.

Canine leproid granuloma syndrome

This is a poorly characterized nodular mycobacterial syndrome in dogs. The pathogenesis of this syndrome is unknown; however, biting flies may be responsible for inoculating novel species of mycobacteria into susceptible dogs. A disease predilection has been noted in short-coated breeds, and Boxers and their crossbreeds are over-represented. This syndrome is common in Australia and Brazil but has a worldwide distribution with reports of disease in New Zealand, South Africa, Europe (Italy) and various regions of the United States such as the central valley of California and Georgia. The organism associated with this syndrome has never been reported to affect any other species, hence no public health risk is believed to exist.

Clinical approach

This syndrome presents with single or multiple firm non-painful nodules, 2–50 mm in diameter, which may ulcerate. Predilection sites include the head and dorsal surface of the pinnae, but lesions may occur on the distal limbs and trunk. Infected dogs appear not to be affected systemically because internal organ and/or lymph node involvement has not been described.

Diagnostic tests: Histopathology of nodules shows variable numbers of acid-fast bacilli surrounded by granulomatous inflammation. Infrequently, fine-needle aspiration of nodules may allow identification of the organisms via cytology. Culture and sensitivity testing are recommended; however, this organism is hard to grow and commonly no mycobacterial organisms are isolated on culture, even though they are evident in the tissues (a negative culture will help to rule out other mycobacterial infections). Although not widely available, a definitive diagnosis is made by gene amplification using *Mycobacterium* specific primers. When obtaining samples, surface cleansing is important to avoid contamination from environmental mycobacteria.

Treatment

Surgical resection or laser ablation of nodules either alone or in combination with antibiotics, such as doxycycline, amoxicillin/clavulanate, cefalexin, enrofloxacin and orbifloxacin, results in a favourable response in most dogs. Spontaneous resolution has been described in up to 86% of untreated dogs, often occurring within 1–3 months. If lesions persist beyond this time period, intervention is recommended. Chronic lesions persist in some dogs despite treatment.

Cutaneous tuberculosis

The causative agents of tuberculosis (*M. bovis, M. tuberculosis* and *M. microti*) may infect dogs and cats. The incidence of infection with *M. bovis* and *M. tuberculosis* in companion animals has decreased in proportion to the decline of disease in humans and cattle. Approximately a third of feline mycobacteriosis cases in the UK are caused by *M. tuberculosis* complex pathogens: *M. microti* has been cultured in 19% of cases and *M. bovis* cultured in 15% of cases. Dogs and cats generally contract *M. bovis* by consuming unprocessed meat or milk. The consumption of a contaminated raw meat-based diet has recently been linked to an outbreak of *M. bovis* in more than 90 cats in the UK (O'Halloran *et al.*, 2019). *M. microti* is carried by wild mice and voles, and cats who hunt these prey species are considered at increased risk of infection. This *Mycobacterium* spp. is not considered zoonotic. Cats are more commonly infected with *M. bovis* and *M. microti* than dogs. *M. tuberculosis* infection is exceedingly rare in dogs and cats, with cats displaying a natural resistance to infection with *M. tuberculosis*, and is contracted via airborne transmission from an infected human.

Clinical approach

The cutaneous lesions present as draining tracts, nodules, plaques, abscesses or ulcers that may be single or multiple, and occur most commonly on the head, neck, tail base and limbs. Cutaneous lesions may also reflect diseased subcutaneous tissues such as lymph nodes. Cutaneous involvement is considered more common with *M. microti* infection; it is unusual with the other forms, in which the respiratory and digestive systems are most commonly affected. Patients are usually systemically ill with variable lymphadenopathy fever, weight loss and anorexia.

Diagnostic tests: Biopsy, culture and compatible history and physical examination findings are needed for diagnosis. Histopathology shows nodular to diffuse pyogranulomatous inflammation with variable numbers of intracellular and extracellular acid-fast bacilli. These organisms are slow growing and may take up to 8 weeks to produce colonies. PCR and interferon-gamma release assay testing may be useful for diagnosis and can be helpful in confirming *M. bovis* infection in cats. Intradermal testing with bacillus Calmette–Guerin (BCG) or purified protein derivative (PPD) is not useful in cats, but may be used in dogs; however, both tuberculous and non-tuberculous mycobacterial infections give positive results with these tests. Intradermal injection with 0.1–0.2 ml of BCG or PPD is best performed on the medial aspect of the pinna. The injection site should be evaluated 48–72 hours later, with resolved erythema at that time compatible with a negative test result. A positive test result manifests as severe persistent erythema with central necrosis progressing to ulceration at 10–14 days.

Treatment

M. tuberculosis infections in animals are notifiable in the UK due to the zoonotic potential. Dogs and cats with tuberculosis caused by *M. tuberculosis* are euthanized and treatment is not recommended. Zoonotic transmission risk for *M. bovis* from cats to humans is considered to be low; however, the risk is still present. It is currently not a notifiable disease, but serious consideration should be given to treatment of affected pets if there are immunocompromised individuals in the household. When treatment is attempted, combination therapy with two or three drugs, such as rifampin, a fluoroquinolone (pradofloxacin) and a macrolide (azithromycin) should be considered; clarithromycin, metronidazole and isoniazid have also been used. Daily treatment is recommended for a minimum of 3 months and for 2 months beyond resolution of clinical signs; if there is pulmonary involvement, the minimum treatment recommendation is 6 months.

Nocardiosis and actinomycosis

Actinomyces spp. and *Nocardia* spp. are actinomycetes that cause disease in dogs and cats. *Actinomyces* spp. are anaerobic actinomycetes, which form part of the normal bacterial flora of the mucous membranes. *Nocardia* spp. are aerobic actinomycetes and ubiquitous soil saprophytes that degrade organic matter and are found in soil, dust, fresh and salt water, faecal matter and on plants. Infections are considered opportunistic and occur via inhalation or wound inoculation. Co-infection with *Actinomyces* spp. and other bacteria is common. Immunocompromised individuals are at higher risk for infection. The use of immunomodulatory medications increases the risk for infection.

Clinical approach

Acute or chronic soft tissue swelling results in a firm to fluctuant, indurated lesion that can be ulcerated or have draining sinuses (Figure 30.2). Draining exudate is pungent, appears serosanguinous to purulent, and may contain macroscopic white, tan or grey granules. Firm lesions may have minimal discharge. Lesions in dogs are typically located in the head/neck region, lateral thoracic wall or flank region, and are usually extensions of cervicofacial, thoracic or retroperitoneal infection with *Actinomyces* spp. Infections involving the extremities and central nervous system (CNS) in the dog are rare. Systemic clinical signs reflect the extent and spread of the infection. The infection may spread via haematogenous or lymphatic dissemination from a primary site, or by direct extension. *Actinomyces* spp. infection in cats is documented infrequently.

Nocardia spp. infection presents in the dog as pulmonary, systemic (or disseminated) and/or solitary cutaneous–subcutaneous nocardiosis. The disseminated form is usually an extension of pulmonary disease. Lesions are similar in appearance to those of *Actinomyces* spp. infection; however, infections may develop on the extremities and involve underlying bone; granules are noted less commonly. Nocardiosis in cats presents most commonly in the cutaneous–subcutaneous form.

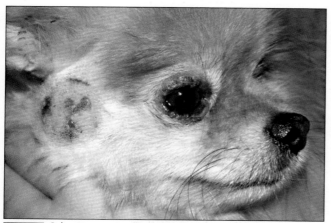

30.2 Subcutaneous swelling and induration with draining tract in a dog infected with *Actinomyces* spp.

Diagnostic tests:

Actinomyces species: On cytological examination, a mixture of bacteria (containing both rods and cocci) is common. Bacteria may be seen individually or in dense aggregates within the granules as Gram-positive, non-acid-fast variably branched filamentous organisms. Diagnosis is confirmed by culture of these organisms (ideally a sample containing granules should be submitted); however, a positive culture may be difficult to obtain or contain only opportunistic bacteria. Co-infection with companion microbes is common as the pathogenicity of *Actinomyces* spp. is dramatically increased in mixed infections. *Actinomyces* spp. are facultative or obligate anaerobes and are best cultured in anaerobic conditions; proper sample handling is critical.

Nocardia species: Cytology of the exudate reveals suppurative to pyogranulomatous, Gram-positive, partially or weakly acid-fast, beaded, branching, filamentous organisms either individually or in loose aggregates. Unlike *Actinomyces* spp. infections, mixed bacterial infections from deeper lesions are rare. The diagnosis is confirmed by aerobic culture. Gene sequencing of the 16s ribosomal deoxyribonucleic acid (DNA) and use of matrix-absorption laser desorption ionization-time-of-flight mass spectrometry (MALDI-TOF MS) can be used to identify *Nocardia* species.

Treatment

Actinomyces *species:* Prolonged courses (usually weeks to months) of antibiotics (usually penicillin G or penicillin V at 40 mg/kg q8h) are usually required. Other antibiotics reported to be effective include erythromycin, clindamycin, ampicillin, minocycline, chloramphenicol and rifampin. Surgical treatment is controversial; however, drainage of abscesses and effusions is recommended in conjunction with antibiotic therapy. Infection of deeper tissues should always be considered. Prolonged antibiotic courses should be extended weeks to months beyond resolution of clinical disease; treatment for more than 12 months may be needed.

Nocardia *species:* Sulphonamides are the antibiotic of choice to treat nocardiosis and prolonged therapy is usually required. Antibiotics in addition to, or other than, sulphonamides may be needed, and antibiotic resistance may develop during therapy. Long-term use of sulphonamides requires monitoring for side effects such as myelosuppression. Antibiotic sensitivity testing of *Nocardia* spp. is technically difficult and should be performed at experienced laboratories, as the different subspecies of *Nocardia* may vary in susceptibility.

Fungal infections

Sporotrichosis

Sporothrix schenckii is a dimorphic fungus of worldwide distribution that exists as a saprophyte in soil and organic matter. Disease occurs more frequently in the Americas, Africa, Japan and Australasia, and is considered rare in Europe. Infection is usually acquired by direct inoculation of the organism into tissues. **Sporotrichosis is a zoonotic disease that can be transmitted from animals to humans.**

Clinical approach

Three different forms of this infection are seen: cutaneous, cutaneo-lymphatic and disseminated. An affected individual may have more than one form of the infection. Dogs most often have the cutaneous or cutaneo-lymphatic form, and the disseminated form is considered rare in this species; the disseminated form is more common in cats.

In dogs, the skin lesions associated with the cutaneous form are mostly multiple firm nodules and plaques that may ulcerate to form draining tracts. They are commonly found on the head, pinnae and trunk, but can occur anywhere on the body. The cutaneo-lymphatic form presents as a nodule on a distal limb with an ascending infection via the lymphatic system. Secondary nodules may develop in association with regional lymph nodes. In most cases, dogs show no signs of pain or pruritus and appear otherwise healthy.

Lesions in cats most often consist of draining wounds and abscesses with associated cellulitis. Disease in cats can range from single skin lesions to a fatal systemic form due to haematogenous dissemination. Lesions, which are sometimes associated with cat fight wounds, are found most commonly on the head, distal limbs and tail head. These lesions may become progressively exudative, with associated crusting, or may ulcerate and exhibit skin necrosis that extends to the underlying soft tissue.

Lymphatic involvement is usually not clinically apparent but is frequently present on post-mortem examination. Grooming behaviour may lead to autoinoculation and the development of additional lesions.

Diagnostic tests: Direct visualization reveals cigar-shaped, round or oval yeast organisms, between 3 and 10 μm in diameter, either extracellularly or within phagocytic cells. Large numbers of organisms are often, but not always, noted in exudates from cats, but consistently low numbers are noted from canine lesions. Organisms may be found in exudate; however, biopsy of early intact nodules is preferred and tissue should be submitted for macerated tissue culture in addition to histopathology. Fluorescent antibody detection on biopsy tissue samples can be helpful in establishing a diagnosis in dogs when the organisms are not detected and fungal cultures are negative. PCR has also been used to detect *S. schenckii* in biopsy specimens. Serological testing for antibodies against *Sporothrix* needs to be interpreted cautiously because positive test results only indicate exposure.

Treatment

Guidelines for antifungal therapy in dogs and cats are given in Figure 30.3. Supersaturated potassium iodide (SSKI) is the preferred therapy for sporotrichosis in dogs;

Disease	Drug	Dose
Blastomycosis	Itraconazole	Dogs: 5 mg/kg orally q24h for 60 days Cats: 5 mg/kg orally q12h for 60 days
	Fluconazole	Dogs: 5 mg/kg orally q12h for 60 days
	Amphotericin B lipid complex	Dogs: 1 mg/kg i.v. 3 times a week. Stop when cumulative dose reaches 12 mg/kg
	Amphotericin B	Dogs: 0.5 mg/kg i.v. 3 times a week. Stop when azotaemic or cumulative dose reaches 4–6 mg/kg, then start azole; or when cumulative dose is 8–10 mg/kg when given alone Cats: 0.25 mg/kg i.v. 3 times a week. Stop when azotaemic or cumulative dose reaches 4 mg/kg
Coccidioidomycosis	Fluconazole	Dogs: 10–20 mg/kg orally q12h for 12 months Cats: 10–15 mg/kg orally q12h or 50 mg/cat orally q12h for 12 months
	Itraconazole	Dogs: 5 mg/kg orally q12h for 12 months Cats: 25–50 mg/cat orally q12–24h for 12 months
	Ketoconazole	Dogs: 5–10 mg/kg orally q12h for 8–12 months Cats: 50 mg/cat orally q12–24h for 12 months
	Amphotericin B	Dogs: 0.4–0.5 mg/kg i.v. q48–72h until cumulative dose is 8–11 mg/kg
Cryptococcosis	Fluconazole	Dogs, cats: 10 mg/kg orally q12h for 6–10 months or until titre decreases to zero Cats: 30–50 mg/cat orally q12h for 6–10 months
	Flucytosine	Dogs: 50–75 mg/kg orally q8h for 1–12 months Cats: 30 mg/kg orally q6h OR 50 mg/kg orally q8h OR 75 mg/kg orally q12h for 1–9 months
	Amphotericin B (deoxycholate)	Dogs, cats: 0.5 mg/kg i.v. 3 times a week until minimum cumulative dose of 10 mg/kg. For dogs – up to 40 mg/kg over a course of several months OR 0.5–0.8 mg/kg s.c. 2–3 times a week. Add each dose to 400 ml of 0.45% saline, 2.5% dextrose. For dogs >20 kg, add amphotericin B to 900 ml of 0.45% saline, 2.5% dextrose Cats: 0.5–0.8 mg/kg i.v. 2 times a week until minimum cumulative dose of 10 mg/kg
	Amphotericin B (lipid complex)	Dogs: 1 mg/kg i.v. 3 times a week. With lipid complex drug, dose per administration and cumulative dose may be slightly increased until a cumulative dose of 8–12 mg/kg has been reached
	Ketoconazole	Dogs: 5–15 mg/kg orally q12h OR 30 mg/kg orally q24h for 6–10 months Cats: 5–10 mg/kg orally q12h OR 10–20 mg/kg orally q24h for 6–10 months
	Itraconazole	Dogs: 10 mg/kg orally q24h for 6–10 months Cats: 10–20 mg/kg orally q12h for 6–10 months; 3.5 kg bodyweight: 50 mg/cat orally q24h for 6–10 months; >3.5 kg bodyweight: 100 mg/cat orally q24h for 6–10 months; ≥3.5 kg bodyweight: 100 mg/cat orally q48h for 6–10 months
	Fluconazole	Dogs: 10–20 mg/kg/d 4–6 months Cats: 20 mg/kg/d 4–6 months

30.2 Antifungal therapy for selected deep fungal infections of the dog and cat. (continues) ▶

Disease	Drug	Dose
Histoplasmosis	Itraconazole	Dogs, cats: 10 mg/kg orally q12–24h for 4–6 months
	Ketoconazole	Dogs: 10–20 mg/kg orally q12h for 4–6 months
	Amphotericin B	Dogs, cats: 0.25–0.5 mg/kg i.v. q48h until cumulative dose of 5–10 mg/kg in dogs and 4–8 mg/kg in cats is reached
Sporotrichosis	Supersaturated solution of potassium iodide	Dogs: 40 mg/kg orally q8h for >2 months Cats: 10–20 mg/kg orally q12h for >2 months
	Ketoconazole	Dogs: 5–15 mg/kg orally q12h for >2 months Cats: 5–10 mg/kg orally q12–24h for >2 months
	Itraconazole: Capsules	Dogs, cats: 5–10 mg/kg orally q12–24h for >2 months Cats: 15 mg/kg orally q24h for >2 months
	Solution	Cats: 1.25–1.5 mg/kg orally q24h for >2 months
	Terbinafine	Cats: 30 mg/kg orally q24h for >2 months

30.3 (continued) Antifungal therapy for selected deep fungal infections of the dog and cat.

however, adverse effects have limited its use. Patients should be monitored for signs of iodism (ocular and nasal discharge, dry hair coat with scaling, vomiting, depression and collapse). Ketoconazole and itraconazole are effective, but the risk of hepatotoxicity exists with both drugs. Cats do not tolerate SSKI or ketoconazole well, so itraconazole is the recommended treatment. Liver enzymes should be monitored monthly whilst the patient is undergoing therapy. Terbinafine can be used in combination with other drugs in resistant cases. Refractory cases have been shown to respond to combination drug therapy or cryotherapy. Dogs and cats should be treated for 30 days beyond clinical cure. **Direct transmission from infected patients to humans is a risk with this disease, especially from cats where large numbers of organisms are noted. All individuals handling these patients should wear gloves and dispose of contaminated material properly. If there are immunocompromised individuals in the household, the affected animal should be removed for the duration of treatment.**

Blastomycosis

Blastomyces dermatitidis is a thermally dimorphic fungus that grows as a saprophyte in the environment, where it exists in a septate mycelial form, as yeasts within infected tissues. It is found in sandy acidic soil with a high organic content. This is primarily a North American disease with the organism endemic to the Great Lakes region and the Ohio, Mississippi and Missouri river valleys, but there have been reports further east into New York State. It has also been identified in Africa, India, Europe and Central America. The mycelial form produces conidia (spores) that are inhaled by the host, then phagocytosed by alveolar macrophages. At body temperature, the spores transform into yeasts with characteristic broad-based budding and double-contoured walls. Direct skin inoculation may also occur. Once infection develops, the organism usually affects multiple organ systems, including the skin.

Clinical approach

Dogs are primarily affected; the infection is rare in cats. Lesions may occur anywhere in the body. Cutaneous lesions should be considered an extension of systemic disease because solitary focal cutaneous lesions are rare. Skin lesions often present as intact or ulcerated nodules or plaques, or as abscesses/masses with tracts draining serosanguineous to purulent exudate. The lesions may appear proliferative. Skin lesions occur in 20–50% of dogs with blastomycosis. Cats have lesions similar to those of dogs, but very few cases have been reported. Common systemic clinical signs include anorexia, weight loss, cough, dyspnoea, ocular disease and lameness.

Diagnostic tests: Diagnosis is made by identification of the budding yeast organism (5–20 μm diameter) on cytology or histopathology; every effort should be made to identify the organisms. Serology can be used to help establish a diagnosis when organisms cannot be identified. The agar gel immunodiffusion test has a sensitivity of 41–90% and specificity of >90% in dogs; thus, a positive test is supportive, but not definitive, for blastomycosis. Serology should not be used to monitor the response to treatment because antibodies may persist in cured animals. Antigen detection from urine may be helpful in diagnosis and monitoring therapy; however, there is cross-reactivity between *Histoplasma* and *Blastomyces*. Culture of specimens is not recommended because the mycelia of *Blastomyces* spp. are highly infectious.

Treatment

Blastomycosis requires systemic therapy (see Figure 30.3). The current treatment of choice is itraconazole; fluconazole treatment is equally effective, and amphotericin B can also be used. However, it should be noted that the absorption of compounded generic itraconazole is not reliable. Affected animals should be treated with antifungal therapy for 4–6 weeks beyond clinical resolution. Relapse after therapy is seen in 20–25% of dogs, which may occur between 6 months and 3 years of age, and some individuals may require maintenance antifungal therapy to keep the disease in remission. Prognosis for recovery is good, but patients with ocular or neurological disease have a poor prognosis for cure. The zoonotic risk is minimal from aerosol transmission of the yeast phase. Penetrating wounds contaminated with organisms have produced infection in humans. Pulmonary disease has occurred in laboratory workers exposed to the mycelial form of the fungus.

Histoplasmosis

Histoplasma capsulatum is a soil-borne dimorphic fungus that grows best in moist, humid conditions and nitrogen-rich organic matter, such as the excrement of bats and birds. The free-living mycelium stage produces micro-conidia and macroconidia, which are the source of infection in dogs and cats. The microconidia are inhaled and then converted into the yeast form at body temperature. This organism and its resulting disease are described most commonly in the Ohio, Missouri and Mississippi river valleys, and the Midwest and Southern United States; however, it is endemic throughout large areas of the temperate and subtropical regions of the world, including Europe.

Clinical approach

Cats present most commonly with disseminated disease and clinical signs of fever, anorexia, weight loss, dyspnoea, ocular disease and depression. Skin lesions are uncommon, but when they do occur, they consist of draining tracts, papules, ulcers and nodules, often on the face, bridge of the nose and pinnae. Lesions may be limited to the skin. Clinical signs of skin disease in dogs are similar to those in cats; however, most dogs present with signs of large bowel diarrhoea, characterized by tenesmus, mucus and fresh blood in the stool.

Diagnostic tests: Direct visualization of the organisms on cytological evaluation of material collected by fine-needle aspiration and exfoliative cytology is considered the 'gold standard' and primary method of diagnosis; histopathology can also be used to diagnose this disease. The organisms appear as round yeast bodies, 2–4 μm in diameter, which are often contained within cells of the mononuclear phagocyte system. The inflammatory response is typically granulomatous to pyogranulomatous. Organisms may also be identified using PCR from infected tissue. A urine *Histoplasma* enzyme immunoassay, which detects the fungal antigen galactomannan, is available for dogs and cats; however, data regarding cross-reactivity with other fungal infections is lacking.

Treatment

Histoplasmosis requires systemic treatment (see Figure 30.3). Itraconazole and fluconazole are the current treatments of choice; fluconazole may be preferred if the eyes or CNS are affected. However, it should be noted that the absorption of compounded generic itraconazole is not reliable. Treatment typically involves a prolonged course of antifungal therapy, often 4–6 months, which should be continued for 4–6 weeks beyond clinical cure. Relapse may occur after cessation of therapy. Monitoring antigen concentrations may be helpful in detecting clinical relapse. Direct transmission of histoplasmosis from companion animals to humans has not been reported. The mycelial form, when grown in the laboratory, is highly infectious.

Cryptococcosis

Cryptococcosis may result from infection with *Crypto-coccus neoformans* or *C. gattii*. It is a saprophytic, yeast-like fungus often associated with accumulations of pigeon droppings. *C. neoformans* has a worldwide distribution and is the most common systemic mycosis of cats. *C. gattii* is usually associated with tropical and subtropical climates; however, it has also been found in some temperate climates in Europe and North America. The prevalence of this disease in cats is equal to or greater than that in dogs.

Clinical approach

Skin or subcutaneous lesions are present in up to 50% of feline cases. Lesions in cats manifest most commonly in the nasal cavity/upper respiratory tract, skin, CNS and eyes. Papules and variably sized nodules, abscesses, ulcers and draining tracts may be present anywhere on the body, but are noted most commonly on the face, pinnae and paws. Classic nasal lesions present in the cat as firm to boggy swellings over the bridge of the nose (Figure 30.4) or a fleshy polyp-like mass in the nostril. Sneezing, with unilateral or bilateral mucopurulent serous to haemorrhagic discharge, is compatible with commonly associated upper respiratory tract infections. Lesions confined to the skin without nasal involvement has been described in cats infected with a capsule-deficient form of *Cryptococcus* spp.

Cryptococcosis is an uncommon disease in the dog. Approximately 20% of cases will present with skin lesions. Lesions can occur anywhere on the body, but abscesses, nodules, papules, ulcers and draining tracts are noted most commonly on the lips, nose and digits, as well as the tongue, gums and hard palate on occasion. The eyes and CNS are also commonly affected. Dogs frequently develop severe disseminated disease. Multifocal cutaneous lesions are consistent with disseminated disease in dogs and cats.

Diagnostic tests: Diagnosis is made by direct visualization of the organism in smears made from exudates or by histopathology of biopsy samples from a lesion. Round to elliptical yeast-like organisms, ranging from 2–20 μm in diameter, are seen. These organisms typically display narrow-based budding and have a thick clear or refractile halo. The associated inflammation is granulomatous to pyogranulomatous. Culture of the organism and fungal susceptibility testing may be helpful in identifying resistant strains. Panfungal PCR may be performed on formalin-fixed paraffin embedded tissues. The latex agglutination test, which detects cryptococcal capsular antigen, is the most widely used serological test. It can be used to confirm the diagnosis and to monitor the response to therapy. Point of care cryptococcal antigen tests may also be useful for more rapid diagnosis; however, they appear to be less sensitive and specific than the latex agglutination test.

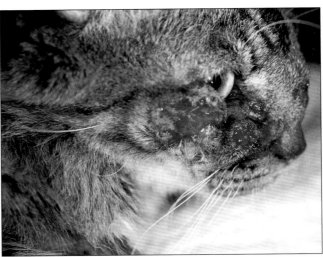

30.4 Cryptococcosis in a cat.
(Courtesy of R Marsella)

Treatment

Cryptococcosis requires systemic treatment (see Figure 30.3). Surgical debulking, prior to medical management, should be considered. Fluconazole therapy is effective; however, resistance has been identified in strains of *C. gattii* from North America. Liposomal amphotericin B may be used alone or in combination with flucytosine, which has been shown to have synergistic activity. Rapid resistance can develop if flucytosine is used alone, but it is mainly used to improve the efficacy of other antifungal drugs. Cutaneous drug reactions may occur 10–40 days after onset of flucytosine therapy in dogs and resolve after therapy is discontinued. Like other deep fungal infections, cryptococcosis typically requires a prolonged course of antifungal therapy. Treatment should be continued for at least 4–6 weeks beyond clinical cure. Relapse may occur after cessation of therapy. Organisms from infected tissues and body fluids do not spread between humans and animals; however, the environmental source of exposure for animals is also a potential source of exposure for humans.

Coccidioidomycosis

Two genetically distinct soil-borne fungi *Coccidioides immitis* and *C. posadasii*, which prefer sandy alkaline soil, low rainfall, elevation and high ambient temperatures, cause infection in endemic areas. These regions include areas of Central and South America, Mexico and the southwestern United States. Arthroconidia are inhaled and result in infection. Primary cutaneous infection is rare. Most inhabitants of endemic areas become infected, but the majority of infections are subclinical.

Clinical approach

Approximately 1–3 weeks after the inhalation of arthroconidia, respiratory signs are noted and are usually characterized by a dry harsh cough or a moist productive cough. Dogs may also exhibit clinical signs of intermittent fever, weight loss, lethargy, lameness and painful/sensitive bony swellings. Ocular disease may also present as uveitis, keratitis and acute blindness. Generalized peripheral lymphadenopathy and gastrointestinal signs are uncommon. Multiple skin lesions consisting of nodules, papules, ulcers, draining tracts and abscesses may be widely distributed on the body and usually result from the systemic hematogenous spread of organisms. Clinical signs in cats are similar to those in dogs; however, respiratory disease is seen less often. Skin lesions, as well as subcutaneous granulomas, draining tracts and abscesses are the most common clinical signs in cats and may occur with or without underlying bony involvement.

Diagnostic tests: Diagnosis is by direct visualization of the organism in a cytological or histopathological specimen. Organisms can be present in either a spherical form (20–200 μm in diameter) or an endospore form (2–5 μm in diameter). Serological tests, by means of agar gel immunodiffusion or antigen enzyme immunoassay, can be used to help confirm the diagnosis and monitor therapy.

Treatment

As with other deep disseminated fungal infections, coccidioidomycosis typically requires a prolonged course of antifungal therapy (see Figure 30.3). Fluconazole is most commonly used due to its high bioavailability and excellent tissue penetration. Other antifungal therapies are less commonly used alone or in combination with fluconazole. Treatment should be continued for 3–6 months beyond resolution of clinical signs and normalization of serological titres; therapy often in excess of 12 months is required. Relapse may occur after the cessation of therapy. Primary pulmonary disease may resolve spontaneously. Spread to humans by direct contact with an infected animal is very rare. However, the mycelial form of this organism grown in the laboratory is highly infectious.

Granulomatous dermatophytosis

For information on dermatophytosis, the reader is referred to Chapter 25.

Zygomycosis

Fungi in the genera *Conidiobolus* and *Basidiobolus* cause infection in immunocompetent patients. Lesions can appear grossly and histologically similar to those caused by oomycetes. These organisms are found in soil and decaying plant matter. In addition, *Basidiobolus* species are isolated commonly from insects and from reptile and amphibian faeces. Infection can result from percutaneous inoculation, direct implantation via trauma or inhalation.

Clinical approach

Lesions may present as non-healing masses that can progress to large boggy proliferative areas with ulceration and draining tracts, and variable degrees of tissue destruction. In dogs, conidiobolomycosis usually presents as ulcerative lesions of the nasopharyngeal region, including the hard palate; however, multifocal nodular draining subcutaneous lesions and pneumonia have also been described. Culture-confirmed infection in cats is lacking, but ulcerative lesions of the hard palate have been described. Basidiobolomycosis presents as ulcerative draining skin lesions in dogs and has also been described as a disseminated disease affecting the abdominal organs, including the gastrointestinal tract.

Diagnostic tests: A definitive diagnosis can only be made by isolating and identifying the pathogen from affected tissues. It is essential to distinguish true infection from contamination with these organisms. Histopathologically, a wide eosinophilic sleeve can be seen surrounding hyphae using routine staining haematoxylin and eosin (H&E), which helps in the detection of these structures.

Treatment

Limited information is available regarding therapy. Current recommendations are for aggressive surgical resection of the infected tissue followed by itraconazole therapy for 2–3 months.

Other mycotic infections

Opportunistic infections with saprophytic fungi that produce non-dematiaceous (non-pigmented) hyphae in the tissues are known as hyalohyphomycoses; infections with fungi that produce dematiaceous (melanin-pigmented) hyphae are known as phaeohyphomycoses. Infections are usually found in immunocompromised individuals in the case of hyalohyphomycosis and disseminated phaeohyphomycosis; however, localized cases of phaeo-hyphomycosis usually occur in immunocompetent individuals. These fungi, of which there are hundreds of different species, are assumed to infect individuals via exposure of wounds to an environmental source, which varies depending upon the species of fungus. Phaeohyphomycosis is considered to involve an emerging group of pathogenic fungi. Phaeohyphomycoses in cats most commonly present in areas of the body that come into contact with soil. Hyalohyphomycoses occur more frequently in dogs than in cats, with young adult large-breed dogs most commonly affected.

Clinical approach

Widespread cutaneous and subcutaneous nodules are assumed to be the result of disseminated disease. Various organ systems may be involved and the clinical signs vary depending upon the system affected. Phaeohyphomycosis may present as singular or multifocal poorly circumscribed ulcerating or fistulating nodules or plaques, and pigmentation may be noted in the affected tissue. Most cases of phaeohyphomycosis have been described in cats, where lesions resembling thick-walled cysts or chronic bacterial infections are present on the head or distal extremities and may evolve over weeks to months. Hyalohyphomycosis occurs more commonly in dogs. The incidence of opportunistic fungal infections is increased substantially in dogs receiving immuno-suppressive therapy, especially if ciclosporin is included in the treatment protocol or when multiagent protocols are used (see Chapter 29).

Diagnostic tests: Phaeohyphomycosis may be diagnosed tentatively by visualization of pigmented hyphae in potassium hydroxide-mounted macerated tissue samples. A definitive diagnosis is made on histology by identifying hyphal elements growing in the tissue. Correlation between culture and histology is essential because these organisms can be found in the ambient environment, and on the skin and hair coats of clinically healthy animals. Sampling must be performed using proper techniques to avoid contamination. Tissue culture is preferred. Molecular identification of cultured isolates is recommended. Sequencing fungal DNA from paraffin-embedded tissue samples has a sensitivity ranging from 54–94%. The organisms that cause opportunistic mycoses are common contaminants, so isolation from non-sterile sites requires further supportive evidence of infection.

Treatment

Surgical excision may be curative for localized disease. Disseminated disease or CNS disease carries a grave prognosis and is more common in immunocompromised individuals. If treatment is attempted, the isolate should be identified and subjected to sensitivity testing *in vitro* to guide formulation of a therapeutic plan. Several pathogens categorized as hyalohyphomycoses are inherently resistant to amphotericin B and itraconazole. Itraconazole and posaconazole are most commonly used to treat phaeo-hyphomycosis; voriconazole is preferred in canine cases involving the CNS. Discontinuation of immunosuppressive medications is recommended.

Oomycete infections

Pythiosis and lagenidiosis

Pythiosis, caused by *Pythium insidiosum*, and lagenidiosis, caused by *Lagenidium* spp., are associated with aquatic pathogens that are members of the order Oomycetes. *Lagenidium* spp. are known to include two morphologically and molecularly distinct, yet unnamed, species. These organisms have a worldwide distribution, but are most common in wet, tropical and subtropical climates. Disease prevalence is increased in the Gulf Coast states of the United States but has expanded to various other locations in the USA, southeast Asia (especially Thailand and Indonesia), eastern coastal Australia, New Zealand, Korea, Japan, the Caribbean and South America. Disease occurs uncommonly in dogs and rarely in cats. Infection usually occurs after exposure to contaminated warm freshwater habitats. In the water, these organisms are flagellate zoospores that are attracted to tissues. The zoospores encyst in tissue, which leads to penetration and tissue invasion. Infections have been described in domestic dogs with no known exposure to water. Certain breeds of dog appear to have a greater tendency to attract zoospores than others.

Clinical approach

Gastrointestinal and subcutaneous forms of pythiosis have been described. Large-breed dogs are frequently affected, and the gastrointestinal form of the disease is most common. Clinical signs associated with the gastrointestinal form relate to the region of the digestive tract that is infected. The subcutaneous form presents most commonly as a non-healing wound or mass on the extremities (Figure 30.5), tail head, ventral neck, perineum or medial thigh. These lesions may progress to large boggy proliferative areas with ulceration and draining tracts. A variable degree of tissue destruction, which may involve the underlying soft tissues, is seen. The lesions are variably pruritic. Cats affected by pythiosis present with subcutaneous masses in the inguinal, tail head and periorbital regions, some of which are highly invasive. In addition, masses with draining nodules and ulcerated plaque-like lesions may be seen on the extremities; and a case with nasal and naso-pharyngeal/retrobulbar lesions has been described.

Clinical signs associated with *Lagenidium* spp. infection range from a uniformly fatal dermatological and disseminated disease caused by *Lagenidium giganteum forma caninum*, to a chronic, ulcerative nodular dermatopathy with a prolonged course confined to local tissue (rarely extending beyond cutaneous and subcutaneous tissues) seen with *Paralagenidium karlingii*. Dogs infected with the aggressive form have multifocal lesions with associated regional lymphadenopathy. Great vessel disease,

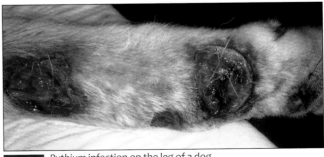

30.5 *Pythium* infection on the leg of a dog.
(Courtesy of R Marsella)

pulmonary lesions, mandibular sialadenitis and hilar masses have also been identified on post-mortem examination of dogs infected with this *Lagenidium* spp.

Diagnostic tests: Histopathology of lesional biopsy samples from individuals affected by either *Pythium* or *Lagenidium* spp. shows a granulomatous to pyogranulomatous infiltrate with numerous eosinophils. Hyphae are most numerous in areas of necrosis and are often surrounded by eosinophilic material. They can be visualized easily with Gömöri methenamine silver (GMS) stain. Cytological examination of macerated tissue fixed with 10% potassium hydroxide may allow visualization of poorly septate wide and branching hyphal elements. Tissue samples submitted for culture will grow *P. insidiosum*; the laboratory should be consulted regarding the handling of submitted tissue. Immunohistochemistry to detect *Pythium* antigen in formalin-fixed paraffin-embedded tissue has test-variable specificity. A highly sensitive and specific serology test based on an enzyme-linked immunosorbent assay (ELISA) is available for *P. insidiosum* at Louisiana State University laboratory and Auburn University, and this may be used for diagnosis and monitoring of therapy. *Lagenidium* spp. can be definitively diagnosed by culture on an amended peptone–yeast–glucose medium, by ribosomal RNA gene sequencing, or by specific PCR amplification. Culture is recommended as this is the only method currently available that is able to differentiate between the two pathogenic variants of *Lagenidium*.

Treatment

Early and complete surgical removal of affected tissue can be curative. Medical therapy with antifungal agents has yielded poor results. Recent combination therapy using itraconazole, terbinafine and anti-inflammatory doses of corticosteroids have been helpful in some cases of gastrointestinal pythiosis. Efficacy of *Pythium* vaccines in dogs (often used in horses) appears to be poor. The prognosis for dogs and cats infected with these organisms is poor.

Parasitic infections

Leishmaniosis

Leishmaniosis is a protozoal infection caused by various *Leishmania* spp. Transmission of this parasite to a vertebrate host occurs when phlebotomine sandflies (*Phlebotomus* in the Old World and *Lutzomyia* in the New World) transmit promastigotes, which transform and multiply in the host as amastigotes. Old World disease occurs in the Mediterranean basin, Portugal, the foothills of the Alps in northern Italy, the Pyrenees in France, northern Spain, the Middle East and some parts of China, but is not strictly limited to these regions, and is mostly caused by *Leishmania infantum*. Clinical cases in non-endemic areas have increased due to large numbers of companion animals travelling to or being imported from endemic areas. In the New World, the disease is endemic to South and Central America, with foci described in the United States (including English Foxhound kennels in the eastern United States). The geographical distribution of this disease is limited to the range of the sandfly vector, except in the United States where the mode of transmission in English Foxhounds remains to be determined. New World disease is most often caused by *L. chagasi* with a seasonal occurrence.

Disease distribution is primarily bimodal, mainly affecting dogs <3 years and >8 years of age. Disease is considered to be common in the dog and rare in the cat, even in endemic areas. However, the advances in feline medicine and the availability of more sensitive and specific diagnostic tests has led to an increase in the number of documented cases of clinical and subclinical infections in cats. Leishmaniosis should be considered for any animal with a travel history to affected areas, particularly imported dogs from regions where the disease is endemic. Domestic and wild rodents as well as other mammals may serve as disease reservoirs; dogs are considered to be a primary reservoir host for human disease in many parts of the world.

Clinical approach

Not all dogs infected with *Leishmania* develop disease. Predisposing factors for disease development include breed, age and genetic background. The type of immune response mounted by each individual determines the course of the clinical disease. Cutaneous lesions are characterized by a dry exfoliative dermatitis with silvery scaling, which may be generalized but typically is most severe on the head, pinnae and extremities. Periocular alopecia is also common. Other frequently seen cutaneous lesions include pustular dermatitis, cutaneous ulcers (Figure 30.6), nodular dermatitis, sterile pustular dermatitis, nasodigital hyperkeratosis and onychogryphosis (Figure 30.7). Depigmentation of the nasal planum and muzzle may also be seen. When cutaneous lesions are found, visceral disease is typically present. Numerous body systems can be involved and the clinical signs exhibited are associated with the affected system(s). Renal failure is an important result of disease progression and the main cause of mortality. The incubation period for this disease can range from weeks to years. Feline leishmaniosis is rare. Lesions similar to the cutaneous ulcerative or nodular lesions in dogs are most often seen on the head and extremities, with rare dissemination. Clinical disease is often associated with immunocompromise in cats.

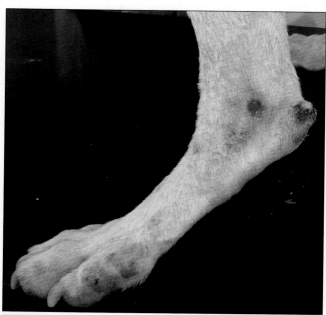

30.6 Cutaneous ulcers and exfoliative dermatitis in a dog infected with *Leishmania*.
(Courtesy of M Saridomichelakis)

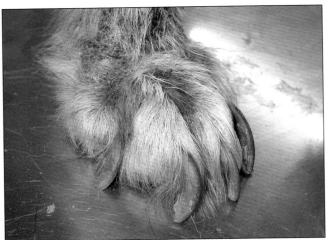

30.7 Onychogryphosis (also known as ram's horn nail) is a nail disorder resulting from slow nail plate growth due to *Leishmania* infection. Note the opaque, yellow-brown thickening of the nail plate with elongation and increased curvature in this dog.
(Courtesy of Photo Archive, Universitat Autònoma de Barcelona)

Diagnostic tests: A definitive diagnosis is made by identifying amastigotes in macrophages or free within the tissues via cytology or histology. Dermal patterns of inflammation are highly variable. Numerous serological tests (e.g. ELISA, complement fixation and indirect fluorescent antibody tests) will identify the presence of antibodies; however, these do not confirm active disease. Quantitative serological tests are recommended. Previous vaccination may need to be considered when interpreting serological test results. PCR amplification of *Leishmania* DNA is possible, and lymph node tissue, conjunctival swabs or bone marrow samples are preferred to blood samples for this test. Oral swabs have also been found to contain *Leishmania* DNA. However, false-positive tests are possible due to DNA contamination and therefore are not recommended as the sole diagnostic technique for confirmation of disease. *Leishmania* organisms can be detected in the urine of up to 85% of clinically affected dogs that show signs of renal insufficiency, which may offer a less invasive test for debilitated patients. The diagnosis of *Leishmania* in cats requires similar diagnostic tests as for dogs, with quantitative ELISAs being most frequently employed. A four-stage clinical grading system based on clinical signs, clinicopathological abnormalities and serological status is shown in Figure 30.8.

Treatment

Meglumine antimonite is most often used for the treatment of leishmaniosis in dogs, at doses ranging from 40–75 mg/kg s.c. q12h to 75–100 mg/kg s.c. q24h; miltefosine may also be used at a dose of 2 mg/kg orally q24h for 28 days. Combination therapy with allopurinol and meglumine antimonite or miltefosine improves the clinical response and is usually the initial approach. Allopurinol at a dose of 10 mg/kg orally q24h is commonly used as long-term therapy. Some antimonial-resistant strains of *L. infantum* have been reported. Treatment rarely results in cure, but it may give a favourable clinical response.

Clinical stage	Serology[a]	Clinical signs	Laboratory findings	Therapy	Prognosis
Stage I: mild disease	Negative to low positive antibody levels	Dogs with mild clinical signs such as peripheral lymphadenopathy or papular dermatitis (Ordeix *et al.*, 2005; Bottero *et al.*, 2006)	Usually no clinicopathological abnormalities observed; normal renal profile: creatinine <1.4 mg/dl; non-proteinuric: UPC <0.2	Scientific neglect[b] Allopurinol alone Allopurinol + meglumine antimoniate or miltefosine	Good
Stage II: moderate disease	Low to high positive antibody levels	In addition to those signs seen in stage I, dogs may present with diffuse or symmetrical cutaneous lesions such as exfoliative dermatitis/onychogryphosis, ulcerations (nasal planum, footpads, bony prominences, mucocutaneous junctions), anorexia, weight loss, fever and epistaxis (Petanides *et al.*, 2008)	Clinicopathological abnormalities such as mild non-regenerative anaemia, hypergammaglobulinaemia, hypoalbuminaemia and serum hyperviscosity syndrome (Petanides *et al.*, 2008) Substages: • Normal renal profile: creatinine <1.4 mg/dl; non-proteinuric: UPC <0.5 • Creatinine <1.4 mg/dl; UPC = 0.5–1	Allopurinol + meglumine antimoniate or miltefosine	Good to guarded
Stage III: severe disease	Medium to high positive antibody levels	In addition to those signs seen in stages I and II, dogs may present with signs originating from immune-complex lesions: vasculitis, arthritis, uveitis and glomerulonephritis	Clinicopathological abnormalities listed in stage II CKD IRIS stage I (UPC >1) or stage II (creatinine 1.4–2 mg/dl)[c]	Allopurinol + meglumine antimoniate or miltefosine Follow IRIS guidelines for CKD[d]	Guarded to poor
Stage IV: very severe disease	Medium to high positive antibody levels	In addition to those signs seen in stage III, dogs may have pulmonary thromboembolism or nephrotic syndrome and end-stage renal disease	Clinicopathological abnormalities listed in stage II CKD IRIS stage III (creatinine 2–5 mg/dl) and stage IV (creatinine >5 mg/dl)[c] Nephrotic syndrome: marked proteinuria UPC >5	Allopurinol (alone) Follow IRIS guidelines for CKD[d]	Poor

30.8 Clinical staging of canine leishmaniosis is based on serological status, clinical signs and laboratory findings. The type of therapy and prognosis for each clinical stage is also shown. [a] Dogs with negative to medium positive antibody levels should be confirmed as infected by other diagnostic techniques such as cytology, histology/immunohistochemistry and polymerase chain reaction (PCR). High levels of antibodies confirm a diagnosis of canine leishmaniosis and are defined as 3–4-fold increase of a well-established laboratory reference cut-off value. [b] Dogs in stage I (mild disease) are likely to require less prolonged treatment with one or two combined drugs (allopurinol, domperidone, meglumine antimoniate or miltefosine) or alternatively monitoring with no treatment. There is limited information on this stage and, therefore, treatment options remain to be defined. [c] iris-kidney.com/guidelines/staging.html. [d] iris-kidney.com/guidelines/recommendations.html. CKD = chronic kidney disease; IRIS = International Renal Interest Society; UPC = urine protein:creatinine ratio.
(Data from Solano-Gallego *et al.*, 2009)

Relapses are common. Owing to the poor prognosis for cure and public health concerns, euthanasia may be indicated in non-endemic areas. Allopurinol at a dose of 10 mg/kg orally q12h or 20 mg/kg orally q24h is the most frequently used treatment in cats and appears to be well tolerated. Meglumine antimonite has also been used. Information regarding pharmacokinetic, pharmacodynamics and drug safety is lacking for cats.

Preventive measures include an integrated approach using a combination of veterinary registered products containing synthetic pyrethroids, permethrin, deltamethrin or flumethrin to repel sandflies, reducing exposure to sandflies and vaccination. Vaccination against *Leishmania* has shown efficacy in decreasing the incidence of clinical disease due to natural *L. infantum* infection in dogs. Dogs should be seronegative prior to vaccination.

Other infections

Protothecosis

Prototheca spp. are saprophytic, achlorophyllous algae found in Europe, Asia and the United States (most commonly in the southeastern USA). *Prototheca* spp. cause infection via the gastrointestinal tract or through contact with traumatized skin or mucosa. These infections are rare in dogs and cats, although immunosuppressed individuals are at high risk.

Clinical approach

The infection in dogs manifests most commonly as disseminated disease. Multiple organs are usually involved with clinical signs, including bloody diarrhoea, weight loss, CNS signs and ocular lesions. Skin lesions present as chronic nodules, draining ulcers and crusted lesions with associated exudation, and are located on the trunk, extremities and mucocutaneous junctions (Figure 30.9).

Diagnostic tests: Tissue samples or exudates will grow *Prototheca* when plated on routine fungal media. Cytology of exudates or tissue aspirates shows granulomatous to pyogranulomatous inflammation with intracellular *Prototheca* organisms, which are round, oval and polyhedral spherules that vary in size; some may contain endospores.

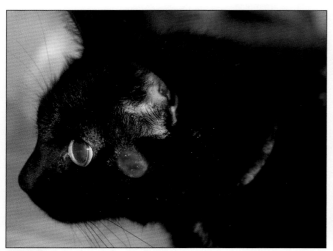

30.9 *Prototheca* infection in a cat.
(Courtesy of R Marsella)

Histopathology shows a nodular to diffuse granulomatous to pyogranulomatous dermatitis and panniculitis with large numbers of *Prototheca* organisms.

Treatment

The preferred treatment for this condition is wide surgical excision. This infection is poorly responsive to medical management, especially if disseminated. Described therapies include:

- Amphotericin B:
  - Dogs: 0.25–0.5 mg/kg i.v. 3 times a week to reach a cumulative dose of 8 mg/kg
  - Cats: 0.25 mg/kg i.v. 3 times a week to reach a cumulative dose of 4 mg/kg.
- Ketoconazole:
  - Dogs: 10–15 mg/kg orally q12–24h.
- Itraconazole: 5–10 mg/kg orally q12h with a fatty meal
- Fluconazole: 2.5–5.0 mg/kg orally, i.v. q12h.

Summary

The geographical distribution of the infectious agents described above, the differential diagnoses of nodules and draining tracts, diseases commonly associated with systemic manifestations and a list of diseases with zoonotic potential are detailed in Figures 30.10 to 30.13, respectively.

Disease	Geographical distribution
Bacterial infections	
Rapidly growing mycobacteria	Southeastern United States; Canada; Australia; Finland; Germany
Feline leprosy	Northwestern United States; Canada; Australia; New Zealand; United Kingdom; the Netherlands; France; Japan; Italy; the Greek islands
Canine leproid granuloma syndrome	United States; Brazil; Australia; New Zealand; South Africa; Europe (Italy)
Fungal infections	
Blastomycosis	Great Lakes region of the United States; Ohio, Mississippi and Missouri river valleys of the United States[a]; Central America; Africa; Europe; India
Histoplasmosis	Ohio, Mississippi and Missouri river valleys of the United States[a]; Europe
Coccidioidomycosis	Southwestern United States; Mexico; Central and South America
Oomycete infections	
Pythiosis	Gulf Coast of the United States; Caribbean, South America[a]; Australia (east coast); New Zealand[a]; southeast Asia (Thailand, Indonesia); Korea; Japan
Lagenidiosis	Southeastern United States
Parasitic infections	
Old World Leishmaniosis	Mediterranean basin; Middle East; Portugal; China
New World Leishmaniosis	Foci in the United States (e.g. English Foxhounds); Central and South America
Other infections	
Prototheca	Southeastern United States; Europe; Asia

30.10 Geographical distribution of infectious agents. [a] Increased incidence of disease in this location.

Bacterial infections

- Deep pyoderma with furunculosis
- Folliculitis and furunculosis
- Foreign body and abscess
- German Shepherd Dog pyoderma
- Actinomycosis
- Nocardiosis
- Atypical mycobacteria (slow growing *Mycobacterium avium* complex and rapidly growing)
- Feline leprosy
- Canine leproid granuloma syndrome
- Cutaneous tuberculosis

Fungal infections

- Dermatophytosis (kerion, mycetoma, pseudomycetoma, Majocchi's granuloma)
- Sporotrichosis
- Blastomycosis
- Histoplasmosis
- Cryptococcosis
- Coccidioidomycosis
- Conidiobolomycosis
- Basidiobolomycosis
- Hyalohyphomycosis
- Phaeohyphomycosis

Parasitic infections

- Leishmaniosis
- Rhabditic dermatitis
- Demodicosis

Other infections

- Prototothecosis
- Pythiosis
- Lagenidiosis

Tissue growths

- Neoplasia (various)
- Histiocytosis
- Nodular dermatofibrosis of German Shepherd Dogs

Deposition of material

- Xanthoma
- Calcinosis cutis
- Calcinosis circumscripta
- Cutaneous nodular amyloidosis

Sterile reactions

- Sterile nodular granuloma/pyogranuloma
- Collagenolytic granuloma
- Eosinophilic furunculosis of the face

Pannicular disease

- Post-injection panniculitis
- Traumatic panniculitis
- Idiopathic sterile nodular panniculitis
- Metatarsal fistulation of the German Shepherd Dog
- Pancreatic panniculitis

30.11 Differential diagnosis for nodules and draining tracts.

- Atypical slow growing mycobacteria (*Mycobacterium avium* complex)
- Feline leprosy[a]
- Cutaneous tuberculosis
- Nocardiosis
- Actinomycosis
- Sporotrichosis[a]
- Blastomycosis
- Histoplasmosis
- Cryptococcosis[a]
- Coccidioidomycosis[a]
- Pythiosis
- Lagenidiosis
- Conidiobolomycosis[a]
- Basidiobolomycosis[a]
- Hyalohyphomycosis
- Prototothecosis

30.12 Diseases with increased incidence of systemic manifestations. [a] Variable or transient systemic disease.

- Cutaneous tuberculosis
- Sporotrichosis (feline)
- Blastomycosis[a]
- Histoplasmosis[a]
- Coccidioidomycosis[a]
- Dermatophytosis
- Leishmaniosis

30.13 Diseases with zoonotic potential. [a] Mycelial form infectious in laboratory culture.

Key points

- Unusual infections should be considered in animals that present with persistent nodules or draining tracts, which do not respond to regular therapy
- Many of these infectious agents require specific cultures or laboratory techniques to confirm their presence; therefore, it is advised to contact the diagnostic laboratory prior to sample submission to discuss the case
- Veterinary staff handling affected animals should wear protective clothing as some of these infectious agents are contagious

References and further reading

Arbona N, Butkiewicz CD, Keyes M and Shubitz LF *et al.* (2019) Clinical features of cats diagnosed with coccidioidomycosis in Arizona, 2004-2018. *Journal of Feline Medicine and Surgery* **22**, 129–137

Bottero E, Poggi M and Viglione M (2006) Lesioni papulari indotte da *Leishmania* spp. in 8 cani giovani. *Veterinaria* **1**, 33–36

Cook A, Cunningham LY, Cowell AK and Wheat LJ (2012) Clinical evaluation of urine *Histoplasma capsulatum* antigen measurement in cats with suspected disseminated histoplasmosis. *Journal of Feline Medicine and Surgery* **14**, 512–515

Cunningham L, Cook A, Hanzlicek AS *et al.* (2015) Sensitivity and specificity of *Histoplasma* antigen detection by enzyme immunoassay. *Journal of the American Animal Hospital Association* **51**, 306–310

Dedeaux A, Grooters A, Wakamatsu N and Taboada J (2018) Opportunistic fungal infections in small animals. *Journal of the American Animal Hospital Association* **54**, 327–337

Dedola C, Zobba R, Pinna Parpaglia ML *et al.* (2014) First report of canine leprosy in Europe: molecular and clinical traits. *Veterinary Record* **174**, 120

Gerontiti S, Oikonomidis IL, Kalogianni L *et al.* (2016) First report of canine systemic cryptococcosis owing to *Cryptococcus gattii* in Europe. *Journal of Small Animal Practice* **58**, 58–59

Greene CE (2012) *Infectious Diseases of the Dog and Cat, 4th edn.* Elsevier Saunders, Philadelphia

Grooters AM, Leise BS, Lopez MK *et al.* (2002) Development and evaluation of an enzyme-linked immunosorbent assay for the serodiagnosis of pythiosis in dogs. *Journal of Veterinary Internal Medicine* **16**, 142–146

Gunstra A, Steurer JA, Seibert RL *et al.* (2019) Sensitivity of serologic testing for dogs diagnosed with coccidioidomycosis on histology: 52 cases (2012–2013). *Journal of the American Animal Hospital Association* **55**, 238–242

Hanzlicek AS, Meinkoth JH, Renschler JS *et al.* (2016) Antigen concentrations as an indicator of clinical remission and disease relapse in cats with histoplasmosis. *Journal of Veterinary Internal Medicine* **30**, 1065–1073

Holbrook ED, Greene RT, Rubin SI *et al.* (2019) Novel canine anti-Coccidioides immunoglobulin G enzyme immunoassay aids in diagnosis of coccidioidomycosis in dogs. *Medical Mycology* **57**, 800–806

Lombardo G, Pennisi MG, Lupo T *et al.* (2012) Detection of *Leishmania infantum* DNA by real-time PCR in canine oral and conjunctival swabs and comparison with other diagnostic techniques. *Veterinary Parasitology* **184**, 10–17

Malik R, Medeiros C, Wigney DI and Love DN (1996) Suspected drug eruption in seven dogs during administration of flucytosine. *Australian Veterinary Journal* **74**, 285–288

Malik R, Smits B, Reppas G *et al.* (2013) Ulcerated and nonulcerated nontuberculous cutaneous mycobacterial granulomas in cats and dogs. *Veterinary Dermatology* **24**, 146–153

Mazepa A, Trepanier LA and Foy DS (2011) Retrospective comparison of the efficacy of fluconazole or itraconazole for the treatment of systemic blastomycosis in dogs. *Journal of Veterinary Internal Medicine* **25**, 440–445

Mourning AC, Patterson EE, Kirsch EJ *et al.* (2015) Evaluation of an enzyme immunoassay for antibodies to a recombinant *Blastomyces* adhesin-1 repeat antigen as an aid in the diagnosis of blastomycosis in dogs. *Journal of the American Veterinary Medical Association* **247**, 1133–1138

Myers A, Meason-Smith C, Mansell J *et al.* (2017) Atypical cutaneous *Cryptococcus* in four cats in the USA. *Veterinary Dermatology* **28**, 405–e97

O'Brien C, Malik R, Globan M *et al.* (2017a) Feline leprosy due to Candidatus '*Mycobacterium lepraefelis*'. *Journal of Feline Medicine and Surgery* **19**, 919–932

O'Brien C, Malik R, Globan *et al.* (2017b) Feline leprosy due to Candidatus '*Mycobacterium tarwinense*'. *Journal of Feline Medicine and Surgery* **19**, 498–512

O'Brien C, Malik R, Globan M *et al.* (2017c) Feline leprosy due to *Mycobacterium lepraemurium*. *Journal of Feline Medicine and Surgery* **19**, 737–746

O'Halloran C and Gunn-Moore D (2017) Mycobacteria in cats: an update. *In Practice* **39**, 399–406

O'Halloran C, Ioannidi O, Reed N *et al.* (2019) Tuberculosis due to *Mycobacterium bovis* in pet cats associated with feeding a commercial raw food diet. *Journal of Feline Medicine and Surgery* **21**, 667–681

Ordeix L, Solano-Gallego L, Fondevila D *et al.* (2005) Papular dermatitis due to *Leishmania* spp. infection in dogs with parasite-specific cellular immune responses. *Veterinary dermatology* **16**, 187–191

Pennisi MG, Cardoso L, Baneth G *et al.* (2015) LeishVet update and recommendations on feline leishmaniosis. *Parasites and Vectors* **8**, 302

Petanides T, Koutinas A, Mylonakis ME *et al.* (2008). Factors associated with the occurrence of epistaxis in natural canine leishmaniasis (*Leishmania infantum*). *Journal of Veterinary Internal Medicine/American College of Veterinary Internal Medicine* **22**, 866–872

Reagan KL, Marks SL and Pesavento PA (2019) Successful management of 3 dogs with colonic pythiosis using itraconazole, terbinafine, and prednisone. *Journal of Veterinary Internal Medicine* **33**, 1434–1439

Reagan KL, McHardy I, Thompson GR and Sikes JE (2019) Evaluation of the clinical performance of 2 point-of-care cryptococcal antigen tests in dogs and cats. *Journal of Veterinary Internal Medicine* **33**, 2082–2089

Simoes D, Dial SM, Coyner KS *et al.* (2016) Retrospective analysis of cutaneous lesions in 23 canine and 17 feline cases of coccidioidomycosis seen in Arizona, USA (2009–2015). *Veterinary Dermatology* **27**, 346–e87

Solano-Gallego L, Koutinas A, Miro G *et al.* (2009) Directions for the diagnosis, clinical staging, treatment and prevention of canine leishmaniosis. *Veterinary Parasitology* **165**, 1–18

Solano-Gallego L, Miró G, Koutinas A *et al.* (2011) LeishVet guidelines for the practical management of canine leishmaniosis. *Parasites and Vectors* **4**, 86

Timm K, Wlle M, Friedel U *et al.* (2019) *Mycobacterium* nebraskense infection in a dog in Switzerland with disseminated skin lesions. *Veterinary Dermatology* **30**, 262–e80

Wilson AG, Kukanich KS, Hanzlicek AS and Payton ME (2018) Clinical signs, treatment, and prognostic factors for dogs with histoplasmosis. *Journal of the American Veterinary Medical Association* **252**, 201–209

Chapter 31

Nutrients and the skin

Rebecca Ricci and Carla Dedola

The importance of nutrients and the skin

The skin is the largest organ of the body and is characterized by an active metabolism and a high nutritional requirement. A proper balance of nutrients is essential for a healthy status and proper function. Thus, it is not surprising that nutrient deficiencies can result in skin disorders. Proteins (amino acids) and lipids (fatty acids) together with micronutrients, such as vitamins and minerals, are all essential for good epidermal health. With the global distribution of high-quality commercial pet food, skin diseases associated with true nutritional deficiency are nowadays a rare event. When detected, they may be due to poor nutrient absorption associated with genetic factors, dietary factors (e.g. ingestion of compounds that prevent absorption of others), gastrointestinal pathology or excessive loss due to the presence of comorbidities. In this chapter, important nutrients for the skin are discussed along with the potential clinical consequences of deficiency. In addition, metabolic diseases leading to skin disorders are also addressed.

Proteins and amino acids

Proteins are complex molecules comprising hundreds to thousands of amino acids, in which the amino group of one amino acid and the carboxyl group of another amino acid are linked together by a peptide bond (Gross *et al.*, 2010). Dietary proteins are required for two main reasons (NRC, 2006):

- To provide amino acids that dogs and cats cannot synthesize (known as 'essential amino acids'), which are required for the synthesis of several body proteins
- To provide non-essential amino acids for maintenance, growth, gestation and lactation.

It has been estimated that normal hair growth and maintenance of the skin barrier account for 25–30% of an animal's daily protein requirement (Muller and Kirk, 2013), with higher requirements needed for hair growth in long-haired small-breed dogs compared with short-haired, large-breed dogs. Hair comprises 95% protein, with a high percentage of sulphur-containing amino acids, therefore, developing new hair, as well as renewing skin,

requires adequate dietary protein in terms of both quantity and quality.

Dogs and cats experience a higher requirement for proteins, amino acids and energy during specific periods of life, such as growth, gestation and lactation (NRC, 2006). Poor skin and coat condition may be observed at these times if inadequate dietary protein, low-quality food or nutritionally unbalanced home-prepared diets are provided (Gross *et al.*, 2010). Severe illness and consequent malnutrition may also result in poor coat quality, weakening of the hair shafts and alterations in the process of keratinization, if appropriate nutritional changes are not instituted. Increased amounts of energy, proteins, specific amino acids and other nutrients are required in animals with severe skin disease to heal and promote recovery (Gross *et al.*, 2010). For example, dogs with severe primary seborrhoea experience a three-fold increase in epidermal cell renewal. Although no studies have evaluated the nutrient requirements of dogs suffering from this disease, it has been observed that the clinical signs worsen significantly in dogs with nutritional inadequacies (Roudebush and Schoenherr, 2010).

Pet food guidelines

The National Research Council (NRC), the European Pet Food Industry (FEDIAF) and the Association of American Feed Control Officials (AAFCO) are the main bodies that provide guidelines for the nutritional requirements of dogs and cats, including minimum and maximum (if any) levels of nutrients for maintenance, growth and reproduction. In the *Nutritional Guidelines for Complete and Complementary Pet Food for Cats and Dogs*, which is based on state-of-the-art knowledge of cat and dog nutrition and reviewed yearly by a Scientific Advisory Board, the FEDIAF provides European pet food manufacturers with nutritional recommendations to ensure the production of well balanced and nutritionally sound pet food. Thus, pet food products must contain nutrient levels that meet those stated in the guidelines. However, it should be noted that pet foods for particular nutritional purposes and some other specialized foods are excluded from the FEDIAF nutritional guidelines

Raw meat-based diets

In recent years, the use of raw meat-based diets (RMBDs) has grown in popularity. Despite this, few studies have investigated their health effects on pets and the advantages of RMBDs have not yet been clearly proven. On the contrary, health concerns related to the consumption of these diets have been widely documented, both in pets and their owners (Freeman et al., 2013; van Bree et al., 2018; Dodd et al., 2019; Morelli et al., 2020), ranging from nutritional imbalances to microbial contamination. In a recent survey (Morelli et al., 2019), it emerged that the main health benefit recognized by 79% (173/218) of RMBD feeders was 'a shinier coat and skin improvement'. Although health benefits may be anecdotally reported by pet owners, they remain unproven and future studies are required to demonstrate the positive impact of feeding RMBDs to pets

Grain-free diets

With the objective of providing pet food products that meet both the nutritional needs of dogs and cats and the increasing requests from owners to provide alternatives to traditional pet foods, manufacturers have recently introduced a variety of different products to the marketplace, including grain-free diets (GFDs). GFDs are marketed as high protein 'ancestral diets' that are healthier than their grain inclusive counterparts (Conway and Saker, 2018) and more respectful of the carnivorous nature of dogs and cats.

GFDs have become quite popular amongst pet owners, as demonstrated in a survey by Morelli et al. (2021) in which 21% (258/1228) of people who were providing a dry food to their dog or cat were feeding a GFD at the time of interview. These findings were echoed in a further survey conducted in the USA by Conway and Saker (2020), in which it emerged that 19.2% (15/78) of people had adopted a GFD for their pet. The potential health benefits of feeding a grain-free *versus* a grain-inclusive diet have not yet undergone scientific evaluation and, therefore, GFDs cannot be considered a useful tool in the management of skin diseases in dogs and cats at this time. Furthermore, there is little evidence that RMBDs or GFDs provide substantial benefits in animals with cutaneous reactions to foods. Recently, there has been increased awareness of a potential link between GFDs with taurine deficiency and dilated cardiomyopathy in the veterinary literature, highlighting the need for additional studies (McCauley et al., 2020; Ontiveros et al., 2020)

Essential fatty acids

Lipids are a group of substances found in plant and animal tissue that are insoluble in water but soluble in common organic solvents such as benzene, ether and chloroform. The dietary intake of lipids supplies energy in the form of essential fatty acids (EFAs), which are required in certain amounts for the proper absorption of fat-soluble vitamins. Dietary fats supply 2.25 times the metabolizable energy of proteins and carbohydrates per gram and, therefore, contribute significantly to the energy density of food.

Most fats in the diet are triglycerides, which comprise three fatty acids attached to a glycerol backbone. Fatty acids consist of hydrocarbon chains with a carboxylic acid group (COOH) at one end and a methyl group at the other. Fatty acids can be classified according to their chain length (short chains having <6 carbon atoms, medium chains having 6–12 carbon atoms and long chains having >12 carbon atoms) or degree of saturation; in this case, those with no double bonds in the hydrocarbon chain are referred to as saturated, chains with one double bond are termed monounsaturated, and chains with more than one double bond are called polyunsaturated. Lipids may be in either a liquid (oils) or solid (fats) state, depending on temperature and fatty acid composition; fats that contain more unsaturated fatty acids have a lower melting point and are in a liquid state at room temperature. On the contrary, fats that contain more saturated fatty acids have a higher melting point and are in a solid state at room temperature.

The carbon atom at the opposite end of the chain from the carboxylic acid group is designated n-1. Nomenclature specifies the number of carbon atoms and the location and number of double bonds (Gross et al., 2010).

- Fatty acids with the first double bond between the third and fourth carbon atoms are in the omega-3 family.
- Fatty acids with the first double bond between the sixth and seventh carbon atoms are in the omega-6 family.
- Fatty acids with the first double bond between the ninth and tenth carbon atoms are in the omega-9 family.

Both omega-6 and omega-3 are essential for dogs and cats. The requirements can usually be met by providing linoleic acid (LA; C18:2 n-6) and alpha-linolenic acid (ALA; C18:3 n-3) in the diet; linolenic acid is considered essential because dogs and cats cannot synthesize it adequately in the body. Dogs, but not cats, are able to elongate and desaturate linoleic acid to form arachidonic acid (AA; C20:4 n-6) (MacDonald et al., 1984), thus arachidonic acid is considered an EFA for cats. However, during growth or reproduction, modest provision of arachidonic acid is also necessary in dogs. It should also be remembered that under certain physiological conditions, other fatty acids are considered conditionally essential.

Although no definitive studies have been carried out on its essential nature in dogs and cats, several alpha-linolenic acid long chain derivatives such as eicosapentaeonic acid (EPA; C20:5 n-3) and docosahexaenoic acid (DHA; C22:6 n-3) have important metabolic implications in nervous tissue (e.g. retinal and brain function), as well as in inflammatory and immune responses (NRC, 2006). Conversion of alpha-linolenic acid to eicosapentaeonic acid occurs in dogs and cats, but conversion to docosahexaenoic acid is limited. Although conversion may be sufficient for maintenance in adult dogs, in growing puppies and kittens, as well as in bitches and queens, C:20 and C:22 n-3 polyunsaturated fatty acid (PUFA) intake is recommended in international nutritional guidelines.

PUFAs are fundamental for maintaining the stability and fluidity of the cell membrane structure, as well as related functions such as transport, metabolic regulation and the transepidermal water barrier (NRC, 2006). EFAs are also precursors of eicosanoids (e.g. prostaglandins, thromboxanes and leucotrienes); these metabolites contain

20 carbon atoms, are synthesized from arachidonic acid by individual cells and act like local mediator molecules. They are widely distributed in the cells and tissues of the body and have wide ranging biological action. Arachidonic acid can either take the cyclooxygenase (COX) pathway, which leads to the production of prostaglandins and thromboxanes, or the lipoxygenase pathway, which results in the synthesis of leucotrienes.

Eicosapentaeonic acid (the arachidonic acid analogue within the n-3 fatty acid family) can compete with arachidonic acid for membrane incorporation, modulating the family of eicosanoids produced. The eicosanoids resulting from omega-3 fatty acid metabolism have reduced pro-inflammatory properties compared with those produced from omega-6 fatty acids. For this reason, feeding omega-3 fatty acids has been recommended in situations where a reduced inflammatory response is desired, for example atopic dermatitis and lupoid onychitis (Hunter et al., 2020).

There are no definitive data regarding the optimal ratio between dietary and supplemental omega-6 and omega-3 fatty acids for dogs and cats. However, the use of dietary omega-3 fatty acids as adjunctive treatment for several clinical disorders has been evaluated in canine dermatoses and, to a lesser extent, in feline skin conditions. In dogs, a beneficial response to the inclusion of omega-3 fatty acids in the diet has been demonstrated in several inflammatory conditions, including atopic dermatitis. Several studies have evaluated the effect of oral EFA supplementation and/or the topical application of products containing EFAs and sphingolipid emulsion in atopic dogs. Both the changes in the composition of the skin barrier and the improvement in clinical signs and pruritus were assessed. Although the results were variable, the studies demonstrated that their use may be beneficial and should be considered as a fundamental part of a multimodal therapeutic approach in atopic dogs; however, there was scant evidence that the use of EFAs would be helpful as a sole therapy (Tretter and Mueller, 2011; Blaskovic et al., 2014; Saevik et al., 2014). In cases of atopy, a daily dosage of 125 mg eicosapentaeonic acid + 0.75 mg docosahexaenoic acid per kg has been recommended (Bauer, 2011).

Low amounts of dietary fat will lead to energy and EFA deficiencies. EFA deficiency is considered an uncommon disorder in dogs, especially when they are fed commercially available complete diets. When detected, the deficiency may have been caused by poor food preservation or inadequate antioxidant (vitamin E) levels within the food, which can result in alteration of the quality of the fat. Concurrent diseases that impair fat absorption, such as intestinal, pancreatic and hepatic conditions, may also interfere with EFA absorption and dogs can eventually show signs of deficiency. The principal cutaneous signs of EFA deficiency are: coarse, dry hair and skin; scaliness; loss of skin elasticity, alopecia; and desquamation. With time, the skin becomes greasy, pruritic and more vulnerable to infection due to the altered surface lipids (Codner and Thatcher, 1990; Roudebush and Schoenherr, 2010).

It has been demonstrated that diet has an important impact on skin health: dietary EFA supplementation has been shown to increase both the serum and cutaneous fatty acid concentrations in dogs (Campbell and Dorn, 1992) and cats (MacDonald et al., 1984). This can lead to a rapid improvement of clinical signs, as linoleic acid supplementation has been shown to reverse cutaneous alterations in cats within a few days (MacDonald et al., 1984). In addition, supplementation with either flax seeds or sunflower seeds for 1 month results in temporary improvement in skin and hair in healthy dogs (Rees et al., 2001).

Vitamins

Vitamin A

Vitamin A (retinol) is a fat-soluble vitamin necessary for normal embryonic development, adult growth and development, proper immune system functioning and vision. It also has a role in the maintenance of a normal epithelial barrier, cell proliferation, differentiation and apoptosis. Deficiency in vitamin A results in clinical signs involving different systems, including reproductive failure, growth disorders, increased susceptibility to infections, xerophthalmia, retinal degeneration and night blindness. Dermatological signs resulting from a lack of vitamin A include hyperkeratosis, excessive scaling, occlusion of sebaceous ducts, poor hair coat and alopecia. Retinoids, a term that encompasses both the natural form of vitamin A and its synthetic derivatives (i.e. tretinoin (all-trans retinoic acid), isotretinoin (13-cis retinoic acid), acitretin (analogue of retinoic acid ethyl ester)), are used therapeutically for skin diseases characterized by epidermal keratinization disorders both alone and in conjunction with other treatments (Mueller and Kirk, 2013).

Vitamin A-responsive dermatosis

In 1983, Ihrke and Goldschmidt described a dermatitis characterized by marked follicular plugging that responded to vitamin A supplementation in Cocker Spaniels. Subsequently, the same condition has been reported in Labrador Retrievers and Miniature Schnauzers, as well as anecdotally in other breeds. The disease is more commonly seen in American Cocker Spaniels and some controversy exists about the distinction between primary seborrhoea and vitamin A-responsive dermatosis, as they may represent the same disease. However, it should be noted that Cocker Spaniels are predisposed to atopic dermatitis and often present with significant scaling associated with secondary bacterial and Malassezia infections.

The most noticeable clinical aspects of this disorder are the severe follicular plugging with a prominent follicular cast and the presence of marked hyperkeratotic plaques, which are mainly localized to the ventral and lateral thorax and abdomen. Alopecia, crusts, scales, poor and dull hair coat, together with ceruminous otitis externa are the other typical cutaneous signs. Histologically, the most striking finding is severe follicular orthokeratotic hyperkeratosis with massive plugs of keratin in the follicle and no or minimal dermal inflammation. Treatment consists of oral vitamin A supplementation at a dose of 10,000 IU per dog (larger breeds may require higher doses) or 625–800 IU/kg q24h, preferably given with a fat meal to increase absorption. It should be noted that these dogs are not vitamin A deficient, but respond to vitamin A therapy. Signs of toxicity or side effects with over supplementation are paradoxically represented by poor coat quality, alopecia and scaling, together with liver disease and keratoconjunctivitis sicca. Vitamin A can affect the tear film, therefore, regular Schirmer tear tests are recommended, especially in breeds predisposed to keratoconjunctivitis sicca.

Vitamin B

B vitamins are water-soluble and most act as cofactors in EFA metabolism (see above). This explains the sparing effect of EFAs on the cutaneous lesions caused by vitamin B complex deficiency. Vitamin B complex deficiency is quite uncommon in dogs and cats fed commercial pet foods because these products are largely supplemented with vitamin B complexes.

The experimental deficiency of riboflavin (vitamin B2) and biotin can cause skin problems in dogs and cats, which manifest as dermatitis, erythema, alopecia and dry exfoliative dermatitis, as well as anorexia, weight loss, cataracts, impaired growth and reproduction and neurological changes (NRC, 2006). Biotin deficiency can be caused by feeding raw egg whites because they contain the glycoprotein avidin, which binds biotin making in unavailable for absorption. Moreover, since part of the biotin requirement can be met by the gut microbial population, the protracted use of oral antibiotics can theoretically cause signs of biotin deficiency.

In one study, 91% of dogs (108/119 cases) with a poor hair coat and skin condition (mainly a dull coat, brittle hair, alopecia, scales and pruritus) that were treated with biotin only (5 mg biotin/10 kg bodyweight/day) for 3-5 weeks showed improvement in the clinical signs or recovered completely (Frigg et al., 1989). It is important to rule out any other diseases that might result in these signs and ensure that the dog is being fed a balanced diet.

Vitamin D

Vitamin D is a fat-soluble vitamin with a well established role in calcium homoeostasis and maintenance of skeletal health. Cats and dogs are reliant on dietary vitamin D because they are unable to produce active vitamin D3 in the skin from isomerization of 7-dehydrocholesterol via ultraviolet (UV) radiation. Vitamin D can be obtained from the ingestion of vitamin D2 (ergocalciferol) or D3 (cholecalciferol) in the diet. Vitamin D2 is obtained from plants, whereas vitamin D3 is highly concentrated in oily fish (e.g. sardines and salmon), egg yolk and liver. Following absorption, vitamin D is either stored in fat or transported to the liver. In the liver, the first hydroxylation of vitamin D occurs and 25 hydroxyvitamin D (25(OH)D) is produced; 25(OH)D can be further hydroxylated by renal 1-alpha-hydroxylase to produce 1,25 dihydroxyvitamin D (1,25(OH)D). 1,25(OH)D is considered the most active vitamin D metabolite. The conversion of 25(OH)D to 1,25(OH)D is regulated by parathyroid hormone, ionized calcium and 1,25(OH)D concentrations (Mellanby, 2016). Serum 25(OH)D is a valid parameter for monitoring the status of vitamin D in the body, although the optimal serum concentration has not yet been defined in companion animals.

It has recently been demonstrated that vitamin D receptors are highly expressed in the kidneys, duodenum, skin, ileum and spleen, and weakly expressed in the colon, heart, lymph nodes, liver, lungs and ovaries. On the contrary, gastric and testicular tissues do not express vitamin D receptors (Cartwright et al., 2018). These results highlight the involvement of vitamin D in numerous biological processes. A vitamin D deficiency has been implicated in cases with gastrointestinal, renal and cardiac diseases, mycobacterial infection, various inflammatory conditions and increased mortality. In addition, previous investigations in human medicine have shown that vitamin D functions as a regulator of cellular growth and differentiation in various tissues; in the skin it suppresses growth and stimulates the terminal differentiation of keratinocytes.

Few studies have investigated the relationship between vitamin D and skin health in dogs and cats. In a recent study (Casini et al., 2020), the concentration of serum vitamin D was measured in 103 Japanese Akitas, which were divided according to their health status into two groups: healthy and pathological. In the latter group, dogs

suffering from chronic diseases such as uveodermatological syndrome, sebaceous adenitis, chronic dermatitis, epilepsy, toxoplasmosis, allergies, enteritis and arthrosis were included. The pathological Akitas showed a significantly lower serum 25(OH)D concentration compared with the healthy control group. In addition, areas of congenital skin depigmentation, similar to that seen with vitiligo, were often present in healthy Akitas of any age without other clinical signs. Dogs with non-congenital depigmentation also formed part of both the healthy and pathological groups of Akitas, and a significantly lower serum 25(OH)D level was detected in healthy depigmented dogs compared with healthy pigmented animals. This reflects an observation in human studies, where a strong correlation between hypovitaminosis D and the autoimmune disease vitiligo was detected (Upala and Snaguankeo, 2016). The Akita study also suggests that skin depigmentation may be associated with low serum vitamin D. In a recent randomized, placebo-controlled, double-blinded cross-over study of the treatment of 23 dogs with atopic dermatitis, cholecalciferol administration alongside other therapies resulted in a significant decrease in pruritus and lesion scores; furthermore, the serum 25(OH)D concentration was shown to be highly correlated with a reduction in pruritus (Klinger et al., 2018).

Vitamin E

Vitamin E (alpha-tocopherol) is one of the most powerful natural antioxidants present in the body. It has an important role in the protection of skin cell membranes against free radicals that are produced during lipid metabolism, as a consequence of exposure to UV radiation and air pollutants, and as a result of skin inflammation secondary to bacterial, yeast or parasitic infection. High levels of PUFAs in the diet can result in high production of free radicals – this is one of the common causes of a relative deficiency in vitamin E. Thus, it is important to ensure that such supplements also contain vitamin E (Hall et al., 2003).

Pansteatitis is a feline disorder caused by a severe deficiency in vitamin E. It is particularly recognized in cats fed exclusively with canned red tuna or supplemented with excessive cod liver oil. The depletion of antioxidants leads to lipid peroxidation, causing necrosis and inflammation of the subcutaneous and intra-abdominal fat. Clinically, multiple firm and painful nodules are detected in the affected tissue both in the abdominal cavity and in the subcutaneous fat. Systemic signs include fever, anorexia, lethargy and intense pain of the affected areas. The diet of the cats should be changed, vitamin E supplemented and glucocorticoids given in severe cases; however, the prognosis is usually poor (Watson et al., 1973; Niza et al., 2003).

Vitamin E is also recognized as having an immunomodulatory and anti-inflammatory function exerted by stabilization of lysosomes, reduction in prostaglandin E2 synthesis and increased production of interleukin (IL)-2, with a deficiency causing T-cell dysfunction. Many anecdotal reports suggest its use at a dose of 400–800 IU/dog orally q12h as an adjunctive therapy together with immunosuppressive drugs for the management of immune-mediated skin diseases such as canine cutaneous lupus erythematosus, sterile panniculitis, dermatomyositis and vasculopathy. Recently, supplementation was assessed in a placebo-controlled study of dogs with atopic dermatitis (Kapun et al., 2014). A reduction in lesion score was documented at a dose of 8.1 IU/kg orally q24h, but there was no effect on pruritus.

Minerals

Zinc

Zinc is an important mineral, which is necessary for numerous metabolic functions. It is primarily incorporated into enzymes. Approximately 20% of the zinc contained within the body is stored in the skin, where it is involved with the keratinization process. Zinc deficiency is thought to result in a decrease in zinc-related lytic enzymes with subsequent disruption of the keratinization process and increase in epidermal turnover rate. This leads to a hyperplastic epidermis with retention of nuclei in a very thick stratum corneum (parakeratosis). Clinically this manifests as crusts, scales and alopecia with a multifocal distribution.

Zinc deficiency can also cause systemic clinical signs proportional to its severity and may include (Gross *et al.*, 2005; Mueller and Kirk, 2013):

- Reduced appetite and anorexia (suggested to be secondary to a decrease in sense of smell and taste)
- Weight loss
- Reduced growth
- Poor wound healing
- Ocular problems (i.e. conjunctivitis and keratitis).

The lack of zinc can arise from:

- Absolute zinc deficiency in the diet
- A genetic defect that impairs zinc absorption, leading to syndrome I zinc-responsive dermatosis and lethal acrodermatitis
- An increased concentration of phytate, calcium and copper in the diet, which reduces zinc absorption
- Severe gastrointestinal diseases that interfere with zinc absorption and utilization.

Absolute zinc deficiency is very rare nowadays due to the accuracy in formulating commercial diets.

Zinc-responsive dermatoses

Syndrome I: This is primarily seen in Nordic breeds such as the Alaskan Malamute, Samoyed and Siberian Husky, although it has been occasionally reported in other breeds. The syndrome can be observed in dogs of all ages, but it is seen more frequently in early adulthood, and is apparently worse during oestrus or other stressful periods. Dogs are usually fed a well balanced diet and the relative deficiency is probably related to an inherited defect in intestinal zinc absorption or metabolism. Cutaneous lesions are characterized by erythema, alopecia, crusts and adherent thick scale, mainly localized around the mouth, eyes, ears, scrotum, prepuce, vulva and pressure points with a bilateral symmetry in distribution (Figures 31.1 and 31.2). Bacterial or *Malassezia* secondary infections are common any may contribute to the presence of pruritus and the worsening of the lesions (Colombini and Dunstan, 1997; White *et al.*, 2011).

Syndrome II: This usually occurs in rapidly growing large-breed dogs fed a diet with a low zinc concentration or over supplemented with substances such as phytate, calcium and other minerals that prevent zinc absorption by chelation (Sousa *et al.*, 1988). The clinical presentation is similar to that described for syndrome I, but with greater severity. Some patient may experience systemic clinical signs such as anorexia, depression, reduced growth and lymphadenopathy (Van den Broek and Thoday, 1986).

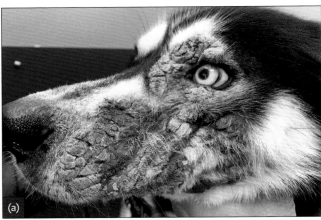
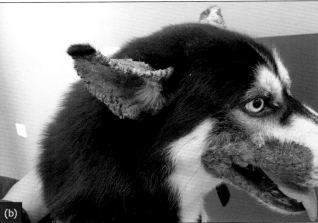

31.1 Zinc-responsive dermatosis: syndrome I. Severe crusting and hyperkeratosis of (a) the muzzle and the periocular areas, and (b) the ear pinna.
(Courtesy of Francesco Albanese)

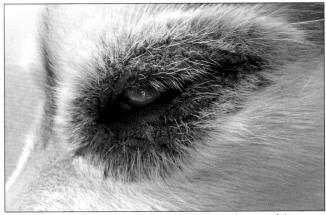

31.2 Zinc-responsive dermatosis: syndrome I. Close up of the periocular hyperkeratotic region of a young Siberian Husky.

Diagnostic tests: The diagnosis of both syndrome I and II is based on the history, clinical signs and histopathological examination of skin biopsy samples. Differential diagnoses that should be ruled out for both syndrome I and II include: dermatophytosis, sarcoptic mange and demodicosis for patients with mild clinical signs; in more severe cases, superficial necrolytic dermatitis, pemphigus foliaceous and systemic or mucocutaneous canine lupus erythematosus should be considered. Histopathological examination reveals a moderate to severe acanthotic epidermis with a multifocal to diffuse, mild to moderate parakeratosis, which can extend into the follicular infundibula. Intraepidermal pustules and the variable presence of serocellular crusting with erosion may be seen and often reflects secondary infection. Dermal inflammation is usually superficial, perivascular to interstitial and comprises lymphocytes, macrophages, eosinophils and neutrophils. The measurement of serum or hair zinc levels does not appear to be valuable for a definitive diagnosis, as many factors (e.g. age, environmental temperature, stress, comorbidities) can influence and alter the results.

Treatment: The majority of dogs affected by syndrome I experience complete resolution of clinical manifestations following zinc supplementation, although a consistent response may take up to 6 months. Life-long zinc supplementation is required with syndrome I and discontinuation or variation in dosage might lead to prompt relapse. In syndrome II, correction of the diet alone is sufficient to yield a complete resolution of the lesions in 2–6 weeks, although the provision of zinc supplements during the first few weeks can help speed up resolution. Three forms of zinc are available – zinc sulphate, zinc gluconate and zinc methionine – with no apparent difference in efficacy (Figure 31.3).

Alternatively, elemental zinc at a dose of 1–2 mg/kg orally q24h can be administered; increasing the dose by up to 50% has been suggested in patients that are refractory to treatment. Vomiting, nausea and decreased appetite are common side effects seen with zinc sulphate; splitting the administration to twice daily with food may ameliorate these side effects. Low dose glucocorticoid treatment may be beneficial in cases not responding to zinc supplementation alone (Burton and Mason, 1998). EFA supplementation has also been shown to improve the response, therefore concomitant administration is recommended. Bitches should be neutered, as a worsening of the condition has been recorded during oestrus, and affected animals should not be used for breeding (White *et al.*, 2011).

Formulation	Daily dose
Zinc gluconate	5 mg/kg
Zinc sulphate	10 mg/kg
Zinc methionine	1.7 mg/kg

31.3 The three forms of available zinc and their suggested daily dose.

Lethal acrodermatitis

Lethal acrodermatitis (LAD) is an autosomal recessive disease affecting Bull Terriers and Miniature Bull Terriers. The disease is considered to be clinically and pathologically similar to an inherited disorder in zinc metabolism, acrodermatitis enteropathica, in humans. However, in contrast to the condition in humans, puppies affected by LAD do not show any improvement following oral or systemic zinc supplementation; furthermore, serum zinc levels in affected patients have been found to be contradictory. Recently, a splice defect in the canine gene encoding the intracellular protein muskelin 1 (*MKLN1* gene) has been identified in both Bull Terriers and Miniature Bull Terriers with LAD. The functions of muskelin 1 are only partially known, therefore, the exact pathogenesis of LAD remains unclear and whether this is truly a nutritional disease is unknown (Bauer *et al.*, 2018). A condition similar to LAD has also been described in a litter of 3-month-old Pharaoh Hound puppies (Campbell and Crow, 2010).

Affected puppies tend to show weakness, stunted growth, and difficulties in swallowing and chewing because of an abnormally arched hard palate. By 6–10 weeks of age, skin lesions start to appear and comprise erythema, tightly adherent scales, erosions or ulcerations with crusts, mainly localized on the feet, distal limbs, elbows, hocks and muzzle. Severe secondary bacterial and/or yeast infections are common. With time, severe hyperkeratosis of the footpads with fissuring of the paw pads and deformed claws is observed. Affected dogs can also suffer from chronic diarrhoea and bronchopneumonia. The prognosis is very poor, and the median survival time is approximately 7 months, with the majority of dogs dying from secondary infections or being euthanised due to a poor quality of life (McEwan *et al.*, 2000). The diagnosis is straightforward, especially when multiple puppies are affected. In isolated cases, pemphigus foliaceus, bacterial or yeast infections and adverse drug reactions should be considered and ruled out. Histopathology is supportive of the diagnosis and is similar to that described in zinc-responsive dermatosis syndromes I and II.

Copper

Copper is an essential trace element and the liver is responsible for both its storage and the excretion of excess amounts in the bile. Copper has a role in many biological functions and is involved in the synthesis of various enzymes. Some of the so-called cuproenzymes are involved in skin functions, including:

- Lysyl oxidase – implicated in the synthesis of connective tissue
- Tyrosinase – catalyses the production of melanin from tyrosine and copper, and activates a thiol oxidase enzyme which is responsible for the formation of keratin filaments.

Cutaneous signs of copper deficiency include alopecia, a dull or rough coat and a greyish appearance of the pigmented hair of the head and muzzle, which may spread over the entire body (Zentek and Meyer, 1991). As modern pet foods are well balanced, copper deficiency is rarely seen in practice.

Metabolic diseases

Superficial necrolytic dermatitis

Superficial necrolytic dermatitis (SND), also referred to as hepatocutaneous syndrome, is a rare metabolic disease recognized in dogs and cats and mainly associated with an underlying hepatopathy of unknown origin. Some patients affected by SND are also diagnosed with concomitant diabetes mellitus and hyperadrenocorticism (Hall-Fonte *et al.*, 2016). A few cases of hepatic disease associated with the ingestion of mycotoxins and chronic phenobarbital administration have been described, and the condition may also be associated with pancreatic glucagonoma (March *et al.*, 2004; Mizuno *et al.*, 2009). The cases reported in cats have been seen in conjunction with pancreatic or hepatic tumours and chronic hepatopathy (Asakawa *et al.*, 2013).

Cutaneous lesions in SND are due to the degeneration of keratinocytes via a pathomechanism that is still not fully understood. An increased hepatic catabolism of amino acids is one of the proposed mechanisms; other suggestions include reduced absorption leading to a general nutritional deficiency and hyperglucagonaemia, although the latter has not been systematically identified in affected dogs (Outerbridge *et al.*, 2002). Cell starvation causes necrosis, epithelial cell death and difficulties in repairing damaged collagen, especially in cutaneous sites exposed to mechanical trauma (i.e. pressure points).

Clinical presentation

Affected dogs are usually old (mean age of 10 years) with no clear breed or sex predilection. However, cases reported in the veterinary literature emphasize that small to medium sized breeds, particularly Shih Tzus, West Highland White Terriers, Jack Russell Terriers and Cocker Spaniels are overrepresented (Hall-Fonte *et al.*, 2016). Skin lesions comprise erythema, scales and exudation, progressing to thick adherent crusts, erosions and ulcers. The distribution is usually symmetrical and the lesions affect the mucocutaneous junctions, pressure points and footpads (Figure 31.4). When dermatological signs become apparent, systemic signs such as weight loss, anorexia and lethargy are already evident. Polyuria and polydipsia may be detected if diabetes mellitus is also present.

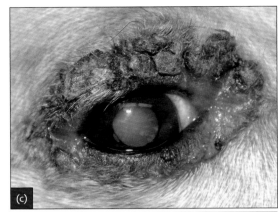

(c)

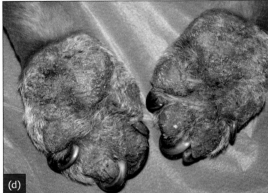

(d)

31.4 (continued) Superficial necrolytic dermatitis. (c) Periocular area and (d) footpads.
(Courtesy of Francesco Albanese)

Diagnostic tests

The main differential diagnoses are pemphigus foliaceous, zinc-responsive dermatoses, leishmaniosis, systemic lupus erythematosus and hyperkeratotic erythema multiforme. Common clinicopathological abnormalities include non-regenerative anaemia and high hepatic enzyme activity, particularly alkaline phosphatase and alanine aminotransferase. In advanced cases, liver enzymes may be normal. The liver shows a distinct hepatic pattern with numerous hypoechoic nodules in a typical honeycomb appearance (Figure 31.5). Cytology of skin samples reveals the presence of a usually quite severe bacterial or yeast infection.

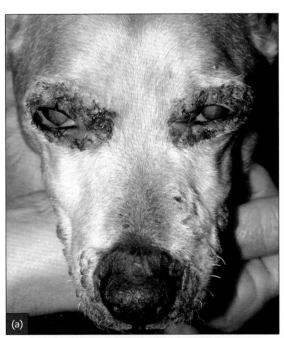

(a)

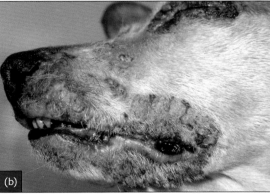

(b)

31.4 Superficial necrolytic dermatitis. (a) Severe crusting and ulceration symmetrically distributed on the muzzle. Close up of the (b) perioral area. (continues)
(Courtesy of Francesco Albanese)

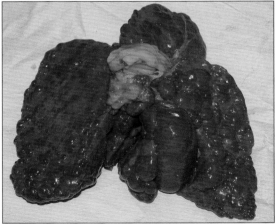

31.5 Gross appearance of the liver of a dog with superficial necrolytic dermatitis. Note the presence of widespread nodules of various sizes.
(Courtesy of Francesco Albanese)

Histopathological examination of skin biopsy specimens shows a pattern that is conventionally defined as 'the French flag', consisting of a diffuse parakeratotic epidermis (red), with inter- and intracellular oedema (white) and hyperplastic basal cell layers (blue).

Treatment

The therapeutic approach should be directed at correcting the nutritional deficiency and supporting liver function by feeding a nutritionally balanced diet with high-quality proteins, together with zinc, EFAs, antioxidants and hepatoprotective agents. Intravenous administration of amino acids appears to be the most effective treatment with an infusion needed approximately every 2–3 weeks. However, this is not uniformly effective and is complicated by the need to deliver the solution via a central line. Most affected dogs survive for <6 months on average, but occasionally longer survival times (≥36 months) may be seen (Hill *et al.*, 2000). Recently, a high-quality nutritionally complete home-cooked prescription diet based on chicken breast and eggs (as sources of high-quality protein) was demonstrated to improve clinical signs and reduce the frequency of intravenous amino acid administration required in a dog with SND (Jaffey *et al.*, 2020).

Xanthomas

Xanthomas (*Xanthós* from the Greek meaning blond) are granulomatous lesions containing lipid-laden macrophages that can occur in the skin and other locations such as the oral mucosa, corneas, internal organs and tendons. Their development has been reported in cats presumably affected by primary hereditary hyperlipoproteinaemia, a disorder caused by defective expression of the enzyme lipase, which is involved in the clearance of lipoproteins rich in triglycerides. Xanthomas have also been reported in animals with spontaneous or drug-induced diabetes mellitus and associated with feeding high fat foods or treats (Chastain and Graham, 1978; Chanut *et al.*, 2005).

Clinical presentation

Lesions consist of white to yellow papules, nodules and plaques that occasionally ulcerate with a consequent discharge of a creamy necrotic substance. The distribution is often symmetrical and typically located in the preauricular and periorbital regions, especially in cats. Other locations such as the pinnae, head, neck and bony prominences of the extremities (Figure 31.6) may be involved.

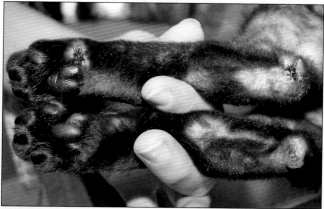

31.6 Multiple xanthomas on the pads of a cat. (Courtesy of Michela DeLucia)

Diagnostic tests

The differential diagnoses include other papular/nodular granulomatous diseases, both infectious (caused by fungi or mycobacteria) and sterile (feline progressive cell histiocytosis and neoplasia). Cytology reveals a granulomatous inflammation comprising macrophages with a foamy cytoplasm, lymphocytes and, rarely, eosinophils and neutrophils. Elevations of both cholesterol and triglyceride levels in conjunction with the clinical signs are highly suggestive of the disease. A definitive diagnosis is confirmed by histopathology, which is characterized by a nodular to diffuse granulomatous inflammation composed of foamy macrophages together with histiocytic giant cells. Eosinophils may be present in high numbers, whilst neutrophils, plasma cells and lymphocytes are less prominent.

Treatment

Correction of the underlying disease results in rapid resolution of the lesions. The institution of an appropriate diet (i.e. low-fat diet) is always recommended as this helps to bring about a complete clinical resolution after approximately 2–4 weeks.

> **Key points**
> - The skin has a high nutritional requirement and can be affected by poor quality diets or systemic disease
> - Certain skin conditions may respond to supraphysiological doses of nutrients that are normally present in adequate quantities in the diet
> - Omega-6 fatty acids are particularly important for skin barrier function and should be supplemented along with omega-3 EFAs

References and further reading

Ackerman L (1987) Nutritional supplements in canine dermatoses. *The Canadian Veterinary Journal* **28**, 29–32

Anderson PJ, Rogers QR and Morris JG (2002) Cats require more dietary phenylalanine or tyrosine for melanin deposition in hair than for maximal growth. *The Journal of Nutrition* **132**, 2037–2042

Asakawa MG, Cullen JM and Linder KE (2013) Necrolytic migratpry erythema associated with a glucagon-producing primary hepatic neuroendocrine carcinoma in a cat. *Veterinary Dermatology* **24**, 466–e110

Bauer A, Jagannathan V, Hogler S *et al.* (2018) MKLN1 splicing defect in dogs with lethal acrodermatitis. *PLOS genetics 2018* **14**, e1007264

Bauer JE (2011) Therapeutic use of fish oils in companion animals. *Journal of the American Veterinary Medical Association* **11**, 1441–1451

Blaskovic M, Rosenkrantz W, Neuber A *et al.* (2014) The effect of a spot-on formulation containing polyunsaturated fatty acids and essential oils on dogs with atopic dermatitis. *Veterinary Journal* **199**, 39–43

Bloom P (2013) Nonsteroidal, non-immunosuppressive therapies for pruritus. *Veterinary Clinics of North America: Small Animal Practice* **43**,173–187

Burton G and Mason KV (1998) The possible role of prednisolone in 'zinc-responsive dermatosis' in the Siberian Husky. *Australian Veterinary Practice* **28**, 20

Campbell GA and Crow D (2010) Severe zinc-responsive dermatosis in a litter of Pharaoh Hounds. *Journal of Veterinary Diagnostic Investigation* **22**, 663–666

Campbell KL and Dorn GP (1992) Effects of oral sunflower oil and olive oil on serum and cutaneous fatty acid concentrations in dogs. *Research in Veterinary Science* **53**, 172–178

Cartwright JA, Gow AG, Milne E *et al.* (2018) Vitamin D Receptor expression in dogs. *Journal of Veterinary Internal Medicine* **32**, 764–774

Casini L, Zago D, Cavicchioli Enand Tomiazzo C (2020) Serum 25-hydroxyvitamin D concentration in Japanese Akita dogs: a survery. *Veterinary and Animal Science* **10**, 1001399

Chanut F, Colle MA, Deschamps JY *et al.* (2005) Systemic xanthomatosis associated with hyperchylomicronaemia in a cat. *Journal of Veterinary Medical Association: A Physiology, Pathology Clinical Medicine* **52**, 272–274

Chastain CB and Graham CL (1978) Xanthomatosis secondary to diabetes mellitus in a dog. *Journal of the American Veterinary Medical Association* **172**, 1209

Cline DJ (1988) Changes in hair color. *Dermatologic Clinics* **6**, 295–303

Codner EC and Thatcher CD (1990) The role of nutrition in the management of dermatoses. *Seminars in Veterinary Medicine and Surgery (Small Animal)* **5**, 167–177

Colombini S and Dunstan RW (1997) Zinc-responsive dermatosis in northen-breed dogs: 17 cases (1990–1996). *Journal of the American Veterinary Medical Association* **211**, 451

Conway DMP and Saker KE (2018) Consumer attitude toward the environmental sustainability of grain-free pet foods. *Frontiers in Veterinary Science* **5**, 170

Dodd S, Barry M, Grant C et al. (2019) Abnormal bone mineralization in a puppy fed an imbalanced raw meat homemade diet diagnosed and monitored using dual-energy X-ray absorptiometry. *Journal of Animal Physiology and Animal Nutrion* doi: 10.1111/jpn.13118

Freeman LM, Chandler ML, Hamper BA et al. (2013) Current knowledge about the risks and benefits of raw meat–based diets for dogs and cats. *Journal of the American Veterinary Medical Association* **243**, 1549–1558

Frigg M, Schulze J and Völker L (1989) Clinical study on the effect of biotin on skin conditions in dogs. *Schweizer Archiv fur Tierheilkunde* **131**, 621–625

Gross KL, Yamka RM, Kim CK et al. (2010) Macronutrients. In: *Small Animal Clinical Nutrition*, eds. MS Hand, CD Thatcher, RL Remillard, P Roudebush and BJ Novotny. Mark Morris Institute, Topeka, Kansas

Gross TL, Ihrke PJ, Walder EJ and Affolter VK (2005) *Skin Diseases of The Dog and Cat. Clinical and Histopathological Diagnosis, 2nd edn*, Blackwell's, Oxford

Hall JA, Tooley KA, Gradin JL et al. (2003) Effects of dietary n-6 and n-3 fatty acids and vitamin E on the immune response of healthy geriatric dogs. *American Journal of Veterinary Research* **64**, 762–772

Hall-Fonte DL, Center SA, MC Donough SP et al. (2016) Hepatocutaneous syndrome in Shih Tzus: 31 cases (1996-2014). *Journal of the American Veterinary Medical Association* **248**, 802–813

Hill PB, Auxilia ST, Munro E et al. (2000) Resolution of skin lesions and long-term survival in a dog with superficial necrolytic dermatitis and liver cirrhosis. *Journal of Small Animal Practice* **41**, 519–523

Hunter E, Foster A, O'Dair H and Place E (2020) Are oral essential fatty acids alone an effective treatment for symmetrical lupoid onychodystrophy / onychomadesis? *Veterinary Record* **186**, 452–454

Ihrke PJ and Goldschmidt MH (1983) Vitamin A-responsive dermatosis in the dog. *Journal of the American Veterinary Medical Association* **182**, 682

Jaffey JA, Backus RC, Sprinkle M et al. (2020) Successful long-term management of canine superficial necrolytic dermatitis with amino acid infusions and nutritionally balanced home-made diet modification. *Frontiers in Veterinary Science* **7**, 28

Kapun Plevnik AP, Salobir J, Levart A et al. (2014) Vitamin E supplementation in canine atopic dermatitis: improvement of clinical signs and effects on oxidative stress markers. *Veterinary Record* **175**, 560

Klinger CJ, Hobi S, Johansen C et al. Vitamin D shows in vivo efficacy in a placebo-controlled, double-blinded, randomised clinical trial on canine atopic dermatitis. *The Veterinary Record 2018* **182**, 406

MacDonald ML, Rogers QR and Morris JG (1984) Nutrition of the domestic cat, a mammalian carnivore. *Annual Review of Nutrition* **4**, 521–562

March PA, Hiller A, Weisbrode SE et al. (2004) Superficial necrolytic dermatitis in 11 dogs with a history of phenobarbital administration (1995–2002). *Journal of Veterinary Internal Medicine* **18**, 65–74

McDonald P, Edwards RA, Greenhalgh JFD et al. (2010) *Animal Nutrition 7th edn*. Blackwell's, Oxford

McEwan NA, McNeil PE, Thompson H et al. (2000) Diagnostic features, confirmation and disease progression in 28 cases of lethal acrodermatitis of bull terriers. *Journal of Small Animal Practice* **41**, 501–507

Mellanby RJ (2016) Beyond the skeleton: the role of vitamin D in companion animal health. *Journal of Small Animal Practice* **57**, 175–180

Miller WH (1989) Nutritional consideration in small animal dermatology. Veterinary Clinics of North America: Small Animal Practice 19, 497–511

Miller WH, Griffin CE and Campbell KL (2013) *Mueller & Kirk's: Small Animal Dermatology, 7th edn*, W.B. Saunders, Philadelphia

Mizuno T, Hiraoka H, Yoshioka C et al. (2009) Superficial necrolytic dermatitis associated with extrapancreatic glucagonoma in a dog. *Veterinary Dermatology* **20**, 72–79

Morelli G, Bastianello S, Catellani P et al. (2019) Raw meat-based diets for dogs: survey of owners' motivations, attitudes and practices. *BMC Veterinary Research* **15**, 74

Morelli G, Catellani P, Miotti Scapin R et al. (2020) Evaluation of microbial contamination and effects of storage in raw meat-based dog foods purchased online. *Journal of Animal Physiology and Animal Nutrition* **104**, 690–697

Morelli G, Stefanutti D, Ricci R et al. (2021) A survey among dog and cat owners on pet food storage and preservation in the households. *Animals* **11**, 273

Morris JG, Yu S and Rogers QR (2002) Red hair in black cats is reversed by addition of tyrosine to the diet. *Journal of Nutrition* **132**, 1646S–1648S

Muller and Kirk's Small Animal Dermatology 7th edn., eds. WH Miller, CE Griffin and KL Campbell. Elsevier, St Louis, MO

Niza M, Vilela CL and Ferreira LMA (2003) Feline pansteatitis revisited: hazard of unbalanced home-made diets. *Journal of Feline Medical Surgery* **5**, 271–277

Nutrient Requirements of Dogs and Cats (2006) National Research Council, The National Academies Press, Washington DC

Outerbridge CA, Marks SL and Rogers QR (2002) Plasma amino acid concentrations in 36 dogs with histologically confirmed superficial necrolytic dermatitis. *Veterinary Dermatology* **13**, 177–186

Rees CA, Bauer JE, Burkholder WJ et al. (2001) Effects of dietary flax seed and sunflower seed supplementation on normal canine serum polyunsaturated fatty acids and skin and hair coat condition scores. *Veterinary Dermatology* **12**, 111–117

Rogers QR and Morris JG (1979) Essentiality of amino acids for the growing kitten. *Journal of Nutrition* **109**, 718–723

Roudebush P and Schoenherr WD (2010) Skin and hair disorders. In: *Small Animal Clinical Nutrition*, eds. MS Hand, CD Thatcher, RL Remillard, P Roudebush and BJ Novtony. Mark Morris Institute, Topeka, Kansas

Saevik BK, Bergvall B, Holm BR et al. (2004) A randomized controlled study to evaluate the steroid sparing effect of essential fatty acid supplementation in the treatment of canine atopic dermatitis. *Veterinary Dermatology* **15**, 137–145

Scott DW and Miller Jr WH (1993) Nonsteroidal anti-inflammatory agents in the management of canine allergic pruritus. *Journal of the South African Veterinary Association* **64**, 52–56

Sousa CA, Stannard AA, Ihrke PJ et al. (1988) Dermatosis associated with feeding generic dog food: 13 cases (1981–1982). *Journal of the American Veterinary Medical Association* **192**, 676–80

Tretter S and Mueller RS (2011) The influence of topical unsaturated fatty acids and essential oils on normal and atopic dogs. *Journal of the American Animal Hospital Association* **47**, 236–240

Upala S and Sanguankeo A (2016) Low 25-hydroxyvitamin D levels are associated with vitiligo: A systematic review and meta-analysis. *Photodermatology Photoimmunology Photomedicine* **32**, 181–190

van Bree FPJ, Bokken GCAM, Mineur R et al. (2018) Zoonotic bacteria and parasites found in raw meat-based diets for cats and dogs. *Veterinary Record* **182**, 50

Van den Broek AHM and Thoday KL (1986) Skin disease in dogs associated with zinc deficiency: A report of 5 cases. *Journal of Small Animal Practice* **27**, 313

Watson A, Servet E, Hervera M et al. (2015) Tyrosine supplementation and hair coat pigmentation in puppies with black coats – A pilot study. *Journal of Applied Animal Nutrition* **3**, e10, doi: 10.1017/jan.2015.8

Watson AD, Porges WL, Huxtable CR and Ilkiw WJ (1973) Pansteatitis in a cat. *Veterinary Journal* **49**, 388–392

Watson TDG (1998) Diet and skin disease in dogs and cats. *Journal of Nutrition* **128**, 2783–2789

White SD, Bordeaux P, Rosychuk RAW et al. (2011) Zinc-responsive dermatosis in dogs: 41 cases and literature review. *Veterinary Dermatology* **12**, 101–109

Yu S, Rogers QR and Morris JG (2001) Effect of low levels of dietary tyrosine on the hair colour of cats. *Journal of Small Animal Practice* **42**, 176–180

Zentek J and Meyer H (1991) Investigations on copper deficiency in growing dogs. *Journal of Nutrition* **121**, S83–S84

Chapter 32

Actinic (solar) dermatoses

Mandy Burrows

Solar dermatitis and solar-induced neoplasia occur in dogs and cats as a consequence of chronic exposure to sunlight and ultraviolet (UV) radiation on non-pigmented, lightly pigmented or damaged (depigmented or scarred) skin that is unprotected by hair. The deleterious effects of UV radiation on the skin depend upon the duration and frequency of exposure, the intensity of solar radiation related to the geographical latitude, and the reactivity of the skin based on skin colour, hair coat density and genetic susceptibility.

Lesions are more common in dogs and cats that sunbathe or that are housed where there is reflective ground cover (including snow) and little sun protection. This is more commonly seen in animals that spend a substantial amount of time outdoors in tropical, subtropical, desert or mountainous regions, and is most problematic in hot sunny climates, such as Australia, California, Florida, Hawaii and South Africa. Many affected dogs are reported to be sunbathers and spend long periods of time in dorsal or lateral recumbency in direct sunlight. The most commonly affected dog breeds are white English Bull Terriers, Dalmatians, Beagles, Fox Terriers, Whippets, white Boxers, American Staffordshire Bull Terriers, Basset Hounds and American Bulldogs. White-haired areas of shorthaired cats are most at risk. Blue-eyed white cats are most susceptible.

Actinic (solar) dermatitis

Clinical presentation

Dogs

The earliest clinical signs are patchy to confluent erythema and scaling affecting non-pigmented skin (Figure 32.1a). With chronic solar exposure, there is marked thickening of erythematous skin and lesions range from focal patches of erythema and crusting to scaly, erythematous papules, and crusted, indurated, linear plaques and nodules (Figure 32.1bc). Erosions and ulcers have adherent haemorrhagic crusts.

Actinic comedones may be present. These are distinctive and occur in non-pigmented lightly haired skin as a consequence of follicular occlusion secondary to dermal fibrosis. They are multiple, grouped, dilated hair follicles that are filled with darkly coloured keratinous or caseous debris (Figure 32.1d). Lesions may not appear follicular but as discrete pigmented subepidermal foci or small nodules. Palpation of comedones in apparently normal skin may reveal irregular firmness and thickening, suggesting

solar-induced changes. Rupture of comedones releases follicular keratin and hair into the dermis, eliciting a foreign body response that then results in a deep furunculosis (Figure 32.1e).

Actinic furunculosis can arise from comedonal rupture and develop in any hair follicle located in a region of solar damage. Intact haemorrhagic bullae are a distinctive feature secondary to actinic comedonal rupture (Figure 32.1f) with crusted erythematous nodules that may be intact or fistulated. The clinical features of both actinic comedones and actinic furunculosis occur in the context of other solar-induced lesions. A coexistent bacterial pyoderma may make the clinical diagnosis more difficult to interpret.

In dogs that sunbathe in lateral recumbency, lesions are commonly observed on the glabrous skin of the ventral and lateral abdomen, as well as the flank folds and inner thighs. Lesions are often found abruptly adjacent to normal, pigmented skin. The hock and distal hind limb, bridge of the nose, pinnae, dorsal muzzle, periorbital regions and tail tip may also be affected (Figure 32.2). Some dogs will lie on one side more frequently and this causes more severe lesions to develop on the side with greatest sun exposure. The ventral region, scrotum and perineal skin are often affected in dogs that sunbathe on their backs or are housed on reflective surfaces.

Cats

The early lesions appear on the margin of the sparsely haired pinnae and are characterized by mild erythema and fine scaling (Figure 32.3a). Advanced lesions consist of severe erythema, alopecia and thickening of the pinnae with peeling, crusting and erosions that are associated with pain, scratching and twitching of the pinnae. With further progression, there is severe crusting, ulceration and haemorrhage, and the pinnal margins may curl (Figure 32.3b). The margins of the lower eyelids, lips, dorsal aspect of the nasal planum and the sparsely haired preauricular region of the face may be similarly affected.

Differential diagnoses

Dogs

For the early stage of solar dermatitis, differential diagnoses include hypersensitivity dermatitis (atopic, dietary, contact irritant, insect), *Malassezia* dermatitis and primary disorders of cornification. However, the pruritus associated with solar dermatitis is usually minimal, unlike that in dogs

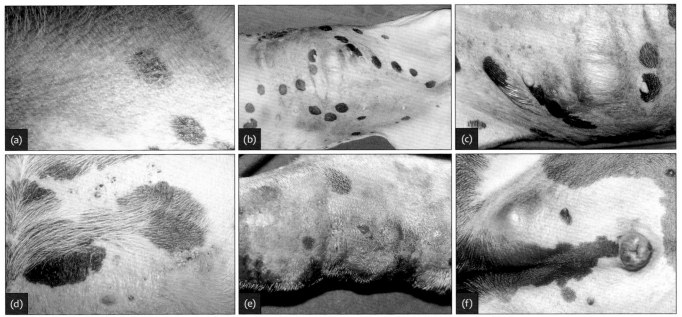

32.1 Canine actinic dermatitis. (a) Erythema and scaling. (b, c) Erythema, indurated plaques and papules. (d) Erythematous plaques and comedones. (e) Furunculosis. (f) Haemorrhagic bullae.
(a, Courtesy of G Burton)

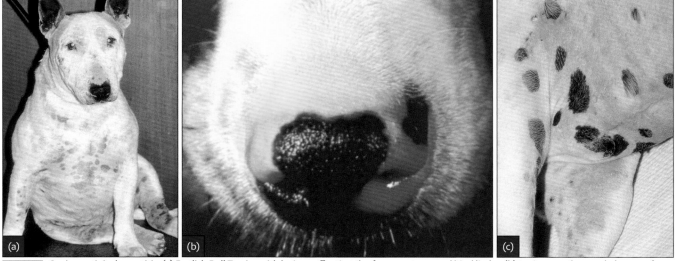

32.2 Canine actinic dermatitis. (a) English Bull Terrier with lesions affecting the face, ventrum and hind limbs. (b) Lesions on the nasal planum of a dog. (c) Lesions on the ventral abdomen and hind limb of a dog.
(b, Courtesy of R Muse)

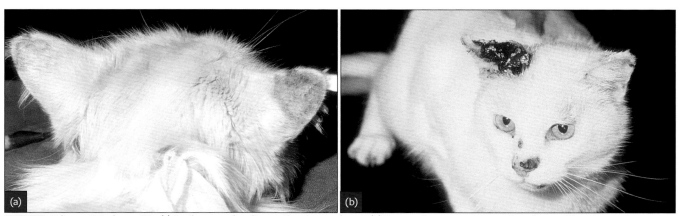

32.3 Feline actinic dermatitis. (a) Erythema and scaling on the pinnae of a cat. (b) Progression to squamous cell carcinoma. There is crusting, erosion and haemorrhage on the pinna and face.
(a, Courtesy of WT Clark)

with allergic dermatitis; this is a major difference between these two differential diagnoses. Some dogs can have solar dermatitis and concurrent allergic skin disease. The differential diagnoses for actinic comedones include other comedogenic disorders such as demodicosis, hyperglucocorticoidism and Schnauzer comedone syndrome. The presence of comedones in a lightly pigmented breed with habitual access to sun exposure, with or without evidence of other solar-induced lesions, should increase suspicion for actinic comedones. The lesions associated with actinic furunculosis need to be differentiated from deep bacterial folliculitis and furunculosis, demodicosis with secondary deep pyoderma, pressure point pyoderma, infections involving systemic or opportunistic fungi, and other nodular tumours (e.g. cutaneous lymphoma, mast cell tumour and metastatic neoplasia).

Cats

Differential diagnoses include facial immune-mediated diseases such as pemphigus foliaceus, systemic and cutaneous lupus erythematosus, vasculitis and drug reactions. In cold climates, cold-agglutinin disease and frostbite also need to be considered. In the cat, other clinical differential diagnoses include dermatophytosis and bowenoid *in situ* carcinoma.

Diagnostic tests

The diagnosis of actinic dermatitis is based on: the correlation of breed, coat colour and length; a history of acute or chronic UV light exposure; and lesion localization to body sites commonly affected by solar damage. The presence of lesions in non-pigmented sparsely haired regions and a history of sun exposure are highly suggestive of solar dermatitis. It is useful to compare adjacent pigmented skin with lesional non-pigmented areas. The pigmented regions are supple on palpation and the skin is a normal thickness, whereas lesional areas are non-pliable with irregular firmness and thickening. The difference in skin thickness may be striking in dogs with coloured spots; unaffected pigmented skin appears thinner than the surrounding affected non-pigmented skin.

Skin biopsy

Definitive diagnosis of actinic dermatitis requires histological evaluation of skin biopsy samples. It is recommended to delay skin biopsy of suspected actinic lesions until the dog has received appropriate topical or systemic antibiotics for at least 3 weeks in order to resolve secondary bacterial pyoderma. This increases the likelihood of targeting solar-induced lesions for biopsy and aids interpretation of the histopathology. Specimens for biopsy should be obtained from different types of lesions and/or different stages of the disease.

Since some of the histological changes can be seen with other skin conditions, one key to achieving a definitive diagnosis from the pathologist is to include a complete history with the biopsy submission form, including signalment, degree of solar exposure, distribution and clinical description of the lesions, response or lack thereof to prior therapies and current medications (e.g. glucocortoicoids) that could affect the histological findings. It is recommended, if possible, that interpretation by a veterinary dermatohistopathologist is sought.

In the early stages of disease, there is a mild superficial perivascular dermatitis (hyperplastic and spongiotic).

Vacuolated keratinocytes with pyknotic nuclei and eosinophilic cytoplasm or 'sunburn cells' are also scattered throughout the epidermis. Epidermal hyperplasia, follicular keratosis and mild superficial dermal fibrosis are features of more chronic solar dermatitis.

In dogs, laminar alteration of collagen begins in the superficial dermis and is characterized by a narrow subepidermal band of homogenous pale-staining hypocellular collagen. This homogenous substance consists of poorly staining collagen fibres separated by a pale ground substance, which is mucin-positive (blue-green) with Alcian blue periodic acid-Schiff (PAS) staining. This is one of the most frequent dermal histopathological changes in dogs with solar dermatitis and may be an indicator of early solar damage (Figure 32.4); it is not common in cats. In conjunction with the laminar alteration of collagen, there may also be superficial laminar fibrosis of varying depth, representing scar tissue subtended by the pale hypocellular collagen layer. True laminar fibrosis is sometimes observed in cats.

In the dog, the dermis typically contains perivascular to lichenoid inflammation, with plasma cells and lymphocytes predominating and accompanied by a variable number of neutrophils, macrophages and eosinophils. Pigmentary incontinence may be present. Lichenoid dermatitis is generally not observed in actinic lesions of cats; inflammation is mild and perivascular. Superficial dermal vessels may be proliferative and ectatic. The dermal inflammation may be accompanied by solar elastosis. In some dogs, actinic comedones or actinic furunculosis may be seen. Actinic comedones are often multiple, with concentric accumulations of pale-staining collagen surrounding dilated, keratin-filled follicles. Deep dermal and diffuse pyogranulomatous folliculitis and furunculosis are common sequelae to comedonal rupture.

Solar elastosis is well recognized in humans with chronic solar exposure and may be seen in dogs or cats. In tissue sections stained with haematoxylin and eosin (H&E), elastosis appears as distinctive, thickened, wavy, basophilic fibres and as black tangled thick elastotic material with Verhoeff's-van Giessen elastin stain. Solar elastosis is not considered a reliable indicator of actinic dermatitis in the dog and cat.

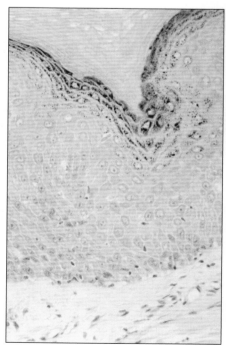

32.4

Histological characteristics of actinic dermatitis. There is epidermal hyperplasia, keratinocyte dysplasia and a subepidermal band of pale-staining collagen. (H&E stain; original magnification X40)

Management

The best treatment for solar dermatitis is prevention. It is important to educate owners of dogs and cats at risk about the need for sun avoidance and protection at an early age. When middle-aged dogs and cats present with chronic actinic dermatitis, many of the changes elicited by exposure to UV light are from previous exposure and thus irreversible, and whilst these cases can be managed, the disease is not curable.

Sun avoidance

Avoidance of direct or reflected sunlight is of paramount importance. Affected dogs and cats should be kept inside from 9 am to 3 pm and should not be permitted to sunbathe near open doors and windows. Normal window glass does not block UV radiation. Total sun avoidance is recommended but unfortunately is not often achievable. For animals that cannot be kept inside, providing generous shade is highly recommended, although UV light can be reflected from grass and sand, as well as water and snow. White concrete floors should be avoided due to their ability to reflect sunlight.

Sun-protective clothing

Sun-protective clothing is strongly recommended. Body suits made from synthetic fabrics (lycra, dacron) with a high sun protection factor (SPF) are mandatory. A dog sun-suit is commercially available (www.designerdogwear. com) or owners may be able to sew a sun-suit for their pets by using sun-protective fabric. In the author's experience, most dogs tolerate the flexible and comfortable protection suits and these have been very successful adjuncts to the management of dogs that cannot be confined inside (Figure 32.5). Nose caps (www.dognoseprotectors.com) can also be useful and are well tolerated.

Sunscreens

For maximal efficacy, sunscreen should be applied 10–15 minutes prior to sun exposure and if solar exposure is unpredictable, it should be applied twice daily. The combined effect of two applications gives on average 2.3 times better protection from ultraviolet radiation (UVR) than a single application. The products should not be 'rubbed in', especially those containing titanium or zinc oxide, as they work best when applied as a thin smear

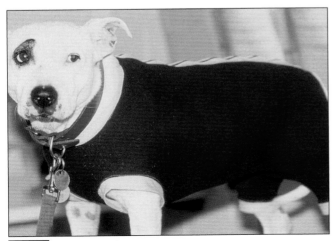

32.5 A sun protection suit.

on the surface of the skin. The author recommends that veterinary practitioners select a waterproof, high-SPF (30 or higher) sunscreen that contains a broad-spectrum UV-absorbing chemical with a combination of titanium or zinc oxide for maximal efficacy. These chemicals should be used cautiously in animals because of the potential for toxicity if ingested. Ingestion of some ingredients may cause adverse gastrointestinal effects, as well as specific toxicities (e.g. zinc toxicity from excessive licking of zinc-based products).

Colourants

Colourants are characterized by their ability to absorb or reflect visible light (400–700 nm). Black absorbs all light; white reflects all light. Pigment application (e.g. ink) may be effective but solvents can cause contact sensitization. Tattooing is ineffective as the ink is deposited in the mid to deep dermis, below the level of UV damage.

Topical treatment

Glucocorticoids: Acute solar dermatitis responds to the application of topical corticosteroids (e.g. 1–5% hydrocortisone ointment or cream every q12–24h for 7–10 days). If systemic therapy is required to reduce erythema, a short course of oral prednisolone (1 mg/kg q24h for 7-10 days) is usually sufficient.

Diclofenac: This is a non-steroidal anti-inflammatory drug (NSAID), which inhibits cyclooxygenase (COX) enzymes. NSAIDs are anti-angiogenic, pro-apoptotic and have anti-carcinogenic properties. Topical 3% diclofenac in 2.5% hyaluronan gel (Solaraze) acts by blocking COX-2, reducing angiogenesis and cellular proliferation and upregulating apoptosis of UV damaged cells. The drug is of moderate efficacy with low morbidity in the treatment of mild human actinic keratoses. There are no studies at present available in veterinary medicine; however, the author has used this product for chronic management of dogs with early and mild actinic dermatitis and has found it effective and well tolerated. The author's recommendation is to apply the topical agent sparingly to affected skin daily for 4 weeks and then once to twice a week for maintenance. Care must be taken to avoid ingestion. The side effects are limited to mild pruritus and irritation at the site of application. Firocoxib, a NSAID that inhibits COX-2, has also been used for the management of actinic dermatitis in dogs at a dose of 5 mg/kg orally q24h (Albanese *et al.*, 2013). The rationale behind this is that the COX-2 pathway has been shown to be upregulated in skin cancer and contribute to the progression of neoplasia.

Imiquimod (5%): This is a topical immune response modifier that induces tumour-specific apoptosis. The drug is of good efficacy with moderate morbidity in the treatment of human actinic keratosis, with the clinical response largely in proportion to the side effects. There are no studies available in veterinary medicine; however, the author has used this product in dogs with moderate actinic dermatitis and actinic keratosis and has found it effective. The author's recommendation is to apply the topical agent to affected skin 2–3 times a week until the lesions resolve, and then repeat treatment as necessary. Care must be taken to avoid ingestion. The side effects in dogs include moderate erythema and mild pruritus and irritation at the site of application.

Oral treatment

Synthetic retinoids: In veterinary medicine, synthetic retinoids have been used with variable success for the treatment of solar-induced precancerous lesions. Isotretinoin acts directly to normalize follicle keratinization, although the mechanism is unclear. There are limited studies available in veterinary medicine regarding the use of etretinate and isotretinoin for actinic dermatitis; however, the author uses isotretinoin at a dose of 1–2 mg/kg orally q24h for 8–12 weeks in dogs with actinic dermatitis and actinic keratosis and has found it effective for some dogs. A Schirmer tear test should be performed prior to and weekly during isotretinoin therapy. Potential side effects include keratoconjunctivitis sicca, vomiting, diarrhoea, musculoskeletal abnormalities, triglyceride elevations and hepatotoxicity, so careful monitoring is necessary. Retinoids are also highly teratogenic. Unfortunately, the cost of retinoids often precludes their use, particularly in larger breeds of dogs. In addition, they are not licensed for use in dogs and subject to prescribing restrictions in some countries.

Vitamin A: Due to the expense of synthetic retinoids, oral vitamin A (a natural retinoid) has been used anecdotally for canine and feline actinic dermatitis but controlled clinical trials and published studies are lacking. The recommended dosage of vitamin A is 800–1000 IU/kg/day for 3 months and then the dose is tapered to three times a week. In addition, some dermatologists advocate using vitamin E at a dose of 400 IU orally q12h and vitamin C at a dose of 500 mg orally q24h for antioxidant effects; however, there are no studies that prove that this is beneficial.

Actinic keratoses

Actinic keratoses are premalignant epithelial lesions that occur in the sparsely haired regions of unpigmented skin in middle-aged to older dogs and cats that are frequently exposed to sunlight. Actinic keratoses can transform to invasive squamous cell carcinoma (SCC).

Clinical presentation
Dogs

Lesions are either single or multiple and are asymptomatic, erythematous, scaly, red to reddish-brown, ill-defined macules that progress to indurated crusted plaques, varying in size from 0.5–5 cm in diameter, and are rough on palpation. Actinic comedones may be present. Palpation of visibly normal skin may detect irregular firmness and thickening. The glabrous skin of the ventral and lateral abdomen and inner thigh is most frequently affected. Induration, erosion, ulceration or increasing diameter of the keratotic lesion should raise the suspicion of evolution into SCC.

Cats

Lesions consist of erythematous plaques with crusting, erosion and superficial ulceration. They affect the margins of the pinnae, nasal planum, preauricular region of the face and dorsal muzzle. The lesions may appear symmetrical.

Diagnostic tests

It is impossible to differentiate premalignant actinic keratosis from solar-induced malignancy without histological evaluation of an incisional or excisional biopsy sample.

The principal histological diagnostic feature of an actinic keratosis is an irregular epidermal hyperplasia and diffuse dysplasia with marked hyperkeratosis or parakeratosis. Dysplasia is characterized by a loss of normal stratification of the epidermis, nuclear atypia, increased mitotic activity and individual keratinocyte dyskeratosis. In dogs, a dense lymphoplasmacytic dermal infiltrate obscuring the dermal-epidermal interface is common, with superficial to deep laminar dermal fibrosis. In the cat, the dermal infiltrate is usually mild and perivascular. Solar elastosis may be seen in dogs and rarely in cats. Actinic keratosis is differentiated from SCC by absence of dermal invasion.

Management

In humans, the most common treatments for actinic keratosis are liquid nitrogen freezing, curettage, electrosurgery, dermabrasion, laser and chemical peels. Medical options include fluorouracil, retinoids, photodynamic therapy, imiquimod, diclofenac and piroxicam. The treatments of choice for actinic keratosis in dogs and cats are excisional surgery, cryosurgery and carbon dioxide laser ablation. In terms of medical management, synthetic retinoids have been recommended. To the best of the author's knowledge, no other medical treatments known to be of benefit in humans have been documented for use in dogs, although veterinary dermatologists regularly use diclofenac and imiquimod for mild and moderate cases, respectively. Solar protection, including sun avoidance, use of solar suits and regular use of sunscreen, may prevent the development of new actinic keratoses.

Squamous cell carcinoma

Cutaneous SCC is a malignant proliferation of the keratinocytes of the epidermis and the most frequently reported malignant epithelial neoplasm of the dog and cat. It is associated primarily with exposure to UV radiation and is usually preceded by actinic (solar) keratoses. Cutaneous SCC is most commonly located in the non-pigmented or depigmented skin in the sparsely haired regions of white dogs and cats in geographical regions characterized by long periods of intense sun exposure. Papilloma virus structural antigens have been demonstrated in 30% of cases of feline UV-induced SCC and 80% of SCC in UV protected skin. However, the role of papillomavirus in the development and progression of these lesions is not conclusive. Abnormalities in the expression of the tumour suppressor gene p53 have been described in both dogs and cats with cutaneous SCC.

Clinical presentation
Dogs

Canine SCC occurs at an average age of 9 years, with no sex predilection. Short-coated breeds with white or piebald hair and skin colour, such as the English Bull Terrier, Dalmatian and Beagle, have the highest incidence of solar-induced SCC. Lesions occur most commonly on the trunk, scrotum and hind limbs and less frequently on the lips, nose and anus. Lesions may be single or multiple. SCC occurs as shallow, crusted ulcers that become deep and crateriform, or as papillary to nodular masses that vary from several millimetres to several centimetres in diameter (Figure 32.6). Erythema, erosion, ulceration, crusting and haemorrhage are often present.

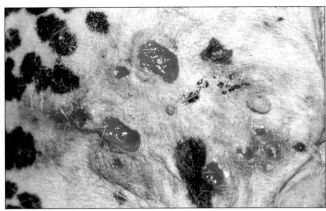

32.6 Actinic keratoses and squamous cell carcinoma. There are multiple ulcerated nodules on the ventrum of this dog.

Cats

Feline SCC occurs at an average age of 11 years, with no breed or sex predilection, and is more frequent in white-haired cats. The most common sites are the pinnae, external nares, preauricular region, eyelids and lips. Feline SCC can be proliferative, but is more commonly seen as an erosive, crusted and indurated lesion that bleeds easily when traumatized. Lesions are multiple in about 45% of affected cats (Figure 32.7).

Diagnostic tests

The diagnosis of SCC requires histological examination of skin biopsy material. Histologically, SCC consists of irregular masses or cords of keratinocytes that proliferate downwards and invade the dermis. Frequent findings include keratin formation, atypia, mitotic figures, intercellular bridges and horn pearls. Solar elastosis may occasionally be seen.

Management

SCC is considered a locally invasive, malignant tumour with a low rate of metastasis. However, metastasis to regional lymph nodes and the lungs can be seen with poorly differentiated neoplasms. In cats, the prognosis correlates with the degree of histological differentiation, and there is a correlation between the histological grade and local invasiveness of the tumour.

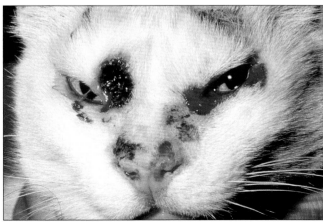

32.7 Feline squamous cell carcinoma. There is crusting, erosion and haemorrhage on the eyelids, pre-auricular region and nasal planum of this cat.

Clinical management of SCC may include:

- Surgical excision
- Cryosurgery
- Electrosurgery
- Hyperthermia
- Radiotherapy
- Chemotherapy
- Photodynamic therapy
- Laser therapy.

Surgery and cryosurgery

Surgery and cryosurgery are the most common therapeutic modalities used and are the most practical for the general practitioner, although there are numerous reports detailing the use of hyperthermia and photodynamic therapy. In general, the outcome for small, superficial, non-invasive lesions that are treated early is favourable. A combination of surgery with radiation therapy or adjuvant chemotherapy may be the best approach for advanced, infiltrative lesions.

Chemotherapy

In general, systemic chemotherapy with various agents has shown little consistent efficacy for the management of canine and feline SCC.

Environmental control

In all cases, avoidance of sunlight is important, as the successful management of SCC does not preclude the development of new lesions in other non-pigmented sites.

Cutaneous haemangioma and haemangiosarcoma

Cutaneous haemangioma is a benign neoplasm arising from vascular endothelial cells and is common in dogs and rare in cats. Cutaneous haemangiosarcoma is a malignant neoplasm of the same cells and is uncommon in both species. Chronic solar irradiation has been implicated as the cause of haemangioma and haemangiosarcoma in the ventral glabrous skin of lightly pigmented, sparsely haired dogs and as the cause of haemangiosarcoma on the pinnae of white-eared cats.

Clinical presentation

Dogs

Cutaneous solar-induced haemangioma and haemangiosarcoma occur in dogs at an average age of 10 years and there is a female sex predilection. Whippets, Dalmatians, Beagles, Bassett Hounds, Salukis, English Pointers, American Staffordshire Bull Terriers and other shorthaired and light-skinned breeds are at increased risk. Lesions are usually located on the ventral abdomen and thorax. Solar-induced haemangiomas are usually well circumscribed round blue to red-black lesions, 0.5-4 cm in diameter, and are dermal to subcutaneous in location (Figure 32.8). Conversely, solar-induced haemangiosarcomas are often multiple, poorly circumscribed, red to blue plaques or nodules, usually <2 cm in diameter and are dermal in location. They are also often associated with haemorrhage and ulceration.

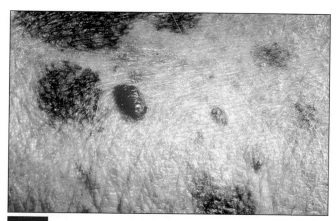

32.8 Solar-induced haemangioma on the ventrum of a dog.

Key points

- Adverse effects of solar radiation are seen on lightly pigmented and sparsely haired areas of the skin
- Early actinic damage can progress to neoplasia, and prevention of sun exposure for animals at risk is recommended
- Squamous cell carcinomas, haemangiomas and haemagiosarcomas can arise from solar damaged skin

Cats

Feline solar-induced haemangiosarcomas usually occur in male cats older than 10 years, with no breed predilection. White cats are predisposed. Lesions are usually solitary, rapidly growing and occur most commonly on the head and pinnae. Dermal haemangiosarcomas are poorly circumscribed, red to dark blue plaques or nodules that are usually <2 cm in diameter.

Diagnostic tests

The diagnosis is confirmed by histological examination of biopsy samples. Haemangiomas are characterized by a proliferation of blood-filled vascular spaces lined by single layers of well differentiated endothelial cells, whereas haemangiosarcomas are characterized by an invasive proliferation of atypical endothelial cells, with areas of vascular space formation. Solar dermatosis and elastosis may be present.

Management

Clinical management of haemangiomas includes surgical excision, cryosurgery, electrosurgery and observation without treatment. The therapy of choice for haemangiosarcomas is radical surgical excision. However, the prognosis for both dogs and cats is poor, with local recurrence and metastasis being common.

References and further reading

Albanese F, Abramo F, Caporali C *et al.* (2013) Clinical outcome and cyclo-oxygenase-2 expression in five dogs with solar dermatitis/actinic keratosis treated with firocoxib. *Veterinary Dermatology* **24**, 606–612

De Berker, McGregor JM and Hughes BR (2007) Guidelines for management of actinic keratoses. *British Journal of Dermatology* **156**, 222–230

Frank LA and Calderwood Mays MB (1994) Solar dermatitis in dogs. *Compendium on Continuing Education for the Practicing Veterinarian* **16**, 465–472

Frank LA, Calderwood Mays MB and Kunkle GA (1996) Distribution and appearance of elastic fibres in the dermis of clinically normal dogs and dogs with solar dermatitis and other dermatoses. *American Journal of Veterinary Research* **57**, 178–181

Gross TL, Ihrke PJ and Walder EJ (2005) *Veterinary Dermatopathology: A Macroscopic and Microscopic Evaluation of Canine and Feline Skin Disease*. Mosby-Yearbook, St Louis

Hargis AM, Ihrke PJ, Spangler WL *et al.* (1992) A retrospective clinicopathologic study of 212 dogs with cutaneous haemangiomas and haemangiosarcomas. *Veterinary Pathology* **29**, 316–328

Kitchell BE, Orenberg EK, Brown DM *et al.* (1995) Intralesional sustained-release chemotherapy with therapeutic implants for treatment of canine sun induced squamous cell carcinoma. *European Journal of Cancer* **31**, 2093–2098

Lana SE, Ogilvie GK, Withrow SJ *et al.* (1997) Feline cutaneous squamous cell carcinoma of the nasal planum and pinnae: 61 cases. *Journal of the American Animal Hospital Association* **33**, 329–332

Marks SL, Song MD, Stannard AA and Power HT (1992) Clinical evaluation of etretinate for the treatment of canine solar-induced squamous cell carcinoma and preneoplastic lesions. *Journal of the American Academy of Dermatology* **27**, 11–16

Miller MA, Ramos JA and Kreeger JM (1992) Cutaneous vascular neoplasia in 15 cats: clinical, morphologic and immunohistochemical studies. *Veterinary Pathology* **29**, 329–336

Peaston AE, Leach MW and Higgins RJ (1993) Photodynamic therapy for nasal and aural squamous cell carcinoma in cats. *Journal of the American Veterinary Medical Association* **202**, 1261–1265

Rosenkrantz WS (1993) Solar dermatitis. In: *Current Veterinary Dermatology*, ed. CE Griffin *et al.*, pp. 309–315. Mosby, St Louis

Ruslander D, KaserHotz B and Sardinas JC (1997) Cutaneous squamous cell carcinoma in cats. *Compendium on Continuing Education for the Practicing Veterinarian* **19**, 1119–1129

Chapter 33

Regional dermatoses

Domenico Santoro and Natalie Barnard

Diseases of the nasal planum

Diseases affecting the nasal planum can vary from benign disorders to more serious immune-mediated conditions. They are uncommon in dogs and cats. In the early stages of disease, the structure of the nasal planum may change, but this is not usually detected by the owner unless they are very astute. Often when the patient is presented to the clinic their clinical signs are advanced. The most common clinical sign seen is depigmentation, which may or may not be associated with ulceration. Once the surface of the epithelium is damaged it makes these patients more susceptible to secondary bacterial infection. Differential diagnoses for diseases affecting the nasal planum in dogs and cats are listed in Figure 33.1.

Clinical approach

History

A thorough dermatological history is essential when investigating these cases. Age of onset, breed and signs of systemic disease all give important clues to help narrow

Dogs
• Mucocutaneous pyoderma
• Discoid lupus erythematosus
• Mucocutaneous lupus erythematosus
• Vitiligo (see Chapter 16)
• Snow nose/Dudley nose
• Hereditary nasal hyperparakeratosis in Labrador Retrievers
• Dermal arteritis of the nasal planum
• Epitheliotrophic lymphoma
• Uveodermatological syndrome
• Squamous cell carcinoma
• Pemphigus foliaceus
Rarely, the following diseases may also cause lesions on the nasal planum:
• Leishmaniosis
• Pemphigus vulgaris
• Superficial necrolytic dermatitis
• Zinc-responsive dermatosis
Cats
• Cryptococcosis
• Herpesvirus dermatitis
• Squamous cell carcinoma
• Pemphigus foliaceus
It should be noted that other types of fungal granuloma can occur on the bridge of the nose, but generally do not affect the nasal planum

33.1 Differential diagnoses of diseases affecting the nasal planum in dogs and cats.

the list of differential diagnoses. For example, in a dog that has travelled abroad and is systemically unwell, leishmaniosis should be high on the list of differential diagnoses. It is also useful to ask owners about the presence of nasal discharge, as nasal lesions can develop secondary to respiratory conditions in some cases.

Physical and dermatological examination

A general physical and dermatological examination should be performed to look for any signs of nasal discharge or respiratory disease. Several of the diseases that can affect the nasal planum are associated with more generalized skin lesions, other mucocutaneous lesions or signs of systemic disease (Figure 33.2). It is also important to identify the primary and secondary lesions present, as primary lesions in particular can provide clues to the underlying pathology.

Diagnostic tests

Cytology: This should be performed in all cases. It will help to detect the presence of bacterial or fungal infection and inflammatory cells, which may give vital clues to the underlying pathology.

Bacterial culture and sensitivity testing: This may be required if bacteria are seen on cytology samples. Generally, a swab should always be sent for culture and sensitivity testing if rod-shaped bacteria are seen on cytology due to the unpredictable sensitivity of these organisms to antibiotics. Culture should also be performed if the condition has failed to respond to suitable empirical treatment.

Skin biopsy: Many of the diseases affecting the nasal planum are diagnosed with histopathology. It is important that any bacterial infection is treated prior to taking biopsy samples, as with many of the immune-mediated diseases the presence of bacterial infection can cloud the histological picture.

- Nasal biopsy samples should always be taken under anaesthesia.
- The skin should not be prepared prior to taking a sample.
- Taking biopsy samples from ulcerated skin should be avoided as a general rule because this is not diagnostic, but an ellipse spanning ulcerated and normal tissue would be useful.

BSAVA Manual of Canine and Feline Dermatology, fourth edition. Edited by Hilary Jackson and Rosanna Marsella. ©BSAVA 2021

Disease	Depigmentation	Crusting	Ulceration	Hyperkeratosis	Other clinical signs
Mucocutaneous pyoderma	x	x	x		May affect other mucocutaneous junctions
Discoid lupus erythematosus Mucocutaneous lupus erythematosus	x	x	x		Distribution can vary with disease
Vitiligo	x				May be depigmentation in other areas
Snow nose/Dudley nose	x				None; localized to nasal planum
Hereditary nasal hyperparakeratosis in Labrador Retrievers			(x) if secondary infection	x	Limited to nasal planum; first noted in young dogs; as the condition progresses fissures, ulceration and erosions may be seen
Dermal arteritis of the nasal planum	x		x		None; localized to the nasal planum
Epitheliotrophic lymphoma	x				Often other clinical signs on the skin, including nodules, erythema, scaling and pruritus
Uveodermatological syndrome	x				Severe ocular lesions, often these cases present with ocular lesions prior to the skin lesions
Squamous cell carcinoma	x		x		None; usually a localized lesion
Leishmaniosis	x				Often systemic signs associated with renal disease, gastrointestinal disease and more generalized skin lesions, such as scaling, nodules and onychogryphosis
Pemphigus vulgaris	x		x		Ulceration of other mucocutaneous junctions; pyrexia and depression are common
Zinc-responsive dermatosis		x		x	Skin lesions may also be noted on elbows and hocks; bilaterally symmetrical
Herpesvirus dermatitis		x	x		Skin signs are often accompanied by signs of ocular and/or respiratory disease

33.2 Dermatological and systemic clinical signs seen in dogs and cats with diseases affecting the nasal planum.

- A sample of a primary lesion, such as an area of depigmentation or crusting, should be taken.
- It is advisable to send samples to a specialist dermatopathologist and include a clinical history.

Blood biochemistry and haematology: This may be useful if there are clinical signs of systemic disease.

Mucocutaneous pyoderma

Pathogenesis

This is a bacterial infection, which can affect the mucocutaneous junction of the nasal planum. It can also affect the mucocutaneous junctions of the lips and perianal skin. The bacterial infection involves the epidermis and follicular epithelium of adjacent haired skin. *Staphylococcus pseudintermedius* is the most commonly isolated pathogen, but other organisms can also be identified.

Clinical presentation

There is no age or sex predisposition. German Shepherd Dogs and their crossbreeds may be at an increased risk. The early clinical signs include swelling, depigmentation and erythema of the skin; the lesions then become crusted, which in turn can lead to fissuring and erosions (Figure 33.3). This appearance mimics immune-mediated disorders, namely, discoid lupus erythematosus or mucocutaneous lupus (see below and Chapter 28). Often a purulent exudate is present beneath the crusted lesions, which is ideal for cytology. In chronic cases, the skin may be depigmented.

Diagnostic tests

Cytology samples will confirm the presence of a bacterial infection. These cases respond to appropriate antibacterial treatment. A swab should be taken for culture

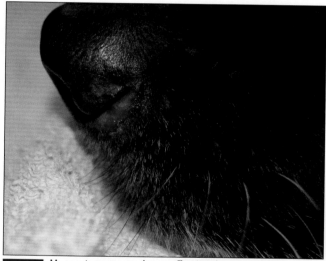

33.3 Mucocutaneous pyoderma affecting the nose of a dog. Note the depigmentation and crusting of the nares.

and sensitivity testing if rod-shaped bacteria are seen on cytology or there is a failure to improve on empirical treatment. Mucocutaneous pyoderma should resolve completely with appropriate antibacterial treatment. If there is only partial improvement and no bacteria are seen on cytology, then a biopsy should be performed to determine whether there is an underlying immune-mediated disease.

Treatment

Systemic antimicrobial treatment is advised; however, these cases are often slow to respond. Topical treatments, such as chlorhexidine gel or fusidic acid, can be used alongside systemic therapy, but application is often challenging or may be removed by the animal during grooming. Systemic antibiotic treatment is often required for a minimum of 3–4 weeks and should be continued beyond resolution of the clinical signs. Relapses are common.

Discoid lupus erythematosus and mucocutaneous lupus erythematosus

Pathogenesis

Cutaneous lupus affecting the nasal planum of dogs can be subdivided into discoid lupus erythematosus (DLE) and mucocutaneous lupus erythematosus (MCLE) (see Chapter 28). These variants have subtle clinical and histological differences. Lupus affecting the nose is rare in cats. Although lesions may be confined to the nose in both variants, other areas of the body may be affected (mucocutaneous junctions with MCLE and, rarely, generalized disease with DLE). Cutaneous lupus is an autoimmune condition and is exacerbated by ultraviolet (UV) light.

Clinical presentation

Initial clinical signs often include depigmentation of the nasal planum, which can become slate grey or blue in colour (Figure 33.4). Lesions often start at the nares or dorsal aspect of the nose and then gradually spread over time to involve more of the nasal planum. There is a loss of the cobblestone appearance of the nose. As the condition progresses, the nasal planum can become erythematous; scaling is also a common feature. Secondary infection is common and can lead to crusting and erosions (Figure 33.5), similar to that seen with mucocutaneous pyoderma (see above). Rarely, lesions can affect the periocular skin (Figure 33.6) or ears.

Diagnostic tests

History and clinical examination are suggestive, but histopathology is diagnostic. It is important that any secondary infections are treated prior to taking skin biopsy samples, as infection can mask the histological features.

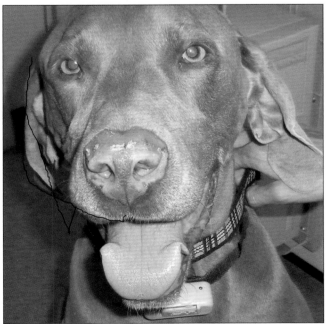

33.4 Dog with discoid lupus erythematosus that presented predominantly with nasal planum depigmentation.

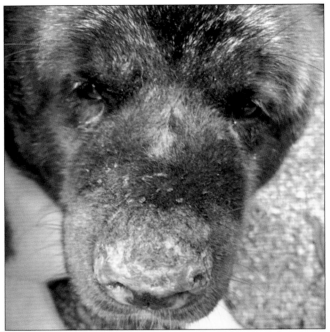

33.5 Discoid lupus erythematosus in a dog. This patient also presented with nasal planum depigmentation, but more severe crusting, erosions and scarring compared with the dog in Figure 33.4.

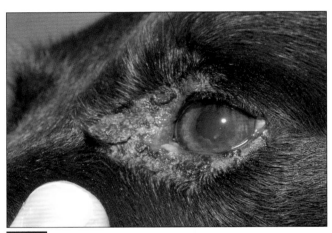

33.6 This dog presented with lesions on the eyelid margins.

Treatment

The prognosis for this condition is good, although many cases require chronic treatment. Systemic and/or topical glucocorticoids appear to be most effective. Topical tacrolimus (0.1%) is a treatment option for localized DLE. For refractory cases, the addition of oral ciclosporin may be required. It is recommended that dogs affected by this condition avoid sunlight or use a sun block on the nose. Dog-specific sun block is available (see Chapter 32).

Hereditary nasal hyperparakeratosis in Labrador Retrievers

Pathogenesis

This is a hyperkeratosis of the dorsal aspect of the nasal planum in Labrador Retrievers and their crossbreeds. This condition is uncommon. An autosomal recessive mode of inheritance has been identified.

Clinical presentation

Clinical signs are generally noted at a young age, typically between 6 and 12 months of age. Affected dogs have a band of tightly adherent keratin on the dorsal aspect of the nose. This may get worse as the dog ages. Often, these patients will have secondary infections and other lesions, such as fissures, ulceration and erosions, may develop. Manipulation of the area of hyperkeratosis can be painful.

Diagnostic tests

History and clinical signs are suggestive, especially if a young Labrador Retriever presents with this condition. Biopsy with histopathology is diagnostic. A genetic test is available to identify affected and carrier individuals.

Treatment

This is a lifelong condition that can only be managed, not cured. The aim of treatment is to hydrate and moisturize the skin on the nasal planum. Topical application of propylene glycol diluted 50:50 with water and applied twice daily may be effective; alternatively, the use of a product containing soybean and cajuputi oil has proved to be effective. If a patient is severely affected, then topical glucocorticoids or tacrolimus may be indicated. However, topical glucocorticoids should not be used for prolonged periods of time as they can cause atrophy of the skin.

Dermal arteritis of the nasal planum

Pathogenesis

This is an immune-mediated condition that causes arteritis of the nasal philtrum. Cases have been described in St. Bernards and other large-breed dogs (see Chapter 28).

Clinical presentation

The characteristic sign is ulceration localized to the nasal philtrum, which can haemorrhage profusely due to arterial bleeding; this can be distressing for owners. Chronic lesions are also associated with depigmentation.

Diagnostic tests

The clinical signs are visually distinctive, with an associated history of profuse bleeding. Although histopathology may provide a definitive diagnosis, this procedure should be weighed against the risk of provoking further haemorrhage.

Treatment

Successful treatment has been reported using oral prednisolone, ciclosporin and topical tacrolimus. Surgery may be indicated for cases that are bleeding profusely or fail to respond to medical management.

Epitheliotrophic lymphoma

Epitheliotrophic lymphoma can cause depigmentation and scaling of the nasal planum (Figure 33.7). It usually affects middle-aged to older patients. Other skin lesions are often present, ranging from generalized erythroderma to nodular or plaque-like lesions. Some patients may also have pruritus and signs of systemic disease. The condition is diagnosed by skin biopsy and histopathology. Treatment with chemotherapy can help some cases, but the prognosis is guarded (see Chapters 16 and 34 for more information).

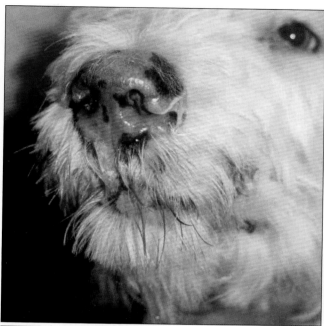

33.7 Canine epitheliotrophic lymphoma causing depigmentation and marked loss of the nasal architecture characteristic of this disease. The depigmentation had developed over 2–3 weeks.

Uveodermatological syndrome

Uveodermatological syndrome (Vogt–Koyanagi–Harada syndrome) is a rare syndrome of granulomatous uveitis and depigmenting skin lesions in dogs that may affect the nasal planum (see Chapter 16 for more information).

Pathogenesis

Uveodermatological syndrome is a genetic condition with an immune-mediated basis.

Clinical presentation

This syndrome is commonly seen in Japanese Akitas, but also reported in other breeds, such as the Alaskan Malamute, Bassett Hound, Chow Chow, German Shepherd Dog and Samoyed. The first clinical sign is usually an acute onset bilateral uveitis (photophobia, blepharospasm, corneal oedema, congestion of the conjunctiva, cataract formation, glaucoma). The dog then develops depigmentation of the hair and skin, usually on the nose, lips and eyelids. The depigmentation may be accompanied by erythema or scaling, but occasionally the lesions may become ulcerated or eroded with crusting on the surface.

Diagnostic tests

History and clinical signs are suggestive. A skin biopsy is required to confirm the diagnosis. Histologically, a lichenoid interface granulomatous dermatitis is present.

Treatment

Treatment of the uveitis takes precedent and this needs to be managed aggressively to prevent blindness; an ophthalmologist should be consulted regarding treatment. Often the skin signs respond well to treatment, while the ocular lesions remain active. Systemic glucocorticoids and systemic azathioprine or ciclosporin are advised in addition to topical ocular therapy. Long-term treatment and monitoring is advised, especially with regard to the ocular lesions.

Squamous cell carcinoma

Squamous cell carcinomas are malignant tumours that originate from skin keratinocytes. They can affect the nasal planum and are more common in cats with hypopigmented noses. Chronic exposure to sunlight is considered a risk factor, although papilloma viruses can also be involved. The lesions are more common in older animals; they often initially present as an area of crusting and scaling, but, as time progresses, the tumour can be either proliferative or ulcerative. Diagnosis is confirmed by histopathology. There are many different treatment options, including surgery, ionizing radiation and chemotherapy (see Chapters 32 and 34).

Pemphigus foliaceus

This autoimmune disease affects both dogs and cats and is discussed in more detail in Chapter 28.

Clinical presentation

The primary lesions seen are pustules, which rupture readily to form multifocal crusts. Distribution is usually symmetrical and can include the nasal planum, footpads and haired skin of the face and pinnae. In some cases, the disease may become generalized.

Diagnostic tests

The diagnosis relies on compatible cytology and histopathology (see Chapter 28 for more information).

Treatment

The reader is referred to Chapter 28 for information on treatment of pemphigus foliaceus.

Zinc-responsive dermatosis

This condition is primarily seen in the Nordic breeds (syndrome I), although various other breeds may also be affected (syndrome II). Crusting affects the nasal planum, mucocutaneous junctions, pressure points and footpads (see Chapter 31 for more information).

Feline herpesvirus dermatitis

Pathogenesis

This condition is caused by feline herpesvirus 1. It is estimated that 80% of cats that recover from the respiratory infection are latent carriers and have the virus present in their trigeminal ganglia. Stress or glucocorticoids may cause a reactivation of the disease and, occasionally, these patients can develop cutaneous and oral ulceration.

Clinical presentation

Ulcerative and necrotizing facial dermatitis and stomatitis are seen in cats with herpesvirus dermatitis. Often crusted lesions affect the nasal planum, bridge of the nose or periocular skin. Beneath the crusted lesions are ulcerated erythematous lesions. Affected patients may or may not have a history of active respiratory infection. Adult cats are more commonly affected.

Diagnostic tests

Cytology of samples collected from beneath the crusted lesions is often strongly eosinophilic, although neutrophils may also be present especially if there is secondary bacterial infection. Histopathology is diagnostic if intra-nuclear viral inclusions are seen. Conventional polymerase chain reaction (PCR) testing of the affected tissue can lead to false-positive results and, if available, quantitative PCR is more reliable. Tissue immunohistochemistry is of limited usefulness but can confirm infection where viral inclusions are seen. Virus isolation can also be used to confirm presence of the virus in affected tissue.

Treatment

Symptomatic treatment and removal of stressors or glucocorticoids will aid resolution of the condition. Regarding specific antiviral treatment, oral famciclovir is the best option (although not licensed for use in this species). There is no evidence to support lysine supplementation in this condition.

Diseases of the paws

Claws and claw folds

The claws and claw folds are highly specialized structures. The claw grows very slowly (0.8–1.9 mm per week) from a particular structure inside the claw fold, called the matrix, which is in direct contiguity with the epidermis of the adjacent skin. The matrix surrounds the claw; however, the dorsal matrix is more active than the ventral one and this determines the curved aspect of the claw in dogs and cats. Any alteration of the matrix results in deformation of the claws.

Anatomically, the claw is composed of three portions: one dorsal surface, two lateral surfaces and one inferior surface. Clinically, the claw appears smooth, hard in consistency and has a variable, but homogeneous, colour (e.g. white translucent, pink or dark). The length of the claw is determined by its intrinsic growth, the environment and the species or breed. For example, small-breed dogs that live almost entirely indoors need more frequent trimming of their claws owing to the lack of natural usage.

Specific terms are used to describe claw abnormalities (Figure 33.8). However, descriptive terminology is lacking for other lesions, such as the presence of a waxy deposit on the base of the claw, abnormal staining or abnormal growth rate. More than one of these abnormalities can be present in the same claw or in different claws in the same patient, as part of the same pathological process. A particular abnormality frequently associated with other claw lesions is inflammation of the claw fold (paronychia). This can be a manifestation of a direct or an indirect stimulus to the claw fold. A list of diseases involving the claw and claw folds can be found in Figure 33.9.

Clinical approach

History: The clinician should consider the generalization of the condition (one claw, multiple claws on one paw, or multiple claws affected on more than one paw) and whether the abnormality is localized to the claw and/or claw fold, if it involves the paws, or if a more general cutaneous and/or systemic disease is present. Where only one or multiple claws of one paw are affected, trauma, infection (e.g. bacterial, fungal and parasitic) and neoplasia should be considered. More generalized paw disease may be associated with skin diseases, such as demodicosis, atopic dermatitis or leishmaniosis.

Term	Definition
Anonychia	Absence of claws (congenital)
Brachyonychia	Short claws
Leuconychia	Whitening of the claws
Macronychia	Unusually large claws
Micronychia	Unusually small claws
Onychalgia	Claw pain
Onychauxis (hyperonychia)	Simple hypertrophy of the claws
Onychia (onychitis)	Inflammation of the claws
Onychocryptosis (onyxis)	Ingrown claw
Onychodystrophy	Abnormal claw formation
Onychogryphosis	Hypertrophy and abnormal curvature of claws
Onycholysis	Separation of claw structure at distal attachment and progressing proximally
Onychomadesis (onychoptosis)	Sloughing of claws
Onychomalacia (hapalonychia)	Softening of claws
Onychomycosis	Fungal infection of claws
Onychopathy (onychosis)	Disease or abnormality of claws
Onychorrhexis	Fragmentation and horizontal separation in claw lamellae at the free edge
Onychoschizia (onychoschisis)	Splitting or lamination of claws, usually beginning distally
Pachyonychia	Thickening of claws
Paronychia (perionychia)	Inflammation or infection of claw folds
Platonychia	Increased curvature of claws in long axis
Trachyonychia	Lustreless, longitudinally ridged, rough-surfaced claws

33.8 Terminology used to describe claw and claw fold diseases.

Diagnostic tests:

Skin scrapings and trichography: The examination of skin scrapings and plucked hairs from affected claw beds and interdigital skin is essential to rule out demodicosis. At this site, trichography is often easier to perform (see Chapter 3). It should be noted that negative findings do not always rule out demodicosis at this body site.

Cytology: Examination of exudates from the dorsal and/or ventral portion of the claw fold is one of the most important diagnostic tests to perform (Figure 33.10). Samples may be collected using a spatula, cotton bud or blunted stick and spread on to a slide.

Culture: Bacterial and fungal culture can be very useful to confirm bacterial, yeast or dermatophyte infection. In the case of bacteria, antibiotic sensitivity testing may be indicated. It should be noted that submission of avulsed claws for dermatophyte culture is unrewarding.

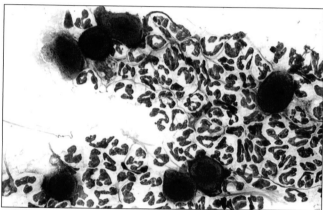

33.10 Cytology of an intact pustule from a case of pemphigus foliaceus. Note the non-degenerate neutrophils and free-floating acantholytic keratinocytes. (Diff-Quik® stain; original magnification X1000)

Claw and claw folds affected	Diseases
Claws on one paw only	• Trauma (physical, chemical, arteriovenous fistula) • Dermatophytosis (*Trichophyton mentagrophytes* or *Microsporum gypseum*) • Fungi (blastomycosis, cryptococcosis, sporotricosis, geotrichosis) • Demodicosis • Bacterial infection (secondary to trauma) • Eosinophilic plaques (cats) • Neoplasia
Claws on multiple paws	• Demodicosis • Neoplasia • Symmetrical onychitis (lupoid symmetrical onychodystrophy) (dogs) • Autoimmune disease (cats: pemphigus foliaceus; dogs: hookworm dermatitis) • Eosinophilic plaques (cats)
Claws on one or more paws associated with generalized cutaneous disease and systemic clinical signs	• Bacterial infection (secondary to trauma, endocrinopathies or viral infections) • Yeast infection (*Malassezia* spp., *Candida* spp.) • Demodicosis • Dermatophytosis • Autoimmune disease (systemic lupus erythematosus, cryoglobulinaemia, drug reactions) • Leishmaniosis (dogs and cats) • Eosinophilic plaques (cats) • Allergies (atopic dermatitis, food-responsive dermatosis (also known as food allergy or adverse food reaction), contact allergy) • Zinc-responsive dermatosis (dogs) • Hookworm and ascarid dermatitis • Vasculitis • Vitiligo • Dermatomyositis (dogs) • Viral infection (distemper, feline leukaemia virus, feline immunodeficiency virus)

33.9 Causes of claw and claw fold disease in dogs and cats.

Biopsy: Obtaining a biopsy sample for histopathology is the only way to make a definitive diagnosis in certain diseases, such as lupoid onychitis, pemphigus foliaceus and neoplasia. Histological examination of the avulsed claw is rarely diagnostic; for this reason, examination of the matrix and claw fold is essential to confirm the diagnosis. Samples should be collected from the animal under anaesthesia.

Performing a claw biopsy

Two techniques have been described in the literature. The first involves the complete excision of the third phalanx, whilst the second (described in 1999 by Mueller and Olivry) is more conservative and is known as onychobiopsy without onychectomy. Although a complete onychectomy may provide the most diagnostic information, it is highly invasive and deforming in some cases. For these reasons, where possible, it is advisable to remove the dewclaw in preference to other claws. The onychobiopsy without onychectomy technique involves longitudinal excision of part of the claw, including the matrix and the claw fold, using an 8 mm biopsy punch. The final result is a section of the entire claw and adjacent structures for histological examination.

As with all skin biopsy specimens, the claw and paronychial skin should be sent to a dermatopathologist. Certain structural changes (e.g. intrakeratinocyte vacuoles, intraepithelial and dermoepidermal clefting, pseudospongiosis and apoptotic keratinocytes) are common features of the architecture of the normal claw and can be very easily mistaken for abnormalities by an inexperienced examiner.

Ancillary tests: Other laboratory tests, such as bloodwork and hormone assays, along with radiography, may be required in certain cases. Radiographs of the affected region are indicated to assess possible local bone involvement when trauma, invasive neoplasia or deep infection (bacterial and/or fungal) are present.

Treatment

The treatment and prognosis vary with the diagnosis. Given that treatment will be administered for several weeks or months, an accurate diagnosis is essential. Furthermore, if damage to the matrix has occurred, focal or diffuse claw abnormalities will be permanent. Appropriate treatment for bacterial, dermatophyte and *Malassezia* infection are discussed in Chapters 8, 21 and 26.

When onychodystrophy is severe enough to cause significant pain and secondary infection, prophylactic trimming and the use of a human acrylic nail cement to fill the claw can be useful. In severe, chronic, medically refractory cases of claw disorders in large-breed dogs, onychectomy should be considered as a reasonable and effective treatment option.

Lupoid onychitis

Clinical presentation

The owner usually reports discomfort affecting one paw manifesting as licking or limping. On initial presentation, there is separation of the claw from the underlying claw bed followed by onychomadesis and subungual haemorrhage,

resulting in deformity of the claw (onychodystrophy) if the condition is not treated (Figure 33.11). Paronychia and a purulent discharge are present if there is a concurrent secondary bacterial infection.

Clinical approach

History: Labrador Retrievers, Greyhounds, German Shepherd Dogs, Bearded Collies and Rottweilers may be predisposed to lupoid onychitis (also known as symmetrical lupoid onychodystrophy), but it can be seen in other breeds and crossbreed dogs. Recently, an allelic mutation in the regions CFA12 and CFA17 has been identified in Bearded Collies affected by lupoid onychitis. There may be a rapid or slow onset of lameness and pain associated with onychomadesis (claw loss), starting on one digit and later involving more or all digits. Generally, it affects young to middle-aged dogs.

Diagnostic tests: The diagnosis is based on the characteristic clinical lesions. Biopsy of the claw bed may confirm the diagnosis.

Treatment

The prognosis is good with treatment, but, infrequently, relapses occur. Treatment options include oral essential fatty acids (omega-3/omega-6) alone or combined with tetracycline, oxytetracycline or doxycycline and nicotinamide. The dose of nicotinamide is 250 mg orally q8h for dogs <10 kg, and 500 mg of each drug orally q8h for dogs >10 kg. Tetracycline is unavailable currently but doxycycline may be used in its place. However, the long-term use of antibiotics should be discouraged and alternative treatment regimens advised.

Recently, the use of an oral fish oil supplement containing 165 mg of eicosapentaenoic acid (EPA)/ml, 106 mg of docosahexaenoic acid (DHA)/ml and 1 mg of vitamin E/ml (each dog received 10 ml q24h) was compared with oral ciclosporin (5 mg/kg q24h) in affected Setter dogs (Ziener and Nødtvedt, 2014). Both therapies resulted in an equally significant improvement of the claws after 6 months of treatments. However, reoccurrence was seen after discontinuation with both therapies.

Other treatment options include the use of systemic glucocorticoids (e.g. prednisolone) at a dose of 1–2 mg/kg orally q24h, oral vitamin E at a dose of 400 IU orally q12h

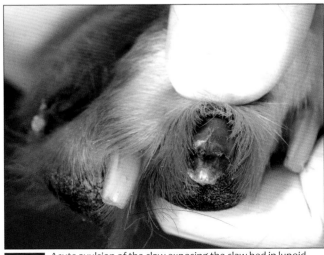

33.11 Acute avulsion of the claw exposing the claw bed in lupoid onychitis.

and pentoxifylline 10–15 mg/kg orally q12h. Some cases have reportedly responded to the exclusive feeding of a novel protein diet.

Treatment should be continued until new claw growth is evident without recurrence of clinical signs and then tapered.

Bacterial onychitis and pododermatitis
Clinical presentation

Dogs and cats generally present with purulent exudate at the claw fold, onychalgia and lameness. Discoloration of the hairs around the claw fold is also present owing to continued licking of the paws. This may be associated with a more general bacterial overgrowth affecting the interdigital spaces, as seen secondary to atopic dermatitis (see Chapters 9 and 21).

Clinical approach

History: The history can be very variable depending on the underlying problem; however, there is often an association with lameness. It is frequently seen as a complication following trauma.

Diagnostic tests: Surface cytology of the affected area indicates the presence of bacteria. Bacterial culture can help in determining the choice of antibiotic, particularly if rods are present or in the case of recurrent nail fold infection. Bloodwork to rule out systemic diseases, such as endocrinopathies (e.g. hyperadrenocorticism, hypothyroidism and diabetes mellitus), may be indicated in some cases. Radiography or computed tomography of the paw may confirm the presence of an arteriovenous fistula or neoplastic process.

Treatment

The prognosis is good if the bacterial infection and underlying disease are treated. Treatment options include systemic antibiotics, based on the results of a bacterial culture or used empirically, and topical antibacterial solutions (e.g. 2–4% chlorhexidine, benzoyl peroxide, ethyl lactate, 2% sulphur or silver compounds).

Malassezia onychitis and pododermatitis
Clinical presentation

Dogs and cats present with mild to severe paronychia associated with a dry (sometimes slightly moist) brown exudate around the claw fold and the claws, which themselves often become brownish red (Figure 33.12).

Clinical approach

History: A history consistent with an allergy is common (e.g. food-responsive dermatosis and/or atopic dermatitis), although this may occur in the context of any systemic or cutaneous disease. Constant licking and chewing of the paws or claws are noted.

Diagnostic tests: The clinical presentation is very characteristic of *Malassezia* infection. In addition, claw fold cytology shows multiple *Malassezia* organisms. Samples for cytology can be obtained via adhesive tape or scraping, with the latter being more sensitive.

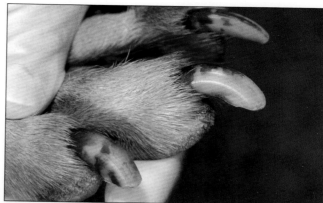

33.12 Brown discoloration of the claw in a case of *Malassezia* paronychia.

Treatment

The prognosis is good if the *Malassezia* infection and underlying allergy are treated. Treatment involves the use of topical and systemic antifungal medications, including azoles (e.g. ketoconazole, itraconazole or fluconazole) and terbinafine. The most commonly used topical treatments include 2% miconazole and 2–4% chlorhexidine solutions. Other options include 2% sulphur or enilconazole solutions.

Paronychia in cats

Occasionally, cats present with erythema, swelling and a paronychial purulent discharge affecting multiple claws. The differential diagnoses for this presentation include feline pemphigus foliaceus (see Chapter 28) and bacterial infection secondary to an underlying systemic disease. The diagnostic work-up should include cytology, bacterial culture and, in older cats, assessment of general underlying health.

Neoplastic disease of the claw folds
Clinical presentation

Cats with metastatic pulmonary adenocarcinomas often have multiple affected claws and a primary lung tumour. Claws are dislocated due to neoplastic growth. In dogs with subungual squamous cell carcinomas or melanomas, single or multiple claw beds may be affected, and metastases to the lymph nodes and body cavities may be present.

Clinical approach

History: Slow onset of swelling, pain and lameness localized to one or more digits.

Diagnostic tests: Surface cytology may indicate secondary infections. Cytology of fine-needle aspirates may suggest neoplasia. Biopsy can be used to confirm neoplastic disease. Thoracic radiography may confirm the presence of primary or secondary neoplasia.

Treatment

The prognosis for cats with metastatic pulmonary adenocarcinomas is poor. For dogs with subungual squamous cell carcinomas or melanomas, radical excision may be curative if no metastases are present. The reader is referred to specialist oncology texts such as the *BSAVA Manual of Canine and Feline Oncology* for a discussion of treatment options.

Diseases of the footpads and interdigital skin

Diseases affecting the interdigital skin are more common in dogs than cats. Pruritus associated with canine atopic dermatitis is one of the most common clinical presentations of pododermatitis seen in practice (see Chapter 9). Other diseases affecting the paws are described below.

Chronic pododermatitis with interdigital furunculosis (interdigital cysts)

This condition occurs in dogs, with a predilection for English Bulldogs, Beagles, Cocker Spaniels and Cavalier King Charles Spaniels. The aetiology of these lesions is multifactorial and can include allergic inflammation, abnormal weight bearing associated with conformation, orthopaedic conditions, obesity, demodicosis and endocrine disease (Figure 33.13). In addition, neoplastic processes and foreign bodies may need to be considered for individual lesions. This condition begins as a sterile process and infection occurs only when the lesions rupture and are subject to trauma (e.g. licking). The lesions originate on the plantar surface of the paw, but rupture as draining sinus tracts in the interdigital spaces. The condition can severely impact on the quality of life of the dog. A thorough evaluation of the contributing causes and appropriate long-term management is indicated (Nuttall, 2019).

Canine pododemodicosis

Chronic demodicosis affecting the pedal tissue results in interdigital folliculitis and furunculosis, usually associated with secondary bacterial infection. Affected dogs often present with swollen paws, lameness and the owners tend to report a constant licking of the paws and reluctance to walk. Clinical signs of alopecia, scaling, draining tracts and swelling of the interdigital tissue may be present. It should be noted that *Demodex* mites may not be found on routine skin scrapes and trichograms, as scarring results in their entrapment deep in the skin. Biopsy samples are required to confirm the diagnosis (see Chapters 7 and 8 for further information).

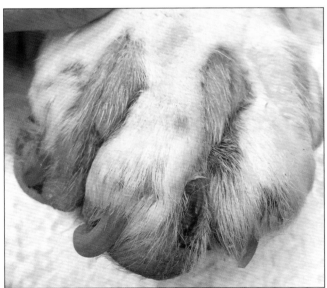

33.13 Marked interdigital swelling associated with furunculosis in an overweight Bulldog with atopic dermatitis.

Feline eosinophilic granulomas

Eosinophilic granulomas can present as interdigital nodules in cats and may be associated with one or more of the feline reaction patterns associated with pruritus (see Chapters 23 and 24). Secondary bacterial infections are common at this site, as is erosion or ulceration. Cytology may confirm the presence of eosinophils, but if there is secondary infection, then neutrophils and bacteria may predominate.

Diseases affecting the footpads

- **Plasma cell pododermatitis** – this is a unique feline disease in which one or more footpads become swollen and may ulcerate. Diagnosis is confirmed by cytology or biopsy; tissue samples from affected areas demonstrate a predominantly plasmacytic infiltrate (see Chapter 24 for more information).
- **Pemphigus foliaceus** – crusts overlying ruptured pustules on the footpads and interdigital skin are clinical features of this disease. This is usually associated with the involvement of other body sites (see Chapter 28).
- **Zinc-responsive dermatoses** – marked thickening and crusting of the footpads, pressure points and mucous membranes is seen with this condition (see Chapter 31).
- **Hepatocutaneous syndrome** – with this disease, crusting develops of the footpads, interdigital skin, mucous membranes and around the genitalia. Affected animals usually have other systemic signs (see Chapter 31).

Diseases of the anal sacs

Anatomy and normal physiology

Anal sacs are present in most carnivores. They are a pair of bilaterally symmetrical skin invaginations that sit at the 4 and 8 o'clock positions in relation to the anus and connect to the anocutaneous junction by a small duct. The duct itself runs between the internal and external anal sphincter muscles. The wall of the anal sacs is lined by squamous cornified epithelium, surrounded by connective tissue in which a large number of epitrichial (apocrine) and sebaceous glands are embedded.

Anal sac secretions comprise a combination of glandular secretions and desquamated corneocytes. The secretions are usually released during defecation. The exact function of the anal sac is unknown, but it is thought to play a role in scent and territorial identification, as the secretions have a very distinct odour due to the breakdown of the cellular contents. The contents are usually cream or brown in colour, but the consistency and colour can vary between animals and even within the same animal. It should be noted that normal anal sac flora includes a range of bacteria (e.g. *Bacillus*, *Escherichia coli*, *Micrococcus*, *Proteus*, *Streptococcus fecalis*).

Differential diagnosis

Anal sac impactions and infections occur fairly commonly in dogs, but are rare in cats. Often impacted anal sacs are mistakenly identified as a cause of perianal pruritus; however, allergic skin disease is usually a more common cause.

It should also be noted that rarely autoimmune conditions (e.g. erythema multiforme and cutaneous adverse drug reactions) may cause skin lesions in the perianal area and on the anus. The differential diagnoses for anal sac disease are summarized in Figure 33.14.

Clinical presentation

Whether anal sac disease is due to impaction, infection, abscess or perianal fistulae, all clinical presentations are very similar.

- Scooting, licking, chewing or rubbing of the perianal skin in dogs. However, it is important to realize that these clinical signs can be seen in any dog with perianal pruritus and may not necessarily be related to anal sac disease. These signs are also associated with atopic dermatitis, food-responsive dermatoses and, in brachycephalic dogs, tail fold dermatitis. Overweight bitches may also scoot due to intertriginous perivulval dermatitis.
- Cats rarely scoot but may overgroom the tail head.
- Reluctance to sit or defecate.
- Tenesmus.
- Constipation.
- Anal discharge; redness and swelling of anal and perianal region.
- Infected anal sacs may occasionally rupture causing cellulitis with localized erythema, swelling and pain. This may also lead to a draining fistula.
- Abscessation of the anal sacs is usually unilateral.
- Often there is a pungent odour from the anal sacs.

Disease	Clinical signs
Anal sac impaction	• Localized pruritus manifested by licking the area or bottom scooting • There may be a history of soft stools that precedes this presentation • Glands usually difficult to express, but contents are normal
Anal sac infection	• Pruritus and scooting • Pain • Erythema • Swelling • Purulent discharge when glands are expressed
Anal sac abscess	• Similar signs to anal sac infection, but the patient may also be pyrexic and systemically unwell • Noticeable swelling • May not be able to manually express the glands due to pain and discomfort • Sometimes the abscess may have ruptured and there may be a discharging sinus tract
Anal furunculosis	• German Shepherd Dogs are predisposed, but the condition has been identified in other breeds • Early lesions are small abscesses around the anus • Ulceration and multiple draining fistulae • Pain • Dyschezia • Rectal examination reveals thickening, which may or may not involve the anal sacs • Chronic scarring and fibrosis may be evident
Anal sac neoplasia	• A nodule is palpable on rectal examination • Middle-aged to older dogs are affected • Polyuria and polydipsia may be present due to malignant hypercalcaemia

33.14 Common causes of anal sac disease and perianal disease in dogs and their associated clinical signs.

Perianal pruritus

It should be remembered that perianal pruritus is a clinical feature in dogs with allergic skin disease and can be due to a cutaneous food-responsive dermatosis or atopic dermatitis. A thorough history and clinical examination should help to identify these patients, as often they have other signs of allergic skin disease. In allergic patients, secondary skin infections are common and may also contribute to the perianal pruritus. Cytology should be used to look for evidence of yeast or bacterial infection; if these infectious organisms are identified they should be treated appropriately

Clinical approach
Physical and dermatological examination

A full general and dermatological examination should be performed. Evaluation of the anal sacs should also be undertaken; this may need to be performed under sedation if the animal is showing signs of pain.

Diagnostic tests

Cytology: Cytology of the anal sac contents may be useful in some cases; however, it should be borne in mind that cytology of the anal sac contents of normal dogs can reveal intracellular bacteria and neutrophils. Therefore, cytology findings should be interpreted in light of the patient's clinical signs.

Treatment
Medical management

Expression of the anal sacs is the most useful treatment to manage this condition. If infection is present, then flushing the anal sacs with saline solution under anaesthesia may also be required. Typically, an antibiotic otic preparation is instilled into the affected sacs.

Surgical management

Surgical removal of the anal sacs is indicated if medical management fails or if the problem becomes recurrent. It is important to identify any underlying cause for the problem before proceeding to surgical removal, as it is not without its risks and complications. Surgical complications can include faecal incontinence, wound break down and dehiscence.

Anal sac impaction

Impaction is the most common problem associated with the anal sacs. It occurs when an anal sac fails to empty, resulting in thicker secretions that cause the anal sac to swell and become painful. Distended anal sacs can be palpated in the 4 and 8 o'clock positions. It is believed to be more common in dogs with soft stools. The exact aetiology of anal sac impaction is unknown, but it is thought to occur secondary to obesity or intestinal disorders, which may affect the consistency of the stool. This can often be a recurring problem for some patients. Manual expression of the anal sacs is the best way to manage impaction; on occasions, sedation may be required to complete this procedure. Manual expression may need to be repeated weekly for 3–4 weeks. Once the anal sacs have been expressed, the clinical signs should resolve, although relapse is common. Dietary changes are indicated if the problem is recurrent and the patient has loose stools or small hard stools. The addition of fibre to the diet may help some patients. Patients with chronically impacted anal sacs may benefit from irrigation and flushing, but there is little in the literature to evaluate the efficacy of this technique.

Anal sac infection

Sacculitis is inflammation or infection within the anal sac that can lead to abscessation and/or fistulation. It is often a sequel to chronic or recurrent anal sac impaction because the retained secretions can cause an inflammatory response within the anal gland, leading to cellulitis and abscess formation. Bacteria can also proliferate within the retained secretions. Allergic skin disease and endocrinopathies may predispose to anal sac infection. It has been suggested that incomplete emptying of the anal sacs may also be a cause of infection. Anal sac abscessation is thought to occur as a sequel to infection and impaction. The ruptured anal sac releases its contents into the surrounding tissue causing cellulitis and, sometimes, fistulae formation. If the anal sacs are chronically infected, then flushing may be helpful. The anal sacs can be flushed with saline or an antiseptic solution. Cytology and culture of the contents may be indicated. Systemic antibiotic treatment is often required in patients with anal sac infection. Anal sac infection is rare in cats.

Anal furunculosis/perianal fistulae

Perianal fistulae are ulcers and sinus tracts that spontaneously occur in the skin around the anus and can be very painful for affected dogs (Figure 33.15). The condition occurs commonly in middle-aged to older German Shepherd Dogs, which are reported to have a genetic susceptibility. Intact male dogs are over-represented. It has also been reported in other mixed and purebreed dogs, such as the Beagle, Border Collie, Irish Setter and Staffordshire Bull Terrier. This disease has an immune-mediated pathogenesis and develops as a consequence of local T-cell-mediated inflammation. Affected dogs have been shown to have increased anti-staphylococcal immunoglobulin (Ig)G compared with normal dogs. An association between anal furunculosis and colitis is recognized, and many patients may have gastrointestinal signs.

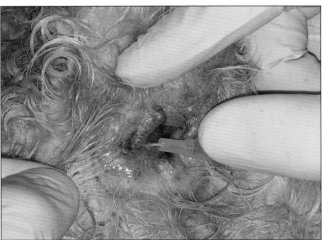

33.15 Perianal fistula on the right-hand side of a dog's anus. The catheter denotes the position of the anal sac.

Clinical presentation

Single or multiple sinus tracts and ulceration may be present. In some cases, the lesions can be extremely large and deep. These lesions do not generally communicate with the rectal lumen. Other clinical signs may include:

- Licking of the perianal area
- Pain
- Abnormal tail carriage
- Gastrointestinal signs (e.g. tenesmus, haematochezia, soft stools, mucus in the faeces and increased frequency of defecation)
- Dyschezia
- Mucopurulent discharge.

Diagnostic tests

The signs are very distinctive and this often facilitates a clinical diagnosis, especially in German Shepherd Dogs. A rectal examination should be performed; this may need to be done under sedation due to the extreme pain that can be associated with the condition. During the rectal examination, anal sac abnormalities such as impaction, infection or rupture may be noted, which can occur secondary to the inflammation and fibrosis caused by the anal furunculosis.

Treatment

Medical management: Medical management is the treatment of choice. The calcineurin inhibitors, namely ciclosporin and tacrolimus, have the most evidence for use. Success rates with ciclosporin can be up to 85%. The main aims of treatment are:

1. To treat the disease with immunomodulatory therapy.
   - **Ciclosporin** – this is generally regarded as the treatment of choice and is used at a dose of 5 mg/kg q12h for the best clinical outcome, although lower doses have been effective in some cases. Once the disease is in remission, which usually takes between 8 and 12 weeks, the medication can be tapered to the lowest effective dose. However, it should be remembered that relapses can occur as the dose is reduced, so owners need to be made aware of this possibility. Ciclosporin can also be used in combination with ketoconazole to reduce the total dose of ciclosporin administered. Patients on combination therapy should be closely monitored.
   - **Topical tacrolimus (0.1%)** – this is an effective treatment, but applying it can be difficult if the animal is in pain. It should be remembered that this treatment is unlicensed, so appropriate consent from the owner should be obtained. Generally, it is used for mild lesions or for severe lesions that are partially in remission to speed up resolution. It can also be used as a longer-term maintenance treatment, alongside or instead of oral therapy.
   - **Prednisolone and azathioprine** – there is minimal evidence for the use of these medications and success rates are generally lower than that for ciclosporin, thus their use is not recommended.
2. To treat any secondary infection with suitable antimicrobials.
   - The perianal skin is often colonized with bacteria due to the location and keeping the area clean is an important aspect of management. Samples for cytology should be obtained. If there are active signs of infection and rod-shaped bacteria are

identified, a swab for culture and sensitivity testing should be submitted to ensure that the correct antimicrobial treatment is instituted.

3. To manage pain.
   - This is an extremely painful condition and so appropriate analgesia should be provided whenever active lesions are present. If there is pain of defecation, then stool softeners (e.g. lactulose) should be considered.

Dietary trials: As there is an association with gastrointestinal disease, dietary trials using a novel or hydrolysed diet are advised in these cases. It is unclear from the literature whether disease remission can be maintained with diet alone.

Surgical management: Surgical management can be considered if medical management fails and may include *en bloc* resection of the lesions with concurrent anal sacculectomy, cryosurgery and laser excision. However, it should be noted that there is a wide range of surgical complications, including dehiscence of the surgical site, recurrence of the lesions, which is likely to be related to failure to control the underlying immune-mediated inflammation, faecal incontinence and strictures.

Anal sac neoplasia

Anal sac neoplasia is uncommon. The two main types of tumour seen in male dogs are adenocarcinomas and perianal adenomas; rarely, squamous cell carcinomas may be encountered. Anal sac adenocarcinomas are more common in older female dogs. Patients with adenocarcinomas often present with constipation, dyschezia and tenesmus due to sublumbar lymph node enlargement or signs associated with hypercalcaemia (polydipsia, polyuria, weakness, vomiting and lethargy). Fine-needle aspiration or excisional biopsy is required for a definitive diagnosis and the treatment of choice is surgical removal. More information on this topic can be found in the *BSAVA Manual of Canine and Feline Oncology*.

References and further reading

Auxilia ST, Hill PB and Thoday KL (2001) Canine symmetrical lupoid onychodystrophy: a retrospective study with particular reference to management. *Journal of Small Animal Practice* **42**, 82–87

Banks WJ (1993) Integumentary system. In: *Applied Veterinary Histology, 3rd edn*, ed. WJ Banks, pp. 298–325. Mosby Yearbook, Inc., St Louis

Bergvall K (1998) Treatment of symmetrical onychomadesis and onychodystrophy in five dogs with omega-3 and omega-6 fatty acids. *Veterinary Dermatology* **9**, 263–268

Boord MJ, Griffin CE and Rosenkrantz WS (1997) Onychectomy as a therapy for symmetric claw and claw fold diseases in the dog. *Journal of the American Animal Hospital Association* **33**, 131–138

Dobson JM and Kascelles BDX (2011) *BSAVA Manual of Canine and Feline Oncology, 3rd edn*. BSAVA Publications, Gloucester

Gross TL, Ihrke PJ, Walder EJ and Affolter VK (2005) Lupoid onychitis. In: *Skin Disease of the Dog and Cat. Clinical and Histopathologic Diagnosis, 2nd edn*, ed. TL Gross *et al.*, pp. 70–72. Blackwell Science, Oxford

Miller WH, Griffin CE and Campbell KL (2013) Diseases of eyelids, claws, anal sacs, and ears. In: *Muller and Kirk's Small Animal Dermatology, 7th edn*, ed. Miller WH *et al.*, pp.724–773. WB Saunders, Philadelphia

Mueller RS (1999) Diagnosis and management of canine claw diseases. *Veterinary Clinics of North America: Small Animal Practice* **29**, 1357–1371

Mueller RS, Friend S, Shipstone MA *et al.* (2000) Diagnosis of canine claw disease – a prospective study of 24 dogs. *Veterinary Dermatology* **11**, 133–141

Mueller RS and Olivry T (1999) Onychobiopsy without onychectomy: description of a new biopsy technique for canine claws. *Veterinary Dermatology* **10**, 55–59

Mueller RS, Rosychuk RA and Jonas LD (2003) A retrospective study regarding the treatment of lupoid onychodystrophy in 30 dogs and literature review. *Journal of the American Animal Hospital Association* **39**, 139–150

Mueller RS, Sterner-Kock A and Stannard A (1993) Microanatomy of the canine claw. *Veterinary Dermatology* **4**, 5–11

Nuttall T (2019) Chronic pododermatitis and interdigital furunculosis in dogs. *Companion Animal* **24**, 194–200

Santoro D, Pease A, Linder KE *et al.* (2009) Post-traumatic peripheral arteriovenous fistula manifesting as digital haemorrhages in a cat: diagnosis with contrast-enhanced 3D CT imaging. *Veterinary Dermatology* **20**, 206–213

Scott DW, Rousselle S and Miller WH (1995) Symmetrical lupoid onychodytrophy in dogs: a retrospective analysis of 18 cases (1989–1993). *Journal of the American Animal Hospital Association* **31**, 194–201

Verde MT and Basurco A (2000) Symmetrical lupoid onychodystrophy in a crossbreed pointer dog: long-term observations. *Veterinary Record* **146**, 376–378

Waisglass S (2018) Claw disease in the dog: Does your patient have symmetrical lupoid onychodystrophy (SLO)? *Canadian Veterinary Journal* **59**, 796–798

Ziener ML and Nødtvedt A (2014) A treatment study of canine symmetrical onychomadesis (symmetrical lupoid onychodystrophy) comparing fish oil and cyclosporine supplementation in addition to a diet rich in omega-3 fatty acids. *Acta Veterinaria Scandinavica* **56**, 66

Key points

- Biopsy is indicated for many diseases affecting the nasal planum. Secondary infections should be managed first
- Dermatophyte (fungal) infection of the claws is rare in dogs and cats
- Chronic interdigital draining tracts in dogs are multifactorial in origin and a thorough investigation is indicated for effective management of this problem

Chapter 34

Neoplastic and paraneoplastic syndromes affecting the skin

Jane M. Dobson and David H. Shearer

Neoplasms of the skin are the most frequently diagnosed tumours of domesticated animals. The prevalence varies depending on the study and geographical location, but in dogs and cats they represent between 25% and 58% of all neoplasms. More than 25 morphologically distinct cutaneous neoplasms have been described. Skin tumours may arise from epithelial elements (epidermis, hair follicles, sweat and sebaceous glands), mesenchymal tissue and melanin-producing cells (Figures 34.1 and 34.2). Skin tumours may also arise from cells of the skin's resident immune system, including cells of macrophage/histiocytic lineage, lymphoid cells, plasma cells and mast cells. In addition, neoplasms of non-cutaneous origin, especially carcinomas, may metastasize to the skin.

Tumours of epithelial origin

• Epidermal cells:
  ◦ Squamous papilloma/papillomatosis
  ◦ Squamous cell carcinoma
  ◦ Multicentric squamous cell carcinoma *in situ* (Bowen's disease)
  ◦ Basal cell tumour (basal cell carcinoma, rare)
  ◦ Keratoacanthoma/intracutaneous cornifying epithelioma
• Follicular hair matrix/follicular epithelial components:
  ◦ Trichoepithelioma
  ◦ Pilomatrixoma
• Sebaceous/hepatoid gland cells/epitrichial/ceruminous:
  ◦ Adenoma/adenocarcinoma

Tumours of mesenchymal origin

• Spindle cell sarcomas:
  ◦ Perivascular wall tumour (haemangiopericytoma, dogs)
  ◦ Peripheral nerve sheath tumour (Schwannoma)
  ◦ Fibrosarcoma (fibroblast origin)
  ◦ Myxosarcoma
• Blood and lymphatic vessels:
  ◦ Haemangioma/haemangiosarcoma
  ◦ Lymphangioma/lymphangiosarcoma
• Adipose tissue:
  ◦ Lipoma/liposarcoma
  ◦ Fibrolipoma
  ◦ Infiltrative lipoma
• Fibrous tissue:
  ◦ Fibroma

Tumours of round cell origin
• Mast cell tumour • Plasmacytoma • Lymphoma • Histiocytic tumours

Tumours of melanocytic origin
Melanoma: • Benign dermal • Malignant

34.1 Neoplasms of the skin.

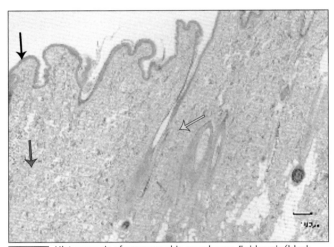

34.2 Histogenesis of common skin neoplasms. Epidermis (black arrow), epithelial: papilloma, basal cell carcinoma, squamous cell carcinoma; dermis (yellow arrow), adnexal lesions, mast cell tumour, melanoma; subcutis (red arrow), mesenchymal: lipoma, sarcoma.
(Courtesy of Dr Fernando Constantino-Casas)

Neoplastic lesions

Clinical approach

Typically, cutaneous neoplasia tends to be seen in the older animal, with a mean age in the dog of 8.3 ± 3.7 years and in the cat of 8.6 ± 4.7 years (Goldschmidt and Shofer, 1992). A notable exception is canine cutaneous histiocytoma (not a true neoplasm), which is most common in dogs under the age of 2 years. Most cutaneous neoplasms in the dog are benign and present as a solitary lesion of the skin with or without involvement of the subcutis. The majority of such neoplasms are slow-growing and not painful. The prevalence of benign skin lesions is far lower in the cat than in the dog, and a higher proportion of skin tumours are malignant in this species.

Most primary cutaneous neoplasms are solitary, but their clinical appearance can vary considerably:

- Exophytic/pedunculated masses (squamous papilloma, sebaceous adenoma) (Figure 34.3)
- Superficial, ulcerated lesions (basal cell carcinoma, squamous cell carcinoma) (Figure 34.4)

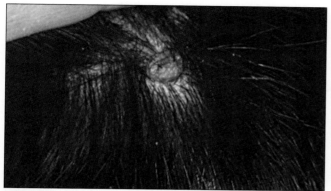

34.3 Nodular sebaceous hyperplasia: one of several similar lesions on the skin of this elderly dog.

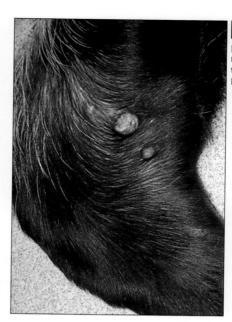

34.5 Mast cell tumour presenting as dermal nodules on the medial thigh of a Labrador Retriever.

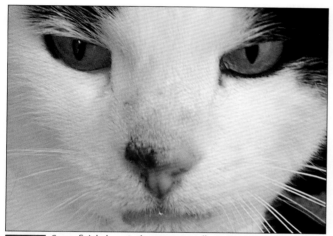

34.4 Superficial ulcerated squamous cell carcinoma on the nasal planum of a cat.

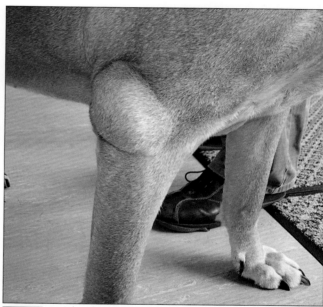

34.6 Peripheral nerve sheath tumour presenting as a subcutaneous mass on the lateral elbow of a dog.

- Dermal nodules ± ulceration (histiocytoma, plasmacytoma, mast cell tumour, basal cell tumours (trichoepithelioma, pilomatrixoma), dermal melanoma) (Figure 34.5)
- Subcutaneous masses (lipoma, fibroma, any of the soft tissue sarcomas) (Figure 34.6).

Neoplastic lesions may also present as multiple skin nodules:

- Epitheliotrophic lymphoma (mycosis fungoides)
- Non-epitheliotrophic lymphoma (primary cutaneous lymphoma) (Figure 34.7)
- Angiotropic lymphoma (lymphomatoid granulomatosis)
- Papillomatosis
- Malignant tumours that metastasize to the skin (carcinoma, mast cell tumour) (Figure 34.8)
- Multicentric squamous cell carcinoma *in situ* (Bowen's disease), especially in old cats
- Basal cell carcinoma in cats may be multicentric
- Feline sarcoma virus-associated fibrosarcoma in cats (very rare).

History and signalment

The age, breed and sex of the animal may be relevant; for example, hepatoid (perianal) adenomas occur more often in male dogs, whilst canine cutaneous histiocytoma tends to occur in young dogs. Certain breeds of dog

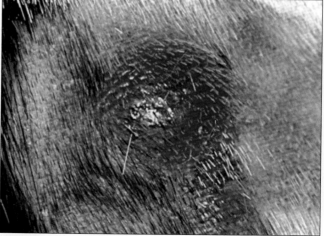

34.7 Primary cutaneous lymphoma forming multiple coalescing dermal nodules.

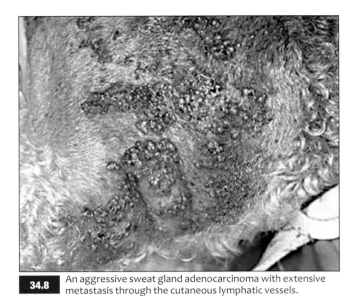

34.8 An aggressive sweat gland adenocarcinoma with extensive metastasis through the cutaneous lymphatic vessels.

are prone to different tumours (e.g. Boxers, Labrador Retrievers and Golden Retrievers are predisposed to mast cell tumours; see Figure 34.5). The duration and progression of the lesion may indicate whether a tumour is benign or malignant (i.e. slow-growing lesions are more likely to be benign).

Clinical examination

The possible histogenesis and phenotype of a skin tumour may be indicated by the location of the tumour within the skin and its appearance. Epithelial tumours tend to be superficial and exophytic, whilst adnexal, round cell and mesenchymal tumours present as endophytic, intradermal or deeper/subcutaneous masses (see Figure 34.2). Ulceration occurs with cutaneous tumours of different types and is not indicative of histogenesis. Cytology and/or biopsy and histopathology are required to confirm the tumour phenotype.

Diagnostic tests

Cytology: Where the lesion is nodular and of sufficient size (>1 cm), cytological examination of fine-needle aspirates is a logical first test (Figure 34.9) and may differentiate: between neoplastic and non-neoplastic lesions; and between round cell, epithelial and mesenchymal neoplasms (Figure 34.10). In some cases, such as mast cell tumours, cytology can be diagnostic.

Biopsy: Histological examination of skin punch or incisional (or excisional) biopsy samples is usually required to provide a definitive diagnosis of histological type and to grade the tumour. These samples may be collected from a sedated patient under local anaesthesia or, depending on body site, may require general anaesthesia. As the majority of skin tumours in the dog are benign, clinical staging (i.e. evaluation of lymph nodes and imaging for more distant metastases) is not indicated until a diagnosis of malignancy is established. Investigations will then be informed by the nature and likely clinical behaviour of the tumour.

Immunohistochemistry (IHC) of formalin-fixed tissue samples, which is routinely undertaken in human medicine, is being used more frequently in veterinary medicine for

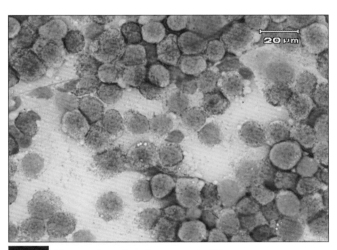

34.9 Fine-needle aspirate from a mast cell tumour.

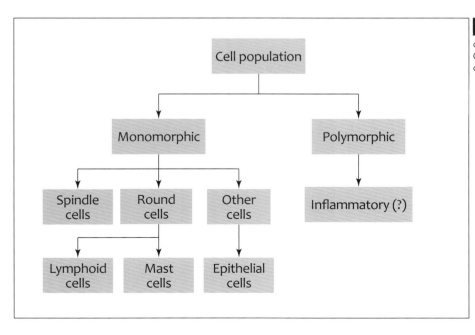

34.10 Cytological examination of fine-needle aspirates from skin nodules can help determine the type of mass present. Once the cell population has been determined, criteria for malignancy can be applied.

the identification of tumour phenotype in both skin and other masses. IHC is particularly useful for the differentiation of round cell tumours, especially lymphoma and histiocytic sarcoma. Clonality testing by polymerase chain reaction (PCR) for antigen receptor rearrangement (PARR) is now routinely employed in the diagnosis of canine and feline cutaneous lymphoma, especially where inflammation is present and the neoplastic cell populations have minimal atypia. This can be performed on formalin-fixed tissue biopsy samples.

Haematology and biochemistry: Routine haematological and biochemical analyses are not generally very helpful in the diagnosis of skin tumours; although, some skin tumours may be associated with haematological or paraneoplastic complications (e.g. mast cell tumours may cause anaemia as a result of gastric ulceration and gastrointestinal blood loss, and hypercalcaemia of malignancy may be associated with carcinomas of the epitrichial (apocrine) glands of the anal sacs in dogs).

Specific tumour types

Epithelial tumours

Most tumours arising from the epidermis and adnexae are solitary, well circumscribed, slow-growing benign lesions that are cured by local surgical excision. Examples of benign and malignant tumours include:

- Squamous cell carcinomas
- Basal cell tumours
- Trichoepitheliomas, pilomatrixomas and tricholemmomas
- Intracutaneous cornifying epitheliomas/keratoacanthomas
- Sebaceous gland tumours
- Hepatoid (perianal) gland adenomas/hyperplasia
- Epitrichial (apocrine) gland tumours (adenomas/adenocarcinomas)
- Atrichial (eccrine) gland tumours (adenomas/adenocarcinomas).

Squamous cell carcinomas

Incidence and epidemiology: Squamous cell carcinoma (SCC) is one of the more common malignant cutaneous tumours in the dog, and the most common in the cat. It usually affects older animals, with a mean age of 9 years (dogs: >6 years; cats: >5 years). There is no known breed predisposition in either species. Prolonged exposure to ultraviolet (UV) light is an important factor in the development of some cutaneous SCCs (see Chapter 32). There is a strong aetiological association with exposure of non-pigmented, lightly haired skin, especially in cats. In addition, papilloma virus structural antigens have been demonstrated in 80% of SCC in cats with UV-protected skin, but in only 30% of UV-induced SCC, suggesting that this virus may play a role in the development of neoplasia.

Clinical presentation: SCCs can occur anywhere in the skin. In dogs, the trunk, legs, scrotum, lips and nail beds are the most frequent sites of occurrence. In contrast, lesions in the cat are more commonly located on the head, nasal planum (see Figure 34.4), pinnae, eyelids and lips.

SCC is a locally invasive tumour that infiltrates the underlying dermal and subcutaneous tissues. Lesions are usually solitary, proliferative or erosive and often associated with ulceration. Metastasis tends to be via the lymphatic route, but the incidence of metastasis is variable. SCCs of the skin are usually well differentiated and slow to metastasize; however, at other sites (e.g. digital claw bed) the tumour may be much more aggressive. Amputation in these cases can still be curative if metastasis has not occurred.

Treatment and prognosis: Wide local surgical excision is the treatment of choice and, in cases where complete excision is achieved, the prognosis is favourable. Local recurrence can occur if the tumour is incompletely excised. SCCs are moderately radiosensitive and radiotherapy (external beam or strontium) may be indicated as an alternative or adjunctive treatment in cases where adequate surgical resection is not possible. Photodynamic therapy has been used successfully for the treatment of early, superficial lesions of the nasal planum in cats. Chemotherapy is not indicated in the management of localized SCCs and its role in the management of metastatic SCCs has not been established.

Basal cell tumours

Incidence: Basal cell tumours are common in both dogs and cats, representing 4–11% of canine skin tumours and 14–34% of feline skin tumours (but it should be noted that accurate figures are quite hard to find for many of these tumours). They affect middle-aged to older animals: mean age of dogs is 6–7 years; mean age of cats is 9 years. No sex predisposition has been reported. Cocker Spaniels, Poodles and Kerry Blue Terriers are reported to be predisposed.

Clinical presentation: Basal cell tumours tend to occur on the head, neck and shoulders. They are usually solitary, discrete, firm, well circumscribed masses (0.5–2.0 cm; although they may sometimes be larger) (Figure 34.11). Lesions may be pigmented or cystic; in cats, basal cell tumours are often heavily pigmented and may be confused on gross inspection with melanomas, which are rare in this species. Recurrence and metastasis are both rare. Occasionally, basal cell tumours can be locally aggressive and invasive.

Treatment: Wide surgical excision is the treatment of choice.

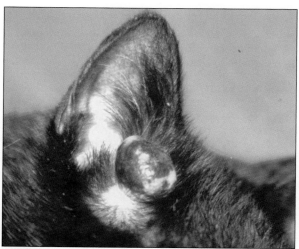

34.11 Basal cell tumour on the head of a cat.
(Courtesy of David Grant)

Trichoepitheliomas, pilomatrixomas and tricholemmomas

These tumours are classified as basal cell tumours with various types of hair follicle differentiation.

Incidence: These tumours occur in cats and dogs >5 years of age. No sex predisposition has been reported. Kerry Blue Terriers and Poodles are predisposed to pilomatrixomas; whereas, Cocker Spaniels and Bassett Hounds are predisposed to trichoepitheliomas.

Clinical presentation: In dogs, lesions occur most frequently on the back, rump and shoulders. In cats, the head is most often affected. They are solitary, well circumscribed, slow-growing, non-invasive dermal lesions. The lesions may attain a large size. Local recurrence and metastasis are rare.

Treatment: Wide surgical excision is the treatment of choice.

Intracutaneous cornifying epitheliomas and keratocanthomas

Incidence: These tumours account for 5% of canine epithelial tumours. They tend to affect older dogs (>5 years of age) but are rare in cats. A possible male predisposition has been identified. These tumours have been recognized in Keeshunds, German Shepherd Dogs, collies, Old English Sheepdogs and Norwegian Elkhounds.

Clinical presentation: Lesions usually occur on the back or tail and are dermal or subcutaneous in origin. They are usually solitary masses, but some dogs have multiple, non-invasive benign lesions characterized by pore opening to the surface, through which grey–brown keratin can be expressed. Multiple lesions have been reported in Norwegian Elkhounds.

Treatment: Wide surgical excision is the treatment of choice. Retinoids have been used in cases with multiple tumours to restrict further development, but no controlled studies on the efficacy of this treatment are available.

Sebaceous gland tumours

There are a number of different types of sebaceous gland tumour, including nodular sebaceous hyperplasia, sebaceous gland adenoma and sebaceous epithelioma (basal cell tumour with sebaceous differentiation).

Incidence: Sebaceous gland tumours are common in dogs, accounting for 6–21% of skin tumours (50% nodular hyperplasia; 30–40% sebaceous epithelioma; 8% sebaceous adenoma; and 1–2% sebaceous carcinoma). These tumours tend to occur in older dogs (mean age 9–10 years old). No sex predisposition has been noted. Cocker Spaniels are predisposed to sebaceous gland tumours, and they are also common in Poodles, Kerry Blue Terriers, Boston Terriers, Beagles, Dachshunds and Bassett Hounds. These tumours are rare in the cat.

Clinical presentation: Lesions occur commonly on the trunk, head, eyelids and lips. Nodular sebaceous hyperplasia and sebaceous adenomas are superficial lesions that may arise at any site. Sebaceous epitheliomas are dermal. Lesions may be solitary or multiple in predisposed animals, and are usually slow-growing, well circumscribed and benign.

Treatment: Wide surgical excision is the treatment of choice in the majority of cases. Nodular sebaceous hyperplasia is common and excision is not required.

Hepatoid gland adenomas and hyperplasia

Incidence and epidemiology: These tumours tend to affect old male dogs (>8 years of age), but up to 25% occur in females. They can occur in both intact and neutered animals. No breed predisposition has been reported, but these lesions are common in Cocker Spaniels, English Bulldogs, Samoyeds and Beagles. Tumour growth is benign and usually androgen-dependent. These tumours are not reported in cats.

Clinical presentation: Lesions usually arise in the perianal skin but may also occur around the base of the tail, prepuce, caudal ventral abdomen and, occasionally, elsewhere. Lesions present as nodules with or without ulceration. In females and neutered males, consideration should be given to androgen production by hyperplastic adrenal glands in the context of hyperadrenocorticism.

Treatment and prognosis: Wide surgical excision is the treatment of choice. The prognosis is good.

Epitrichial gland tumours

Incidence: Epitrichial gland tumours are uncommon in dogs and cats, and usually affect animals >10 years old. No sex predisposition has been reported in either species. Golden Retrievers, Cocker Spaniels and German Shepherd Dogs may be predisposed.

Clinical presentation: In dogs, lesions tend to occur on the head, neck, dorsal trunk and limbs; whereas, the head, pinnae, neck, axillae, limbs and tail are more commonly affected in cats. Lesions are usually solitary. Adenocarcinomas occasionally metastasize to the lymph nodes, lungs and bones.

Treatment: Wide surgical excision is the treatment of choice.

Atrichial gland tumours

Incidence: Atrichial gland tumours are rare in dogs and cats.

Clinical presentation: Lesions commonly affect the footpads and digits. These tumours are often malignant and rapidly metastasize to the local lymph nodes.

Treatment: Wide surgical excision, castration and oestrogen therapy are the treatments of choice. It should be noted that oestrogen therapy has a transient effect, with recurrence of lesions following withdrawal.

Round cell tumours

Round cell tumours include:

- Histiocytic disease complex:
  - Canine cutaneous histiocytomas
  - Reactive histiocytosis
  - Histiocytic sarcomas (local and disseminated).
- Tumours of lymphoid origin:
  - Primary cutaneous lymphomas

- Epitheliotrophic lymphomas
- Lymphomatoid granulomatosis/angiotrophic lymphomas.
- Plasmacytomas
- Mast cell tumours (see below)
- Canine transmissible venereal tumours.

Histiocytic disease complex

There are a number of proliferative disorders of histiocytes (dendritic cells of the monocyte–macrophage family) recognized in the dog, ranging from non-neoplastic reactive, through benign to highly malignant lesions. Proliferative histiocytic conditions have also been described in the cat, although they are less well defined in this species.

Canine cutaneous histiocytomas:
Incidence: Canine cutaneous histiocytoma (CCH) is a benign cutaneous tumour that is unique to the skin of the dog and represents up to 10% of all canine cutaneous tumours. Canine cutaneous histiocytoma is more common in young dogs with 50% of these tumours occurring in animals <2 years of age.

Clinical presentation: The tumour arises typically on the head (especially the pinna), the limbs, feet and trunk and presents as a solitary, rapidly growing, well circumscribed, intradermal lesion (Figure 34.12). The surface may become alopecic and ulcerated. Boxers and Dachshunds are reported to be predisposed to CCH. Histological sections show infiltration of the epidermis and dermis by histiocytic tumour cells. Numerous mitotic figures and an indistinct boundary give this lesion the appearance of a highly malignant neoplasm.

Treatment: Despite the histological appearance and the rapid growth rate, CCH is a benign reaction that usually regresses spontaneously. Regression is associated with infiltration of the tumour by cytotoxic T-cells, which are often seen along the tumour base in histological sections.

Reactive histiocytosis:
Reactive histiocytoses represent a group of histiocytic skin lesions that are rare and not fully understood, including cutaneous reactive histiocytosis and systemic reactive histiocytosis. It seems likely that these conditions are not actually neoplastic, but rather a manifestation of dysregulation of the immune system.

Cutaneous histiocytosis:

- **Incidence:** Bernese Mountain Dogs, Rottweilers, Golden Retrievers and Labrador Retrievers are predisposed.
- **Clinical presentation:** This condition involves diffuse or nodular infiltration of the dermis by histiocytes (activated interstitial dendritic cells) admixed with lymphocytes, neither of which have the cytological features of malignancy. The condition manifests as dermal nodules and plaques, which can occur at any site, but often around the face and nares (Figure 34.13). Lesions tend to wax and wane.
- **Treatment:** Immunosuppressive treatment (high doses of glucocorticoids and other immunosuppressive drugs) may be effective; however, the condition tends to regress spontaneously and recrudesce irrespective of treatment.

Systemic histiocytosis:

- **Incidence and epidemiology:** This has been reported to be familial in the Bernese Mountain Dog, but may occur in any breed. Other predisposed breeds include Golden Retrievers, Labrador Retrievers and Rottweilers.
- **Clinical presentation:** In this condition, the lesions are not confined to the skin and may affect other organs, as well as the ocular and nasal mucosae. Clinical signs include lethargy, anorexia, weight loss, respiratory stertor, conjunctivitis, episcleritis, lymphadenopathy, papules, plaques and nodules. This tends to be more of a progressive disease, although the lesions may also wax and wane.
- **Treatment:** This condition may respond to immunosuppressive treatment with high doses of glucocorticoids or other immunosuppressive drugs.

Histiocytic sarcoma complex: This condition is currently referred to as localized and disseminated histiocytic sarcoma (the latter formerly termed malignant histiocytosis), although it is recognized that these are likely two ends of a

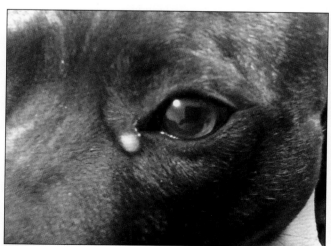

34.12 Canine cutaneous histiocytoma. This lesion, located at the medial canthus of the left eye in a young Staffordshire Bull Terrier, shows the typical appearance.

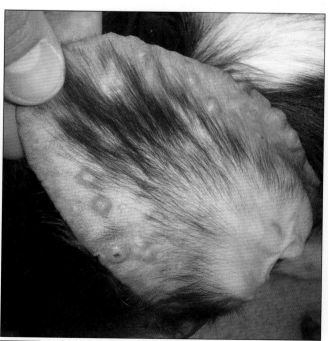

34.13 Multiple dermal nodules of cutaneous histiocytosis on the pinna of a young spaniel.

spectrum of malignant histiocytic disease, with different manifestations in different breeds of dog. Although the localized form presents as a single mass lesion, it is locally invasive with a high rate of distant metastasis, initially to the local, regional lymph node and then to multiple visceral sites. Disseminated histiocytic sarcoma is an aggressive multisystem disease with multiple visceral tumour masses, often involving the spleen, liver, lungs and bone marrow.

Localized histiocytic sarcoma:
- **Incidence:** This is a rare condition. Bernese Mountain Dogs, Rottweilers, Golden Retrievers, Labrador Retrievers and Flat-coated Retrievers appear to be predisposed.
- **Clinical presentation:** A solitary soft tissue mass is usually seen, which may be subcutaneous or arise in deeper tissues, at periarticular sites and in internal organs (especially the spleen). These tumours usually behave in a locally aggressive manner and have high metastatic potential, particularly in Flat-coated Retrievers.
- **Treatment:** Wide surgical excision is the treatment of choice. Where complete surgical resection is not possible, adjunctive local radiotherapy may decrease the risk of recurrence.

Disseminated histiocytic sarcoma:
- **Incidence:** This is also a rare condition. Bernese Mountain Dogs, Rottweilers and retrievers appear to be predisposed.
- **Clinical presentation:** The lesions in this condition are multifocal or metastatic to other organs. Disseminated histiocytic sarcoma usually presents with multifocal lesions that involve the spleen, liver, lymph nodes, lungs, bone marrow, skin, subcutis and brain. Clinical signs reflect the organs involved but are often vague and non-specific (e.g. lethargy and weight loss). Lymphadenopathy, hepatomegaly, splenomegaly, anaemia, other cytopenias and hypoproteinaemia may be detected.
- **Treatment and prognosis:** The response to chemotherapy with lomustine (CCNU) has been reported, but at best is brief. The prognosis is grave and many dogs are euthanased upon diagnosis due to the morbidity associated with the disease.

Tumours of lymphoid origin

These tumours include epitheliotrophic (T-cell) lymphoma and non-epitheliotrophic, primary cutaneous lymphoma (may be B- or T-cell).

Clinical presentation: Cutaneous lymphoid tumours present as (multi)focal or generalized skin conditions. The clinical appearance of the lesions can be variable, therefore, cutaneous lymphoma should be considered as a differential diagnosis for many ulcerative, crusting, pruritic and nodular skin conditions. The first signs of epitheliotrophic lymphoma may be subtle mucocutaneous depigmentation (Figure 34.14a) progressing to generalized scale and pruritus (Figure 34.14b). Foci of erythroderma, crusting, ulcerated lesions, multiple dermal nodules (Figure 34.14c) or erythematous plaques may feature in both epitheliotrophic and non-epitheliotrophic lymphoma in the dog.

Cats may present with a single plaque that may be pruritic. Lymph nodes may become involved as the disease progresses. Fine-needle aspirate cytology may be

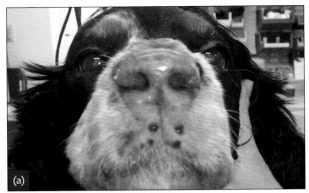
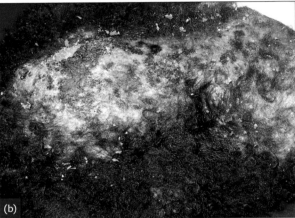
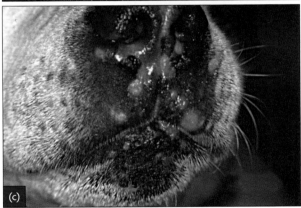

34.14 (a) Epitheliotrophic lymphoma causing depigmentation of the nasal planum and mucocutaneous junctions of the lips. (b) Generalized epitheliotrophic lymphoma in a Miniature Poodle with pruritus, scaling, erythroderma and ulceration along the dorsum. (c) Epitheliotrophic lymphoma giving rise to multiple non-pigmented nodules in the muzzle/nasal tissues. This dog also had nodules on the eyelids, digits and perianal region.

indicative of a diagnosis of a round cell or lymphoid tumour. Histological examination of incisional or excisional biopsy material is required for a final diagnosis. With epitheliotrophic lymphoma, the neoplastic lymphoid cells show a trophism for the epidermis (Figure 34.15). Epitheliotrophic lymphoma in dogs and cats is almost invariably T-cell in origin; therefore, IHC is not especially useful for diagnosis or guidance of therapy. Clonality by PARR can be very useful in cases with a lot of concurrent inflammation and minimal cellular atypia. Non-epitheliotrophic lymphoma can be of B- or T-cell origin.

Treatment: Chemotherapy is the treatment of choice for lymphoma, but both forms of cutaneous lymphoma have proven difficult to treat with conventional chemotherapeutic

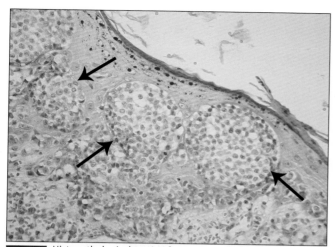

34.15 Histopathological section from a case of epitheliotrophic lymphoma showing aggregates of neoplastic lymphocytes (arrowed) within the epidermis (Pautrier's microaggregates or microabscesses).

protocols. They show poor initial response rates and short remission times with conventional chemotherapeutic protocols based on vincristine, cyclophosphamide and prednisolone. Lomustine (CCNU) has been reported to have some efficacy in the treatment of epitheliotrophic lymphoma, usually in conjunction with prednisolone (Risbon *et al.*, 2006). However, lomustine (CCNU) is a potent anticancer drug with potentially severe toxicity (myelosuppression, hepatotoxicity), and the advice of a clinical oncologist should be sought before its use. There are also some reports in the literature about the use of retinoids to treat epitheliotrophic lymphoma, but again these drugs are best used under the advice of a specialist. Surgical resection or radiotherapy may be indicated for localized lesions, but the disease is rarely solitary.

Prognosis: Non-epitheliotrophic lymphoma is an aggressive disease that progresses rapidly to involve the lymph nodes and other organs and is ultimately fatal. Epitheliotrophic lymphoma is a much more chronic disease that may wax and wane over a period of months before the true tumour stage develops and disseminates to other organs.

Plasmacytomas

Plasmacytoma is usually a solitary skin tumour of the dog that comprises a proliferation of mature plasma cells. Cutaneous plasmacytoma in dogs is generally not associated with a bone marrow-derived tumour of plasma cells (e.g. myeloma), but in cats it is more likely to be an extramedullary manifestation of myeloma.

Incidence: The condition is common in dogs, but rare in cats. It usually affects older dogs (mean age 9 years). No sex or breed predispositions have been reported.

Clinical presentation: The lesions are usually solitary and present as a well defined, raised red or ulcerated mass. The lesions may also affect the mucocutaneous junctions and, occasionally, arise in the gingiva.

Treatment and prognosis: Behaviour is benign and surgical resection is usually curative. Metastasis does not occur, although a second tumour at a different site may arise in a small percentage of cases.

Mast cell tumours
Canine mast cell tumours

Canine mast cell tumours show tremendous diversity in gross appearance, clinical behaviour, rate of metastasis and response to treatment, as a result of which they present considerable prognostic and therapeutic problems. The following is a brief overview of canine mast cell tumours (for a more detailed review, see Warland *et al.*, 2015).

Clinical presentation: There is no typical presentation for a canine mast cell tumour. The gross appearance can mimic any other cutaneous tumour, and mast cell tumours should be considered in the differential diagnosis of any skin tumour in the dog. Low grade, well differentiated mast cell tumours usually present as solitary, slow-growing, dermal nodules (Figure 34.16a). Tumours can ulcerate through the skin and, in some cases, the local release of histamine from tumour cells may cause the lesion to fluctuate in size and appear red or oedematous at times. More aggressive mast cell tumours may present as large, ill defined soft tissue masses, and some may be surrounded by satellite nodules as the tumour spreads through the surrounding cutaneous lymphatic vessels (Figure 34.16b).

Paraneoplastic syndromes: Solitary and metastatic mast cell tumours can have local or systemic effects via the release of histamine and other vasoactive amines from the tumour cells. Local histamine release may be associated with oedema and erythema of the tumour and adjacent

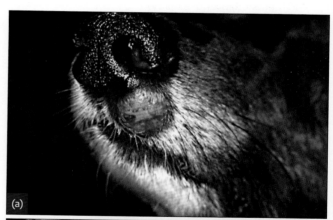

(a)

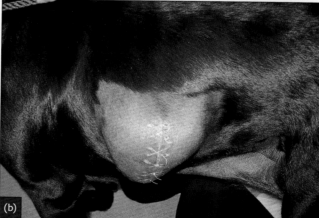

(b)

34.16 (a) Mast cell tumour presenting as a well circumscribed, erythematous dermal nodule on the lip of a dog. (b) Grade III mast cell tumour showing extensive mass/swelling on the flank of a Labrador Retriever.

tissues. Systemically, histamine may also be associated with gastroduodenal ulceration, leading to anorexia, vomiting, melaena, anaemia and, in some cases, perforation and sepsis. One author [DS] has seen several examples of local and distant paraneoplastic eosinophilic folliculitis and furunculosis, which have resolved spontaneously once the offending tumour has been excised.

Diagnostic tests:

Biopsy and fine-needle aspiration: Mast cells can be readily identified by fine-needle aspirate cytology (see Figure 34.10) and this simple technique should be performed prior to surgical removal of any cutaneous lesion. Mast cell tumours cannot be graded (see below) accurately on cytology alone, although some indication of the degree of differentiation of the tumour cells may be possible. Thus, excisional biopsy samples should be submitted for histological grading and assessment of the margins of surgical excision.

Staging: Malignant mast cell tumours may metastasize either by the lymphatic route or haematogenously. In most cases, the first sign of metastasis is enlargement of the local lymph node. Discrete pulmonary metastases are rare; disseminated mast cell tumours more commonly form metastatic deposits or infiltrates in the spleen and liver. Local and regional lymph nodes should always be evaluated by palpation, radiography, ultrasonography and/or cytology as appropriate. Ultrasonographic evaluation of the liver, spleen and kidneys is valuable in the staging of high-grade tumours (see below); radiography of the thorax is less useful. The skin is a potential site for mast cell tumour metastasis, and skin nodules should be investigated by fine-needle aspiration or biopsy.

Haematology: Routine haematological assessment may indicate anaemia caused by blood loss from a bleeding intestinal ulcer. It is rare to see circulating mast cells (mastocytosis), even on buffy coat smears, but eosinophilia may be a feature of widespread metastatic mast cell tumours.

Treatment and prognosis:

Mast cell tumours can vary in behaviour from slow-growing, low grade tumours that follow a benign course to rapidly growing, invasive, highly malignant tumours, and many stages in-between. Histological grading based upon the degree of cellular differentiation, the mitotic index and the invasion of adjacent tissues has been shown to be of prognostic value. Three

histological grades of mast cell tumour were originally described (Patnaik *et al.*, 1984.; Figure 34.17):

- **Well differentiated tumours** (grade I) are generally of low grade/benign nature and carry a favourable prognosis
- **Moderately differentiated tumours** (grade II) are intermediate both in their histological appearance and also in behaviour
- **Poorly differentiated tumours** (grade III) are invasive with a high rate of metastasis and a poor prognosis.

Unfortunately, many mast cell tumours are designated grade II, where the prognosis is difficult to predict. As a result, a two-tier grading system has been introduced to eliminate the intermediate category (Kiupel *et al.*, 2011). A number of additional prognostic markers, such as measurements of cell proliferation (e.g. mitotic index, Ki67, AgNORs and pattern of cKIT staining), can be performed on tissue biopsy samples, which can help to predict the likelihood of metastasis. The mitotic index seems to be one of the most reliable prognostic indicators (a mitotic index >5–7 predicts a poor outcome).

Surgical resection is the treatment of choice for the majority of canine mast cell tumours. Neoadjuvant treatment with prednisolone may help to reduce the tumour mass, making a surgical approach more feasible. For those tumours sited on the lower limbs, where adequate surgical margins cannot be achieved, cytoreductive surgery followed by adjuvant radiotherapy has proved a successful treatment strategy. Although widely reported, chemotherapy is only indicated for the management of high-grade mast cell tumours, and those grade II tumours that are truly inoperable or metastatic. Chemotherapy protocols described for the treatment of inoperable or high-grade canine mast cell tumours are detailed in Figure 34.18.

Protein tyrosine kinases are enzymes involved in cell signalling pathways that regulate key cell functions, such as proliferation, differentiation, migration, activation and survival. Activation of these enzymes by point mutation or overexpression is associated with various forms of cancer. In canine mast cell tumours, cKIT mutations have been documented. Masitinib and toceranib phosphate are tyrosine kinase inhibitors that have been developed for the veterinary market, specifically for the treatment of non-resectable mast cell tumours in dogs; clinical studies have shown both drugs can control and shrink non-resectable mast cell tumours, especially those with cKIT mutation. A

Histological grade	Clinical presentation	Treatment and prognosis
Grade I – well differentiated	Usually solitary, slow-growing, well circumscribed dermal mass	Wide local surgical resection provides a favourable prognosis with a 95% 12-month survival
Grade II – intermediate differentiation	Usually slow-growing dermal or subcutaneous mass. Can range from firm and nodular to soft and fluctuant in character. May even appear similar to lipoma in consistency	Wide local resection with generous (1–2 cm) margins around the tumour is required. Deep margins are also important, but as mast cell tumours do not usually invade through fascial planes, resection to a clean fascial plane deep to the tumour is usually adequate. Postoperative radiotherapy may be indicated for tumours on lower limbs where surgical margins cannot be achieved. Approximately 90% 12-month survival. A small proportion of grade II tumours metastasize to local lymph nodes and other organs. Mitotic index, polymerase chain reaction for cKIT mutation and Ki67/AgNOR expression may be helpful in predicting prognosis for grade II tumours
Grade III – poorly differentiated	Usually fast-growing, invasive, diffuse tumours that can attain large size. Clinical behaviour is aggressive, with early lymph node metastasis and distant dissemination	Surgical resection if lesion is solitary, but prognosis poor due to malignancy with 6–46% of animals surviving >12 months. Various chemotherapy regimes have been reported to achieve moderate short-term responses (Figure 34.18). Tyrosine kinase inhibitors are authorized for the treatment of non-resectable canine mast cell tumours (Hahn *et al.*, 2008; London *et al.*, 2009)

34.17 Mast cell tumours by grade.

Protocol	Comment	Reference
Vinblastine and prednisolone	Approximately 45–50% overall response rate; moderate toxicity; neutropenia; gastrointestinal	Thamm et al., 1999, 2006; Vickery et al., 2008
Lomustine (CCNU)	44% overall response rate; myelosuppression; gastrointestinal; hepatotoxicity	Rassnick et al., 1999
Vinblastine and lomustine (CCNU)	57% overall response rate; 54% toxicity; myelosuppression	Cooper et al, 2009
Vinblastine/ cyclophosphamide/ prednisolone	64% overall response rate; moderate neutropenia	Camps-Palau et al., 2007
Chlorambucil and prednisolone	38% overall response rate; no toxicity	Taylor et al., 2009
Masitinib	55% overall response rate; diarrhoea and vomiting most common side effects	Hahn et al., 2008
Toceranib phosphate	42.8% overall response rate; anorexia, diarrhoea and vomiting most common side effects	London et al., 2009

34.18 Chemotherapy protocols for the treatment of mast cell tumours.

new protein kinase C activator, tigilanol tiglate, designed for intralesional injection, may also be an option for small tumours where resection is not possible.

Feline mast cell tumours

In cats, mast cell tumours are most commonly found in the skin but have also been documented in the spleen and intestine. These visceral lesions may be associated with secondary cutaneous lesions, which may give rise to confusion in respect of prognosis.

Presentation and behaviour: Mast cell tumours are the fourth most common skin tumour in the cat, exceeded only by basal cell tumours, fibrosarcomas and SCCs (Ho et al., 2018). Feline cutaneous mast cell tumours most commonly arise on the head, neck and trunk of middle-aged to older cats (median age 10 years; range <1–20 years). No sex predisposition has been reported. Several breeds are at increased risk of developing mast cell tumours, including Siamese, Burmese, Maine Coon, Ragdoll, Oriental Blue, Russian Blue and Havana. Feline mast cell tumours are usually solitary, quite well circumscribed nodular or plaque-like lesions, often hairless and less frequently ulcerated. Some cats present with or develop multiple lesions.

Diagnosis and histological features: Feline mast cell tumours can be diagnosed by cytological evaluation of fine-needle aspirates from the mass. Cells are characterized by typical metachromatic staining cytoplasmic granules. Histologically, tumours are classified as well differentiated mastocytic, pleomorphic mastocytic and atypical (histiocytic).

Well differentiated mastocytic tumours are the most common histological type (approximately 60%) and comprise circumscribed, non-encapsulated masses of solid sheets of uniform round cells with few mitoses.

Pleomorphic mastocytic tumours are less common (<28%) and contain a population of more pleomorphic mononuclear or multinucleated cells, which infiltrate the dermis and subcutis. Mitotic rate is usually low.

The atypical form accounts for 10–20% of all feline mast cell tumours and is most common in younger cats (<4 years of age). These tumours usually occur on the head, sometimes in groups of small papulonodular lesions, which spontaneously regress over time (4–24 months reported).

Feline mast cell tumours are now graded into Group 1 (benign) and Group 2 (malignant) on the basis of mitotic count and cell morphology according to Sabattini and Bettini, 2018.

Treatment and prognosis: Surgery is the treatment of choice for solitary cutaneous mast cell tumours in cats; most are well differentiated, benign in nature and are cured by surgical excision. A small proportion of feline mast cell tumours do recur; completeness of surgical excision as assessed by histopathology has not been shown to predict or correlate with recurrence rate. Cats with stage I–III disease rarely die from mast cell tumours and most enjoy long-term survival with surgery alone. For this reason, the need for chemotherapy is questionable in most cases of feline mast cell tumours and should only be considered for those lesions that show aggressive behaviour.

Lomustine (CCNU) has been reported to achieve response rates (complete remission and partial response) in 50% of cats in one study, which included 10 of 26 cats with cutaneous tumours (Rassnick et al., 2008). Other chemotherapeutic agents that have been used in the treatment of feline mast cell tumours include vinblastine, cyclophosphamide, chlorambucil and mechlorethamine; however, large-scale prospective studies to support such use are lacking.

A mutation of the cKIT tyrosine kinase receptor, similar to that described in some canine mast cell tumours, has been reported in feline cutaneous mast cell tumours (Rodriguez-Carino et al., 2009), which suggests that the receptor tyrosine kinase inhibitors (masitinib and toceranib phosphate) may have a role in the management of selected feline mast cell tumours, but no large-scale, prospective study has yet been performed to validate the potential of these drugs.

Visceral mast cell tumours: Lymphoreticular mast cell tumours are seen occasionally in cats. The presenting signs are usually vomiting and anorexia.

Mesenchymal and spindle cell tumours

Mesenchymal and spindle cell tumours include:

- Spindle cell tumours/spindle cell sarcomas (fibrosarcomas, myxosarcomas, canine perivascular wall tumours, peripheral nerve sheath tumours)
- Haemangiomas
- Haemangiosarcomas (primary cutaneous haemangiosarcomas)
- Lipomas/infiltrating lipomas
- Fibromas/dermatofibromas/collagenous naevi.

Spindle cell tumours and sarcomas

Incidence: These are common tumours in both dogs and cats. They tend to occur in older animals (mean age in dogs is 8.6 years; mean age in cats is 9.2 years), but may affect young animals of either species. No sex predisposition has been reported in dogs or cats. Retriever breeds may be at increased risk in the dog. Spindle cell tumours may be subdivided according to their supposed tissue of origin (as detailed above); however, their clinical appearance and behaviour is similar.

Clinical presentation: Lesion localization may vary with tumour type; for example, perivascular wall tumours most commonly arise on the limbs, whereas fibrosarcomas occur most frequently on the limbs, head and trunk. An association between fibrosarcomas and vaccine/injection sites has been recognized in cats (Figure 34.19). Lesions may be dermal, subcutaneous or arise in the deep fascia. Most tumours in this group present as solitary, slow-growing masses. They often give the appearance of being well circumscribed or even encapsulated, but in fact are very infiltrative in their pattern of growth. There is a low rate of metastasis.

Treatment: Wide surgical excision is the treatment of choice; however, masses are often incompletely excised at surgery, leading to high rates of local recurrence. In sites where adequate (especially deep) margins of excision cannot be achieved, an intentional cytoreductive surgery followed by adjuvant radiotherapy can result in long-term control of such tumours (Demetriou *et al*., 2012). However, there is a mounting body of evidence to suggest low rates of recurrence for many such tumours following marginal excision (Bray *et al*., 2014).

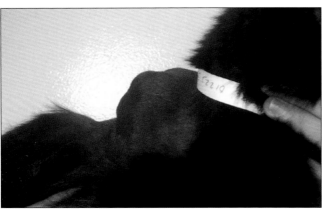

34.19   Injection site sarcoma in the subcutaneous tissue of the dorsal neck in a cat.

Haemangiomas

Incidence and epidemiology: Haemangiomas are relatively common tumours in dogs and cats. They tend to occur in older animals (mean age in dogs is 8.7 years). There have been no reported sex or breed predispositions, but Boxers, German Shepherd Dogs and Golden Retrievers may be at increased risk. There is a possible association with exposure to sunlight, especially in short-haired breeds.

Clinical presentation: Lesions commonly occur on the limbs, trunk and tail. They are usually solitary, although multiple masses have been reported. They tend to present as soft, fluctuant dermal or subcutaneous masses; more superficial lesions may be blue to red–black.

Treatment and prognosis: Wide surgical excision is the treatment of choice. Solitary lesions are amenable to resection and the prognosis is good.

Haemangiosarcomas

Incidence and epidemiology: Haemangiosarcomas are relatively common in the dog and cat. They tend to occur in older animals: mean age in dogs is 9.6 years; mean age in cats is 9.4 years. No sex predisposition has been reported. In the dog, haemangiosarcoma of the skin is distinct from that of internal viscera (spleen and heart); however, haemangiosarcomas arising in the internal viscera may metastasize to the skin, so it is important to ascertain that a cutaneous lesion does not represent metastatic disease from a distant primary site. German Shepherd Dogs are at increased risk of visceral haemangiosarcomas, but cutaneous haemangiosarcomas appear to be more common in other breeds, including Irish Wolfhounds, Whippets and Golden Retrievers.

Clinical presentation: Tumours may arise at any site (the trunk and limbs are equally represented) and may be cutaneous or subcutaneous. In dogs, cutaneous haemangiosarcomas are usually quite well differentiated, well circumscribed tumours with low rates of metastasis. However, tumours that are sited in the subcutis tend to be more locally aggressive and carry a higher risk of metastasis. In the cat, haemangiosarcomas may be locally infiltrating, leading to problems of local recurrence.

Treatment and prognosis: Wide surgical excision is the treatment of choice. Cutaneous haemangiosarcomas in dogs are amenable to surgical excision and carry a favourable prognosis.

Lipomas

Incidence and epidemiology: Lipomas are common tumours in the dog and occur occasionally in the cat. They tend to occur in older animals: mean age in the dog is 8.8 years. A predilection in bitches (entire and neutered) and neutered tomcats has been reported. Obesity may also be a predisposing factor for the development of these tumours.

Clinical presentation: Lesions are most commonly located on the abdominal or thoracic wall. They may be solitary or multiple, dermal or subcutaneous, usually soft, mobile, well circumscribed, encapsulated tumours. The infiltrating variant is not encapsulated and infiltrates widely through the connective tissue and muscle. Metastasis does not occur with either form.

Treatment and prognosis: Wide surgical excision is the treatment of choice. Surgical resection for the encapsulated form is curative. Surgical resection is often not effective in eradicating the infiltrative form of lipoma and local recurrence rates are high.

Fibromas, dermatofibromas and collagenous naevi

Incidence: These tumours are relatively uncommon in dogs and uncommon in cats. Tumours that have an histological appearance of fibromas are uncommon in cats and represent well differentiated fibrosarcomas (Goldschmidt and Shofer, 1992). They tend to occur in older dogs (mean age 8.4 years). No sex or breed predisposition has been reported.

Clinical presentation: Lesions occur most commonly on the head and limbs. They are solitary, intradermal or subcutaneous, soft to firm masses. The overlying epithelium may be hyperplastic.

Treatment and prognosis: The clinical behaviour of these tumours is benign. Wide surgical excision is the treatment of choice and the prognosis is good.

Melanocytic tumours

Incidence

Melanocytic tumours are relatively uncommon tumours of the skin in the dog and are very rare in the cat.

Clinical presentation

Grossly, these tumours may appear as flat, plaque-like to domed masses, up to 2 cm in diameter, sited within the dermis. They are usually dark brown to black and quite well defined. Malignant tumours may attain a larger size, contain less pigment and frequently ulcerate. In the cat, cutaneous melanoma must be distinguished from the much more common pigmented basal cell tumour.

Treatment and prognosis

The tumour site seems to be an important factor that affects the behaviour of cutaneous melanoma. Most melanocytic tumours of canine skin are solitary, slow-growing lesions that follow a benign course. Tumours that arise on the digits and mucocutaneous junctions (e.g. eyelids and lips) are more aggressive and behave in a similar manner to oral mucosal melanoma, with a high incidence of metastasis to local lymph nodes and via the blood to the lungs and other organs. Tumours with three or more mitoses per 10 high-powered fields on histopathology are usually considered malignant. Ki67 (proliferation assay) is also used along with mitotic count to differentiate benign from malignant canine melanocytic tumours.

Wide surgical excision is the treatment of choice for benign dermal melanoma, and the prognosis following complete surgical excision is good. Tumours may recur locally if excision is incomplete. Surgical excision is also indicated for local control of malignant tumours, but the prognosis in such cases is guarded to poor because of the high incidence of metastasis. These tumours are not considered to be chemosensitive. A xenogeneic plasmid deoxyribonucleic acid (DNA) vaccine (Oncept®, Bohringer Ingleheim) (based on a human tyrosinase antigen) is available on restricted licence in North America; to date the licence only covers treatment of dogs with the oral/mucosal form of melanoma, although its use as an adjunct to surgery (amputation) has been reported in cases of canine digital melanoma (Manley et al., 2011).

Paraneoplastic syndromes affecting the skin

Tumours can cause systemic or metabolic disturbances through the production of hormones or hormone-like substances that act on organs at sites distant to the primary tumour. The resulting clinical syndromes are termed paraneoplastic syndromes. The most commonly recognized paraneoplastic syndrome in the dog is hypercalcaemia of malignancy, which is associated most frequently with lymphoma or carcinoma of the epitrichial glands of the anal sacs. Mast cell tumours may result in local paraneoplastic dermatitis, swelling and pruritus. Very few cutaneous tumours cause paraneoplastic syndromes, but a small number of cutaneous paraneoplastic syndromes have been reported in dogs and cats. These conditions (summarized in Figure 34.20) are rare, but their recognition can be important for the early diagnosis of the underlying neoplasm (Turek, 2003).

Key points

- Cutaneous neoplasms are common in dogs and cats and fine-needle aspirate cytology should be performed on any mass
- Paraneoplastic skin disorders are rare, but recognition can be important to localize and identify the underlying neoplasm
- Cutaneous lymphomas in dogs and cats can have a variable presentation and biopsy should be considered for any unusual cutaneous presentation in the older animal

Cutaneous syndrome	Clinical signs	Underlying neoplastic condition
Feline paraneoplastic alopecia	Non-pruritic, progressive alopecia involving the limbs and ventrum	Pancreatic carcinoma that has usually metastasized to the liver and other distant sites by the time of diagnosis (Brooks et al., 1994; Tasker et al., 1999). Also reported in biliary carcinoma
Feline thymoma associated exfoliative dermatitis	Non-pruritic, generalized scaling and erythema on the head and pinnae, which may progress to general distribution	Thymoma in cats (Scott et al., 1995; Forster-Van Hijfte et al., 1997)
Feminization syndrome	Bilateral flank alopecia	Oestrogen-secreting Sertoli cell tumour in male dogs
Nodular dermatofibrosis (Renal cystadenocarcinoma and nodular dermatofibrosis (RCND))	Multiple firm, well-circumscribed cutaneous nodules, usually affecting the extremities but can be diffuse	Bilateral renal tumours, renal cystadenoma or cystadenocarcinoma and uterine leiomyomas (Moe and Lium, 1997). Autosomal dominant inheritance in German Shepherd Dogs. The mutation in a tumour suppressor gene results in tumour formation. Cutaneous nodules usually preceed this by a number of years
Paraneoplastic pemphigus	Erosive and ulcerative oral lesions	Mediastinal lymphoma (Lemmens et al., 1998)
Sterile nodular panniculitis	Nodules with sinus tracts and ulceration	Bile duct carcinoma leading to pancreatic necrosis (Paterson, 1994)
Superficial necrolytic dermatitis (necrolytic migratory erythema, hepatocutaneous syndrome)	Ulcerative dermatosis resembling human necrolytic migratory erythema. Erythema, crusting, exudation, ulceration and alopecia on feet, pressure points, flank, muzzle, perineum and external genitalia. Often symmetrical. Hyperkeratosis and fissuring of the footpads with symmetrical erythema, ulceration and crusting of the face, feet and external genitalia	Glucagon-secreting pancreatic carcinoma (Gross et al., 1990). More commonly associated with end-stage hepatic disease and concurrrent diabetes mellitus (see Chapter 31) (Bond et al., 1995)

34.20 Paraneoplastic conditions that affect the skin.

References and further reading

Bond R, McNeil PE, Evans H and Srebernik N (1995) Metabolic epidermal necrosis in two dogs with different underlying diseases. *Veterinary Record* **136**, 466–471

Braund KG (1990) Remote effects of cancer on the nervous system. *Seminars in Veterinary Medicine and Surgery (Small Animal)* **5**, 262–270

Bray J.P., Polton GA, McSporran KD *et al.* (2014) Canine soft tissue sarcoma managed in first opinion practice: outcome in 350 cases. *Veterinary Surgery* **43**, 774–782

Brooks DG, Campbell KL, Dennis JS *et al.* (1994) Pancreatic paraneoplastic alopecia in three cats. *Journal of the American Animal Hospital Association* **34**, 557–563

Camps-Palau MA, Leibman NF, Elmslie R *et al.* (2007) Treatment of canine mast cell tumours with vinblastine, cyclophosphamide and prednisolone: 35 cases (1997–2004). *Veterinary and Comparative Oncology* **5**, 156–167

Cooper M, Tsai X and Bennett P (2009) Combination CCNU and vinblastine chemotherapy for canine mast cell tumours: 57 cases. *Veterinary and Comparative Oncology* **7**, 196–206

Demetriou JL, Brearely MJ and Constantino-Casas F (2012) Intentional marginal excision of canine limb sarcoma followed by radiotherapy. *Journal of Small Animal Practice* **53**, 174–181

Forster-Van Hijfte MA, Curtis CF and White RN (1997) Resolution of exfoliative dermatitis and Malassezia pachydermatis overgrowth in a cat after surgical thymoma resection. *Journal of Small Animal Practice* **38**, 451–454

Goldschmidt MH and Shofer FS (1992) *Skin Tumours of the Dog and Cat.* Pergamon Press, Oxford

Gross TL, Ihrke PJ and Walder EJ (1992) *Veterinary Dermato-pathology. A Macroscopic and Microscopic Evaluation of Canine and Feline Skin Disease.* Mosby-Year Book, St Louis

Gross TL, O'Brien TD, Davies AP and Long RE (1990) Glucagon producing pancreatic endocrine tumours in two dogs with superficial necrolytic dermatitis. *Journal of the American Veterinary Medical Association* **197**, 1619–1622

Hahn KA, Oglivie G, Rusk T *et al.* (2008) Masitinib is safe and effective for the treatment of canine mast cell tumors. *Journal of Veterinary Internal Medicine* **22**, 1341–1349

Henry C and Herrera C (2013) Mast cell tumours in cats: clinical update and possible new treatment avenues. *Journal of Feline Medicine and Surgery* **15**, 41–47

Ho NT, Smith KC and Dobromylskyj MJ (2018) Retrospective study of more than 9000 feline cutaneous tumours in the UK: 2006-2013. *Journal of Feline Medicine and Surgery* **20**, 128–134

Kiupel M, Webster JD, Bailey KL *et al.* (2011) Proposal of a 2-tier histological grading system for canine cutaneous mast cell tumors to more accurately predict biological behavior. *Veterinary Pathology* **48**, 147–155

Lemmens P, de Bruin A and de Meulemeester J (1998) Paraneoplastic pemphigus in a dog. *Veterinary Dermatology* **9**, 127–134

London CA, Malpas PB, Wood-Follis SL *et al.* (2009) Multicenter, placebo-controlled, double blind, randomized study of oral toceranib phosphate (SU11654), a receptor tyrosine kinase inhibitor, for the treatment of dogs with recurrent (either local or distant) mast cell tumour following surgical excision. *Clinical Cancer Research* **15**, 3856–3865

Manley CA, Leibman NF, Wolchok JD *et al.* (2011) Xenogeneic murine tyrosinase DNA vaccine for malignant melanoma of the digit of dogs. *Journal of Veterinary Internal Medicine* **25**, 94–99

Mellor PJ, Haugland S, Smith KC *et al.* (2008) Histopathologic, immunohistochemical and cytologic analysis of feline myeloma-related disorders: further evidence for primary extramedullary development in the cat. *Veterinary Pathology* **45**, 159–173

Moe L and Lium B (1997) Hereditary multifocal renal cystadenocarcinomas and nodular dermatofibrosis in 51 German Shepherd Dogs. *Journal of Small Animal Practice* **38**, 498–505

Paterson S (1994) Panniculitis associated with pancreatic necrosis in a dog. *Journal of Small Animal Practice* **35**, 116-118

Patnaik AK, Ehler WJ and MacEwan EG (1984) Canine cutaneous mast cell tumor: Morphologic grading and survival time in 83 dogs. *Veterinary Pathology* **21**, 469–474

Rassnick KM, Moore AS, Williams LE *et al.* (1999) Treatment of canine MCT with CCNU (lomustine). *Journal of Veterinary Internal Medicine* **13**, 601–605

Rassnick KM, Williams LE, Kristal O *et al.* (2008) Lomustine for treatment of mast cell tumors in cats: 38 cases (1999–2005). *Journal of the American Veterinary Medical Association* **232**, 1200–1205

Risbon RE, deLorimer LP, Skorupski K *et al.* (2006) Response of canine cutaneous epitheliotrophic lymphoma to lomustine (CCNU): a retrospective study of 46 cases (1999–2004). *Journal of Veterinary Internal Medicine* **20**, 1389–1397

Rodriguez-Carino C, Fondevila D, Segales J and Rabanal RM (2009) Expression of KIT receptor in feline cutaneous mast cell tumors. *Veterinary Pathology* **46**, 878–883

Sabattini S and Bettini B (2019) Grading cutaneous mast cell tumors in cats. *Veterinary Pathology* **56**, 43–49

Scott DW, Yager JA and Johnson KM (1995) Exfoliative dermatitis in association with thymoma in three cats. *Feline Practice* **23**, 8–13

Tasker S, Griffon DJ, Nuttal TJ and Hill PB (1999) Resolution of paraneoplastic alopecia following surgical removal of a pancreatic carcinoma in a cat. *Journal of Small Animal Practice* **40**, 16–19

Taylor F, Gear R, Hoather T and Dobson J (2009) Chlorambucil and prednisolone chemotherapy for dogs with inoperable MCT: 21 cases. *Journal of Small Animal Practice* **50**, 284–289

Thamm DH, Maudlin EA and Vail DM (1999) Prednisolone and vinblastine chemotherapy for canine mast cell tumor – 41 cases (1992–97). *Journal of Veterinary Internal Medicine* **13**, 491–497

Thamm DH, Turek MM and Vail DM (2006) Outcome and prognostic factors following adjuvant prednisone/vinblastine chemotherapy for high-risk canine MCT: 61 Cases. *Journal of Veterinary Medical Science* **68**, 581–587

Turek MM (2003) Cutaneous paraneoplastic syndromes in dogs and cats: a review of the literature. *Veterinary Dermatology* **14**, 279–296

Vickery KR, Wilson H, Vail DM and Thamm DH (2008) Dose-escalating vinblastine for the treatment of canine MCT. *Veterinary and Comparative Oncology* **6**, 111–119

Warland J, Brioschi V, Owen L and Dobson J (2015) Canine mast cell tumours: decision-making and treatment. *In Practice* **37**, 315–332

Weiss DJ, Evanson OA and Sykes J (1999) A retrospective study of canine pancytopenia. *Veterinary Clinical Pathology* **28**, 83–88

Yager JA and Wilcock BP (1994) *Color Atlas and Text of Surgical Pathology of the Dog and Cat.* Mosby-Year Book, St Louis

Index

Page numbers in *italic* refer to figures